SIXTH EDITION

Language and Communication Disorders in Children

Deena K. Bernstein
*Lehman College,
City University of New York*

Ellenmorris Tiegerman-Farber
Adelphi University

Boston   New York   San Francisco
Mexico City   Montreal   Toronto   London   Madrid   Munich   Paris
Hong Kong   Singapore   Tokyo   Cape Town   Sydney

Executive Editor and Publisher: Stephen D. Dragin
Editorial Assistant: Anne Whittaker
Marketing Manager: Krista Clark
Production Editor: Gregory Erb
Editorial Production Service: Omegatype Typography, Inc.
Composition Buyer: Linda Cox
Manufacturing Manager: Megan Cochran
Electronic Composition: Omegatype Typography, Inc.
Interior Design: Omegatype Typography, Inc.
Photo Researcher: Kate Cebik
Cover Designer: Elena Sidorova

For related titles and support materials, visit our online catalog at www.pearsonhighered.com.

Between the time website information is gathered and then published, it is not unusual for some sites to have closed. Also, the transcription of URLs can result in typographical errors. The publisher would appreciate notification where these errors occur so that they may be corrected in subsequent editions.

Library of Congress Cataloging-in-Publication Data

Bernstein, Deena K. (Deena Kahan)
  Language and communication disorders in children / Deena K.
Bernstein, Ellenmorris Tiegerman-Farber. —6th ed.
        p.   cm.
  Includes bibliographical references and index.
  ISBN-13: 978-0-205-58461-1 (pbk.)
  ISBN-10: 0-205-58461-6 (pbk.)
  1. Language disorders in children.   2. Communicative disorders in
children.   I. Tiegerman-Farber, Ellenmorris.   II. Title.
  RJ496.L35B47 2009
  618.92'855—dc22

                                             2008009329

Printed in the United States of America
10   9   8   7   6   5   4   3   2   1   RRD-VA   12   11   10   09   08

Allyn & Bacon
is an imprint of

www.pearsonhighered.com

ISBN-10: 0-205-58461-6
ISBN-13: 978-0-205-58461-1

About the Authors

Deena K. Bernstein received her B.A. from Brooklyn College, her M.A. from Temple University, and her PhD from the Graduate Center of the City University of New York. She was the Graduate Program Director of Speech Pathology at Lehman College/CUNY and is presently a professor and chair of the department of speech-language-hearing sciences at that institution. Her works have been published in the *Journal of Remedial & Special Edition, Folio Phoniatrica, Topics in Language Disorders, Journal of Applied Psycholinguistics, Journal of Educational Research,* and *Language, Speech, & Hearing Services in the Schools.* Dr. Bernstein has made numerous professional presentations at state, national, and international meetings, and she has been a reviewer for many peer-reviewed journals, including *Psychology in the Schools, Communication Disorders Quarterly, Journal of Speech & Hearing Research,* and the *American Journal of Speech Pathology.* She holds specialty recognition in child language and has been a member of ASHA and the Council for Exceptional Children for more than twenty-five years.

Ellenmorris Tiegerman-Farber received her M.S. from Brooklyn College, her MSW from Adelphi University, and her PhD from the Graduate Center of the City University of New York. She served on the faculty at Adelphi University in the departments of communication disorders and psychology for twenty-three years. In 1985, she started the School for Language and Communication Development (SLCD) for children with language and autism spectrum disorders. SLCD serves approximately 400 children from Long Island and New York City in preschool, elementary, middle, and high school programs. Dr. Tiegerman-Farber has written several other textbooks, including *Language Disorders in Children; Real Families, Real Issues, and Real Interventions; Collaborative Decision Making: The Pathway to Inclusion;* and *Language and Communication Intervention in Preschool Children* (with Dr. Christine Radziewicz). Dr. Tiegerman-Farber is married to Joseph Farber, an attorney, and they have six children.

Contents

CHAPTER 5

Understanding the Nature and Scope of Language Learning Disability: Characteristics, Frameworks, and Connections   206

Cheryl Smith Gabig

CHAPTER 6

Mental Retardation/Intellectual Disability   246

Robert E. Owens, Jr.

CHAPTER 10 Planning Language Intervention for Young Children   436

CHAPTER 11 Making Sense of Language Learning Disability: Assessment and Support for Academic Success   496

Preface

Language and Communication Disorders in Children has proceeded through six editions in the last twenty years. Each edition refined its predecessor by adding new theoretical and practical knowledge. In this vein, the present edition reflects the most current clinical, educational, and legislative changes that have impacted the professions of special education and speech-language pathology since the last edition.

This volume continues to follow a tripartite structure that users of our text have found valuable. Part I (Chapters 1 and 2) presents the fundamentals of language and communication development. Part II (Chapters 3–8) describes language disorders across clinical populations. Part III (Chapters 9–12) discusses the principles and general guidelines for assessment and intervention.

A number of noteworthy improvements distinguish this edition. In addition to the reorganization and inclusion of updated information in all the chapters, there are four new chapters. In Part II, Chapter 4, Liat Seiger-Gardner and Diana Almodovar address communicative impairments in preschool populations with special emphasis on the child with SLI (specific language impairment). In Chapter 5, Cheryl Smith Gabig presents an overview of language learning disabilities. In Part III, there are two new chapters. In Chapter 9, Ellenmorris Tiegerman-Farber discusses the expanded role of the speech-language pathologist, as well as the changes that have affected the delivery of services in school settings. In Chapter 11, Sylvia Diehl and Elaine R. Silliman describe the supports necessary to ensure academic success for children with language learning disabilities.

Examples and case studies abound in Parts II and III. They effectively illustrate how to apply clinical constructs to the actual evaluation and remediation of language difficulties for children with communication disorders.

In this new edition, there is increased emphasis on the use of augmentative and alternative communication (AAC) with infants and toddlers, emergent literacy, and children with specific language impairments. Emphasis is also given to adolescent language development and the literacy challenges of language learning-disabled school-age children. Lastly, evidence-based strategies for assessment and intervention are highlighted, as is the ever-changing role of the speech-language pathologist in the schools.

The study of language and communication disorders touches the heart of human experience—the ways children learn language and ways to help children who do not. This book will challenge you to apply theories of child and language development to the rewarding experience of providing language intervention to children with language and communication disorders. We sincerely hope it will motivate you to keep abreast of new research in clinical and educational practice.

From Deena K. Bernstein

Acknowledging those who make a text a reality is a risky venture, because one runs the risk of inadvertently omitting someone who deserves thanks. However, it would be remiss of me not to acknowledge the major participants in this endeavor. I begin with the professionals at Allyn & Bacon. Steven Dragin and his editorial assistant, Anne Whittaker, deserve a special thanks for all their efforts, as does the production staff of Omegatype Typography, who so efficiently helped make this edition a reality.

We also wish to thank our reviewers, whose suggestions and recommendations substantially improved and enhanced this edition: Mary Beth Armstrong, University of Montevallo; Lisa Bedore, University of Texas at Austin; Bernard Grela, University of Connecticut; Janet L. Patterson, University of New Mexico; and Terry Saenz, California State University, Fullerton.

All the contributors to this text deserve a special thanks. For those who previously participated, you have our thanks for your patience during the reworking of the manuscript. For our new contributors, Liat Seiger-Gardner, Diane Almodavar, and Cheryl Smith Gabig, please accept a special salute for working under the constraints of tight deadlines.

To my husband and best friend, Josh, for his invaluable support over the years, and to my children, Ariella, Chaim Zanvil, and Yakov, who have taught me the lessons of patience and perseverance, I am forever grateful.

This book is dedicated . . .

To the memory of my parents,
Pearl (Chaya Peryl) and Julius (Yuda) Kahan,
for whom the love and understanding of children
were overriding values
and
In honor of their great-grandchildren,
Chaya Peryl, Yuda, Moshe D, Tsvi H, Shoshana Bernstein
and
Bracha and Benjamin Z. Isaac Losice

From Ellenmorris Tiegerman-Farber

As always, I dedicate this textbook to my family . . .

To my husband Joseph Farber—
You are my soul mate and I thank God for you every morning. I could not have reached for the "stars" without you.

To my parents, Morris and Rita Jacobs—
SLCD could not have started without your house. It has taken fifteen years for me to pay back a debt of gratitude—a house for a house.

To my children, Leslie, Dana, Douglas, Jeremy, Andrew, and Jonathan—
You have taught me to be your mother and I love it.

To my grandchildren, Lindsey, Brandon, Gabriel and Olivia—
How wonderful that you are here and that there will be, I am sure, another eight to make an even dozen!

And . . .

To the parents of SLCD—
Never forget the silence, and always cherish your children's words.

To Dr. Christine Radziewicz, Dr. Jeffrey Kassinove, Christine Austin, Alicia Sabatino, Karen Katzman, and Dr. Helene Mermelstein—
I could not have done this without your loyalty and support. I will always be committed to all of you wherever life takes me.

To Senator Dean Skelos, Deputy Majority Leader of the New York Senate—
You are the Champion of SLCD and the staunchest supporter of children with special needs in New York State. This school would have never survived without you.

PART 1

The Nature of Language and Language Development

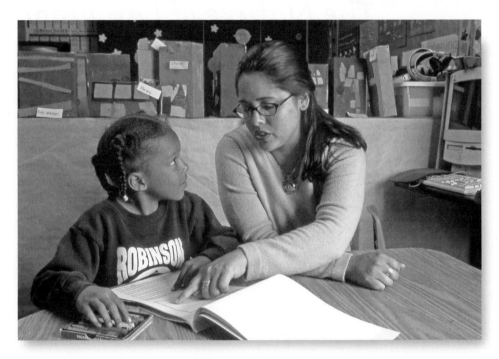

CHAPTER 1

The Nature of Language and Its Disorders

Deena K. Bernstein
Lehman College, City University of New York

When you finish this chapter, you should be able to

- Describe the nature of language, its subsystems, and their interrelationship.
- Discuss various approaches to language acquisition.
- Distinguish between an etiological-categorical approach to language disorders and the developmental-descriptive model.
- Define a language disorder.

Most children acquire language naturally and, for the most part, without any formal instruction. Some children, however, experience serious difficulties in their acquisition of language. These children are language disordered. To overcome their disorders, such children require the assistance of various professionals, including speech-language pathologists, psychologists, and, in the school setting, special educators and resource room teachers.

The multidisciplinary nature of the study of language disorders is one reason for the complexity of the discipline. Speech-language pathology, special education, sociolinguistics, linguistics, psycholinguistics, and psychology, the disciplines that study language, have their own respective inventories of terms and methods. Diversity of terms, constructs, and even attitudes and biases pervades the study of language and its disorders. A cursory perusal of the writings in this field is enough to convince the student of this diversity.

A second reason for the complexity in studying language disorders relates to the complexity of language itself. Although in the first decade of this century we program computers to process information so that they can control a factory, cook a meal, and even fly a plane, we have not yet succeeded in programming a computer to simulate the generative nature of human language. This may happen someday, but for the present, language remains too complex for reduction to a simpler format by programming. Comprehending language, theoretically, is a formidable task. Applying theories pragmatically to assess and to provide remediation to individuals who are language disordered is even more complex.

The centrality of language in the human experience is a third factor that complicates the study of language disorders. Language is crucial to all social and educational functioning. Parents are most concerned that their children acquire language because they recognize that a language deficit may have a serious effect on future educational, social, and vocational opportunities. "Language," it has been said, "may be the most distinctive attribute of human beings; its acquisition is an integral part of human development. It is not surprising that how language is learned and taught are major issues in education and other human service fields" (McCormick & Schiefelbusch, 1984, p. 2).

This first chapter consists of fundamental information on three interrelated subjects relevant to language: the components or elements of language, perspectives on language acquisition, and approaches to language disorders in children. These areas were chosen because speech-language pathologists and special educators must possess a clear understanding of the nature of language and how it is acquired if they are to provide appropriate interventions for children with language and communication disorders.

We will begin, however, by exploring the differences between three seemingly similar but in reality different terms—*communication, speech,* and *language.* We will then further explain the notion of *language* by providing an explanation of its components.

Communication, Speech, and Language

To the average person, the terms *communication, speech,* and *language* are synonymous. Professionals in the field of speech-language, who spend years studying and treating language-disordered children, often must go into lengthy descriptions of their chosen field of specialization to explain why their area of interest does not include correcting stuttering or improving diction. Confusion about the focus of speech-language specialists probably results from confusion of these terms. To the specialist, these terms are very different and denote different aspects of development.

COMMUNICATION

Communication is the process by which individuals exchange information and convey ideas (Owens, 1990). It is an active process requiring a sender who *encodes,* or formulates, a message. It also requires a receiver who *decodes,* or comprehends, the message. Each partner must be alert to the needs of the other to ensure that messages are effectively conveyed and understood.

Although we may primarily use speech and language to communicate, other aspects of communication may enhance or distort the linguistic code. *Paralinguistic cues,* which include intonation patterns, stress, and speech rate, can signal the attitude and emotions of the speaker and alter the linguistic information. Consider the difference that stress makes in the meaning a speaker wishes to convey when uttering the following:

She grabbed the money from him.

She grabbed the *money* from him.

She grabbed the money from *him.*

Or consider the effect a rising intonation would have on the following sentence:

John kissed her on the lips.

In addition to paralinguistic cues, *nonlinguistic cues* also contribute to the communication process. Nonlinguistic cues include gestures, body movements, eye contact, and facial expressions, which can add to or detract from the linguistic message. All of us are familiar with the individual who looks at us as we talk and may intermittently nod his or her head, indicating to us active involvement in the communication process. Conversely, the individual who does not make eye contact often communicates a lack of interest or involvement in the communicative interaction, and we in turn may diminish our communication with him or her.

SPEECH

Speech is one of the modes that may be used for communication. It is the oral verbal mode of transmitting messages and involves the precise coordination of oral neuromuscular movements in order to produce sounds and linguistic units.

Although we use speech primarily for the purpose of communication, it is not the only means available to us. Writing, drawing, and manual signing are other modes of communication. Individuals select a mode depending on the context, their needs, the needs of the decoder, and the message they wish to transmit.

For some children with disabilities, acquiring speech is not a realistic goal. The limited physical control some children have over the speech mechanism makes it unlikely that they can learn to produce recognizable speech. However, many of these children can acquire the ability to communicate if they are given alternative means. In recent years, a number of alternative and/or augmentative communication systems have been designed for them. These systems allow the child to transmit messages without using speech. Beukelman and Mirenda (2005) and Reichle, Halle, and Drasgow (1998) describe a number of these systems (Blissymbolics, American Sign Language, computer-operated systems, etc.). Romski, Seveiki, Cheslock, and Barton (2006) describe the use of augmentative and alternative communication (AAC) and emerging language intervention, while Strum and colleagues (2006) describe using augmentative communication to assess and provide reading instruction to children with severe speech and physical impairments (SSPIs). In addition, Owens (Chapter 6), Tiegerman-Farber (Chapter 7), and Radziewicz and Antonellis (Chapter 8) also discuss the use of nonspeech modes in the intervention programs for children with mental retardation, autism spectrum disorder (ASD), and hearing impairment. Lastly, Robinson and Robb (Chapter 3) describe the use of AAC for facilitating communication for toddlers and very young children.

LANGUAGE

Language is a socially shared code, or conventional system, that represents ideas through the use of arbitrary symbols and rules that govern combinations of these symbols. There are hundreds of languages, each with its own particular symbols and rules. Language exists because language users have agreed on the symbols and rules to be used. Because these symbols are shared, language users can employ them to exchange information and ideas. The linguistic code allows language users to represent an object, an event, or a relationship with a symbol or a combination of symbols.

Language encompasses complex rules that govern sounds, words, sentences, meaning, and use. These rules underlie an individual's ability to understand language

(language comprehension) and his or her ability to formulate language (language production). An individual's implicit knowledge about the rules of his or her language is called *linguistic competence*. A person who possesses linguistic competence has the knowledge needed to be a language user. He or she knows the rules about sounds and their combination; he or she knows what makes sense and what doesn't. He or she can understand and create an infinite number of sentences and can use language in a variety of social settings. Even though he or she cannot state the rules explicitly, the language user behaves in a way that demonstrates that he or she knows them. Although children give evidence of knowing the rules of language at quite an early age, how this rule learning occurs is still being investigated.

In sum, native speakers/listeners of a language learn a linguistic rule system. This rule system can be divided into three major components: form, content, and use. These components are described more thoroughly in the next section.

The Components of Language

Language is a complex combination of several component rule systems. Bloom and Lahey (1978) have divided language into three major components: form, content, and use.

FORM

Form includes the linguistic elements that connect sounds and symbols with meaning. Included in linguistic form are rules that govern sounds and their combination (phonology), rules that govern the internal organization of words (morphology), and rules that specify how words should be ordered to produce a variety of sentence types (syntax).

Phonology

Phonology is the system of rules that govern sounds and their combination. Each language has specific sounds, or phonemes, that are characteristic of that language. Phonemes are combined in specific ways to form linguistic units known as words.

A **phoneme** is the smallest linguistic unit of speech that signals a difference in meaning. The words *bat* and *pat* differ from each other in only one way—their initial sound. Because this initial sound difference produces two different words, the difference is a meaningful one. Therefore, /b/ and /p/ are, by definition, two different phonemes. Phonemes are classified by their acoustic properties (the pattern of their sound waves), their articulatory properties (where in the oral cavity they are produced, or place of articulation), and their production properties (manner of articulation).

The use of phonemes is governed by two sets of rules. One set describes how sounds can be used in various word positions. These are called *distributional rules*. In English, for example, the *ng* sound, as in the word *long*, is a single phoneme that never appears at the beginning of a word. The second set of rules determines which sounds may be combined. They are called *sequencing rules*. In English, for example, the sound sequence *rs* may not appear in the same syllable. In sum, phonological rules govern sounds and their distribution and sequencing within a language.

Morphology

The second component of language—**morphology**—governs word formation. Morphological rules are concerned with the internal structure of words and how they are constructed from morphemes. **Morphemes** are the smallest linguistic unit with meaning (and cannot be broken into any smaller parts that have meaning). Words consist of one or more morphemes. Each of the words *ball, toy,* and *play* consists of one morpheme that can stand alone. Morphemes that can stand alone are called *free morphemes. Bound morphemes* cannot stand alone and are always found attached to free morphemes. They are affixed to free morphemes as prefixes (*un*happy) or suffixes (tall*est*). Bound morphemes that modify tense, person, or number are called *inflectional morphemes.* Examples of inflectional morphemes include the plural *s* (cat*s*), the past tense *ed* (play*ed*), and the possessive *'s* (Joan*'s*).

Bound morphemes can also be used to change one word into another word that may be a different part of speech. For example, *ness* changes the adjective *sad* into the noun *sadness.* In this case, bound morphemes are called *derivational morphemes,* because they are used to derive new words.

One task for the student of language development and disorders is to determine whether children have knowledge of morphology and to what extent it resembles the rule system of adults.

Syntax

Syntax is the rule system that governs the structure of sentences. It specifies the order words must take and the organization of different sentence types. It allows the individual to combine words into phrases and sentences and to transform sentences into other sentences.

A competent language user can take a basic sentence such as "The boy hit the ball" and transform it into a number of different sentence types.

> Did the boy hit the ball? *(interrogative)*
>
> The ball was hit by the boy. *(passive)*

Knowledge of the syntactic system allows a speaker to generate an almost infinite number of sentences (from a finite group of words) and to recognize which sentences are grammatical ("The boy hit the ball") and which sentences are not ("Ball the boy the hit").

Syntactic rules have two additional functions: They describe parts of speech (noun—*house;* verb—*hit;* adjective—*red*) and sentence constituents (noun phrases, verb phrases).

> Lightning *hit* (verb) the *red* (adjective) *house* (noun).
>
> *The boy* (noun phrase) *hit the ball* (verb phrase).

As children produce longer sentences, they begin to build sentences according to syntactic rules. They learn how to construct negative sentences, questions, and imperatives. Later, they add complex structures such as compound sentences and embedded forms. The development of syntax begins at about 18 months and continues for many years. Chapter 2 discusses syntactic growth during the preschool and school years.

CONTENT

The **content** component of language involves meaning. It maps knowledge about objects, events, and people, and the relationship among them. Included are the rules governing **semantics,** that subsystem of language that deals with words, their meanings, and the links that bind them. It encompasses meanings conveyed by individual words and the speaker's or listener's mental dictionary (called a *lexicon*).

Words are used differently by young children than they are by adults. A very young child may use a word that occurs in the adult linguistic system, but that word may not mean the same thing to him as to the adult. A 2-year-old may say the word *doggie,* but his word may refer to sheep, cows, and horses as well as to a dog. Alternatively, a 2-year-old may use the word *doggie* to refer to a particular dog without knowing it refers to a whole class of animals. Studying children's semantic system involves, in part, examining their understanding and use of words. Lexical acquisition is discussed more fully in Chapter 2.

The content component of language maps an individual's knowledge not only of objects ("big car") but also the relationship that exists between objects, events, and people. Note the use of the following semantic relations in the utterances of three 18-month-old toddlers, Benjy, Eli, and Yuda:

Context	Utterance	Semantic Relation
Mother and child sitting on the floor. Child pushes car and says:	"Push car"	Action–object
Mother and child are sitting in the kitchen. Mother is eating a cookie. Child says:	"Mommy eat"	Agent–action
Mother and child are in the kitchen. The child has just finished the milk in her cup. She points to the milk container on the table and says:	"More milk"	Recurrence

A more complete account of the meanings (semantic relations) children convey in their early utterances is given in Chapter 2.

Although most meaning is literal, it can sometimes be nonliteral. For example, if we talk about the "dance of life," we do not mean *dance* in the literal sense. Our meaning is figurative; that is, we are speaking of life in terms of patterns, grace, movement, and change.

Similarly, if I said, "I had a ball," you might infer that I had a good time. The word *ball* is used here in its nonliteral sense. However, note that a literal meaning is also possible (e.g., "I possessed a volleyball," or a baseball or basketball). Which meaning is appropriate will depend on the context and what has already been said.

In sum, meaning in language is conveyed through the use of words and their combinations. Content maps an individual's knowledge about objects, relationships, and concepts. This knowledge is derived from experiences and is a result of one's cognitive development. Lastly, it is important to remember that meaning can be both literal and nonliteral and is dependent on linguistic and nonlinguistic contexts.

USE

The **use** component of language encompasses rules that govern the use of language in social contexts. These rules are also called **pragmatics** and include rules that govern the reason(s) for communicating (called *communicative functions* or *intentions*) as well as rules that govern the choice of codes to be used when communicating (Bloom & Lahey, 1978).

The functions of language relate to the speaker's intention or goal. Greeting, asking questions, answering questions, requesting information, giving information, and requesting clarification are examples of language functions.

In addition to coding communicative intentions, speakers must use information regarding the listener and the nonlinguistic context to achieve their communicative intention. They must choose from alternative forms of a message the one that will best serve their communicative intention. Speakers must take into account what the listener already knows and does not know about a topic, as well as information about the context. The selection of the words and sentences to use to formulate a message depends on this information. For example, knowing the age and occupation of various listeners influences the choice of words with which to greet them. It is appropriate to say "Hi ya" to a 3-year-old and "How do you do?" to a school principal. The form of the message is also influenced by whether the topics of the message are present in the situation in which the utterance is used. For example, whether a speaker says "The doll is on the floor" or "It's over there" depends on whether the doll and the floor are in the immediate vicinity.

Lastly, pragmatics encompass rules of conversation or discourse. Speakers must learn to organize their conversations to make them coherent. They must learn how to enter, initiate, and maintain conversations. They must learn how to take turns, how to respond appropriately, and how to tell a cohesive narrative. An individual who is armed with these skills is said to be an effective communicator.

Correspondence and Integration of the Components of Language

We began this introductory chapter by defining language and by discussing the components that constitute it. The components of language and their subsystems are depicted in Table 1.1. Although the components of language appear as distinct entities, Bloom and Lahey (1978) have pointed out that they are indeed interrelated (see Figure 1.1).

How a child integrates linguistic components is best exemplified by the 2½-year-old child who looks through a window into the yard while her mother sits in the

Table 1.1   **Language Is**

Components	Linguistic Subsystems
Form	*Phonology* Rules that govern speech sounds and their combination *Morphology* Rules that govern the organization of words *Syntax* Rules that govern word order, sentence structure, and organization of different sentence types
Content	*Semantics* Rules that govern meaning (words and their combinations)
Use	*Pragmatics* Rules relating to the use of language in social contexts

Figure 1.1   **Bloom and Lahey's Model of Language**

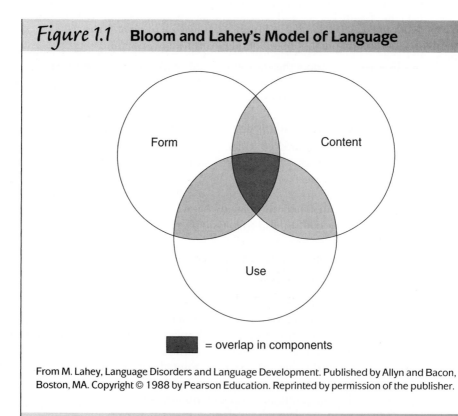

◼ = overlap in components

From M. Lahey, Language Disorders and Language Development. Published by Allyn and Bacon, Boston, MA. Copyright © 1988 by Pearson Education. Reprinted by permission of the publisher.

same room reading a book. As the child sees a kitten in the yard, she says to her mother, "Look, baby cat." The child has accomplished three things with this statement. First, she has linguistically coded two communicative intentions (getting attention and describing) by saying "look" and by describing what she sees. Next, she has linguistically coded knowledge about the animal she sees. Finally, she has expressed an utterance containing an acceptable word order. In sum, the child has communicated successfully by integrating pragmatic, syntactic, and semantic rules.

By taking the example a step further to a 3-year-old, we are able to demonstrate the child's integration of phonology and morphology with pragmatic, syntactic, and semantic rules. Both mother and her 3-year-old child are gazing through a window as two puppies are playing in the yard.

Mother: What do you see?

Child: Two puppies.

As in the previous case, the utterance codes knowledge about the animals and contains appropriate word order. In addition, the latter utterance contains the morphological ending that codes plurality. Using phonological rules, the child "knows" that the *s* in *puppies* is pronounced as a *z* because it follows a vowel, in contrast to the *s* in *cats,* which is pronounced as *s.*

Whereas the integration of form, content, and use is observed in the language of nondisabled children, a disruption of the components is often found in the language of children with disabilities. For example, many hearing-impaired youngsters produce language that possesses content but may be deficient in linguistic form. Their vocabulary and their communicative ability may be age appropriate, but their phonological, morphological, and syntactic skills often lag behind. Note the errors (indicated by bracketing) in the sample of David, a 5-year-old who has a hearing impairment:

Ye[s]terday I give it to . . . to . . . What[′s] hi[s] name? Oh, Bob? Right. He[′s] not in my cla[ss]. He's on my bu[s]. Why he can't come with me?

Or consider the following utterances produced by Sean, an 11-year-old child on the autism spectrum. Note the inappropriateness of his utterances and the lack of meaning in his sample. Also note the lack of errors in linguistic form.

Clinician: Sean, how are you today?

Sean: Fine, oh so fine, so very very fine and on my mind.

Clinician: Your class went on a trip yesterday. Tell me about it.

Sean: A trip, a trip. Yesterday, today, tomorrow. Hot dogs dogs—all kinds of dogs—bow-wow. It's October and Halloween. Pepsi the choice of a new generation; Coca-Cola red, white, and blue . . . and soup is good food, too.

The terms and concepts outlined thus far are basic to the study of language and its disorders. Because an understanding of typical language development is crucial to the student who will undertake intervention with language-disordered children, the following section outlines four theoretical perspectives on language acquisition. As this review is merely introductory, the beginning student is strongly urged to supplement it with references noted in the text.

Perspectives on Language Acquisition

Four multidisciplinary approaches to the study of language acquisition have predominated the literature in the past two decades: the behavioral, the psycholinguistic/syntactic, the semantic/cognitive, and the pragmatic. Each approach is summarized in terms of essential elements, emphasizing background, limitations, and contributions. Owens (2005), Nelson (1998), Bohannon and Bonvillian (2001), Berko Gleason (2001), and McCormick and Schiefelbusch (1990) provide more detailed descriptions of these approaches for interested readers.

BEHAVIORAL APPROACH

Background

The behavioral approach to language development was first presented by B. F. Skinner in *Verbal Behavior* (1957). Language learning, according to this approach, depends on environmental variables, which are mastered by imitation, practice, and selective reinforcement. The result is the acquisition of language through the gradual accumulation of vocal symbols and sequences of symbols. Within the process, parents and significant others are crucial because they model the appropriate utterances that children imitate and practice. By rewarding children's correct productions, parents shape children's utterances until they are grammatical and acceptable. In short, children learn language because their verbal behavior is selectively rewarded by others in the environment (Skinner, 1957). Variations on this theme are provided by Osgood (1963), Mowrer (1954), and Staats (1963).

Limitations

Chomsky (1959) faulted Skinner on three counts, the first being that Skinner attempted to explain the process of language acquisition while ignoring the content being learned. Chomsky said, "There is little point in speculating about the process of acquisition without a much better understanding of *what* is acquired" (p. 55).

Second, Chomsky pointed out that children seem to acquire a verbal repertoire far too quickly to depend on environmental conditioning mechanisms alone. Third, Chomsky argued that children produce utterances they never heard adults use—utterances such as "I goed" and "mouses."

Contributions

Although in the early 1960s criticism was leveled at the behavioral school for overemphasizing parental input, recent researchers have revised their thinking to acknowledge its importance in language development. Studies by Snow (1972), Newport (1976), and others have clearly shown the positive effects of parental linguistic input to children's language development. Another contribution made by the behaviorists to the field of speech-language pathology has been to delineate "systematic training designs and their applications to nonspeaking individuals" (McCormick & Schiefel-busch, 1984; Sandall, Hemmeter, Smith, & McLean, 2005; Schiefelbusch & Bricker, 1981). Structured behavioral techniques are commonly used in speech-language therapy and provide a basis for many intervention programs used with language-disordered children.

PSYCHOLINGUISTIC/SYNTACTIC APPROACH

Background

In the late 1950s and early 1960s, linguists, particularly Noam Chomsky, hypothesized that the human brain contains a mental plan to understand and generate sentences (Chomsky, 1957, 1965). This mental plan incorporates the necessary "electronic cir-cuitry" for children to internalize the knowledge necessary for deriving sentences.

Proponents of the psycholinguistic/syntactic approach hold that children have an innate predisposition to apply linguistic rules and that the human infant is "prewired" for language acquisition. According to Chomsky, a baby is born with an innate linguistic mechanism (called the *language acquisition device* [LAD]) that is ac-tivated by exposure to linguistic input. The LAD contains two parts: a set of rules or general principles for forming sentences, and procedures for discovering how these principles are to be applied to the child's particular language.

The child's LAD processes information from the linguistic environment and gen-erates hypotheses about the rules of his language. Using the concept of the prepro-grammed LAD, Chomsky was able to explain the seemingly miraculous ability of very young children to acquire language easily and rapidly and to produce an infinite number of novel yet grammatical utterances.

More recently, Chomsky (1981, 1999) revised his ideas of grammar and syntax to account more for language rules and well-formedness as well as for language learn-ability. The result is called *government-language binding theory* (GB theory). Chom-sky's goal was to present a theory that could account for the constraints on the kinds of hypotheses a child can form about the structure of his or her language no matter what language the child is learning. Government-binding theory attempts to account for the diversity of human languages and to explain the development of grammar by children on the basis of limited input. Chomsky (1999) called the resultant principles *universal grammar*. (For a more complete account of GB theory, see Bohannon & Bonvillian, 2001; Cairns, 1996; Leonard & Loebb, 1988; Nelson, 1998; Owens, 2005).

Limitations

Child development specialists (Schlesinger, 1977; Sinclair-deZwart, 1973) argue that Chomsky treats language learning as if it occurred independently of cognitive devel-opment. Citing Piaget's work, Sinclair-deZwart (1973) said that language develop-ment is dependent on cognitive development. Schlesinger (1977) pointed out that it is very difficult to ascertain from Chomsky's model precisely what children are born "knowing," as opposed to what they "come to know," and how this knowledge even-tually gets linked to words and phrases.

Semanticists (Fillmore, 1968) fault Chomsky by arguing that language depends more on underlying semantic representation than on syntactic rules. Sociolinguists challenge Chomsky's assertion that linguistic input is too fragmented, confused, and unsystematic to facilitate children's acquisition of language. Their data (Nelson, 1973b; Newport, 1976; Phillips, 1973; Snow, 1972) show that parental input enhances language learning. Chapter 2 details the nature of parental input and its facilitating effect on language development.

Contributions

Although the psycholinguistic/syntactic approach is currently viewed as being inadequate to explain language development, Chomsky's work provided the impetus for much in-depth research on the language acquisition process. Investigators began to search for developmental patterns that crossed cultural boundaries. More important, they began to realize the value of naturalistic observations (McCormick & Schiefelbusch, 1984). A host of studies on both normal and disordered language were published in the 1960s (Braine, 1963; Brown & Bellugi, 1964; Brown & Fraser, 1964; Menyuk, 1964), and studies comparing normal and language-disordered children's acquisition of morphology and syntax continue to be published (Hansson & Nettelbladt, 1995; Johnston & Schery, 1976; Leonard, 1992). Last, an alternative view of language learning evolved in contrast to the behaviorists' view, with the result that we currently view the child as being active and creative, rather than passive, in the language acquisition process (McLean & Snyder-McLean, 1999).

SEMANTIC/COGNITIVE APPROACH

Background

With the publication of Bloom's *Language Development: Form and Function of Emerging Grammars* (1970), there appeared a new focus in the study of language development: the meanings conveyed by children's utterances rather than their syntax.

In her seminal study of children's language at the early multiword stage, Bloom (1970) found that one of her subjects used "Mommy sock" on two different occasions. She used it once while she was picking up her mother's sock and once while her mother was putting a sock on her (the child's) foot. Although the form of the child's utterance was the same in both contexts, the *meanings* the child conveyed were clearly different. On the first occasion, she conveyed possession. The sock she was holding belonged to her mother. On the second occasion, the child's utterance conveyed a meaning found between an actor who was doing an action (Mommy) and an object (sock). Bloom concluded that children's language maps meanings. The meaning categories that children use to code relationships among entities found in the world were termed *semantic relations* by Bloom. Bloom further postulated that children express meanings long before they know anything about syntax and that the meanings they convey are based on their cognitive knowledge.

Following Bloom, the cognitive prerequisites for language acquisition became the subject matter of much research. The works of Piaget (1952, 1954, 1964) were reexplored, and the search began for linkages between the concepts attained in early cognitive development and early linguistic constructions (Sinclair-deZwart, 1973).

The evidence (K. Nelson, 1973a) tends to show that children begin to use language expressively to talk about what they know and that this knowledge is related to their sensorimotor experiences. A fuller account of the cognitive prerequisite for language acquisition is found in Chapter 2. Rees (1980) best captured the essence of the semantic/cognitive approach when she said that "children say only what they know how to mean" (p. 21).

Limitations

The semantic/cognitive approach to language development highlights the importance of meaning and cognition. However, it does not explain why some children, in spite of age-appropriate cognitive abilities, lag in their linguistic development (Cromer, 1974). It seems that conceptual abilities are not the only abilities important for language learning but that these other abilities are not accounted for in the semantic/cognitive approach.

Three other criticisms of the semantic/cognitive view have been offered. Bowerman (1978) pointed out that the semantic/cognitive approach does not answer the question of *how* children acquire language, nor does it explain the relationship between later developing cognitive abilities and corresponding linguistic attainments. Schlesinger (1977) observed that the semantic/cognitive approach ignores the role of linguistic input to the language acquisition process. How could a child learn language without being exposed to it? Last, McLean and Snyder-McLean (1999) argued that an adequate description of language acquisition must include formulations about the nature and purposes of children's social communicative interactions. They maintained that the social environment of the child is crucial to language development.

Contributions

The semantic/cognitive approach to language development is set against a background of overall development; hence, it gave impetus to multifaceted research on (1) the cognitive prerequisites of language (Bowerman, 1974; Sinclair-deZwart, 1973), (2) the universality of children's cognitive experiences resulting in a universality in their coding of meaning, and (3) the relationship between language and thought (Cromer, 1974; Miller, 1981; Rice, 1983). The role of imitation and play was reexamined (Bates, Benigni, Bretherton, Camaioni, & Volterra, 1979; Sinclair-deZwart, 1973; Westby, 1980) because scholars believed it was rooted in children's symbolic functioning. Last, the importance of contextual support (that is, the nonlinguistic context) was highlighted as being important to understanding the meanings children convey.

THE PRAGMATIC APPROACH

Background

Because communicative intentions are expressed in social contexts, the pragmatic approach views language development within the framework of social development. According to Bruner (1974/1975), children learn language in order to socialize and to direct the behavior of others. Social interaction and relationships are deemed crucial because they provide the child with the framework for understanding and formulating linguistic content and form.

Within the pragmatic model, caretaker–child interactions are considered to be the originating force for language learning (Rees, 1978). As caretakers respond to infants' early reflexive behaviors and their gestures, the infants learn to communicate **intentions.** Infants refine these communication skills through repeated communicative interactions with caretakers.

McLean and Snyder-McLean (1978, 1999) summarized the pragmatic model in four major statements:

1. Language is acquired if and only if the child has a reason to talk. Herein it is assumed that the child has learned that he can influence his environment through communication.
2. Language is acquired as a means of acknowledging already existing communication functions.
3. Language is learned in dynamic social interactions involving the child and the mature language user in his environment. The mature language user facilitates this process.
4. The child is an active participant in this transactional process and must contribute to it by behaving in a way which allows him to benefit from the adult's facilitating behavior.

The pragmatic model spawned a range of new research efforts. Expanding on the work of Searle (1965), Dore (1975), Halliday (1975), and Bates (1976) formulated a classification system for categorizing children's communicative intentions, and Bruner (1974/1975), Bates (1976), and others examined the role of parents and caretakers in the language acquisition process.

Limitations

The explanation of language acquisition by the pragmatic approach leaves two major questions unanswered:

1. How do communicative intentions become linked to linguistic structures?
2. How do children acquire symbols for referents?

Two further limitations relate to the newness of the pragmatic view. One, present researchers cannot agree on a common system for classifying communicative intentions; and two, a system for assigning a specific intention to children's utterances has not yet emerged.

Contributions

The pragmatic view highlights the social aspect of language and places language use in center stage. It specifies the contribution of environmental linguistic input and the role of caregiver modeling and feedback. In addition, it has stimulated research on the conditions and contexts in which communication develops (Bates, 1976; Bruner, 1974/1975), and has identified the social prerequisites of language acquisition (see Chapter 2). All of these contributions are aspects of a general communication background established well before children learn to use language expressively.

APPROACHES TO LANGUAGE ACQUISITION REVISITED

The four approaches to language acquisition—behavioral, psycholinguistic/syntactic, semantic/cognitive, and pragmatic—contribute to our understanding of language development and enable us to appreciate the complexity of language in the absence of a full-blown model. The need for a complete model of language acquisition, however, remains. Future research may indeed provide it, pending the successful integration of constructs developed in the four approaches reviewed here. This need for integration is best summarized by McLean and Snyder-McLean (1978):

> By nature of its content, language carries within it the products of the cognitive developmental domain; by nature of its function, language carries within it the products of social development; by nature of its form, language carries within it the complex products of all the inputs identified . . . plus the effect of the nature and functions of human physiological and neurological systems. (p. 43)

For the present, without a full model of language, we may view each approach as best describing one or more of the phases in development. As the normal child passes through these phases, different aspects of language acquisition may be emphasized. In the earliest stage of development (infancy), emphasis may be on pragmatic development. In the early preschool years, emphasis may be on syntactic development. Understanding the process of normal language acquisition provides the reader with a firm basis for understanding language disorders.

Approaches to Language Disorders

There are two major approaches to the study of language disorders in children: the etiological-categorical and the descriptive-developmental. In this section, we define each approach and identify the respective strengths and limitations of each. In conclusion, we present a working definition of language disorders as proposed by the American Speech-Language-Hearing Association (ASHA, 1980).

ETIOLOGICAL-CATEGORICAL APPROACH

The traditional approach to child language disorders involves the classification of disorders by their causes, or *etiology*. Each etiological category summarizes a cluster of behaviors that differentiates language-disordered children from their normally developing peers.

The use of etiological typologies grew out of the early work of McGinnis (1963) and Myklebust (1954). The etiological categories used by Myklebust (1954) included (1) mental retardation, (2) deafness and hearing impairment, (3) emotional disturbance and autism, and (4) childhood aphasia and neurologically based disorders. A fifth category, culturally and socially deprived, was later added, reflecting the political-social climate of the 1960s (Kamhi, 1990).

McCormick and Schiefelbusch (1984) classified language disorders into five etiological categories:

1. *Language and communication disorders associated with motor disorders.* Included in this category are children who possess motor deficits, as well as language disorders due to brain pathology (e.g., cerebral palsy) or damage to the nervous system (e.g., spina bifida). Children in this category possess motor difficulties and may have mental retardation, have visual and hearing impairments, and have seizure disorders. Because of the simultaneous multiple disabilities of these children and the space constraints of this text, we will not discuss this category. Instead, the reader is referred to Cruickshank (1976), McDonald and Chance (1964), and Mysack (1971) for a fuller account of this group.

2. *Language and communication disorders associated with sensory deficits.* Included in this category are children who have hearing and visual impairments. Because data on the language deficits of the blind are very scanty (Bernstein, 1978), we will discuss only hearing impairments as they relate to language disorders (see Chapter 8).

3. *Language and communication disorders associated with central nervous system damage.* Damage may be either mild or severe. Children are generally classified as learning disabled when the damage to the central nervous system is mild. When the damage to the central nervous system is severe, however, they are classified as developmental aphasics. Differentiating aphasics from other severely language-disordered children is both difficult and complex (McCormick & Schiefelbusch 1984). Hence, we limit our discussion to the language disorders associated with learning disabilities (see Chapters 5 and 11).

4. *Language and communication disorders associated with severe emotional-social dysfunctions.* Included in this category are children who are classified as psychotic, schizophrenic, and/or autistic. These children experience a profound disruption in the development of their verbal and nonverbal interaction skills. Considerable research on this disruption has been carried out in the area of autism spectrum disorders (ASD) and is reported in Chapter 7.

5. *Language and communication problems associated with cognitive disorders.* Included in this category are children who are classified as having mental retardation. The cognitive disabilities of children in this group vary according to the level of retardation. Chapter 6 discusses mental retardation and the language deficits associated with it.

Primary and Secondary Language Disorders

Another categorical classification system has also been proposed for childhood language disorders. Bernstein and Seiger-Gardner (in press) divide childhood language disorders into two categories: primary and secondary. A *primary language disorder* is said to exist when a language deficit cannot be accounted for by a peripheral sensory deficit such as a hearing loss, a cognitive deficit such as mental retardation, a social impairment such as ASD, or a harmful environmental condition such as parental drug abuse. This type of language disorder is presumed to be due to impairment of the central nervous system and would include children who are classified as having specific language impairment (SLI) when in preschool, or as having a language learning disability (LLD) when they reach school age (Owens, Metz, & Hass, 2007). The nature of SLI and LLD are described more fully in Chapters 4 and 5.

A *secondary language impairment* includes disorders that are associated with and presumed to be accounted for by sensory (hearing loss), cognitive (mental retardation), or social (ASD) impairment. These are discussed more fully in Chapters 6, 7, and 8.

Strengths of the Etiological-Categorical Approach

Etiology is a convenient way of comparing and distinguishing children with ASD, learning disabilities, mental retardation, and hearing impairment. Each classification is like a label that summarizes how a child is similar to or different from other children both within and across the disability categories.

A second and practical advantage of the etiological-categorical classification is that often a diagnostic label is needed for a child to receive appropriate services in schools. In many states today, children are placed in special education programs for speech, language, and resource services based on their diagnostic label. Furthermore, special education programs often are tailored to the etiology of a language disorder. Thus, one finds programs for children with ASD, hearing impairment, or mental retardation. In this context, it is understandable that a child must be so labeled in order to be admitted to the appropriate program.

Some advocacy groups have argued vociferously for the continuance of a categorical classification because they believe that it is better to be labeled and receive attention and services than to be ignored. This has been especially true of advocacy groups for the severely developmentally delayed: children with autism and children with mental retardation.

A third advantage of the etiological-categorical approach is that it provides speech-language pathologists with clues as to what type of remediation might be indicated and the modalities to be used during intervention. For example, knowing that a child possesses cognitive deficits, as in mental retardation, suggests remediation that focuses on teaching the concepts that language codes and on providing the child with redundant and repetitive cues to support the language being taught. Knowing that a child has a hearing impairment may lead the speech-language pathologist to search for alternative or augmentative systems to teach language. This may involve teaching some form of manual communication (e.g., sign language) or combining manual and spoken language (e.g., total communication).

Because much of the research concerned with language and communication disorders has focused on groups of children within etiological categories, five chapters— 4, 5, 6, 7, and 8—are devoted to explaining these findings. This information should be helpful to speech-language pathologists working in educational or clinical settings in which diagnostic labels are used.

Caution, however, is called for on two accounts: (1) There exists considerable overlap among categories, and (2) not all children within a diagnostic category possess similar abilities.

Limitations of the Etiological-Categorical Approach

Drawbacks of the etiological-categorical approach were highlighted by Bloom and Lahey (1978), who pointed out that a particular diagnostic label does not tell the speech-language pathologist what the child really knows about *language* and what he or she needs to learn. Moreover, it is rare to find a child who fits neatly into one diagnostic category. For example, it is not uncommon to find a child who has both mental retardation and a hearing impairment or a child who has mental retardation and also has autistic characteristics. In a similar vein, a categorical label implies that there is only *one* cause of the language disorder. This is rarely the case. Although a single factor may appear to be in large part responsible for a language disorder, there are almost always several contributing factors.

A second critique of the etiological-categorical approach has been made by Naremore (1980, 1995), who argued that assessment and intervention are not helped by categorizing. She stated that it would be difficult to find a procedure to assess a group of children defined as having either mental retardation or hearing impairments. Within the group, assessment must be customized to each child, with the aim of maximizing the resulting information and the understanding of that child's linguistic system and performance. The goal is to describe the child's linguistic behavior and to prescribe the specific methods and materials for improving his or her linguistic skills.

A third critique of the etiological-categorical model has been made by Kamhi (1990). He noted that an unfortunate outcome of this approach is that it serves "to divide treatment domains" (p. 73). He also pointed out that, in most instances, "speech-language pathologists are the most qualified professionals to treat language disorders *regardless* of etiological type" (p. 73).

THE DESCRIPTIVE-DEVELOPMENTAL APPROACH

The descriptive-developmental approach *describes* rather than classifies language disorders in children. It involves comparing the language-disordered child's ability to comprehend and formulate language with that of nondisabled children. It assumes that a child with a language disorder needs to learn what the nondisabled child needs to learn at some point in development (Naremore, 1980). McCormick and Schiefelbusch (1984) summarized this point of view:

> There is every reason to think that children with deficient language: (a) need language learning experiences as rich as those provided normal language users, (b) will attend to, understand and talk about many of the same objects, events and relations as typical learners, and (c) want and need to experience the same control over their environment as their more competent peers at the same stage of development. (p. 36)

According to the descriptive-developmental approach, a language disorder is "any disruption in the learning or use of the conventional system of arbitrary signals used by persons in the environment as a code for representing ideas about the world for communication" (Bloom & Lahey, 1978, p. 290). Disruptions occur in form, content, or use or in the interactions among them. Based on this construct, Bloom and Lahey (1978) differentiated five types of language disorders in children:

1. Children who exhibit difficulties in learning linguistic form. Included are children whose primary difficulty is in understanding and using phonological, morphological, and syntactic rules.

2. Children who exhibit difficulty in conceptualization and formulation of ideas about objects, events, and relations. Their primary difficulty is related to the semantic component—language content.

3. Children who exhibit difficulties in language use. Included are children who cannot adjust their language to meet listeners' needs, who do not use language to convey a range of communicative functions, and who have difficulties in understanding and speaking in certain contexts. Their primary deficit is in the area of pragmatics.

4. Children who exhibit difficulties in integrating form, content, and use. Bloom and Lahey (1978) termed this group of children as having association problems.

5. Children who exhibit language and communication skills that are similar in all ways to those of younger, typically developing children. Delayed language development is their primary disability.

Strengths of the Descriptive-Developmental Approach

The descriptive-developmental approach focuses on identifying the strengths and weaknesses of children with language deficits. It allows the speech-language pathol- ogist to describe children's language behaviors and to target those areas needing remediation.

Rather than labeling a child, this noncategorical approach is instructionally relevant. It zeroes in on those areas of language that pose difficulty for the child and gives the speech-language pathologist a teaching plan and sequence.

Limitations of the Descriptive-Developmental Approach

Although the descriptive-developmental approach overcomes some of the limitations of the etiological-categorical approach, three problems still prevail:

1. It does not present the clinician with clear-cut procedures as to how to teach those areas needing remediation. Although form, content, and use are useful constructs for understanding language and its disorders, the therapeutic contexts and procedures in which form, content, and use should be taught are not delineated.

2. It assumes that the administration of therapy to a language-disordered child is based on his linguistic disability and is irrelevant to his age or total environment. The descriptive-developmental approach has been criticized by Brown, Nietupski, and Hamre-Nietupski (1976), who have questioned whether it is useful to teach a 16-year-old adolescent with a mental disability, who has the developmental skills of a 2-year-old, the same vocabulary as one might teach a nondisabled 2-year-old. A strict adherence to the developmental approach without regard to the domestic, educational, and vocational settings in which the child must ultimately function is to Brown and his colleagues not educationally sound.

Brown and colleagues (1976) advocated an ecological perspective to intervention. The clinician is asked to search the relevant environments in which the child must function for clues as to what to teach. This might be considered the epitome of customized therapy.

3. The descriptive-developmental approach ignores the practical problems faced by educators in states where a disability label is mandatory for special class placement and/or the receipt of related services (Hobbs, 1978).

Language Disorders: A Definition

Because of the limitations described in both the traditional etiological-categorical approach and the descriptive-developmental approach, it is obvious that neither provides a complete definition. We present, then, ASHA's definition of language disorders as an alternative:

> A language disorder is the abnormal acquisition, comprehension or expression of spoken or written language. The disorder may involve all, one, or some of the phonologic, morphologic, semantic, syntactic, or pragmatic components of the linguistic system. Individuals with language disorders frequently have problems in sentence processing or in abstracting information meaningfully for storage and retrieval from short and long term memory. (ASHA, 1980, pp. 317–318)

According to the definition, impairment is in language comprehension (understanding), expression (formulation), or a combination of both. These deficits may be noted in listening and speaking or in reading and writing. Children who have language disorders may have difficulty in processing linguistic information, organizing and storing it, or retrieving it from memory. In short, ASHA's definition informs us about three important guidelines for considering language disorders: the components of language that might be impaired, the modalities that might be impaired, and the processes that might be impaired.

Summary

In this chapter, we have described the nature of language and its subsystems. After defining language, we went on to explain the various approaches to language acquisition. The discussion began with the behavioral approach and proceeded through the approaches of the psycholinguistic/syntactic, semantic/cognitive, and the pragmatic. Lacking a full-blown model, we integrated the several approaches to language acquisition by suggesting that normal language acquisition is a temporal process emphasizing different dimensions of language development at different stages of chronological development. Apropos is the comment of Owens (1984), who concluded his monograph on language development by saying, "A teacher or speech-language pathologist has to rely upon many sources of information" (p. 334). These sources of information equate with the various approaches to language development. On a practical level, this means that the speech-language pathologist "should be a behaviorist, a pragmatist, a cognitivist, a linguist, a developmentalist, and an optimist in order to put together an effective means of teaching language to children" (Schiefelbusch, 1978, p. 461).

A discussion of language disorders followed, with a review of two different approaches to language disorders: the etiological-categorical and the descriptive-developmental. Each approach was shown to have advantages as well as disadvantages. Unable to reconcile the differences, we presented an alternative—ASHA's approach to defining language disorders—in an attempt to summarize those impairments in the linguistic system that account for language disorders.

The following eleven chapters will elaborate and detail the preliminary discussions and definitions presented here. As you study them, do not hesitate to refer to the terms and definitions outlined in this introductory chapter. This will significantly contribute to a better understanding of communication acquisition and its disorders.

Study Questions

1. List at least five ways of communicating that you have used. Be specific.
2. What is the relationship of speech to language? Is language part of speech or is speech part of language?
3. a. Define each of the following systems of language:
     - (i) phonology
     - (ii) morphology
     - (iii) syntax
     - (iv) semantics
     - (v) pragmatics
   b. How do each of the above subsystems fit into Bloom and Lahey's (1978) model of form/content/use?
4. Discuss the strengths and weaknesses of each of the following perspectives in language acquisition:
   a. the behavioral perspective
   b. the psycholinguistic/syntactic perspective
   c. the semantic/cognitive perspective
   d. the pragmatic perspective
5. Compare and contrast the etiological-categorical classification of language disorders with the descriptive-developmental approach. What are the contributions and limitations of each approach?

References

ASHA Committee on Language, Speech and Hearing Services in the Schools. (April, 1980). Definitions for communicative disorders and differences, *ASHA, 22,* 317–318.

ASHA Committee on Language. (June, 1983). Definition of language, *ASHA, 25,* 44.

Bates, E. (1976). *Language and context: The acquisition of pragmatics.* New York: Academic Press.

Bates, E., Benigni, L., Bretherton, I., Camaioni, L., & Volterra, V. (1979). *The emergence of symbols: Cognition and communication in infancy.* New York: Academic Press.

Berko Gleason, J. (2001). *The development of language.* Boston: Allyn & Bacon.

Bernstein, D. K. (1978). *Semantic development of congenitally blind children.* Unpublished doctoral dissertation, City University of New York.

Bernstein, D. K., & Seiger-Gardner, L. (in press). Promoting communication development. In S. Raver (Ed.), *Introduction to early childhood special education: Strategies and practices.* Boston: Pearson.

Beukelman, D. R., & Mirenda, P. (2005). *Augumentative and alternative communication: Supporting children and adults with complex communication needs* (3rd ed.). Baltimore: Paul H. Brookes.

Bloom, L. (1970). *Language development: Form and function of emerging grammars.* Cambridge, MA: MIT Press.

Bloom, L., & Lahey, M. (1978). *Language development and language disorders.* New York: Macmillan.

Bohannon, J., & Bonvillian J. (2001). Theoretical approaches to language acquisition. In J. Berko Gleason (Ed.), *The development of language* (5th ed.). Boston: Allyn & Bacon.

Bowerman, M. (1974). Discussion summary—Development of concepts underlying language. In R. Schiefelbusch & L. Lloyd (Eds.), *Language perspectives—Acquisition, retardation and intervention.* Baltimore: University Park Press.

Bowerman, M. (1978). The acquisition of word meaning: An investigation in some current conflicts. In N. Waterson & C. Snow (Eds.), *The development of communication.* New York: Wiley.

Braine, M. (1963). The ontogeny of English phrase structure: The first phrase. *Language, 39,* 1–13.

Brown, L., Nietupski, J., & Hamre-Nietupski, S. (1976). The criterion of ultimate functioning and public school services for severely handicapped students. In M. A. Thomas (Ed.), *Hey, don't forget about me!* Reston, VA: Council for Exceptional Children.

Brown, R., & Bellugi, U. (1964). Three processes in the child's acquisition of syntax. *Harvard Educational Review, 34,* 133–151.

Brown, R., & Fraser, C. (1964). The acquisition of syntax. In U. Bellugi & R. Brown (Eds.), *The acquisition of language. Monographs of the Society for Research in Child Development, 92.*

Bruner, J. (1974/1975). From communication to language: A psychological perspective. *Cognition, 3,* 225–287.

Cairns, H. (1996). *The acquisition of language.* Austin, TX: Pro-Ed.

Chomsky, N. (1957). *Syntatic structures.* The Hague: Mouton.

Chomsky, N. (1959). A review of Skinner's "Verbal Behavior." *Language, 35,* 26–58.

Chomsky, N. (1965). *Aspects of the theory of syntax.* Cambridge, MA: MIT Press.

Chomsky, N. (1981). *Lectures on government and binding: The Pisa lectures.* Dordecht, the Netherlands: Foris.

Chomsky, N. (1999). On the nature, use and acquisition of language. In W. Ritchie & T. Bhatia (Eds.), *Handbook of child language acquisition.* New York: Academic Press.

Cromer, R. (1974). The development of language and cognition: The cognitive hypothesis. In D. Foss (Ed.), *New perspectives in child development.* New York: Penguin Education.

Cruickshank, W. (1976). *Cerebral palsy: A developmental disability.* Syracuse, NY: Syracuse University Press.

Dore, J. (1975). Holophrases, speech acts, and language universals. *Journal of Child Language, 2,* 21–40.

Fillmore, C. (1968). The case for case. In E. Bach & R. Harmes (Eds.), *Universals in linguistic theory.* New York: Holt, Rinehart & Winston.

Glennon, S., & DeCoste, D. (1997). *Handbook of augmentive and alternative communication.* San Diego, CA: Singular.

Halliday, M. (1975). *Learning how to mean: Explorations in the development of language.* New York: Edward Arnold.

Hansson, K., & Nettelbladt, U. (1995). Grammatical characteristics of Swedish children with SLI. *Journal of Speech-Hearing Research, 38,* 559–598.

Hobbs, N. (1978). Classification options: A conversation with Nicholas Hobbs on exceptional child education. *Exceptional Children, 44,* 494–497.

Johnston, J., & Schery, T. (1976). The use of grammatical morphemes by children with communication disorder. In D. Morehead & A. Morehead (Eds.), *Normal and deficient language* (pp. 239–258). Baltimore: University Park Press.

Kamhi, A. (1990). Language disorders in children. In M. Leahy (Ed.), *Disorders of communication.* London: Whurr.

Leonard, L. (1992). The use of morphology by children with specific language impairment: Evidence from three languages. In R. Chapman (Ed.), *Processes in language acquisition and disorders* (pp. 186–201). Chicago: Mosby-Yearbook.

Leonard, L. B., & Loebb, D. F. (1988). Government binding theory and some of its applications: A tutorial. *Journal of Speech and Hearing Research, 31,* 515–524.

McCormick, L., & Schiefelbusch, R. L. (1984). *Early language intervention.* Columbus, OH: Merrill/Macmillan.

McCormick, L., & Schiefelbusch, R. L. (1990). *Early language intervention* (2nd ed.). Columbus, OH: Merrill/Macmillan.

McDonald, E. T., & Chance, B. T., Jr. (1964). *Cerebral palsy.* Englewood Cliffs, NJ: Prentice Hall.

McGinnis, M. (1963). *Aphasic children: Identification and education by association method.* Washington, DC: Alexander Graham Bell Association for the Deaf.

McLean, J., & Snyder-McLean, L. (1978). *A transactional approach to early language training.* Columbus, OH: Merrill/Macmillan.

McLean, J., & Snyder-McLean, L. (1999). *How children learn language.* San Diego, CA: Singular Publishing.

Menyuk, P. (1964). Syntactic rules used by children from preschool through first grade. *Child Development, 35,* 533–546.

Miller, J. (1981). *Assessing language production in children.* Baltimore: University Park Press.

Mowrer, O. (1954). The psychologist looks at language. *American Psychologist, 9,* 660–694.

Myklebust, H. (1954). *Auditory disorders in children: A manual for differential diagnosis.* New York: Grune & Stratton.

Mysack, E. (1971). Cerebral palsy speech syndromes. In L. E. Travis (Ed.), *Handbook of speech pathology and audiology.* Englewood Cliffs, NJ: Prentice Hall.

Naremore, R. (1980). Language disorders in children. In T. Hixon, L. Schriberg, & J. Saxman (Eds.), *Introduction to communication disorders.* Englewood Cliffs, NJ: Prentice Hall.

Naremore, R. (1995). *Language intervention with school-aged children.* San Diego, CA: Singular.

Nelson, K. (1973a). Some evidence of the cognitive primacy of categorization and its functional basis. *Merill-Palmer Quarterly, 19,* 21–39.

Nelson, K. (1973b). Structure and strategy in learning to talk. *Monographs of the Society for Research in Child Development, 38.*

Nelson N. W. (1998). *Childhood language disorders in context: Infancy through adolescence.* Boston: Allyn & Bacon.

Newport, E. (1976). Motherese: The speech of mothers to young children. In J. Castellan, D. Pisoni, & G. Potts (Eds.), *Cognitive theory* (Vol. 2). Hillsdale, NJ: Lawrence Erlbaum Associates.

Osgood C. (1963). On understanding and creating sentences. *American Psychologist, 18,* 735–751.

Owens, R. E. (1984). *Language development: An introduction.* Columbus, OH: Merrill.

Owens, R. E. (1990). Communication, language, and speech. In G. Shames & E. Wiig (Eds.), *Human communication disorders* (3rd ed.). Columbus, OH: Merrill/Macmillan.

Owens, R. E. (2005). *Language development: An introduction* (6th ed.). Boston: Allyn & Bacon.

Owens, R. E., Metz, L., & Haas, A. (2007). *Introduction to communication disorders: A lifetime perspective* (3rd ed.). Boston: Allyn & Bacon.

Phillips, J. (1973). Syntax and vocabulary of mothers' speech to young children: Age and sex comparisons. *Child Development, 44,* 182–185.

Piaget, J. (1952). *The origins of intelligence in children.* New York: International Universities Press.

Piaget, J. (1954). *The construction of reality in the child.* New York: Basic Books.

Piaget, J. (1964). Three lectures. In R. Ripple & U. Rockcastle (Eds.), *Piaget rediscovered.* Ithaca, NY: Cornell University Press.

Rees, N. (1978). Pragmatics of language. In R. Schiefelbusch (Ed.), *Bases of language intervention.* Baltimore: University Park Press.

Rees, N. (1980). Learning to talk and understand. In T. J. Hixon, L. D. Shriberg, & J. H. Saxon (Eds.), *Introduction to communication disorders.* Englewood Cliffs, NJ: Prentice Hall.

Reichle, J., Halle, J., & Dragsow, E. (1998). *Implementing augmentative communication systems.* In A. Wertherby, S. Warren, & J. Reichle (Eds.), *Transitions in prelinguistic communication* (pp. 417–436). Baltimore: Paul H. Brookes.

Rice, M. (1983). Contemporary accounts of the cognition-language relationship: Implications for language clinicians. *Journal of Speech and Hearing Disorders, 48,* 347–359.

Romski, M. A., Sevcik, R. A., Cheslock, M., & Barton, A. (2006). The system for augmenting language: AAC and emerging language intervention. In R. McCaulay & M. Fey (Eds.), *Treatment of language disorders in children: Conventional and controversial intervention.* Baltimore: Paul H. Brookes.

Sandall, S., Hemmeter, M., Smith, B., & McLean, M. (2005). *DEC recommended practices: A comprehensive guide for practical application in early intervention/early childhood special education.* Longmont, CO: Sopris West.

Schiefelbusch, R. (1978). Summary and interpretation. In R. Schiefelbusch (Ed.), *Bases of language intervention.* Baltimore: University Park Press.

Schiefelbusch, R. L., & Bricker, D. D. (Eds.). (1981). *Early language: Acquisition and intervention.* Baltimore: University Park Press.

Schlesinger, I. (1977). The role of cognitive development and linguistic input in language acquisition. *Journal of Child Language, 4,* 153–169.

Searle, J. (1965). What is a speech act? In M. Black (Ed.), *Philosophy in America.* New York: Allen & Unwin; Cornell University Press.

Sinclair-deZwart, H. (1973). Language acquisition and cognitive development. In T. E. Moore (Ed.), *Cognitive development in the acquisition of language.* New York: Academic Press.

Skinner, B. F. (1957). *Verbal behavior.* New York: Appleton-Century-Crofts.

Snow, C. (1972). Mothers' speech to children learning language. *Child Development, 43,* 549–566.

Staats, A. W. (1963). *Complex human behavior.* New York: Holt, Rinehart & Winston.

Strum, J., Spadorcia, S., Cunningham, J., Cali, K., Stables, A., Erickson, K., Yoder, D., & Koppenhaver, D. (2006). What happens to reading between first and third grade? Implications for students who use AAC. *Augmentative and Alternative Communication, 22,* 21–36.

Westby, C. (1980). Assessment of cognitive and language abilities through play. *Language, Speech and Hearing Services in Schools, 111,* 154–168.

CHAPTER 2

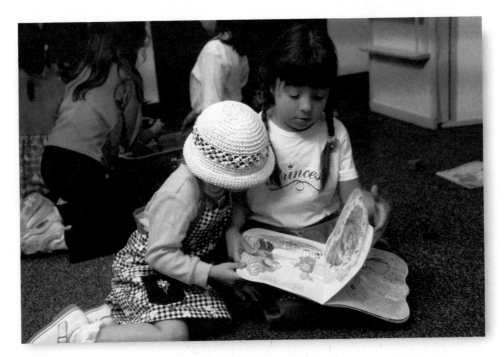

Language Development

A Review

Deena K. Bernstein
Lehman College, City University of New York
Sandra Levey
Lehman College, City University of New York

When you finish this chapter, you should be able to

- Describe the prelinguistic abilities of young children.
- Explain the role of the environment in language development.

- Describe the development of form, content, and use in preschool and school-age children.
- Trace the development of literacy skills.

The acquisition of speech, language, and communication is a complex process. It begins in infancy and continues to change throughout life. In Chapter 1, we discussed the nature of speech, language, and communication and showed how they are different but interdependent. This chapter presents a general overview of language development from birth through the school-age period. We include a review of the linguistic forms, meanings, and communicative functions acquired by children and adolescents. The following aspects of language development are its focal points:

1. the cognitive and social prerequisites for language acquisition
2. the prelinguistic development of infants and toddlers
3. the growth of phonological, morphological, syntactic, semantic, and pragmatic development from toddlerhood through the school-age years
4. the development of literacy skills

For a more detailed discussion of language development, the reader is referred to Berko Gleason (2001), James (1990), McLaughlin (1998), McLean and Snyder-McLean (1999), N. W. Nelson (1998), and Owens (2005).

Language Development: An Overview

Children come to the language acquisition process biologically equipped to learn language. However, they are not passive (Hirsh-Pasek & Golinkoff, 1997; Karmiloff-Smith, 1995; Sokolov & Snow, 1994). The literature shows that active learning begins early in children's development. For example, by 1 to 4 months, infants are able to detect intonational changes in speech patterns (Jusczyk, 1992), and they can recognize the connection between mouth movements and the sounds connected with these movements by 18 to 20 months (Kuhl & Meltzoff, 1997). Caretaker input, social interaction, play, and cognitive development all play a role in language development.

The preschool period, from 2 to 5 years of age, is a period of rapid growth in all areas of language: phonology (sequencing speech sounds to produce words, phrases, and sentences), syntax (sentence structure), semantics (meaning), and pragmatics (language use). Children begin to produce two-word utterances at age 2, but by age 5, they are producing lengthy sentences that contain information about the past and the future. Children have a 200- to 300-word vocabulary at 24 months and a vocabulary of approximately 2,000 words by age 5. They have mastered most sounds by 4 years of age. By 3 to 4 years of age, children are able to adjust their messages to accommodate to a listener's knowledge and status (child versus adult) and to use more polite forms to make requests.

Language development continues through the school-age years. These years are characterized by growth in all aspects of language: form (phonology, morphology, and syntax), content (semantics), and use (pragmatics). In addition, there is an increased awareness of language, which is necessary to develop more abstract language abilities.

During the school-age years, children also master new forms and learn to use these forms as well as existing structures to communicate more effectively. They learn to clarify messages and to monitor communications that indicate the success or failure of their communicative efforts. They expand the range of their communicative functions as they learn to use language in the classroom. In this environment, children must negotiate their turns by seeking recognition from the teacher and responding in a highly specific and precise manner to teachers' questions. During the school-age years, children also develop metalinguistic skills that enable them to think and talk about language. Metalinguistic skills help them master two important language skills: reading and writing.

Learning to read and write requires that children build on their previous language skills, such as their knowledge that speech sounds (phonemes) correlate with written letters (graphemes), and then they begin to communicate in this new mode.

It is important for the reader to keep in mind that (1) children's rate of language development shows variation due to differences in intellect, learning style, ethnicity, and socioeconomic factors (Owens, 2005); (2) the later stages of language development depend on the earlier ones; (3) language growth is a gradual process; and (4) phonological, morphological, syntactic, semantic, and pragmatic acquisition in spoken language are related to the acquisition of written language. Knowledge of these later areas of development is vital to our understanding of older children who exhibit deficits in reading and writing (Beck & Juel, 1995; Butler, 1999; Catts, 1991, 1996; Greene, 1996; Henry, 1993; Rubin, Patterson, & Kantor, 1991; Wallach, 1984) (see also Chapters 5 and 9).

In the next section, we will focus on some of the underpinnings of language acquisition, including children's cognitive development and interaction with the environment.

Cognitive Development

Early **cognitive development** involves a process by which children construct and reconstruct a representation of the entities and the events around them (Witt, 1998). Initially egocentric (centered around themselves), this egocentrism disappears as children become more aware that they are separate from the world, that they are not the cause of all activities, and that objects have properties separate from their own perception of their activity with these objects. Cognitive development is also tied to linguistic interaction with adults and siblings, and to activities in the environment.

According to Piaget (1954), children are viewed as having psychological structures (*schema*) that allow them to process information. These schemas change in response to the environment (*adaptation*). When confronted by a novel object or action, the child can either fit that novel event into a preexisting schema (*assimilation*) or be required to change the existing schema if that novel event does not fit into it (*accommodation*). Thus, children assimilate novel events into preexisting schema or accommodate preexisting schema to meet the demands of new situations. *Equilibrium* (cognitive balance) is the goal and is achieved through assimilation or accommodation.

Piaget (1954) identified four cognitive stages that begin at birth and continue until maturity (Table 2.1). The sensorimotor period is divided into six stages.

At stage 1 (birth to 1 month), children demonstrate accommodation or modification of a scheme (sucking) in response to environmental stimuli. In response to environmental experience, infants become more efficient at locating the nipple.

At stage 2 (1 to 4 months), there is an increase in eye–hand coordination, visual tracking of moving objects, and localization to sound. Primitive anticipation appears: The infant is now able to identify a wider set of signals that are associated with an event. For instance, a child will perform suckinglike movements when held by the mother, prior to presentation of the nipple. At an earlier stage of cognitive development, children begin sucking only when the nipple is placed in their mouths.

At stage 3 (4 to 8 months), children are (and will remain for a long time) egocentric, the cause of all actions. Imitation appears at this stage and represents the child's attempt to understand; to interact with the world. Children are now able to anticipate the path of a moving object; to reach for an object, even if it is partially hidden; and to manipulate this object.

At stage 4 (8 to 12 months), children are able to anticipate events; to establish a goal with a means to obtain that goal (means–end behavior); to imitate a wider set of

Table 2.1   Piaget's Stages of Cognitive Development

Stage	Age (years)	Characteristics
Sensorimotor period	(0–2)	Children become aware of the world and, at the end of this stage, use words to refer to entities, properties, and actions.
Preoperational thought	(2–7)	Children become aware of space, time, and quantity concepts and relationships.
Concrete operations	(7–11)	Children develop logical thought processes.
Formal operations	(11–15)	Children develop logical abstract thought.

actions; to understand that an object remains the same even when it is viewed from a different perspective, such as upside down or empty (object constancy); to understand that actions have a cause (causality); and to remember that an object exists even when it is removed from sight (object permanence). Increased but limited short-term memory is evident (Owens, 2005), and egocentrism is decreased.

At stage 5 (12 to 18 months), children experiment, explore, and use earlier established schemes or patterns of behaviors to solve new problems. In this manner, older schemes are modified. Children are now interested in producing new behaviors. Symbolic behaviors appear with the appearance of first words.

At stage 6 (18 to 24 months), children solve problems through thought rather than through physical means. They produce labels for objects or actions, even when the referent is not immediately present. Deferred imitation may also appear; that is, children can observe an action, store it in memory, and reproduce this action later.

Role of the Environment in Language Development

Although children may possess the genetic underpinnings for language development (Berko Gleason, 2001), language acquisition depends in no small measure on the interaction of the child with people and events in the environment. Recent literature describes the role of the environment in language acquisition, specifically the influence of adult–child interaction (Sokolov & Snow, 1994).

Caretaker–child interaction differs from the language used in adult–adult and adult–older child interaction in a number of ways: shorter sentences, simplified syntax, focus on objects or activities with which the child is engaged, the adult's repetition of his or her own utterances, repetition of the child's utterances, a higher pitch, exaggerated intonation patterns, increased pause duration between separate utterances, and a greater number of questions and commands (James, 1990; Owens, 2005). Adult-to-child speech efforts are also characterized by focus on the here and now. In fact, it was found that 90 percent of maternal input to younger children is focused on events and objects in the immediate environment (Ninio & Snow, 1996).

As noted previously, cognitive development is dependent on interaction with others and on interaction with the environment. Children assimilate or interpret events such as parental responses to their cries or demands. Children receive specific input relative to language from adults, and they attend to this information (Sokolov & Snow, 1994). The adult-to-child communication patterns presented in Table 2.2 are hypothesized to facilitate language development.

The style of adult-to-child interaction differs from culture to culture (Sokolov & Snow, 1994), and two basic interactive approaches have been proposed by Snow, Perlmann, and Nathan (1987). In the first interactional style, parents provide *discourse frames* for children by being responsive to children's actions, gestures, and vocalizations, thus providing children with a rich source of information about the language system through contingent input. In the second approach, parents present

Table 2.2   **Adult-to-Child Interaction Patterns**

Adult Pattern	Description	Example
Expansion	Verbal responses that increase the length or complexity of the child's utterance	*Child:* That doggie. *Adult:* Yes, that's a doggie or Yes, that's a big doggie.
Expatiations	Verbal responses that add new but relevant information to the child's utterance	*Child:* It fell down. *Adult:* Yes, it fell down because it was too close to the end of the table.
Vertical structuring	Questions are posed to fill in the pieces of an utterance; the adult then produces the entire utterance	*Child:* That moose holding up a hammer. *Adult:* What would happen if he dropped it? *Child:* It would fall on his toe. *Adult:* If moose dropped the hammer, it would hit his toe.
Prompts	Comments and questions that extend what the child has said	*Child:* He was scared of that monster. *Adult:* What did he think the monster would do to him?
Repetition	Repeating the child's utterance	*Child:* Big bird eating. *Adult:* Big bird eating.
Recast	Providing a model of the adult form of the child's utterance	*Child:* That my ball. *Adult:* That's my ball.

Adapted from Gillam (1999) and Strapp (1999). Copyright Gillam, R. B. (2000). Used by permission.

children with *predictable texts* based on the repeated presentation of familiar materials, allowing children to recognize and to internalize the structure of these texts, found in book reading or storytelling. Whichever approach is used, children benefit by gaining information about language.

The influence of adult input to children is found in the difference between the first words produced by English-speaking children and Chinese-speaking children. For example, nouns are more prevalent in adult-to-child interaction by English-speaking adults (Owens, 2005), whereas adult-to-child interaction by Mandarin Chinese–speaking adults consists mainly of verbs (Tardif, 1995; Tardif, Shatz, & Naigles, 1997). Consequently, the first words produced by English-speaking children are mainly nouns (Gentner, 1982; K. Nelson, 1973), but the first words produced by Mandarin Chinese–speaking children are nouns and verbs. Similar results were found for Korean-speaking children, whose parents use more words for activities than words for objects (Choi, 2000; Choi & Gopnik, 1995). These differences suggest that adult-to-child speech plays a significant role in some aspects of language development.

Infant and Toddler Early Communication

Infants possess innate abilities that prepare them for learning language. Some investigators argue that there is a connection between the sounds produced in infancy and early words. This view assumes that babbling is related to later speech production and constitutes a form of practice that contributed to language development (Stoehl-Gammon & Cooper, 1984). During babbling, the child stores the associations between oral–motor movements and sounds. Later in development, the child is able to draw on this behavior to produce meaningful speech.

Infants are capable of producing intentional communication. This means that they are able to use communication to indicate specific wants and needs. In infancy, intentionality is signaled by the use of gesture and/or vocalization coupled with eye contact, and by persistent attempts to communicate a request (James, 1990).

The sounds produced by infants from birth to 1 month of age consist of crying and vegetative sounds, such as clicks and burps (McLaughlin, 1998). Vowel-like sounds are also produced, termed *quasi-resonant nuclei* (Oller, 1978). At this stage of development, infants are able to discriminate between their mother's and another mother's voice and between utterances in a foreign language and their mother's language (Jusczyk, 1992).

Between 1 and 6 months of age, cooing, laughter, squealing, and growling appear. Cooing consists of vocalic sounds, sometimes produced in combination with the back consonants, /k/ and /g/, in consonant–vowel (CV) forms. In addition, infants are able to detect changes in intonation and to detect and recognize the occurrence of the same syllable in different utterances.

By 4 months of age, infants are able to match some vocalizations with corresponding facial shapes and show a preference for infant-directed speech (e.g., exaggerated intonation patterns, slower speech production, and higher pitch). They are also able to follow their mother's eye gaze or direction of pointing (Owens, 2005).

At 4 to 6 months of age, marginal babbling appears and consists of vowels, CV (/ba/) and VC (/ab/) forms. Reduplicated babbling, which appears at 6 to 8 months of age, consists of the alternation of consonants and vowels (*babababab*). Vocal play also emerges at this stage, and there is an increase in the variety of sounds that the child produces. Infants at this stage are now able to distinguish between words produced in their native language and words produced in a foreign language, based on the difference in prosodic features.

Variegated babbling appears at 8 to 10 months of age. This consists of strings of alternating consonants and vowels (*babigabadidu*). Babbling now corresponds to the intonation patterns of the adult language, but a decline occurs in the ability to detect phonetic contrasts and phonetic cues in foreign languages (Werker & Tees, 1984). This change correlates with the emergence of first words and suggests that discrimination has become more focused on the language spoken in the infant's environment.

At 8 to 12 months of age, echolalia appears. This is characterized by a parrotlike imitation of another's speech (McLaughlin, 1998). For example, the child may attempt to imitate the adult's utterances as well as the adult's tonal quality and gestures.

At 9 to 12 months of age, jargon emerges. Jargon consists of strings of syllables that mirror the stress patterns of adult speech, but these speech efforts are unintelligible.

Sounds that are consistent relative to a specific context emerge at 9 to 10 months of age. At this stage, children may produce one sound to indicate a request and a distinctly different sound to indicate refusal or rejection. These sounds are labeled *phonetically consistent forms* (PCFs), *vocables,* or *performatives* (James, 1990). PCFs and performatives are the consistent production of sounds to match a particular request within a context, such as *ah* to request being picked up by an adult and *uh* to request food items. While children produce sounds or sound sequences to communicate their intentions, sometime these are paired with gestures or with pointing.

Semantic Development

Semantics is the component of language concerned with meaning. Meaning can be conveyed through language at the word, sentence, and discourse levels, with *discourse* defined as a continuous stretch of speech, such as conversation. The meanings of some words can also be derived from the nonlinguistic context.

VOCABULARY DEVELOPMENT

Children's first words are produced at around 12 months of age. Their early word meanings consist of labels for familiar entities, action, and properties in the child's environment. An investigation of English-speaking children's first words (K. Nelson, 1973) revealed that the majority of them are nouns, such as *mommy* and *ball* (65 percent), followed by action words such as *go* and *up* (13 percent), modifiers such as *hot* and *mine* (9 percent), personal–social words such as *bye-bye* and *no* (8 percent), and function words such as *what* (4 percent). Nelson, Hampson, and Shaw (1993) also found that many of these first words could be considered either nouns or verbs (*drink*).

Children's early word meanings often do not correspond to adult meanings. For example, children may use the word *dog* to label other four-legged animals (sheep, cows, pigs, and horses). The use of a word to extend beyond the category for that word is called *overextension.* Notice that in the case of *dog,* the overextension that is produced by the child is related to the target word in terms of perceptual similarity (shape or movement). A child may also use the label *hat* to refer to a hat, a scarf, a ribbon, and a hairbrush. This overextension is related to the target word in terms of its function (Peccei, 1999).

Some researchers hypothesize that children produce overextensions because the target word has not yet been acquired and the child chooses the word that best fits that target. Another explanation offered is that children use overextension as a device for requesting the correct label for the target. In either case, overextension is a frequent pattern in acquisition until around 3 years of age. As children develop their semantic abilities, their meanings will more closely resemble the adult targets.

Young children have an expressive vocabulary of one or more words at 12 months, a 4- to 6-word vocabulary at 15 months, a 20-word vocabulary at 18 months, and a

Table 2.3   **Relational Words: One-Word Utterances**

Category	Meaning	Example
Existence	The child notes an object	Points or says *that* or *what that?*
Nonexistence	The child notes that an entity is absent	Says *no* or *gone*
Disappearance	The child notes that an entity has disappeared	Says *gone* or *all gone*
Recurrence	The child requests reappearance or notes that an entity reappears	Says *more*

Adapted from R. E. Owens, *Language Development.* Copyright © 2001 by Allyn & Bacon. Reprinted/adapted by permission.

200- to 300-word vocabulary at 24 months. Children's receptive vocabulary generally exceeds their expressive vocabulary. For example, when children have an expressive vocabulary of 10 words, they are usually able to comprehend at least 50 words.

RELATIONAL MEANING

In addition to acquiring lexical knowledge that specifies referents, children acquire meanings that code relationships among people, objects, and events. Later, these relationships are coded in children's simple sentences. The semantic relations that appear when children are at the one-word stage are shown in Table 2.3.

As children develop cognitively, the relationships they map and the forms they use to express these relationships become increasingly complex. The study of early semantic development by Brown (1975) revealed that children consistently produced certain semantic roles. These are presented in Table 2.4.

Pragmatic Development

Children's increase in social awareness is evidenced in the uses to which they put their developing language skills. Children at the one-word stage use language to communicate three main functions: regulating others' behavior, establishing joint attention, and social interaction (James, 1990). Children between 1 and 2 years of age increase the variety of communicative intents to include regulation intents (gaining attention, requests, and calling), statement intents (naming, description, and giving information that is beyond the here and now), exchange intents (descriptions of activities, intent to carry out an action, refusal, and protest), and conversational intents (imitation, answer, conversational responses, and questions) (McShane, 1980).

Children's early attempts to communicate their intentions have also been described by Halliday (1975). According to this researcher, the function of toddlers' early communicative intentions are (1) the *instrumental* function, used to obtain a

Table 2.4   **Semantics Roles Underlying Children's Early Language**

Semantic Role	Definition/Example
Nomination	Labeling an animate or an inanimate object: *doggie, ball*
Existence	Noting the existence of an animate or an inanimate entity: *mommy, that shoe*
Agent	Recognition that an animate initiated an activity: *daddy throw*
Object	Recognition that an inanimate is receiving the force of an action: *cut bread*
Possession	Recognition that an object belongs to or is in the frequent presence of someone: *mommy shoe*
Location	Recognition of a spatial relationship between two objects: *doggie bed*
Experiencer	Recognition that animate was affected by an event: *baby fall*
Attribution	Recognition of properties not inherently part of the class to which the object belongs: *baby cry*
Denial	Rejection of a proposition: *no bed*
Nonexistence	Recognition of the absence of an object that was once present: *cookie all gone*
Rejection	Prevention or cessation of the occurrence of an activity or the appearance of an object: *no more throw*
Instrument	awareness that an inanimate was causally involved in an activity: *car bump*
Recurrence	awareness of the potential for marking the reappearance of an object or reenactment of an event: *more cookie*
Notice	recognition that an object has appeared or some event has occurred: *hello daddy*

Adapted from R. E. Owens, *Language Development*. Copyright © 2001 by Allyn & Bacon. Reprinted/adapted by permission; and J. S. Peccei, *Child Language*. Copyright © 1999 by Routledge. Reprinted by permission.

goal and to have wants and needs met (the child holds out a cup and says *more*); (2) the *regulatory* function, used to control others' behaviors (the child gives a ball to an adult to request play and says *ball*); (3) the *interaction* function, used to obtain joint attention (the child calls *mama*); and (4) the *personal* function, used to express feelings or attitudes (the child says *yum* while eating a cookie) (Halliday, 1975).

Dore (1978) discussed the early communicative intentions produced by infants and toddlers at the prelinguistic and the one-word utterance stage. He labels these primitive speech acts as shown in Table 2.5. Whichever taxonomy one uses, it is now clear that babies understand that their words will produce responses from others; they have become active communicators.

Table 2.5   **Primitive Speech Acts**

Speech Act	Nonlinguistic Aspect	Example
Requesting action	Gesture, attends to adult	Cannot reach a toy, utters *uh, uh* while reaching for the toy
Protesting	Resists, attends to adult	Cries and resists being dressed
Requesting answer	Addresses adult, gesture	Holds out a toy and produces label with a rising intonation, awaits adult response
Labeling	Attends to entity	Touches doll's nose and says *nose*
Answering	Addresses adult	Adult points to a picture of a cow and asks "What's that?"; the child answers *moo*
Greeting	Attends to adult or entity	Child says *hi* when sees adult
Repeating	Attends to preceding utterance	Adult says *book*; child says *book*
Practicing	Not addressed to adult	Child practices words or phrases
Calling	Addresses adult and expects a response	Child calls *mama* from another room

Adapted from R. E. Owens, *Language Development*. Copyright © 2001 by Allyn & Bacon. Reprinted/adapted by permission.

Phonological Development

Children produce their first words with recognizable meaning between 1 and 1½ years of age. Toddlers' abilities to make themselves understood is often limited by their difficulty in producing sounds and the sound sequences that constitute words. Unfamiliarity with the child's manner of speaking or with the nonlinguistic context often makes it difficult to recognize /gɔgi/ for *doggie* or /dus/ for *juice*.

Children's acquisition of speech sounds is orderly, but a great deal of variability is shown by them in their acquisition of particular sounds. Figure 2.1 shows the age at which most children acquire specific consonants.

In the process of learning the sound system of a language, children often simplify the adult word targets. The simplifications children use as they attempt to produce adultlike speech are called **phonological processes.** Phonological processes may consist of substitution of one sound for another (*tat* for *cat*), the omission of a sound or a syllable (*nana* for *banana*), the distortion of a sound (a sound produced incorrectly), or the addition of a sound (*buhlack* for *black*).

Toddlers' productions of words are often characterized by the following phonological processes: reduplication, unstressed syllable deletion, final consonant deletion, and cluster reduction (Owens, 2000). These are defined in Table 2.6 (p. 40).

The phonological processes listed in Table 2.6 are part of the typically developing child's speech and may persist for many years. Researchers believe that the presence of phonological processes in children's speech may be due to either their

Figure 2.1 **Normative Articulation Data**

The left-hand margin of each bar represents the age at which 50 percent of the children in a normative study used the specified sound correctly. The right-hand margin shows the age at which 90 percent of the children used the sound correctly.

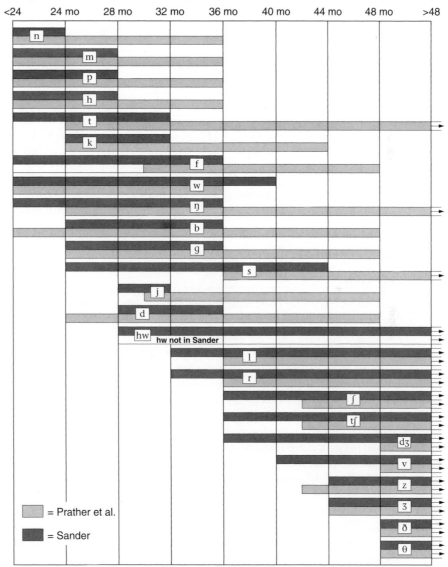

Adapted from J. E. Bernthal & N. W. Bankson, *Articulation and Phonological Disorders.* Copyright © 1998 by Allyn & Bacon. Reprinted/adapted by permission; and Prather, Hedrick, and Kern (1975). Articulation development in children aged two to four years. *Journal of Speech and Hearing Disorders, 40,* 186. © American Speech-Language-Hearing Association. Reprinted with permission.

Table 2.6   **Common Phonological Processes of Toddlers**

Process	Example
Reduplication: the first syllable of a word is repeated and is substituted for subsequent syllables in the word.	*Cracker* becomes *caca* /kækæ/.
Final consonant deletion: the final consonant of a word is deleted (CV/CVC).	*Bed* becomes *be* /bɛ/.
Cluster reduction: one or more consonants from a target consonant cluster is deleted.	*Please* becomes *pease* /piz/.
Deletion of unstressed syllables: a simplification.	*Giraffe* becomes *raffe* /ræf/.

Adapted from R. E. Owens, *Language Development*. Copyright © 2001 by Allyn & Bacon. Reprinted/adapted by permission.

difficulty in perceiving the adult target or to their limited ability to produce the adult target, and its presence often interferes with their speech intelligibility.

Preschool Language Development: An Overview

As children advance from simple one- and two-word utterances, their utterances become longer and more complex. They gradually elaborate the way they say things by adding more detail and by adding and filling in words and word endings that were missing in their early utterances. Whereas children at 18 months are producing such utterances as *mama, milk, close it, sock off,* and *more juice,* as their language abilities grow, their language samples consist of two- and three-word utterances that include articles (*a, the*), prepositions (*in, on*), pronouns (*I, he*), auxiliary verbs (*is, are*), noun endings (such as *-s* to indicate plurality), and verb endings (such as *-ed* to indicate past tense). Examples of such utterances include *want a cookie, block in box, he is bad, more cookies,* and *door opened.*

In the preschool period, children's vocabulary continues to grow and they learn many new word meanings. They learn new concepts and how to code these concepts linguistically. As they develop cognitively, they begin to refer to objects, actions, people, and events that are displaced in terms of time and place, and they transform their ideas into sentences by using a variety of sentence types.

During this period, children also learn more complex ways to use language socially and begin to develop discourse skills, such as participating in conversations; giving instructions; providing descriptions about objects, events, and people; and relating personal experiences and simple stories. Lastly, during this period, they learn about the nature of print. The emergence of preliteracy skills during the preschool years lays the foundation for their development of reading and writing.

It is important to note that children's development of language during this period is related to their cognitive development. We now turn our attention to this area and its relationship to play skills and language development.

COGNITION, PLAY, AND LANGUAGE

According to Piaget (1954), the preoperational stage of development occurs between 2 and 7 years of age. Symbolic functioning appears and is represented by symbolic play and further language development.

Patterson and Westby (1998) provide a description of symbolic or pretend play development that occurs during this period. At around 18 months, play consists of activities that are familiar to children, such as pretending to sleep or to drink. This period is followed at 19 to 22 months by the extension of these activities to another entity or person, with children pretending to feed a doll or imitating adult activities. At 24 months of age, children begin to perform sequences of familiar activities, such as baking a cake, and between 24 and 30 months, they include dolls in their pretend activities, ascribing needs to the doll (hungry, tired, or sick), and placing the doll in the role of agent (walking the doll rather than carrying it).

The scope of play expands at about 30 months as children begin using a wider set of less frequently occurring activities in their play activities: going to the store, going to the doctor, or going to visit a relative are play sequences that are often observed. Play behaviors that are episodic and consist of multischeme sequences emerge at about 3 years of age. These multischeme sequences may include going to the store to buy groceries, cooking and serving dinner, or having a birthday party. Ascribing emotional states to dolls (or stuffed toys) and talking for a toy appears at 3 to 3½ years of age. By 3½ to 4 years of age, children begin to take on different roles in play activities. These roles expand to include fantasy characters, police and fire fighters, and more familiar family roles. Their play may involve imaginary friends, or they may take a multifaceted role, such as a mother who goes to work. By 5 years of age, children do not need props to engage in play, and they can use language alone to maintain play activities. Their play consists of complex sequences that include dialogue.

Patterson and Westby (1998) argue for a relationship among cognition, pretend play, and language development. They assert that the emergence of first words co-occurs with the emergence of pretend (symbolic) play because pretend play demonstrates a child's ability to separate an object from an immediate context. Thus, a child may use a block to represent a train or a telephone and a word to represent an object or action that is removed from the immediate context. Over time, as children develop cognitively, their play becomes increasingly sophisticated.

THE DEVELOPMENT OF SYNTAX AND MORPHOLOGY

Children begin to produce two-word utterances at about 18 months of age. This stage is characterized by utterances such as *see boy, see sock, push it, close it , allgone milk, I sit, I see, boot off, mama come, milk cup, dry pants, change diaper, more juice, other bib,* and *do it* (O'Grady, 1997). Children at this stage are remarkably accurate in producing the correct syntactic form. For example, children place modifiers in the correct position preceding common nouns (*big doggy*) and preceding indefinite pronouns (*big one*). They do not make errors by placing the modifier preceding a definite pronoun (**big he*) (P. Bloom, 1990).

As children advance from simple two-word utterances, their utterances become longer and more complex. They elaborate their utterances by adding more details, such as words and suffixes (inflectional and derivational morphemes) that were missing in their early utterances. Words take the form of articles (*a, the*), prepositions (*in, on*), pronouns (*I, he*), and auxiliary verbs (*is, are*). Inflectional morphemes take the form of the plural *-s* attached to nouns to indicate plurality, the possessive *'s* to indicate possession, the present progressive *-ing* attached to verb stems to indicate present and ongoing action, and the past-tense marker *-ed* to indicate prior activity. The inclusion of these forms acts to expand young children's utterances, making their utterances more adultlike and less telegramatic. They progress from producing utterances such as *more milk* at 12 to 18 months to utterances such as "I want more chocolate milk" at 24 to 36 months.

Young children's sentences frequently are produced with subject drop, or omission of pronouns in the initial position in utterances—for example, *want cookie, give cookie,* and *go car*. Subject drop will persist until children's mean length of utterance (MLU) is increased (Valian, 1991), their preference for a strong–weak stress pattern is lost (Gerken, 1991), or they are able to produce verb tenses (Hyams, 1992).

By age 4, most children's syntax is adultlike (Gopnik, 1997), but language continues to develop and to be refined throughout childhood and adulthood. Children learn how to transform their ideas into sentences, and they begin to use a variety of sentence types. Their utterances contain expanded noun phrases ("Gimme *the big red ball*") and verb phrases ("He pushed me *down the steps*"). Utterances also consist of negative sentences ("I *won't* do it"), yes/no questions ("*Can* you cut the cake?"), and *wh-* questions ("*What* will I do later?"). Causal constructions ("He didn't get a prize *because* he was bad"), conditional constructions ("*If* I do my homework, I'll get to watch TV"), and temporal constructions ("*When* he comes, he'll get a surprise") are also evident.

BROWN'S STAGES

Brown's pioneering work, *A First Language* (1975), demonstrated that children's acquisition of syntactic structures is not as much a function of their chronological development as it is a function of the average number of morphemes per utterance that they produce. This measure is called **mean length of utterance** (MLU). In a longitudinal study of three children, Adam, Eve, and Sarah, Brown found that utterance length and the mastery of grammatical forms varied greatly with age. For example, Sarah and Adam progressed from MLU of less than 2.0 to MLU of 4.0 in fifteen months. It took Eve less than eight months to make this progress. Major linguistic changes take place as MLU increases. These changes are characterized by certain MLU stages, outlined in Table 2.7.

Stage I is characterized by single-word utterances and early multiword combinations that follow semantic rules. Examples of utterances during this period include *more* and *mommy*. Later in this stage, children produced two-word utterances such as *drink milk, gimme juice,* and *push car*.

Table 2.7 **Brown's Stages**

Linguistic Stage	MLU	Approximate Chronological Age (months)	Characteristics
I	1.0–2.0	12–26	Use of semantic rules
II	2.0–2.5	27–30	Morphological development
III	2.5–3.0	31–34	Development of a variety of sentence types: negative, imperative, interrogative
IV	3.0–3.75	35–40	Emergence of complex constructions: coordination, complementation, relativization
V	3.75–4.5	41–46	
VI	4.5+	47+	

Adapted from Brown (1975).

Stage II is characterized by the appearance of grammatical morphemes. Children expand and modify their linguistic productions by including morphological endings such as *-ing*, the plural *-s*, and the prepositions *in* and *on*. Utterances such as *Jimmy eating*, *Put ball in*, and *See cats* are characteristic of this stage. At Brown's Stage II (at approximately 2 to 2½ years of age), American English–speaking children begin filling out their short, immature sentences by incorporating one or more of the fourteen grammatical morphemes studied by Brown. Grammatical morphemes begin to emerge in Stage II, but many are not mastered (used correctly 90 percent of the time) until after Stage V.

The fourteen morphemes studied by Brown are obligatory, meaning that their use is required. The absence of a particular morpheme in a child's utterance at a certain stage of development may mean that either it has not yet been acquired or it may indicate a developmental delay. Table 2.8 lists the order of emergence of these fourteen grammatical morphemes.

The three children studied by Brown (1975) were remarkably consistent in the order in which they acquired morphological endings and function words. These results were confirmed in a later study of morphological development of twenty-one children (de Villiers and de Villiers, 1978). A more recent study of morphological development in forty-two children (Lahey, Liebergott, Chesnick, Menyuk, & Adams, 1992) found that variability among children was higher until MLU reached 3.5 or 4.0, or until children were 35 months of age. In addition, the order of acquisition differed somewhat from earlier studies: The contractible copula ranked higher and the past irregular ranked lower in comparison to Brown's (1975) results. In addition, mastery of certain morphemes was found to be slower than previously described.

Table 2.8   **Order of Emergence of 14 Grammatical Morphemes***

Grammatical Morphemes	Examples	Age of Mastery (months)
1. Present progressive verb ending -*ing*	Mommy push*ing*. Johnny throw*ing*.	19–28
2. Preposition *in*	Put *in* box.	27–30
3. Preposition *on*	Put *on* table.	27–30
4. Plurals (regular) (-*s*)	Eat cookie*s*. More block*s*.	24–33
5. Past irregular verbs (*came, fell, broke, went*)	He *went* outside. Johnny *broke* it.	25–46
6. Possessive noun ('*s*)	Jimmy'*s* car. Mommy'*s* coat.	26–40
7. Uncontractible copula (*be* as the main verb: *am, is, are, were, was*)	He *was* bad. They *are* good.	27–39
8. Articles (*a, the*)	Billy throw *the* ball. Give me *a* big one.	28–46
9. Past regular (-*ed*)	He jump*ed*. She push*ed* me.	26–48
10. Third-person singular regular	He cook*s*. Johnny goe*s*.	26–46
11. Third-person singular irregular	He *has* books. She *does* work.	28–50
12. Uncontractible auxiliary (*be* verbs preceding another verb: *am, is, are, was, were*)	The boys *are eating*. The baby *is crying*.	29–48
13. Contractible copula	I'*m* good. She'*s* nice.	29–49
14. Contractible auxiliary	I'*m* eating. She'*s* jumping. They'*re* playing.	30–50

*Used correctly 90% of time in obligatory contexts.
Adapted from Brown (1975).

A burst of syntactic development occurs in Stage III. Utterance length continues to grow as children begin to use simple declarative sentences, imperatives, *wh-* questions, and simple negative sentences. During this period, children begin to use a variety of sentence types. Examples of utterances characteristic of this stage include "Jimmy hit the ball," "Will I eat?" "The boy is not eating," and "Push the truck."

Stage IV is marked by the emergence of complex constructions, although the mastery of syntax continues beyond this stage. Children exhibit the use of noun- and verb-phrase elaborations as well as compound and complex sentences. Examples of utterances produced at Stage IV and beyond include "Daddy is cooking and Mommy is writing," "The first boy is nice," "Jill wants to buy the dress with the green band," "She likes to eat chocolate ice cream," and "I want to push the red truck."

PRONOUN ACQUISITION

Learning the English pronominal system is a very complex process (P. Bloom, Barss, Nicol, & Conway, 1994; Dale & Crain-Thoreson, 1993; Oshima-Takane, Takane, & Shultz, 1999; Ricard, Girouard, & Decarie, 1999; Rispoli, 1998). In the case of *I* and *you,* the child must learn to understand that the referent changes, depending on the changing role of speaker and listener in a communicative interaction. Learning also requires understanding that a pronoun may refer to a previously mentioned word or an entity—for example, "Sue bought a dress; *it* was expensive." The meaning of a sentence that contains a pronoun often cannot be understood without referring to a preceding sentence. This use of a pronoun in reference is known as **anaphoric reference** and is discussed more fully later in this chapter.

Some pronouns appear in Brown's Stage II, whereas others emerge much later. In general, the earliest pronouns to emerge usually involve the child as subject (*I, mine, my, me*). Other subjective pronouns emerge later (*he, she, they*). Objective pronouns (*him, her, them*) follow and are acquired earlier than possessive pronouns (*his, her, theirs*). Reflexive pronouns (*himself, herself, themselves*), the last to emerge, are usually not mastered until after age 5. Table 2.9 presents the general order of pronoun acquisition.

ADJECTIVE AND NOUN SUFFIXES

During the preschool years, children acquire some additional suffixes for adjectives and nouns. The adjectival comparative *-er* and the superlative form *-est* emerge between 3 and 5 years of age (McLaughlin, 1998). Children add these forms to adjectives

Table 2.9 **Development of Pronouns within Brown's Stages**

Brown's Stages	Pronouns
I	I, mine
II	My, me
III	He, she, we, you, your
IV	They, his, hers
V	Their, our, ours, theirs
V+	Herself, himself, themselves

Adapted from Haas and Owens (1985) and Owens (1988). Reprinted by permission.

to create the words *nicer, biggest,* and *smallest.* Comparatives and superlatives that are exceptions to the rule (*better, best*) usually take longer to acquire. Derivational noun suffixes are usually understood by children by age 5 and mastered somewhat later. Thus, by age 5, children understand and produce such words as *hitter* and *teacher* (which contain the derivational noun suffix *-er*), whereas they acquire words that contain the derivational *-ist* morpheme somewhat later (*pianist, cyclist*).

PHRASE AND CLAUSE DEVELOPMENT

Whereas words are made up of morphemes, sentences are composed of phrases and clauses. There are two major types of phrases: noun phrases and verb phrases. A **noun phrase** must contain a noun and may contain optional elements that modify the noun, such as a determiner (*the*) or adjectives (*big, pretty*). A **verb phrase** must contain a verb and may contain other optional elements, such as adverbs (*fast, slowly*) and another noun phrase (*in the morning, at school, a cookie*). An example of a sentence that contains all of these elements is "The little dog slowly ate the big cookie in the kitchen."

There are four types of noun phrase modifiers:

1. *Determiners* include articles (*a* and *the*), possessive pronouns (*my, your*), demonstratives (*this, that*), and qualifiers (*any, some*). They are always the first element in a noun phrase (*the* boy, *my* book, *some* toys).
2. *Adjectivals* include adjectives (*little, big*), ordinals (*first, last*), and quantifiers (*two, few*). They modify nouns (*two* dresses, *big* boy).
3. *Initiators* include *all, only, both,* and *just,* which limit or quantify nouns and must precede a determiner (*only* the boy, *all* the girls).
4. *Postmodifiers* follow the main noun. They may include prepositional phrases (the toy *on the floor* is broken) and clauses (the boy *who came to my house*).

Although noun phrases emerge at Brown's Stage II, the greatest surge in their development occurs at Stage IV, when sentences that contain seven words may be produced. At this stage, semantics, pragmatics, syntax, and morphology have become more adultlike (Norris, 1998). Early modifier types are determiners and adjectivals; initiators and postmodifiers appear later in development. By late Stage IV, noun-phrase elaboration appears in both subject and object positions and includes the use of almost all the modifier types mentioned previously.

A verb phrase must contain a main verb and may contain some optional elements. In the sentence "The girl is pushing the boy," *is pushing the boy* is the verb phrase. It contains the auxiliary verb *is,* the main verb *push,* and the optional present progressive form *-ing.* Optional elements of verb phrases include progressive constructions (is eat*ing*), modals (words that indicate mood or attitude, e.g., *may, must*), and perfective constructions (used to specify a single-occurring, nonhabitual action, e.g., *has seen, has eaten*). Verb-phrase elaboration emerges at Brown's Stage II (with the marking of the present progressive) and continues through Stage V. Modals emerge at Stage IV, and both the contracted and perfective ("I *have* eat*en* dinner") constructions at Stage V (Norris, 1998).

In contrast to a phrase, a **clause** is a group of words that contains both a subject and a predicate. Some clauses can stand alone and can function as simple sentences ("Billy walks," "Mary ate"). Sentences that are made up of two or more main clauses are called *compound sentences* ("John drank and Mary ate"). These structures usually emerge at Brown's Stage IV (Norris, 1998). Complex sentences are made up of one main clause and one subordinate clause ("The dress *that we bought yesterday* was pretty"). The embedding of subordinate clauses appears late in language development, usually at early Stage V.

Generally, *intransitive clauses* (clauses containing a verb that cannot take a direct object, such as "The girl walked") appear in children's declarative sentences before *transitive clauses* (clauses that take a direct object, such as "The boy drank milk"). *Equative clauses,* containing a copula and complement ("Sam is the teacher") emerge last (Dever, 1978). The interaction between syntax and verb identity may affect the difficulty with acquisition of transitive clauses. The first verbs produced by young children describe simple actions such as *eat, read, do,* and *fix* (Bloom, Lightbown, & Hood, 1975).

Gleitman and Gleitman (1994) point out that verb learning occurs when children become aware of syntactic (sentence) structure. In terms of the nature of verbs, the verb *hit* is a two-argument verb (expressing a relationship between two things) and consequently requires a transitive clause: for example, "Daddy hit the ball." In contrast, the verb *cries* is a one-argument verb and is found in intransitive structures: for example, "Mary cries." These factors may explain acquisition in terms of argument structure requirements and the stages of verb acquisition.

SENTENCE DEVELOPMENT

One of the most basic syntactic rules states that every sentence must contain a noun phrase and a verb phrase. Thus, the only required syntactic elements of a sentence are a subject and a predicate. By the end of Brown's Stage II or early Stage III, children have mastered this rule and can understand and produce simple, active declarative sentences such as "The boy hit the ball." Children then begin to modify this basic sentence pattern. They produce a variety of sentence types, including the negative, interrogative, and imperative sentence forms. The emergence of the adultlike form of sentence types is evident within Brown's Stage III. Table 2.10 presents the acquisition of sentence forms within Brown's stages of development. A more detailed account of the development of each sentence type follows.

The Development of Negative Sentence Forms

L. Bloom (1991) found that children at the one- and two-word utterance stage express three types of negation: (1) **nonexistence** (*Allgone juice*—when there is no more juice in the cup), (2) **rejection** (*No milk*—as the child rejects the offer of milk), and (3) **denial** (*Not a book*—as mother points to a truck and says, "This is a book").

Table 2.10   **Acquisition of Sentence Forms within Brown's Stages of Development**

Stage	Negative	Interrogative	Embedding	Conjoining
Early I (MLU: 1–1.5)	Single word—*no, all gone, gone;* negative + X	Yes/no asked with rising intonation on a single word; *what* and *where*		Serial naming without *and*
Late I (MLU: 1.5–2.0)	*No* and *not* used interchangeably	*That* + X; *What* + noun phrase + (doing)?	Prepositions *in* and *on* appear	*And* appears
Early II (MLU: 2.0–2.25)		*Where* + noun phrase + (going)?		
Late II (MLU: 2.25–2.5)	*No, not, don't,* and *can't* used interchangeably; negative element placed between subject and predicate	*What* or *where* + subject + predicate	*Gonna, wanna, gotta,* etc., appear	
Early III (MLU: 2.5–2.75)				*But, so, or,* and *if* appear
Late III (MLU: 2.75–3.0)	*Won't* appears; auxiliary forms *can, do, does, did, will,* and *be* develop	Auxiliary verbs begin to appear in questions (*be, can, will, do*)		
Early IV (MLU: 3.0–3.5)			Object noun phrase complements appear with verbs such as *think, guess, show*	Clausal conjoining with *and* appears (some children cannot produce this form until late V); *because* appears
Late IV (MLU: 3.5–3.75)	Adds *isn't, aren't, doesn't,* and *don't*	Begins to invert auxiliary verb and subject; adds *when, how, why*		
Stage V (MLU: 3.75–4.5)	Adds *wasn't, wouldn't, couldn't,* and *shouldn't*	Adds modals; stabilizes inverted auxiliary	Relative clauses appear in object position; multiple embeddings by late V; infinitive phrases with same subject as the main verb	Clausal conjoining with *if* appears

| Post-V (MLU: 4.5+) | Adds indefinite forms *nobody, no one, none,* and *nothing;* has difficulty with double negatives | Relative clauses attached to the subject; embedding and conjoining appear within same sentence above an MLU of 5.0 | Clausal conjoining with *because* appears with *when, but,* and *so* beyond MLU of 5.0; embedding and conjoining appear within same sentence above an MLU of 5.0 |

From Owens, 1988; reprinted by permission.

Three phases of negative construction development have been described (Bellugi, 1967; L. Bloom, 1991; Peccei, 1999). Table 2.11 illustrates the development of the negative sentence form.

In Phase I, the negative element is placed outside of the sentence (*no bed*). Drozd (1995) describes the use of presentence *no* as a metalinguistic exclamatory negation. In this case, the child is responding to an adult utterance ("Do you want to go to bed?") and repeating most of this adult utterance (*no bed*). O'Grady (1997) proposes a trigger for the child's utterance. When adults frequently say "No, don't touch that," the position of the negative (*no*) cues the child to produce this negative element in sentence-initial position (*no touch*).

In Phase II, children transfer the *no* marker to its correct position before the verb ("I no want milk"). The negative form *not* also appears in this phase ("He not big"). In Phase III, when MLU is greater than 4.0, the negative contractible forms *can't* and *don't* emerge ("I don't have a cookie").

Indefinite negative words such as *nobody, no one,* and *nothing* present the young language learner with difficulty. Young children often say "I want anything," when they mean "I want nothing" (Seymour & Roeper, 1999). Older, school-aged children

Table 2.11   **Development of the Negative Sentence**

Phase	Description	Example
I	The negative marker appears outside the sentence.	*No* the girl running.
II	The negative marker occurs before the verb.	The girl *not* running.
III	The auxiliary is added and completes the transformation to the adult form.	The girl is *not* running.

might say "I don't got no books," and even adults might say "I don't see nobody." Although these sentences may be judged to be ungrammatical, double negatives are considered grammatical in many other languages and dialects (Peccei, 1999).

The Development of the Interrogative Sentence Form

There are two types of questions: **yes/no questions** ("Do you want a cookie?") and *wh-* **questions** (which begin with *who, what, when, where, why,* or *how*). Yes/no questions require that the listener simply answer the question with either a *yes* or a *no* word. *Wh-* questions are more complicated because they require that the listener provide additional information. For example, *where* questions demand information about location, *when* questions demand temporal information, and *who* questions demand information about people.

To form correct yes/no questions, children must learn to invert the subject and the auxiliary verb ("Is the boy eating?"). To form correct *wh-* questions, they must learn to (1) transpose the subject and the auxiliary verb and (2) add the *wh-* form at the beginning of the sentence ("What is the boy eating?"). Children go through four phases as they develop the ability to formulate questions (L. Bloom, 1991; Klima & Bellugi, 1966).

- *Phase 1*—use of rising intonation and some *wh-* forms (MLU 1.75 and 2.25). In this first phase, children typically ask yes/no questions by adding a rising intonation to the end of their utterances. Examples of such question forms are "Johnnie eat?" "Baby drinking?" and "Go outside?" To ask *wh-* questions, young children simply attach a *wh-* word to an assertion and produce questions like "Where doggie?" and "What dat?" These *wh-* questions are used in routines in which children generally ask for the names of objects, actions, or locations, such as the location of an object that has disappeared. *Where* and *what* questions are the more prominent *wh-* questions used during this phase. At this phase, children do not respond appropriately to any of the *wh-* questions.

- *Phase 2*—use of a greater variety of *wh-* questions (MLU 2.25 to 2.75). Children in this phase continue to ask yes/no questions by using rising intonation. Children ask *wh-* questions by adding the *wh-* form at the beginning of the question but fail to use the auxiliary verb. Children are able to provide appropriate answers to *what, who,* and *where* questions. Examples of *wh-* questions that characterize this period include:

  Where my truck?

  Why you pushing it?

  What the man doing?

- *Phase 3*—limited use of inversion (MLU 2.75 to 3.5). Auxiliary + verb inversion appears when children's MLU is at 3.5 morphemes (O'Grady, 1997). In this phase, children regularly invert the subject and verb to produce yes/no questions but fail to do so in all *wh-* questions. Examples of questions that characterize this period are as follow:

  Will I go?

  What the boy is riding?

- *Phase 4*—use of inversion in positive *wh-* questions (MLU 3.5+). In this last stage, children invert the subject and the auxiliary verb when asking positive *wh-* questions but still have difficulty with negative *wh-* questions. Examples of *wh-* questions of this period are the following:

> What is the boy eating?
>
> Where are you going?
>
> Why I can't do that?

What, where, and *who* questions are mastered before *why, how,* and *when* questions (L. Bloom, 1991; Ervin-Tripp, 1970). In the case of the former, the *wh-* words that introduce the questions can be recovered from a sentence—for example, "John (*who*) ate pizza (*what*) in his house (*where*)"—whereas the words *why, how,* and *when* require additional information that must be recovered from context or discourse—for example, "Why did John do it?" and "When will you go?" Thus, *what, where,* and *who* forms code cognitively simpler ideas involving objects, people, or places (Norris, 1998), whereas *when, why,* and *how* forms involve the need to consider intentionality and planning. The order of acquisition of questions is summarized in Table 2.12.

L. Bloom, Merkin, and Wooten (1982) hypothesize an interaction between *wh-* questions and verbs. They argue that young children between 22 and 36 months of age use questions with the verbs *do, go,* and *happen* because these verbs have a general use within a wide range of activities, such as doing things, going places, and things that are happening. In contrast, the later-occurring *why* and *how wh-* questions are used with descriptive verbs with a more limited range of use, such as *sing* and *fix*.

The Development of Imperative Sentence Forms

The imperative sentence requests, demands, commands, or insists that a listener perform some action. At the prelinguistic level, infants request and demand by pointing

Table 2.12 Order of Acquisition of *Wh-* Questions

Type	Example
What	What is the girl eating?
Where	Where is the ball?
Who	Who is pushing the truck?
When	When will you go?
Why	Why is it dark?
How	How did it break?

From S. Ervin-Tripp, "Discourse agreement: How children answer questions," In J. R. Hayes (Ed.), *Cognition and the development of language,* Copyright © 1970 by John Wiley & Sons, Inc. Reprinted by permission of John Wiley & Sons, Inc.

and gesturing. As they develop into toddlers, they begin to employ the imperative form to request, demand, and command. At Brown's Stage I, children produce forms that sound like imperatives because they often omit the subject (subject drop), even when it is required (*touch doggy*).

In imperative sentences, the subject *you* is understood and not included in the surface form of the sentence, and the verb is uninflected. Examples of imperative sentences are "Gimme milk," "Push the truck," and "Pass the butter, please." True imperatives begin to appear at Brown's Stage III, when the omission of the subject in the surface form reflects the mastery of the rule of subject deletion in imperatives.

THE DEVELOPMENT OF COMPLEX SENTENCES

Children begin to combine more than one semantic/syntactic relation in a single utterance when their MLU increases beyond 3.0. Their utterances reflect the elaboration or specification of agent–action–object interactions, and sentence construction advances from a linear ordering of words to a hierarchical ordering within and among sentence elements. Children learn to use complex sentences that allow the expression of old functions and new ideas with increasing clarity (Tyack & Gottsleben, 1986).

Coordination

The complex construction that emerges first in children's language is **coordination.** There are two types of coordination constructions: sentential coordination and phrasal coordination. In **sentential coordination,** two events are combined into one sentence by the conjunction *and* ("John went to the doctor *and* his sister stayed home"). In **phrasal coordination,** the connective *and* is also used, allowing the speaker to delete a redundant element. In the sentence, "Jane went to the movies and ate popcorn," the word *and* allows for the deletion of *Jane* from the second phrase ("Jane went to the movies and ____ ate popcorn"). Lund and Duchan (1993) suggest that semantic and cognitive complexity affect children's learning of complex sentence structures such as coordinated structures. Children must determine the grammatical relations within sentences and the deletion of one or more elements in the sentence.

The earliest use of coordination by children is in stereotypic phrases (*bread and jam, milk and cookie*) that are present in young children's utterances as responses to routine questions such as "What do you want to eat?" Both types of coordination are acquired at the same time (L. Bloom, Lahey, Hood, Lifter, & Fiess, 1980). Children 2½ to 3 years of age use both sentential and phrasal coordinations appropriately when the communicative context is set up to elicit them: sentential coordination for events at different times and places; phrasal coordination for events at the same time and place (Owens, 2005).

L. Bloom (1991) focused on semantic considerations in the acquisition of coordinated sentences and found the following order of acquisition of *and* coordinations:

1. **Additives**—the use of *and* to connect two propositions that go together ("Mother is baking a cake and Daddy is reading").
2. **Temporal**—the use of *and* to designate a sequential ordering of events ("Mommy will mix the batter and put it in the oven").

3. **Causal**—the use of *and* to indicate that one event led to another ("She put a bandage on and it made her feel better").
4. **Adversative**—the use of *and* to indicate a contrast relationship ("This goes in here and that goes there"). Often the connective used in this instance is *but*.

Complementation

There are several types of complement structures in English. **Complementizers** in English consist of words such as *that* (e.g., "I said *that* I would call him"). Other examples of sentences with complement constructions are "I want *to buy a red lollipop*," "Show me *where this one goes*," and "Look at *what she's doing*." In each of these sentences, the main portion of the sentence is coupled with a clause that modifies the verb.

L. Bloom, Lifter, and Hafitz (1980) studied complement constructions and found that the order of emergence is based on the semantics of the verb. The first complements to emerge in children's speech contain state verbs, verbs that express a feeling or intention. *Like, want,* and *need* are state verbs and take the complement *to* ("I want to go home" and "I like to get dirty"). The next complement to emerge is attached to notice verbs, such as *see, look,* and *watch*. These verbs are followed by the complement *what* ("Look at what he's doing").

The third complement to emerge is attached to knowledge verbs such as *know* and *think*. These are followed by the complement *that* or *what* ("I know what to do" and "I think that one is good").

The last complement to emerge is attached to speaking verbs, such as *ask, tell,* or *promise*. Speaking verbs require the complement construction *to* plus a verb. Sentences such as "Ask Mary to come inside" and "John promised to leave" are examples of sentences with speaking verb complements. L. Bloom, Lifter, and Hafitz (1980) concluded that the acquisition of complement constructions is a function of semantic constraints: these verbs are used to qualify the degree of certainty or uncertainty of a proposition (i.e., "I know what to do" versus "I *think* I know what to do").

Relativization

Complex sentences can be formed by adding **relative clauses,** which restrict or qualify the meaning of another portion of the sentence. Relative clauses usually begin with complementizers (*that*) or relative pronouns (*who, which, whom, whose*). Relative clauses are of two types: objective and subjective. Objective relative clauses modify the object of the sentence, as in "That picture is about some birds *that got all smeared up*." An example of a sentence with a subjective relative clause is "The girl *who lives down the block* is my cousin."

Children are reported to produce sentences that contain objective relative clauses before subjective relative clauses, such as "The book [that you want] is on the table" (Menyuk, 1977). The objective relative clause develops after 5 years of age, whereas the relative clause that is part of the subject phrase of the sentence is rare even at 7 years of age. O'Grady (1997) argues that interpretation of relative clause constructions requires determining (1) the role of a gap (a missing noun phrase) and (2) the reference of this gap. Preschool children interpret the sentence "The lion [that the horse kisses __ __] knocks down the duck" as "The lion [that ___ ___ kisses the horse] knocks down the duck." In this example, the broken lines mark the gap, or the missing noun phrase *the lion*. In the previous example, children have difficulty determining the subject of the action *kisses* but have less difficulty with sentences such as "The dog [that ___ ___ jumps over the pig] bumps into the lion." In both examples, children identify the first noun as the subject of the relative clause.

PRESCHOOL CHILDREN'S PHONOLOGICAL DEVELOPMENT

The phonological patterns of preschool children can be classified into two basic categories (Bernthal & Bankson, 1998): **whole-word processes** (simplifications of words, syllables, or contrasts between sounds) and **segment-change processes** (changes in sounds). Examples of these processes follow.

Whole-Word Processes

Children frequently simplify words by reducing them to either the basic consonant–vowel (CV) syllable or to CVCV structure. Four processes that accomplish this simplification are **reduplication, final consonant deletion, cluster reduction,** and **unstressed syllable omission** (see examples in Table 2.6). Additional processes that affect word production include the following:

- **Epenthesis** occurs when children insert a segment in a word. An example is the production of /bəlæk/ for *black*.
- **Metathesis** consists of the reversal of two segments in a word. An example is the production of /bæksɪt/ for *basket*.

Segment-Change Processes

A number of rule-governed segment changes are common in the speech of preschoolers. These changes are classified according to the place or manner of production of the speech sounds:

- **Fronting**—This process occurs when children replace palatal and velar sounds (made in the back of the mouth) with alveolar sounds (made in the front of the mouth). Examples are the production of /tʌp/ for *cup* and /dʌn/ for *gun*. Fronting of velars is usually suppressed by 2½ to 3 years of age, and velar consonants are usually established in children's speech by age 4 at the latest.
- **Stopping**—Instead of producing fricatives (sounds that are made by passing air through a narrow constriction, thereby creating a hissing sound) or affricates (sounds that combine a popping sound and a fricative), children substitute a plosive (a popping sound). The use of the stopping process results in productions such as /dut/ for *juice* and /bæn/ for *van*. Stopping begins to disappear for most fricatives and affricates by 2½ to 3 years of age.
- **Gliding**—Children substitute glides (sounds that are produced during the movement of articulators from one vowel position to another) for liquids (sounds with vowel-like quality of little air turbulence). Examples of gliding are

the production of /wæbɪt/ for *rabbit* and /jaɪt/ for *light*. This process may persist for many years.

ASSIMILATION PROCESSES

Another group of processes are those in which two phonemes within a word become alike:

- **Consonant harmony**—a process in which consonants within a word become more alike in terms of place or manner of articulation. An example of consonant harmony is the production of /gɔgi/ for *doggy*.
- **Prevocalic voicing**—a process in which unvoiced consonants are affected by the following vowel and take on the voicing feature of the vowel. The result is the production of /dʌb/ for *tub*.

Unstressed syllable deletion, final consonant deletion, velar fronting, consonant assimilation, reduplication, and prevocalic voicing should disappear by 3 years of age. Cluster reduction, epenthesis, gliding, and stopping may persist after 3 years of age.

PHONOLOGICAL PROCESSES: LANGUAGE DIFFERENCES

Some of the phonological processes found in typically developing 3- to 4-year-old Spanish-speaking children of Puerto Rican descent consist of the following (Goldstein & Iglesias, 1996):

- Word-final /s/ and /n/ may be deleted: /pæ/ for *pan*.
- The glide /j/ is produced as the voiced alveo-palatal affricate /dʒ/: /dʒo/ for *yo*.
- The labiodental fricative /f/ becomes a bilabial fricative /ɸ/ in initial and medial positions in words: /kaɸɪ/ for *coffee*.

Phonological processes found in speakers of African American English (AAE) include the following (Goldstein, 2000):

- devoicing of final consonants: /pɪk/ for *pig*
- diphthongs often neutralized to vowel form: /aɪ/ for /a/
- final stops devoiced and followed by glottal stop: /bætɪ/ for *bad*
- final stops devoiced: /bæt/ for *bad*
- final consonant deletion of nasals and stops: /pæ/ for *pan*
- stopping in word-initial position: /d/ for /ð/: /de/ for *they*
- intervocalic production of /f/ for /θ/ v for /ð/: /brevɚ/ for *brother*
- final production of /f/ for /θ/ and v for /ð/: /bæf/ for *bath*
- postvocalic liquids deleted: /mo:/ for *more*
- substitution of /k/ for /t/ in initial consonant clusters: /skrit/ for *street*
- metathesis: /æks/ for *ask*
- initial unstressed syllable deletion: /baut/ for *about*

Children's development of phonological and speech production skills plays an essential role in their ability to communicate, especially with unfamiliar listeners. Some phonological difficulties appear only when children produce longer sentences, possibly as a result of the increased demands on sound sequencing when producing longer sentences.

Preschool Semantic Development

Semantics is the component of language concerned with meaning. Without meaning, there would be no point to language. People talk in order to express meaning, and they listen in order to discover the meaning of what others say. Meaning can be conveyed through language at the word, sentence, and discourse levels. The meanings of some words can also be derived from the nonlinguistic context.

LEXICAL MEANING

The most familiar sense of meaning is **lexical meaning.** It is concerned with the meanings of words and the characteristics of the category to which a word belongs. The preschool period is one of rapid lexical growth. Vocabulary increases markedly during the second year of a child's life (Golinkoff, Mervis, & Hirsh-Pasek, 1994). At 3 years of age, preschool children have an expressive vocabulary of 900 to 1,000 words. By age 4, their expressive vocabulary is 1,500 words, and at 5, it is over 2,000 words (Owens, Metz, & Haas, 2000).

As children develop, they become better able to define words. For example, during the late preschool period and into the early school years, children's word definitions are concrete and consist primarily of a referent's appearances and function. Later in development, children's definitions are more abstract and include synonymy (i.e., words with similar features, such as *sick* and *ill*), explanation (i.e., giving the reason for an action), and specifications of categorical relationships (i.e., placing entities in categories, such as *dog* and *bird* in the category *animal*). Lexical growth is a gradual process and continues for many years.

RELATIONAL MEANING

In addition to acquiring lexical knowledge that specifies referents, children acquire meanings that code relationships among people, objects, and events. The **relational meanings** that were coded at the early stage of language development also appear in the language of preschool children. These relationships are now conveyed at the sentence level (also called *intrasentence meaning*).The early relational meanings (or semantic content categories) of existence, nonexistence, and recurrence that are evident in children's early language are coded during this period, not with single words but with multiword combinations and simple sentences (see Table 2.13). As children develop cognitively, the semantic relations they express include the coding of concepts of space, time, causation, and sequencing of action using more complex linguistic forms and a variety of sentence types.

CONTEXTUAL MEANING: THE ROLE OF DISCOURSE

Context affects many aspects of language, including language meaning. The **linguistic context,** or discourse, provides information necessary to derive intrasentence meaning.

Table 2.13   **Semantic Relations (Intrasentence Meanings) Expressed by Two- to Four-Year-Olds**

Semantic Relation	Age	Example
Coordination	2.0	My car . . . truck.
Sequence	2.0	Bye-bye, Mommy, Daddy, Joey.
Causality (logical)	2.0	I can't do it. It too long.
Reasons	2.4	You hit me because you don't like me.
Temporality	2.8	Now I wash my hands, then I eat. When he goes to school he goes on the bus.
Conditionality	3.4	I wear this while walking.
Temporal sequence	3.5–4.0	I will make a tree after I finish this.

Adapted from Miller (1981).

The influence of the linguistic context on meaning can be understood by examining the following sentence:

He bought it.

It is not possible to derive the meaning of this sentence without knowing something about the previous linguistic context, which supplies the information of whom *he* refers to and what *it* is. Within the context of the following discourse, however, the meanings of *he* and *it* become clear:

Tom: John saw a red Jaguar at a car dealer yesterday.

Susan: What happened?

Tom: He bought it.

In the discourse, the pronouns *he* and *it* are used to refer to something that had already been identified linguistically. The use of a pronoun to refer to a previously mentioned referent is called **anaphoric reference**. Anaphoric reference, as well as other linguistic devices, helps bind discourse so that its meaning is better understood. Collectively, these are called **cohesive devices** because they provide the glue for intersentence meaning. Table 2.14 defines some cohesive devices and gives examples of each. Although there is limited information about preschool use of coherence devices, researchers have concluded that the ability to use pronouns anaphorically is a developmental achievement related to children's linguistic, cognitive, and social awareness (Cairns, 1996; Chien & Wexler, 1990).

CONTEXTUAL MEANING: THE ROLE OF THE NONLINGUISTIC CONTEXT

In addition to the linguistic context, the **nonlinguistic context** gives clues about the meaning of words whose referents shift with the perspective of the speaker and the

Table 2.14   **Cohesive Devices**

Type	Definition	Example
Personal pronouns	Substitute for noun	*I, you, she, it,* etc.
Demonstrative pronoun	Deictic (pointing) words	I'll take *this/that* one.
Anaphoric reference	Pronoun used to refer to a previously established entity	Mary is happy. *She* passed the test.
Cataphoric reference	Pronoun used to refer to a coming event	*Here* comes a surprise.
Verb ellipsis	Deletion of information available in the discourse	Do you like cake? I do. (*like cake*)
Nominal ellipsis	Deletion of information that is available in the discourse	Where is he? (*He is*) here!
Conjunctions	Conjoining elements	*and, or, but*
Lexical cohesion	Synonyms referring to previously mentioned entities	A lion appeared. The *beast* roared.
Comparative references	Comparison between entities	*Bigger than . . .*

Adapted from Halliday and Hasan (1976).

timing of the utterance. Consider the sentence "I want you to go there tomorrow." The meanings of *I, you, there,* and *tomorrow* depend on who is speaking, who is listening, where the speaker is when the sentence is uttered, and when the sentence is spoken. Words whose meaning shifts as the nonlinguistic context changes are called **deictic terms.** Thus *I, you, here, there, today,* and *tomorrow* express the deictic relationship of person, place, and time, respectively.

Studies have examined children's development of person, place, and time deixis. In general, pronoun deixis (*I/you, me/my,* and *my/you*) is acquired before the contrasts *this/that, these/those, here/there,* which refer to spatial concepts (McLaughlin, 1998). Last to emerge is temporal deixis (*today, tomorrow*). Children may have difficulty with the difference between *this* and *that* at 4 years of age, and some deictic contrasts present difficulty even for 7-year-olds (Owens, 2005).

SEMANTICS: LANGUAGE DIFFERENCES

Goldstein (2000) points out that lexical differences exist among dialects, with similar words having different meanings. For example, the word *bomba* means *balloon* in some dialects of Spanish but *bomb* in others. Stockman (1999) summarized the four types of meaning relationships that can exist among different dialects and languages: (1) identical words (no differences), (2) different words and different referents for these words, (3) different words for the same referents, and (4) different referents for the same forms. These differences should be considered when evaluating children with different cultural and linguistic backgrounds.

Preschool Pragmatic Development

As noted earlier in the chapter, language is learned within a social context. As children interact with their caretakers (and later with their peers), the uses to which they put language continually multiply. The intentions they code increase, and they learn to become more aware of social settings and the interactors within those social settings.

During the preschool period, children learn to describe objects and events removed from the immediate context. They relate personal experiences and use language effectively to convey their wants and needs. In addition, they become more aware of the general conditions governing cooperative conversations. They learn to take turns in a conversation, to stick to the conversational topic, and to contribute new and relevant information to the discourse. Although these abilities emerge in the preschool period, they continue to grow through the years as children mature cognitively and socially.

THE ELABORATION OF COMMUNICATIVE FUNCTIONS

In addition to the early communicative functions outlined in a previous section (also see Table 2.5), children expand their repertoire of language use. Dore (1978) explored children's use of language during the preschool years. He found that the communicative intentions coded by 2- to 5-year-olds included the following:

1. requesting information by asking a variety of questions ("Can I go now?" "Is he eating candy?" "Where are you going?" "Why can't I have it?")
2. responding to requests by answering questions or supplying information ("It's in my closet," "I wasn't the one who broke the cup," "I don't want to")
3. describing events, objects, or properties ("There's a red truck," "He's building it slowly," "That's a truck with a crane")
4. stating facts, feelings, attitudes, and beliefs ("It happened yesterday," "I feel sick," "I don't like her," "Ghosts are not real")

The internal cognitive and social changes that take place in children influence the ways they use language. For example, young preschoolers use language to direct themselves and to instruct others, as well as to report on present and past experiences (Hulit & Howard, 1997). Older preschoolers, however, add more complex communicative functions; they use language to reason, to think, and to solve problems (Tough, 1979). Consider the following script:

Ari (age 5):   If the roof isn't strong enough, he'll fall in.

Eli (age 5):   I think the tape will fix it. Yep, I'll get the tape.

Sheri (age 5½):   If you put the block here and I put my block there, it will hold everything up.

In the later preschool years, children also use language to tease, annoy, complain, criticize, and threaten. These communication functions are observed not only as they interact with caretakers and siblings but also as they interact with their peers. Consider the following utterances produced by 5-year-olds:

Teasing: You're a fatso.

Annoying: I'll do it again and again.

Complaining: You always give the big one to him.

Criticizing: Your picture is yucky.

Threatening: Give it back or I'll tell Mommy.

During this period, children express a wide variety of communicative intentions with expanding linguistic forms.

CONVERSATION SKILL DEVELOPMENT

In general, children learn language within a conversational context. Preschool children acquire many conversational skills, but much of their conversation concerns the here and now. Their conversations are very short, and the number of turns they take in a conversation are limited.

Topic maintenance in preschoolers usually occurs only when the communicative partner's previous utterance consists of a topic-sharing response to the child's prior utterances (L. Bloom, Rocissano, & Hood, 1976). Young children (2½ to 3) are good at introducing new conversational topics in which they are interested, but they have difficulty sustaining that topic beyond one or two turns. Although they learn to acknowledge their communicative partner, they often fail to wait for their conversational turn and to build a bridge for the next speaker's turn.

Between 3 and 4 years of age, children seem to gain a better awareness of the social aspects of conversation. They begin to adapt their language to the needs of their listeners. With the realization that other people's perspective must be taken into account (called *presuppositional ability*) comes language that is adapted to the listener. That is not to say that preschoolers are always successful in getting their messages across. They are often unable to reformulate their messages in response to a facial expression of miscomprehension and must be asked specifically to clarify their messages. The most common way preschoolers clarify or repair their messages is simply to repeat what they have said (McLaughlin, 1998):

Child (age 3½) to mother: He took it away from me.

Mother: What?

Child: He took it away from me.

Mother: What?

Child: He took it away from me (in a louder voice).

Mother: Who did what?

Child: John took away my book!

The inability to respond to a nonspecific request for clarification is characteristic of preschoolers. The ability to respond more appropriately does not develop until the school-age years (Owens, 2005).

Lastly, during the preschool period, children begin to manifest the ability to understand and to use indirect requests. Consider the sentence "It's awfully hot in here." While this sentence might be a statement, it is usually uttered when a request for action is intended by a speaker (for the listener to open the window). The ability to understand and to use indirect requests advances as children mature socially and linguistically. Between 3 and 4 years of age, children seem to gain a better awareness of the social benefit of using indirect requests (Ervin-Tripp, 1980; Ninio & Snow, 1996; Wells, 1985). A typical indirect request of a 4-year-old is "Mommy, can I have a cookie please?"

In the next section, we will examine preschoolers' development of a different discourse skill: their ability to tell narratives.

NARRATIVE DEVELOPMENT

The *narrative* is a form of discourse. Narratives differ from conversations in that a listener response is not required. When producing a narrative, the speaker produces a monologue throughout and must presuppose the information needed by the listener. The speaker must present all the information in an organized way and must introduce and organize sequences so that events are related and lead to some conclusion. There are a number of different types of narratives. Narratives include sharing and recounting of personal events and experiences, self-generated stories, telling and retelling of familiar tales, and the retelling of stories from movies, books, and television shows.

Research has shown that 2-year-olds incorporate dialogue that accompanies familiar everyday routines into their speech. This type of narrative is called a *script* and is used by young children to talk about events that occurred to them (Owens, 2005; Tiegerman-Farber, 1995). However, it is not until the age of 4 that they are able accurately to describe event sequences, called a *plan* (Karmiloff-Smith, 1986).

Narratives contain principles and structure that give them cohesiveness (McLaughlin, 1998). Around 3½ years of age, preschool children produce **protonarratives**, which are stories about recent events. The organizational structure is a set of unrelated elements (**heaps**), which emerges at 30 months of age.

In general, two types of strategies are used by preschool children for organizing their narratives: chaining and centering. Children of 3 years of age use **chaining** (a narrative that relates to a central topic with no particular temporal order) when producing a narrative. At around 4 years of age, children produce narratives with increased organization that follow a central theme, which is called **centering**. By age 5, 75 percent of typically developing children use both strategies. Below are examples of typically developing preschoolers retelling a story and recounting a birthday experience:

Child (age 3) retelling a story: There was this magician. He had a hat and rabbits came from the hat. The end.

Child (age 5):   I had a birthday party. All the children came to my party. Everybody sang "Happy Birthday to You." I got presents. We ate cake.

By the time they enter school, children acquire the basic elements of narratives and can share their experience and recount familiar events sequentially. In the school-age years, as their linguistic abilities and knowledge of the world develops, they learn to understand and produce more complex narrative forms.

Emergent Literacy

Recent research has begun to highlight the importance of the preschool years in laying the foundation for children's development of reading and writing abilities (Butler, 1999; Snow, Scarborough, & Burns, 1999). There are strong indications that listening/speaking and reading/writing share, at least in part, a linguistic base, although they differ in other ways. The importance of this information for speech-language pathologists and educators who work with preschool children lies in the fact that delays in the comprehension and formulation of oral language fore-shadow difficulties in reading and writing that will appear during the school years (Butler, 1999).

The term that has often been used for the knowledge that preschoolers acquire about print before learning to read is called **emergent literacy.** Studies of emergent literacy have taken numerous directions. Some investigators have concluded that during the preschool period, children acquire the following knowledge and skills:

- master the convention of print (how to hold a book, awareness that the organization of English print is from left to right and top to down, scribble writing)
- learn to name and write letters
- recognize that print represents meaningful ideas
- acquire an understanding of the structure of written language (that stories are organized in a particular way)
- develop a print-related vocabulary (understanding and using words such as *read, write, story, page*)
- acquire the rudimentary skills of phonological awareness (that words consist of discrete units)

Other researchers have focused on the print literacy environment of the young child, particularly in the child's home. They have found that the availability of print in the home (books, posters, magazines, postcards, and nameplates), as well as print artifacts (crayons, pencils, and markers), have a positive correlation with literacy acquisition (Zeverbergen & Whitehurst, 2003). Most of the literacy events that occur in the lives of preschool children are embedded in ongoing real-life family experiences. Caretakers use techniques such as semantic contingency (staying on a topic introduced by a child), scaffolding (structuring the linguistic and nonlinguistic context to facilitate the child's success), and routines (highly predictable situations that occur frequently) to help facilitate an appreciation for literacy experiences (Snow, Perlmann, & Nathan, 1987). Justice and Ezell (2000) found that book reading by parents significantly enhanced children's early literacy development. In addition to the contribution of shared book reading to the future success of children's learning to read (Anderson, Hiebert, Scott, & Wilkinson, 1985; Zeverbergen & Whitehurst, 2003), book reading also contributes to increased vocabulary development (Elley, 1989; Jenkins, Stein, & Wysocki, 1984; Wasik & Bond, 2001) and narrative development (Harkins, Koch, & Michel, 1994; Zeverbergen & Wilson, 1996).

Speech-language pathologists often counsel parents and/or educators about the importance of including book reading in their interaction with children. When doing so, they should emphasize the importance of using an animated, dramatic, and lively reading style (DeTemple & Snow, 2003; Wasik & Bond, 2001). An effective method of book reading that incorporates interaction is found in a *dialogic reading* approach (Zeverbergen & Whitehurst, 2003). This approach involves two assignments, two to three weeks apart, when book reading with 2- and 3-year-olds. The first assignment consists of these elements (p. 179):

1. Ask *what* questions.
2. Follow answers with questions.
3. Repeat what the child says.
4. Help the child as needed.
5. Praise and encourage.
6. Follow the child's interests.
7. Have fun.

The second assignment consists of the following elements (pp. 179–180):

1. Ask open-ended questions.
2. Expand what the child says.

The elements of dialogic reading approach differ when book reading with 4- to 5-year-olds (p. 180):

1. Completion prompts ("When the frog came home again, everyone was   .")
2. Recall prompts ("What happened when the big frog bit the little frog?")
3. Open-ended prompts ("Now you tell me about the next page.")
4. *Wh*- prompts, using *what, where,* and *why* and *how* questions ("Why was the big frog mean to the little frog?" and "How did the little frog feel?")
5. Distancing prompts ("Did you ever go to the zoo and see a real frog?")

When researching the impact of interactive book reading intervention with 2-year-olds from low-income backgrounds, Valdez-Menchaca and Whitehurst (1992) found that children's MLU, sentence complexity, vocabulary variety, and expressive and receptive language skills had improved. Thus, the combination of book reading and structured interaction has been found to have positive effects on language development and to provide support for reading skills.

Most research has focused on literacy socialization in middle-class mainstream families, regardless of ethnicity. Not all families, however, are alike even when they have similar cultural and sociolinguistic histories (Heath, 1996). There may be culturally based differences in literacy events, parental guidance, and the preliteracy expectations of parents for their preschool children (Nelson, 1993). In spite of the diverse approaches to literacy activities found in different cultures, the outcome is the same: Children can develop literacy abilities (Heath, 1996).

PHONOLOGICAL AWARENESS

During the preschool period, children begin to develop an awareness of the sound structures of words. This skill is known as **phonological awareness** (Justice & Scheule, 2004). Armed with this ability they learn (1) that words are composed of segments, (2) that these segments have distinctive features, the phonetic properties that act to provide contrasts between sounds (e.g., the voicing difference that distinguishes /p/ and /b/), and (3) that letters represent sounds in words (Ball, 1997; Snowling, Hulme, Smith, & Thomas, 1994; Torgesen 1999).

At this stage of development, the child can segment syllables into words (*ba-na-na*), rhyme ("What rhymes with *cat*? Do *cat* and *bat* rhyme?"), blend sound segments ("What word is /k/-/æ/-/t/?"), segment sounds in words ("What is the first/last sound in *cat*?"), manipulate sounds (Delete the first sound in the words *smart/mart*, *spark/park*, and *stop/top*), match words on the basis of initial phonemes ("What words have the same first sound: *toy, take,* or *chair*?"), produce alliteration ("*big bad bugs bite boys*"), and choose a target word from a set based on the difference in final or beginning sounds (*doll, dog,* or *toy*?). Preschoolers are able to engage in sound play, repair speech errors, recognize rhyme, and segment syllables (Kamhi & Catts, 1991), while later developing skills consist of segmenting sounds in words and matching words on the basis of initial phonemes.

The relationship of phonological awareness and reading has been discussed by many researchers (Jorm & Share, 1983; Bryant, Bradley, MacLean & Crossland, 1989; Torgesen, 1999), and a correlation between deficits in phonological awareness and reading difficulties has been found (Ball, 1997; Shaywitz, Fletcher, Holahan, & Shaywitz, 1992; Snyder & Downey, 1997; Swanson, Mink, & Bocian, 1999; Westby, 1998). The deficits in phonological awareness evidenced in children with language learning and reading difficulties are discussed more fully in Chapters 4, 5, and 11.

During the preschool years, children's utterances are observed to increase in length and complexity. From a MLU of 2.0 and continuing beyond a MLU of 4.0, children learn several linguistic subsystems simultaneously. They master the phonological system, develop grammatical morphemes, and understand and produce a variety of sentence types. They acquire more abstract meanings and the ability to map these onto linguistic structures. They elaborate their use of language to suit a variety of social contexts and to describe events and personal experiences as well as sequences and outcomes. Finally, they begin to gain knowledge about print, even though they may not actually learn how to decode print until they are formally taught to do so in school. Although each component of language has been discussed separately, language form (phonology, morphology, and syntax), content (semantics), and use (pragmatics) are interrelated in development.

School-Age Language Development: An Overview

Although children's language has reached a measure of complexity by age 5, much communicative development is yet to come. Vocabulary continues to grow throughout the school years (Johnson & Anglin, 1995; McGhee-Bidlack, 1991). Children begin to use nonliteral language such as jokes, riddles, and metaphors in middle childhood (Bernstein, 1986, 1987; Nippold, Leonard, & Kail, 1984) and to comprehend sentences that contain verbs such as *promise* and *ask* (Chomsky, 1969; Eisenberg & Cairns, 1994).

During the school-age years, the cognitive and social changes that take place in children influence the ways that they use language. They expand their pragmatic and discourse skills, their conversational abilities become refined, and they are better able to plan, organize, and sequence their ideas into more coherent and cohesive complex narratives. Lastly, during this period, children also develop the ability to think and talk about language (called *metalinguistic ability*) and master language in another mode by learning to read and write. Although language development continues as children mature cognitively and socially, a good deal of language learning has already been mastered by the time the child enters first grade.

During the early and later school-age years, the cognitive and social changes that take place in children influence the way they use languages. For example, they are able to do the following:

- ignore distractions and irrelevant information
- more effectively reason and problem solve
- expand their pragmatic and discourse skills
- refine their conversational abilities
- plan, organize, and sequence their ideas into more complex narratives

Recent research has turned its attention to the language abilities evidenced by older school-age children—the early and later adolescent. The World Health Organization (WHO, 2005), as well as Breinbauer and Maddaleno (2005), divide this period into three subperiods:

1. *Preadolescence:* 9–12 years of age for females and 10–13 years of age for males
2. *Early adolescence:* 12–14 years of age for females and 13–15 years of age for males
3. *Later adolescence:* 14–19 years of age for females and males

All researchers agree that adolescence is characterized by an interrelationship among various factors—biological, psychocultural, and psychological (Larson & McKinley, 2003)—and that language continues to develop and become more complex throughout adolescence and into adulthood (Nippold, 2000).

SYNTACTIC AND MORPHOLOGICAL DEVELOPMENT

In the realm of morphology and syntax, school-age language development consists of simultaneous expansion of existing forms and acquisition of new ones. Children continue to expand their sentences by elaborating noun phrases and verb phrases. They expand their understanding and use of conjoined sentences with the addition of *therefore, although,* and *unless,* which are used to join clauses ("I went to the store, *although* my brother was supposed to go"). Correct interpretation of the words *if* and *although* may not occur until age 11, and *unless* may not be understood completely until age 15 (McLaughlin, 1998).

Children's use of embedding expands with their comprehension of more syntactically complex embedded sentences; their understanding will depend on the place and type of embedding used. Embeddings may occur in the center of the sentence or at the end. The two clauses of the embedded sentence may share the same subject or object—called **parallel embedding**—or they may not—called **nonparallel embedding.** The comprehension of embedded sentences progresses from the easiest to the most difficult, reflecting the child's cognitive development. Table 2.15 outlines the order in which various types of embedded sentences are acquired.

Several morphological structures emerge during the early school-age years. Gerunds, which are verbs to which *-ing* has been added to produce a form that fulfills a noun function (e.g., *to fish* becomes *fishing;* "Fishing is fun"), emerge after Stage V (Owens, 2005). Derivational morphemes first appear in the late preschool years with the adjectival comparative *-er* (*bigger*) emerging between 4 and 5 years of age and *-est* (*biggest*) emerging between 5 and 6 (Norris, 1998). The derivational suffix *-er* (*farm + er*), used to change a verb to a noun, emerges in the late preschool years. The derivational morpheme *-ist* emerges at 7 years of age, and the derivational suffixes *-ful, -less, -ly, -ness, -al,* and *-ance* emerge during the school-age years (Wiig & Semel, 1984). By the end of second grade, children comprehend irregular noun and verb agreement ("The fish are eating" versus "The sheep is sleeping"), the implicit negative form ("Find the one that is neither red nor blue"),

Table 2.15   Development Sequence of Embedded Sentence Comprehension

Type	Example
Parallel center embedding—same subject (*girl*) serves both clauses.	The girl who bought the dress went to the party.
Parallel ending embedding—same object (*gift*) serves both clauses.	He gave me a gift that I don't like.
Nonparallel ending embedding—the object of the main clause (*boy*) is the subject of the embedded clause.	She hit the boy who ran away.
Nonparallel central embedding—the subject of the main clause (*cat*) is the object of the embedded clause.	The cat that was chased by the dog ran up a tree.

Adapted from Abrahamsen & Rigrodsky (1984), Lahey (1974), and Owens (1996).

and several verb tenses, such as the past participle (*had eaten*) and the perfect (*has been eating*).

Although children 5 to 7 years of age are able to use most elements of noun and verb phrases, they frequently omit them. Even at age 7, they will omit some elements (articles) while expanding others, such as double negatives. In addition, school-age children may still have difficulty with some prepositions, verb tense, and plurals (Menyuk, 1969). Lastly, irregular past tense verbs that form past tense by vowel and (sometimes) consonant change present adolescents and even adults with difficulty (Nelson, 1998) (e.g., *lie–lay–lain* and *swim–swam–swum*)(McLaughlin, 1998).

During the preschool years, reversible passive sentences ("The boy was hit by the ball") are difficult for children to understand and produce because the passive sentence violates the child's strategy of determining *who did what to whom* from the word order. Children do not fully comprehend passives until 5½ years of age, and full passives are not produced until around 7½ to 8 years of age (Owens, 2005).

Other linguistic forms are acquired during the school-age years, such as the ability to distinguish between mass and count nouns. **Mass nouns** are nonindividual, homogeneous substances such as *water, sand,* and *money.* **Count nouns** are heterogeneous individual objects such as *a glass, a toy,* or *a house.* Mass nouns differ from count nouns in that the former cannot accept the plural morpheme *-s* (apple*s* versus sand*s*). Mass nouns take different quantifying modifiers (*much* and *little*) than those taken by count nouns (*many* and *few*).

By early elementary school, children have learned most of the correct noun forms, so that constructions like *monies* and *mens* are rare. Early on, children discover a way around the quantifier question by using *lots of* with both types of nouns; however, children are able to use the correct quantifier (*some* and *any*) with mass nouns (*salt* or *sand*) by age 4 (Owens, 2005). *Many* then appears with plural count nouns, as in *many houses.* *Much* is usually learned by late elementary school, although even 9-year-olds may have difficulty with this form. Full mastery is not accomplished until adolescence (McLaughlin, 1998), when children attach the correct quantifier to the noun (*much* + a mass noun).

At nine years of age, syntactic skills increase with the acquisition of derivational suffixes (Tyler & Nagy, 1989). Examples consist of the morphemes *-ness, -er, -ize, -men, -ity, -ify, -ous,* and *-ive,* while use and comprehension is achieved at age 12. At 9 to 10 years of age, children are able to produce nonreversible passive structures (Baldie, 1976), use noun phrase elaboration in object position, and produce modal auxiliaries, which allows children to produce more complex syntactic structures and indirect requests. Here are some examples of these structures:

Nonreversible passive structure: The ball was thrown by the boy.

Noun phrase elaboration in object position: The boy on the bike is my brother.

Modal auxiliaries: I can/did/may/might ride a bike.

Indirect request: Could you loan me your book?

At about 9 years of age, children produce irregular verbs and reflexive pronouns with greater accuracy, as well as the passive structure using *got* or *was* (Werner &

Kresheck, 1983). Syntactic complexity is increased by the use of coordinating, subordinating, and intersentential conjunctions, while noun phrase elaboration continues with the addition of multiple modifiers for nouns and verbs. Examples of these structures include the following:

Irregular verbs: I drank the milk.

Reflexive pronouns: She wet herself.

Passive structure: The car got/was hit by the train.

Conjunctions: She listened to the rain when she slept in the attic.

Noun phrase elaboration: He wanted to buy the new, bright, shiny bike

At 10 to 11 years of age, children use reversible and nonreversible passives and adverbial conjuncts to enhance narrative and conversation (Scott, 1984). Children also begin to increase their use of mental term verbs (Greenhalgh & Strong, 2001). At 11–13 years of age, instrumental nonreversible passives appear (Baldie, 1976), the use of modals increase in both production and in written text (Hunt, 1965), and the use of perfect and passive structures increase by the time children enter the twelfth grade. Examples of these structures are noted below.

Adverbial conjuncts: Then, the boy was able to follow the rainbow.

Reversible passive: The boy was kissed by the girl.

Irreversible passive: The window was broken by the boy.

Mental terms: I think he understands me.

Instrumental nonreversible passive: The glass was broken by a ball.

Perfect aspect: I have eaten all the cookies.

Passive voice: The girl was kissed by the boy.

SYNTAX AND MORPHOLOGY: LANGUAGE DIFFERENCES

There are differences between the morphological and syntactic rules of Spanish and English (Goldstein, 2000). Spanish is a subject-drop language; therefore, the sentence "Tengo un gato" [have a cat] is considered grammatical. In contrast to English, with fixed word order, word order in Spanish is not fixed—for instance, "Los niños tienen dos gatos" [The boys have two cats] and "Tienen dos gatos los niños" [Have two cats the boys]. Unlike English, articles and adjectives agree with nouns—*el perro* [the dog] but *los perros* [the dogs]. These differences are often reflected in the English utterances of Spanish-speaking children when attempting to master English morphology and syntax.

According to the rules of African American English (AAE), certain inflectional morphemes need not necessarily be produced (possessive *-s,* plural *-s,* regular past

-*ed*, and third-person -*s*) (Goldstein, 2000; Haynes & Shulman, 1998). Statements may not be reversed to form questions ("What it is?"); double negatives ("Nobody don't never like me") and pronominal appositions ("Daddy he mad") are also produced. MLU differences also are present among different languages and dialects. For example, a Standard American English (SAE) speaker might produce eight morphemes in the sentence "Two cats are in John's house" (*two, cat, -s, are, in, John, -'s,* and *house*), but an AAE speaker might produce the same sentence with five morphemes, as in "Two cat in John house" (*two, cat, in, John,* and *house*) (Seymour & Roeper, 1999). These differences between AAE and SAE may lead an educator to believe that an AAE speaker has a language disorder rather than a language difference.

Because the rules of AAE require that redundant and repetitive information be avoided, certain morphemes (i.e., plural -*s*, possessive *'s*, and the auxiliary verb *are*) are omitted because this information is signaled by the preceding words (i.e., *two* + *cat* and *John* + *house*). Although both speakers may be typically developing children of the same age, an educator or a therapist may incorrectly judge the lower MLU to indicate a language delay. Because MLU differences can be found between SAE and AAE speakers, as well as speakers of other languages, speech-language pathologists must be cautious when using only MLU to determine language development for children with dialectal differences or for those children whose first language is not SAE. For a more detailed discussion of differences in language development, the reader is referred to Taylor and Leonard (1999), Haynes and Shulman (1998), Goldstein (2000), and also Chapter 12.

School-Age Semantic Development

During the school-age years, children increase the size of their vocabulary and the specificity of their word definitions. By 6 years of age, children's expressive vocabulary is at 2,600 words and receptive vocabulary is between 20,000 and 24,000 words (Owens, 2005). However, adding lexical items is only a portion of the change that occurs in a child's vocabulary growth.

During the school-age years, children's ability to add new dimensions to their existing lexicon also increases. Differences between the abilities of older and younger school-age children become evident when defining words. Whereas preschoolers define words narrowly in terms of their own experience, school-age children define words using more socially shared meanings (McLaughlin, 1998). Their definitions not only include the meaning of a word learned in early childhood (*block*) but also new (and in some cases nonliteral) meanings of this word ("Walk around the block," "Don't block the entrance," "A block of text"). In high school, adolescents' definitions are abstract and/or represent a concept of function modified by perceptual attributes. The definitions of upper-high-school students (as well as of adults) tend to be descriptive, having concrete terms of reference to specific instances used to modify a concept, and contain synonyms, explanations, and categorizations (Johnson & Anglin, 1995).

Vocabulary knowledge is highly correlated with general linguistic competence and academic aptitude. Acquiring a broad vocabulary allows a child not only to understand and express more complex ideas with greater facility but also to achieve a higher degree of competence in reading and writing.

VOCABULARY DEVELOPMENT

By the fourth grade, children have acquired and are able to understand more abstract vocabulary items (Miller & Gildea, 1987), such as *dizzy, tangle, dodge, distance,* and *swift.* By the time children enter the sixth grade, they understand approximately 50,000 vocabulary items (Owens, 2005). Arlin (1983) reports that children understand that the spatial terms *in* and *on* can also relate to temporal concepts (*in the morning; on Sunday*) by 10 to 11 years of age.

At about 6 to 8 years of age, children respond with syntagmatic responses to word association tasks (e.g., *boy* for the stimulus *tall*) (McNeill, 1970). Paradigmatic responses appear by 9 years of age, when children are able to respond with the word *high* for the stimulus *tall* (Brown & Berko, 1960; Ervin, 1961). Word definition skills increase by 9 years of age, with definition more frequently based on function than category (Al-Issa, 1969). For example, the word *apple* would be defined as "something to eat," rather than with the category label "fruit." While a great deal of word knowledge is acquired during the school-age years, vocabulary continues to increase throughout the lifespan.

DEVELOPMENT OF NONLITERAL MEANING: FIGURATIVE LANGUAGE

Nonliteral meaning adds richness and depth to language by communicating indirectly what would otherwise be communicated directly. Consider the meaning in the metaphor "Her eyes were ice" or in the proverb "The early bird catches the worm." Metaphors, idioms, proverbs, and jokes are examples of nonliteral language—language that has meaning that goes beyond the words of the sentence. The understanding and use of nonliteral meaning depend on the ability to disregard literal interpretation and to rely on nonreferential, abstract, general meaning.

Metaphors

Studies dealing with children's comprehension and use of nonliteral language have focused on **metaphors,** which use a likeness to stand for a word, a referent, or an idea ("He has a heart of stone"). When metaphoric language is marked by the connective *as* or *like,* it is called a **simile** ("It is as light as air").

The ability to comprehend metaphoric language emerges early and continues to develop with time (Bernstein, 1987; Nippold, 1985, 1991, 1998; Nippold, Leonard, & Kail, 1984). Although 3-year-old children may have some understanding of metaphor, they are unable to identify and to explain metaphors until about 7 years of age (Kogan & Chadrow, 1986; Vosniadou, Ortony, & Reynolds, 1984).

Metaphor comprehension requires the understanding that language can associate domains. For example, 5- to 7-year-old children have difficulty equating the physical and psychological domains and will interpret the metaphor "She is a cold person," in physical terms—that is, the person is cold because of temperature or location in a cold place (Owens, 2005). Children do so because they do not understand the psychological meanings of words such as *sweet, cold,* and *bright* until they are 7 to 8 years of age (Westby, 1998). Children are able to understand cross-sensory metaphors ("Her perfume was bright as sunshine"), which associate perceptual domains, more easily than metaphors that associate the psychological-physical domains ("The prison guard was a hard rock") (Winner, Rosentiel, & Gardner, 1976).

Similarity metaphors, in which objects are compared based on shared features ("The stars are a thousand eyes"), are comprehended more easily than *proportional metaphors,* in which three objects are mentioned and a fourth must be inferred to complete a proportion ("My head is like an apple without a core"). Performance on each of the more difficult metaphor types increases with age. Billow (1975) suggested that the precise understanding and use of metaphors are related to children's cognitive development.

Idioms

Figurative, nonliteral expressions that express complex ideas in colorful and concise ways are called **idioms.** Included in different idiomatic types are semantically based idioms that can be assigned to various categories (foods—*sour grapes;* animals—*dark horse;* colors—*in the red*). Idiom comprehension develops and improves throughout childhood, adolescence, and into the adult years (Nippold, 1988, 1991; Nippold & Martin, 1989; Nippold & Taylor, 1995). Although preschoolers comprehend the nonliteral meanings of some idioms, their literal interpretation predominates through childhood and even adolescence (Nippold & Martin, 1989).

Proverbs

Another form of nonliteral language, proverbs, are more abstract than metaphors. In a **proverb,** the domain that is the topic is never mentioned. Wise sayings that express truths are such proverbs as "Don't put all your eggs in one basket" and "A stitch in time saves nine." Preadolescents are generally unable to interpret proverbs, and it is not until adolescence or adulthood that proverbs are understood (Owens, 2005). Nippold (2000) found that proverb understanding improved with grade level, with 60 percent accuracy for sixth-graders, 73 percent accuracy for tenth-graders, and 81 percent for twelfth-graders. Because proverbs are encountered in political speeches, literature textbooks, and other forms of discourse (Nippold, 2000), targeting the comprehension of proverbs can be an important goal when working with adolescents.

Humor

We often infer information about children's semantic knowledge (or lack of knowledge) from the riddles and jokes they understand and tell. The source of humor in riddles and jokes is largely semantically based. Humor in riddles and jokes can depend on understanding words that sound the same but are spelled differently (*bear/bare*) or words that sound the same and are spelled the same way but have more than one meaning (*glasses, tie*). The comprehension of humor often depends on perceiving the incongruity among the meanings of homonyms or multiple-meaning words (*bank*) (Bernstein, 1986).

Children's understanding of jokes and riddles depends on their metalinguistic skills and their ability to comprehend four types of linguistic ambiguity (Westby, 1998): (1) phonological ambiguity ("Why did the clock go to the doctor? Because he was tick."); (2) lexical ambiguity ("What happened to the girl's feet? She had bare feet."); (3) surface-structure ambiguity, based on a figurative versus literal interpretation of a word ("Tell me, how long are trains? Six letters."); and (4) deep-structure ambiguity, based on two diverse meanings for a phrase ("Call me a cab. You're a cab."). Phonological ambiguity is understood at 6 or 7 years of age, followed by the understanding of lexical ambiguity. The comprehension of surface-structure and deep-structure ambiguity occurs later in development.

School-Age Pragmatic Development

The development of pragmatics in the preschool years sets the stage for later changes. During the school years, children learn to be skilled conversationalists and more effective communicators as they become increasingly sensitive to what their listeners need to know. Throughout the school years, children increase their range of communication functions and learn how to become good conversational partners, how to make indirect requests, and how to process the language of the classroom. During this period, children learn to organize and plan narratives and can relate stories in a coherent and cohesive manner. Last, they add various means of conveying their intentions, including greater use of indirect expressions.

EXPANSION OF COMMUNICATIVE FUNCTIONS

In addition to the wide variety of communicative functions that preschoolers use, the changing world of the school-age child requires using language in a wider variety of social contexts. Children's social-emotional and cognitive skills enable them to expand their repertoire of language use. White (1975) maintained that the school-age child displays the following communicative abilities:

1. gaining and holding adults' attention in a socially acceptable manner
2. directing and following peers
3. using others, when appropriate, as resources for assistance or for information
4. expressing affection, hostility, and anger, when appropriate
5. expressing pride in themselves and their accomplishments
6. role-playing
7. competing with peers in storytelling

In addition, school-age children are able to use language to think critically and to reason. This ability is discussed in a later section.

THE DEVELOPMENT OF NARRATIVES

By the time children are in school, they exhibit a storytelling talent; that is, they can communicate information through coherent and cohesive units called narratives. A **narrative** is a form of discourse. It is an uninterrupted stream of language modified by the speaker to capture and hold the listener's interest and attention (Owens, 2005). Narratives differ from conversations in a number of ways. When producing a narrative, the speaker produces a monologue throughout and must presuppose the information needed by the listener. In addition, the speaker must present all the information in an organized way and introduce and organize the sequences of events so that the elements of the narrative are related and lead to some conclusion.

As toddlers, children are exposed to narratives, or stories, in picture books and on television, and as noted previously, they are able to produce narratives by age 4. By first grade, demands are placed on children to relate narratives, to participate in show-and-tell, to relate vacation activities or holiday experiences, or to retell a story heard previously. Later, these activities appear in the form of written assignments such as "My Summer Vacation," "How I Spent the Holidays," and a synopsis of a book.

A perspective on the natural structure of narrative is seen in the work of Stein and Glenn (1979), who describe a model of story structure that follows certain rules. According to this model, stories have an internal structure. They contain statements that are logically connected to reflect causal and temporal relationships and contain principles that promote structure and cohesion. Stein and Glenn maintain that stories are made up of various categories, units, and rules. Category definitions and the rules of the story grammar model are shown in Table 2.16.

When competent storytellers structure their information, they ensure a full understanding of the story. When children hear stories in which the information sequences are inverted (for example, they are told the consequence unit before the initiating event), they remember the events less well than if the story is told to them in the order given by the model. If children are given individual narrative statements and asked to make up a story, the sequence of their stories correlates highly with the

Table 2.16 **Story Grammar Model**

Initiating Event	Action or occurrence that influences the main characters (rain, storm, earthquake): the perception of an event (thunder), a physiological state (hunger, thirst, fatigue)
Internal Response	A character's emotional status relative to the initiating event; a reference to motivation or purpose
Plan	The character's strategy for solving a problem or obtaining a goal
Attempt	The actions used to solve the problem or to obtain the goal
Consequence	Success or failure in the attempt to solve the problem or to obtain the goal
Resolution	The character's feelings, thoughts, or actions in response to the consequences; success or failure of the protagonist
Ending	The conclusion of the story: a summary of the story or a moral

From *Introduction to Language Development*, 1st edition, by McLaughlin © 1998. Reprinted with permission of Delmar a division of Thomson Learning. Fax 800-730-2215.

sequence predicted by the story grammar model. In addition, when asked to retell a story, children are most likely to include the setting unit, initiating event, and the consequence unit.

Although children use the schematic knowledge of story grammars to understand stories and to formulate narratives, there are developmental differences between the abilities of younger and older children (Westby, 1998). The following characteristics are more likely found in the stories of 10-year-olds:

1. greater detail in setting information
2. goal directed episode: centering (central character) and chaining (one activity the cause of another); story grammar components appear for initiating event, response, and consequence
3. complete episodes: character goals and intentions described; story grammar components present for initiating event, internal response, plan, attempt, and consequence
4. in general, less extraneous detail

By the late elementary school, children's narratives consist of elaborated stories that contain these elements:

1. multiple episodes: story with chapters, each chapter consisting of minimal story grammar structure
2. complex episodes: multiple plans and multiple attempts because of obstacles to obtaining a goal
3. embedded episodes: one episode embedded in another

School-age children also include reference to emotional states, double meanings, mystery, attitude statements, and story evaluations in their narratives (Crais & Lorch, 1994). The older adolescent storyteller not only utilizes the above abilities but also employs argumentation and dramatization and includes asides and morals in the narrative (Larson & McKinley, 1995).

CONVERSATIONAL SKILLS

Children learn language within a conversational context. Although preschool children acquire many conversational skills, much of their conversation centers on the here and now. However, they must learn about the conventional routines of conversation, such as taking turns (being a sender or a receiver), clarifying or repairing their message, and maintaining a topic. These skills are refined during the school-age years.

Two processes enable the child to become a more effective communicator: neo-egocentrism and decentration. **Neo-egocentrism** is the ability to take the perspective of another person. (This ability has also been called *presuppositional ability*.) In general, as a communication task becomes more difficult, the young child is less able to take a speaker's perspective. As the child matures cognitively and socially and gains greater facility with language structure, he or she can concentrate more effectively on the audience. Being able to shift perspective enables the child to consider what the listener knows (and needs to know) when he or she constructs a message. This ability is refined during the school years. Being neo-egocentric also allows the child greater facility in the use of deictic terms. You will recall that the understanding and use of these terms depend on the nonlinguistic context—the perspective of the speaker and the listener. The acquisition of deictic terms begins in the preschool period and advances during the school years.

Decentration is the ability to consider several aspects of a problem simultaneously. This cognitive achievement allows the child to move from one-dimensional descriptions of objects and events to coordinated, multiattributional ones. The child recognizes that many dimensions can be used to describe an object or an event and adjusts his or her messages accordingly (Owens, 1996). Whereas a younger child's descriptions are more personal and do not consider the information that must be available to the listener, a school-age child's messages are more accurate because the child considers the listener's perspective and provides more extensive information.

By the time children reach Piaget's concrete operational stage, they perceive the needs of their listeners and make undifferentiated adaptations in their communication to satisfy those needs. In settling peer disputes, children give reasons for disagreements involving their own feelings and beliefs about an event or an action. In the stage of formal operations, children adapt to their listeners' needs in a differentiated manner by negotiating, justifying, and stating reasons for their positions. Table 2.17 summarizes the different communication strategies used by children in Piaget's preoperational, concrete, and formal operational stages. Note the differences between older and younger children's communicative strategies.

CLARIFICATION

Successful conversation involves coordinated interaction between speakers and listeners, and when misunderstandings occur, speakers must repair their messages. During the school-age years, children repair and clarify their messages using a variety of strategies (Konefal & Folks, 1984). Whereas 6-year-olds will elaborate some elements in their repetitions and provide more information to a listener, 9-year-olds are capable of addressing the source of the communicative breakdown and can produce background and context and define terms to provide additional clarification (Owens, 2005). Nine-year-olds not only elaborate their repetitions, but they also seem capable of addressing the perceived source of communication breakdown. Last, they are sensitive to cues that indicate the failure of the communicative attempt and can talk about the process of conversational repair (Brinton, Fujiki, Loeb, & Winkler, 1986; Crais & Lorch, 1994; Hulit & Howard, 1997).

TOPIC MAINTENANCE

Much of the control of conversation during the young school-age years is exercised by adults, who ask children many questions. As noted previously, preschool children maintain a topic by repeating the information in the adult utterance, but older children provide additional information in their responses (Brinton & Fujiki, 1984).

During the school-age years, approximately 60 percent of children's peer interactions are effective. This is because children of this age have developed metalinguistic

Table 2.17   **Communication Strategy Development: An Overview**

Cognitive Stage	Strategy	Examples
Preoperational (ages 2–7)		
Early	Self-oriented perception Nonadaptation to listener	*Context:* Jim and John in sandbox. John wants to play with the pail and shovel. Jim is playing with it.
		John: Gimme pail and shovel.
Late	Perception of listener Nonadaptation to listener	*Context:* Sue and Jean are in the yard. Sue has been riding the bike for five minutes.
		Jean: Now *I* want to ride the bike!
Concrete (ages 7–11)	Perception of listener Undifferentiated adaptation to listener	*Context:* Bill and Sam are on the playground.
		Bill: Please, pretty please, can I try your baseball glove?
		Context: Linda borrowed Stacy's pen.
		Linda: I'm sorry I broke your pen.
Formal (ages 11–14)	Perception of listener Differentiated adaptation to listener needs	*Context:* Jason and Peter are on the playground.
		Jason: If you'll let me try your mitt, I'll let you try my head-to-head football game. (Jason takes the game out of his pocket.)
		Context: Lisa has returned from school. Her mother is upset.
		Lisa: I know you're upset, but the English teacher assigned a composition about El Salvador for tomorrow, and I stopped off at the library to get some books to do the research.

skills, or the ability to reflect on effectiveness of the language used in conversation. The greatest change occurs during the years from late elementary school to adulthood (Brinton & Fujiki, 1984; N. W. Nelson, 1993). A related decrease in the number of different topics introduced or reintroduced occurs. Thus, the school years bring a growing adherence to the concept of conversational relevance and topic maintenance. Although 8-year-olds can sustain a topic through a number of conversational turns, their topics tend to be concrete. Discussions involving abstract topics usually are not sustained until age 11 (Owens, 2005).

CODE SWITCHING

When 8-year-olds talk to their peers, they speak differently than when addressing infants or adults. When speaking with infants, school-age children tend to reduce the length and complexity of their utterances, appearing to understand that very young children require a different form of interaction. Among adults, school-age children vary their codes for parents and for those outside the family. In general, parents are usually the recipients of demands, whining, and short (less conversational) narrative (Owens, 2005). It is not surprising that parents are often shocked when their child, who talks to them with language that is less than polite and informative, is described by other adults as charming, entertaining, and interesting.

During the later school age years, conversation becomes more demanding. It is an important medium for adolescents' social interaction and the establishment of friendships (Nippold, 2000; Whitmire, 2000). During conversation, adolescents add information during their turn and can shade from one topic to another (Larson & McKinley, 1995). During this period, the adolescent can make transitions between formal and informal language, relying more on formal registers with not only adults but their peers as well (unless particularly close to the peer). Modification of the verb phrase is key in switching between informal and formal codes ("Pass me my pen," as opposed to "Would you pass me my pen?")—a skill that the adolescent masters.

Because communication among adolescents requires more sophisticated linguistic and pragmatic skills, they are able to generate multiple arguments with greater facility by the eleventh and twelfth grades while incorporating politeness to create a more successful communicative interaction (Larson & McKinley, 2003). Nippold (1998) found that adolescents demonstrate the ability to resolve conflicts by using improved perspective taking, consideration of long-term consequences, and compromise. Lastly, conversation directed to peers by adolescents usually involves more expressed feelings than conversation directed toward adults (Larson & McKinley, 1995).

INDIRECT REQUESTS

Another dimension of pragmatic development that occurs during the school-age years is the ability to use indirect requests. The development of indirect requests is particularly noteworthy because it represents the child's growing awareness of both socially appropriate requests and the communication context (Hulit & Howard, 1997).

Indirect requests are first produced in the preschool years; the proportion of their occurrence to direct requests increases between the ages of 3 and 5 (Garvey, 1977). This proportion does not change markedly between ages 5 and 6 (Levin & Rubin, 1982). In general, the 5-year-old gets what he or she wants by asking for it *directly*. By age 7, however, the child gains greater facility with indirect forms (Garvey, 1975; Grimm, 1975). Flexibility in the use of indirect requests continues to increase with age. For example, Ervin-Tripp (1980) found that the proportion of hints ("That sweater would go so nicely with my new skirt") increases from childhood through adulthood.

ABSTRACT REASONING

As children progress through the grades, their developing cognitive and linguistic skills allow them to reason more effectively. While young children will reason by just saying "Because," older children understand that this explanation is insufficient. By the time children have reached adolescence, their abstract reasoning is evident in their use of both deductive and inductive reasoning. Deductive reasoning is reflected in the ability to solve syllogisms. Here is an example of a syllogism:

Major premise: All men are mortal.

Minor premise: Socrates is a man.

Conclusion: Socrates is mortal.

Inductive reasoning is reflected in the ability to determine if the premises of an argument support the conclusion. An example of an inductive reasoning task is found in the following example:

All observed crows are black.

Therefore,

All crows are black.

Accuracy for solving syllogisms increases with age: 60 percent accuracy for 8-year-olds; 77 percent for 13-year-olds; and 84 percent for 16-year-olds (Nippold, 1998). Similar development also has been shown in the realm of inductive reasoning skills.

PRAGMATICS: LANGUAGE DIFFERENCES

Researchers have shown that cultural differences can affect pragmatic skills (Taylor, 1999). For example, African American English (AAE) speakers view direct or personal questions as inappropriate and tolerate interruption in conversation. AAE speakers are said to prefer indirect eye contact to direct eye contact while listening to a speaker, whereas Spanish language users view lack of eye contact as inappropriate. Finally, hand shaking with persons of the opposite sex is not customary for Asians and Asian Americans.

In addition to cultural nonverbal communication differences, Haynes and Shulman (1998) report that narratives vary in different cultures. For example, when producing stories, Spanish-speaking children use articles and nouns *(a girl)*, pronouns *(he)*, ellipsis ("She went to school, ate her lunch"), and demonstratives *(this)* for cohesion (Owens, 2005). On the other hand, AAE narrative style employs anecdotes that are more personal, and prosody is used more often than semantic or syntactic cues for cohesion. For more information on cultural and linguistic differences, see Chapter 12.

LANGUAGE IN THE CLASSROOM

The language of the classroom differs from that used in informal social interactions. In the classroom, children are expected to process the language of the teacher and the language of the textbooks. As the grade level increases, so does the complexity of the language students are expected to process (Nelson, 1986; Chapters 5 and 11).

Children with language abilities commensurate with the linguistic demands of the classroom do well in school. However, children who have linguistic deficits have difficulty in the classroom that can affect them emotionally and socially (Gerber, 1981; N. W. Nelson, 1985, 1993).

The language of the classroom differs in several ways from that used in informal social interaction and the language of the home. Children of preschool age receive their major linguistic input from caretakers and can rely on the familiarity of the home context to help them understand what is expected of them. Because language at home depends heavily on context, children can act appropriately by following familiar routines, even if they understand only a little of what is presented to them linguistically. In addition, interactions between children and caretakers during the preschool years are dyadic; if children misunderstand the language directed to them, their caretakers repair the message.

Language in the classroom, however, is highly **decontextualized;** that is, it is not presented in the context that is related to the topic discussed. This removes the contextual cues that the child can rely on to better understand classroom language. In addition, in school, as children advance through the grades, teachers use longer sentences, more complex syntactic structures, more rapid speaking rates (Cuda & Nelson, 1976; N. W. Nelson, 1986, 1993), and the number of opportunities to obtain clarification is decreased (McLaughlin, 1998). Lastly, textbook language is expository, more varied in content, and less predictable (Westby, 1998). A description of expository text and the development of its comprehension is presented later in this chapter.

Because of the increased linguistic demands of the classroom, children with language deficits cannot derive maximal benefit from classroom instruction. In educational settings, the speech-language pathologist can provide the classroom teacher with strategies to help support the academic success of children with language difficulties (see Chapters 5 and 11).

Development of Metalinguistic Abilities

During the preschool period, children view language as a means of communicating. They do not focus on the manner in which language is conveyed. During the school-age years, children begin to reflect on language as a decontextualized object. This is called **metalinguistic ability** and enables children to think and to talk about language—that is, to treat language as an object of analysis and to use language to talk about language. The development of metalinguistic abilities is most obvious during middle childhood, between 5 and 8 years of age.

Van Kleeck (1982) identified three important aspects of metalinguistic development: (1) recognizing that language is an arbitrary conventional code, (2) recognizing that language is a system of units and rules for combining those units, and (3) recognizing that language is used for communication.

1. *Language is an arbitrary conventional code.* Understanding that language is an arbitrary conventional code includes understanding that words are arbitrary labels, separate from the objects or events they represent. Young children do not recognize the arbitrary nature of language; thus, they tend to treat words as though they were part of their referents. For example, a 4-year-old might say that the word *jet* is a big word because jets are big and that *ant* is a short word because ants are short. In contrast, a 7-year-old is likely to say that the word *jet* is a small word because it does not have many letters.

Evidence of the arbitrary nature of language can also be seen in children's ability to recognize ambiguity—that is, that words and sentences can have more than one meaning. An example of ambiguity detection involves the recognition that the sentence "The duck is ready to eat" could mean either (1) the duck (that is in the field) is ready to eat some grass or (2) the duck (which has been cooked) is ready to be served for dinner. Surface- and deep-structure ambiguity, such as in sentences that allow for more than one interpretation ("She fed her dog biscuits"), are not understood until 11 or 12 years of age (Westby, 1998).

Children's awareness of the arbitrary nature of words is reflected in rhyming and word play. In this case, children are able to understand that words are composed of segments and that these segments can be manipulated. Another metalinguistic skill that depends on the awareness that language is an arbitrary code is the ability to understand that different sentence forms can convey the same meaning. This ability is called **recognizing synonymy.** An example of recognizing synonymy would be realizing that the following sentences describe the same event: "The girl chased the boy," "The boy was chased by the girl," and "It was the girl who chased the boy." Children are unable to recognize synonymy until the early to middle elementary school years (Tunmer, Pratt, & Herriman, 1984).

2. *Language is a system of units and rules.* The awareness that language is a system of units is demonstrated by children's ability to break down larger linguistic units into smaller parts. This ability allows the child to divide the sentence "The dog chased the cat" into five words. It also enables the child to break down the word *cat* into three phonemes. The ability to segment words into their component sounds is a result of the child's phonological awareness. It is characterized by the ability to rhyme, to segment words into syllables and sounds, to manipulate sounds, and to blend sounds (Goswami & Bryant, 1990). Three-year-old children are able to break words into syllables but not into segments, but six-year-old children are able to accomplish both tasks. Researchers have found a strong relationship between early rhyming abilities and later phonological awareness (Ball, 1997; Blachman, 1991; Bryant, MacLean, & Bradley, 1990; Catts, 1996; Hatcher, Hulme, & Ellis, 1994; MacLean, Bryant, & Bradley, 1987; Shaywitz, Fletcher, Holahan, & Shaywitz, 1992; Snyder & Downey, 1997; Swanson, Mink, & Bocian, 1999; Torgesen, Wagner, & Rashotte, 1994; Westby, 1998).

The recognition that linguistic rules must be used to combine syntactic units also emerges during the early school years (Owens, 2005). This is illustrated by children's awareness that the utterance "The cat chasing the dog" is ungrammatical and that to make it grammatically acceptable one must add an auxiliary verb (*is* or *was*), change the progressive form to the third-person singular (*chases*), or use the past tense of the verb chase (*chased*).

3. *Language is used for communication.* As noted in a previous section, preschool-age children demonstrate some awareness of the social rules for language use at age 3

to 4, but it is not until the early elementary school years that they can judge the adequacy and appropriateness of their messages—what constitutes good communication. They can judge if an utterance is appropriate for a specific listener or setting and are aware that they should be polite to achieve their goals.

Metalinguistic abilities emerge about the same time children are learning to read, and it has been suggested that metalinguistic awareness and reading development are related (Blackman & James, 1985; Catts, 1996; Saywitz & Wilkinson, 1982; Tunmer & Bowey, 1984; van Kleeck, 1995). However, research has also shown that some children with language disorders demonstrate deficits in metalinguistic abilities (Kamhi & Koenig, 1985; Wallach & Butler, 1994; van Kleeck, 1995), and that metalinguistic and language processing deficits underlie reading disabilities (Brady & Shankweiler, 1991; Catts, 1996; Catts & Kamhi, 1987; Fletcher et al., 1994; Vellutino, Scanlon, Small, & Tanzman, 1991). Smith-Gabig (Chapter 5) and Diehl and Silliman suggest that speech-language pathologists need to assess metalinguistic abilities in school-age children suspected of having a language disorder or a reading disability.

READING DEVELOPMENT

Reading is a complex process that is not totally understood by development and educator professionals. However, it is now recognized that literacy is built on a foundation of intact language skills and that there is a relationship among phonological awareness, verbal memory and retrieval, and learning to read.

It is beyond the scope of this chapter to detail reading models and the cognitive processes that underlie this area of development. However, because reading is a language-based process and speech-language pathologists target linguistic intervention in their therapy with children who have language learning or reading disabilities, their understanding of the links among oral language, reading, and reading difficulties is crucial.

Five stages of reading development have been proposed by Chall (1983). At the prereading stage, from birth to 5 or 6 years of age, children establish the understanding that print has meaning. They also learn to perceive the differences or the contrasts between sounds, to recognize and discriminate between the letters of the alphabet, and to scan print. By 4 years of age, children are able to recognize their names in print and some words in signs and labels (Dickinson, Wolf, & Stotsky, 1993). The word *stop* and the *M* symbol for McDonald's restaurant are recognized at an early age.

The first stage of reading development, from 5 to 7 years of age, consists of learning phoneme–grapheme correspondence rules. However, often there is a lack of correlation between sounds and written segments, such as the association of the grapheme *a* with at last three different sounds (*hat, came,* and *lawn*). This makes the mastery of some sound–letter correspondences difficult for children. Early on, children concentrate on decoding single words in simple stories. At this stage, children rely on the visual configuration of a word in order to recognize it. They pay particular attention to the first letter of the word and to word length while ignoring the order of the letters. Children at this stage learn letter–sound correspondence rules, recognize their importance, and are able to sound out novel words by using the phonetic approach. In addition, they learn that text provides messages and does more than just describe pictures (Ferreiro & Teberosky, 1982).

First-grade readers begin to use text to analyze unknown words. Whenever they read a word incorrectly, it is because they do not know that particular word. Instead, they substitute another word that makes sense in that context. Torgesen (1999) presents three facts regarding context: (1) skilled readers do not rely solely on context (Share & Stanovich, 1995), (2) poor readers rely on context more than good readers (Briggs, Austin, & Underwood, 1984), and (3) context is not adequate for word identification.

The second stage of reading development, from 7 to 9 years of age, involves consolidating the knowledge gained in the earlier stages. Children learn to use their knowledge of decoding skills and story structure to increase their understanding of written materials. They are able to recognize words based on orthographic configuration or spelling patterns and are able to use information about the phonological composition of words to aid them in decoding. However, at this stage, many children with reading difficulties are unable to make use of phonological material or the composition of words to aid them in coding.

In the third stage, from 9 to 14 years of age, decoding abilities are automatized and children are now able to focus on the comprehension of reading material (Kamhi & Catts, 1991). The fourth stage, from 14 to 18 years of age, finds that lower-level skills are firmly established. Adolescents must now use higher-order skills, such as inference and the recognition of the author's viewpoint, to assist them in comprehending the written material. The final stage, from 18 years of age and up, finds readers able to deal with multiple points of view. Since vocabulary skills are now well developed, the ability to read critically and to understand more abstract written materials increases.

PREDICTORS OF READING SKILLS: PHONOLOGICAL AWARENESS AND LANGUAGE ABILITIES

There are two important predictors of good reading skills: (1) phonological awareness and (2) good language skills, with an integral relation between the two (Lewis, Freebairn, & Taylor, 2000; Roth & Troia, 2006; Rescorla, 2002; Schwartz, 1994; Wagner, Torgesen, Laughon, Simmons, & Rashotte, 1993). Several longitudinal studies of children's literacy development across a number of different languages have found that certain aspects of phonological awareness predict good reading skills (Chiappe, Siegel, & Wade-Woolley, 2002; McBride-Chang & Kail, 2002; Muter & Diethelm, 2001; O'Connor & Bell, 2004; Schatschneider, Fletcher, Francis, Carlson, & Foorman, 2004). These aspects include rapid letter naming, knowledge of letter sounds, phoneme segmentation, vocabulary, spelling, blending sounds to form words, and word recognition skills. These skills allow children to recognize known words with speed and accuracy and to identify unfamiliar words (Ball & Blachman, 1991; O'Connor, Jenkins, & Slocum, 1995; Torgesen, Morgan, & Davis, 1992).

The language skills that support reading are age-appropriate vocabulary (McGregor, 2004), morphology (Carlisle, 2004), syntax (Scarborough, 1990; Scarborough & Dobrich, 1990; Scott, 2004), and word recognition skills (Bialystok, 2002; MacDonald & Cornwall, 1995; Snowling, 1991; Vellutino & Scanlon, 1987).

COMPREHENSION OF EXPOSITORY TEXT

Expository text presents explanations, descriptions, and information that is found in textbooks, reports, newspapers, and magazines. Expository text requires that the reader comprehend unfamiliar and factual information, the writer's perspective, and the use of logical-deductive inference to determine meaning (Catts & Kamhi, 1999).

The structure of expository text can consist of descriptions, sequences/procedures, comparisons/contrasts, problems/solutions, and arguments (Westby, 1998). Examples of these structures are shown in Table 2.18. A single expository text may present more than one type of structure (Westby, 1998), requiring the reader to be able to

Table 2.18 **Characteristics of Expository Texts**

Text Pattern	Text Function	Key Words
Description	The text tells what something is.	Is called, can be defined as, is, can be interpreted as, is explained as, refers to, is a procedure for, is someone who, means
Collection/enumeration	The text gives a list of things that are related to the topic.	An example is, for instance, another, next, finally, such as, to illustrate
Sequence/procedure	The text tells what happened or how to do something or make something.	First, next, then, second, third, following this step, finally, subsequently, from here . . . to, eventually, before, after
Comparison/contrast	The text shows how two things are the same or different.	Different, same, alike, similar, although, however, on the other hand, contrasted with, compared with, rather than, but, yet, still, instead of
Cause/effect explanation	The text gives reasons for why something happened.	Because, since, reasons, then, therefore, for this reason, results, effects, consequently, so, in order to, thus, depends on, influences, is a function of, produces, leads to, affects, hence
Problem/solution	The text states a problem and offers solutions to the problem.	A problem is, a solution is

From Communicative refinement in school age and adolescence, C. E. Westby (1998). In W. O. Haynes and B. B. Shulman (Eds.), *Communication development: Foundations, processes, and clinical applications.* Baltimore, MD: Lippincott Williams & Wilkins. Copyright © 1998 Lippincott Williams & Wilkens. Reprinted by permission.

follow the flow of ideas and understand the content (Larson & McKinley, 2003). Expository text is also characterized by the use of connectives (e.g., *before, after, when, therefore*) that help provide organization. Thus, focus, attention, and memory are required to support the comprehension of expository text. The ability of school-age children to understand expository text plays a significant role in their academic success.

READING PROCESSES

Theoretical positions that attempt to explain the processes involved in reading follow two major approaches: the bottom-up approach (perceptual and phonemic processes) and the top-down approach (cognitive processes). These processes are viewed as being interactive, with a third- or fourth-grade reader using the bottom-up strategy for reading words in isolation and the top-down strategy for text (Owens, 2005).

The Bottom-Up Approach

The **bottom-up approach** defines reading as the "translation of written elements into language" (Perfetti, 1984, p. 41). Bottom-up theories emphasize lower-level perceptual and phonemic processes and their influence on higher cognitive functioning. According to this view, knowledge of the perceptual features of letters and of their correspondence to sounds assists in word recognition and decoding. The bottom-up theory assumes that the child must learn to decode print into language. That is, the child must be able to divide each word into phonemic elements and learn the alphabetical letters (graphemes) that correspond to these phonemes. Only when this process is automatic can the child give sufficient attention to the meaning of the text. If the child gains automaticity processing at the visual and auditory levels, he or she will more easily master the other stages of processing written materials.

According to bottom-up theory, each word acts like a switchboard that activates the visual, auditory, and semantic features of that word. If the reader has enough information from these features, the information is automatically presented to the other parts of the system for processing. In sum, the bottom-up theory of reading emphasizes that lower-level processes (perceptual and phonological stages) critically influence all further stages of processing.

The Top-Down Approach

In contrast to bottom-up theories, theories that subscribe to the **top-down approach** emphasize the cognitive task of deriving meaning from print. This approach has been termed the *problem-solving model* (Owens, 2005). Higher cognitive functions, such as concepts, inferences, and levels of meaning, influence the processing of lower-order information. The reader generates hypotheses about the written material based on his or her world knowledge, the content of the material in the text, and the syntactic structures used. Sampling of the reading confirms or disconfirms the hypotheses.

The Interactive Approach

The interactive approach to explaining the reading process incorporates portions of both bottom-up and top-down models (Rumelhart, 1977; Stanovich, 1980). According to this view, top-down and bottom-up processes provide information to the reader simultaneously at various levels of analysis. This information is then synthesized. The processes are interactive and relative reliance on each varies with the skills of the reader and the material that is being read.

It has been proposed that by third or fourth grade, children rely on a bottom-up strategy when reading isolated words and a top-down strategy when reading text. Context supports the more rapid, top-down processes; when such support is lacking, the slower, bottom-up processes are used. Although variations on bottom-up and top-down models of reading abound, all researchers agree that learning to read requires the integration of multiple sensory, perceptual, linguistic, and conceptual processing strategies.

PHONOLOGICAL DECODING

Investigators now believe that stage theories offer an oversimplification of reading development for two reasons: (1) Children follow different paths, and (2) not all words are read with the same approach at each stage (Catts & Kamhi, 1999; Share & Stanovich, 1995). Early reading skills begin with the decoding of the correspondence between sounds and letters as children become aware of spelling regularities. Later reading skills are characterized by the rapid recognition of high-frequency words, while low-frequency words require the phonetic decoding skills developed earlier. Thus, there are differences in the strategies used for decoding familiar and unfamiliar words as reading skills develop over time.

WRITING DEVELOPMENT

Phonological abilities also play a role in writing development (Lewis, O'Donnell, Freebairn, & Taylor, 1998). Consistent with reading development, phonological awareness is considered a strong predictor of spelling success (Nation, 2005; Nation & Hulme, 1997). The awareness of the correspondence between sounds and letters is necessary for translating the speech sounds (phonemes) to written letters (graphemes). Learning to spell also involves morphological knowledge (Kamhi & Hinton, 2000). For example, children must learn that the past -*ed* morpheme has different phonological realizations, such as *pitched* (/t/), *dragged* (/d/), and *ticketed* (/ɪd/).

The development of writing abilities follows five stages (Henderson & Beers, 1980; Owens, 2005): the preliterate stage, the letter-name stage, the within-word stage, the syllable juncture stage, and the derivational constancy stage. Written language is initially represented by drawing, followed by scribbling, followed by attempts to represent letters, followed by inventive spelling, and culminating in conventional writing patterns.

In the preliterate stage, children draw, scribble, begin to write some letters, and talk about the writing project at hand. Writing and drawing are differentiated by 3 years of age (Owens, 2005). In the letter-name stage, children use invented spellings. In this stage, children rely on phonological knowledge, with each written letter representing a speech sound. The sound that children hear is matched to the letter, and their writing reflects this match. Initially, children represent the entire word with the first letter and pay little attention to the other letters of the word. For example, DRLM or DBC may represent *daddy* or MBRS may represent *mommy* (Owens, 2005). This is similar to the initial stage of reading, in which the child pays attention to only the first letter.

Next, children represent syllables, often without vowels. For example, *girl* might be written as GRL or *boy* as BY. In the final stage of inventive spelling, phonemic spelling, children are aware of the alphabet and the correspondence of graphemes to phonemes. Words such as *cat, it,* and *me* are spelled correctly, but words such as *knife, night,* and *soup* are not. Examples of spelling development are also shown in the attempts to spell *dragon* by different children at different grades: MPRMRHM (kindergarten), GAGIN (first grade), and DRAGUN (second grade). The sentence YUTS A LADE YET FEHEG AD HE KOT FLEPR is an example of invented spelling that represents the sentence "Once a lady went fishing and she caught Flipper" (Temple, Nathan, Temple, & Burris, 1993). Finally, children are aware of the sound–symbol correspondence and can produce sentences like HE HAD A BLUE CLTH to represent "He had a blue cloth" (Owens, 2005).

In the letter-name stage, children are not concerned with finding a sound–letter match, but in the within-word pattern stage, they rely on standard orthographic patterns to write. They also begin to recognize the correct spelling of grammatical endings and sound–spelling differences. In addition, better-developed aspects of a child's spelling, handwriting, and sentence structure will often deteriorate when new levels of complexity are introduced, such as changes from print to script or the introduction of greater complexity.

At the syllable juncture stage, children are aware of stress patterns in words, and at the derivational constancy stage, they attend to root forms of words. The formal instruction of school brings mastery of the conventional spelling system. In addition, during the school-age years, children begin to pay attention to format, spacing, and punctuation when producing a written piece of work. In the third or fourth grade, their increased syntactic knowledge allows them to write using complex clauses and phrases and to revise and proofread their written work. By the end of elementary school, the complexity of typically developing children's written language surpasses that of their spoken language (Gillam & Johnston, 1992).

In the higher grades, adolescents are asked to create narratives, summaries, creative pieces such as fiction, descriptions of events, and informational reports (Scott, 1984; Scott & Erwin, 1992). In some cases, 44 percent of classroom time may be devoted to writing tasks in the higher grades (Applebee, 1984).

While grapheme–phoneme relations are essential factors in reading skills, phoneme–grapheme relations are factors in spelling (Larson & McKinley, 2003). Note-taking skills must also be present to support academic progress in the higher grades, including attention, focus, working memory, sentence processing, vocabulary, direction following, simultaneous processing of visual and auditory information, and auditory discrimination (Ratner & Harris, 1994).

Syntactic skills also play a role in written language. Growth in syntactic skills is most apparent in writing persuasive essays, rather than in less formal writing tasks, such as narratives (Nippold, 2000). Persuasive writing involves the need to take a position, to convince a reader of that position, to be aware of a reader's knowledge of the topic at hand, and to develop an argument in a logical and coherent manner (Nippold, 2000).

Finally, spelling development requires that children be able to establish the phonological structure of words and determine which graphemes represent sounds in words. This will enable them to write more complex and abstract written texts in later grades (Apel, Wolter, & Masterson, 2006; Silliman, Bahr, & Peters, 2006).

Summary

During the preschool and school-age years, language development increases significantly. By kindergarten, children have acquired much of the mature language user's form. Development continues as children add new forms and gain new skills in transmitting messages. During the school-age years, children expand their sentences, their vocabulary, their ability to reason, and their mastery of nonliteral language. Their conversational abilities increase with their social skills, and they become good storytellers. Once children have gained a working knowledge of spoken language, most of them adapt to the new mode of written language (reading and writing) with relative ease. Their metalinguistic abilities enable them to decontextualize language and use their knowledge to understand language in the classroom.

However, for children with language learning difficulties, the school years pose special problems. Their needs must be met by a variety of specialists who assess their skills and integrate programming so that they can fully benefit from classroom instruction (see Chapters 5 and 11). We conclude this chapter with a quotation from Rees (1980):

> For professionals in the area of communication disorders, it is recognized that only the most complete understanding possible of the nature and growth of child language will suffice as basic information with which to approach clinical problems. Normal language development provides not only the base of reference against which to evaluate the communicative functioning of the clinical subject, but also guidelines for assessment and intervention. (p. 38)

Information about language development in typically developing children provides the speech-language pathologist with a framework for understanding the assessment and remediation of language disorders in children. Because new knowledge is continuously emerging about the stages, strategies, and processes of normal language development, what we "do today will be replaced tomorrow by wiser principles and improved techniques" (Rees, 1980, p. 38).

Study Questions

1. Describe the prelinguistic abilities of young children.
2. Explain the importance of environmental interaction in language acquisition.
3. What are the major communicative intents coded by young children?
4. Outline the semantic relations found in preschool children and give examples of each.
5. Describe the phonological processes observed in preschoolers' language, and explain which phonological processes should disappear by 3 years of age.
6. What are the main characteristics of each of Roger Brown's (1975) stages of language development?
7. Describe the literacy events that support emergent literacy.
8. Compare the pragmatic skills of preschool- and school-age children.
9. Trace narrative development from the preschool years through the school-age years. What major changes take place?
10. List the metalinguistic abilities that are related to the development of reading. Also briefly describe the bottom-up and top-down theories of reading and the stages in the development of reading abilities.
11. Describe the development of writing abilities.
12. Trace the syntactic achievements of the preschool- and school-age children.

References

Abrahamsen, E., & Rigrodsky, S. (1984). Comprehension of complex sentences in children at three levels of cognitive development. *Journal of Psycholinguistic Research, 13,* 333–350.

Al-Issa, I. (1969). The development of word definition in children. *Journal of Genetic Psychology, 114,* 25–28.

Anderson, R. C., Hiebert, E., Scott, J., & Wilkinson, I. A. G. (1985). *Becoming a nation of readers. The report of the Commission on Reading.* Washington, DC: National Institute of Education.

Apel, K., Wolter, J., & Masterson, J. (2006). Effects of phonotactic and orthotactic probabilities during fast mapping on 5-year-olds' learning to spell. *Developmental Neuropsychology, 29*(1), 21–42.

Applebee, A. (1984). *Contexts for learning to write.* Norwood, NJ: Ablex.

Arlin, M. (1983). Children's comprehension of semantic constraints on temporal prepositions. *Journal of Psycholinguistic Research, 12,* 1–15.

Baldie, B. (1976). The acquisition of the passive voice. *Journal of Child Language, 3,* 331–348.

Ball, E., & Blachman, B. (1991). Does phoneme awareness training in kindergarten make a difference in early word recognition and developmental spelling? *Reading Research Quarterly, 26,* 49–66.

Ball, E. W. (1997). Phonological awareness: Implications for whole language and emergent literacy programs. *Topics in Language Disorders, 17,* 14–26.

Bankson, N. W., & Bernthal, J. E. (1998). Analysis and interpretation of assessment data. In J. E. Bernthal & N. W. Bankson (Eds.), *Articulation and phonological disorders* (4th ed., pp. 270–298). Boston: Allyn & Bacon.

Beck, I., & Jeul, C. (1995). The role of decoding in learning to read. *American Educator, 19*(2), 8–13.

Bellugi, U. (1967). *The acquisition of negation.* Doctoral dissertation, Harvard University.

Berko Gleason, J. (2001). *The development of language* (5th ed.). Boston: Allyn & Bacon.

Bernstein, D. K. (1986). The development of humor: Implications for assessment and intervention. *Topics in Language Disorders, 4,* 65–73.

Bernstein, D. K. (1987). Figurative language: Assessment strategies and implications for intervention. *Folia Phoniatrica, 39,* 130–144.

Bernthal, J. E., & Bankson, N. W. (Eds.). (1998). *Articulation and phonological disorders* (4th ed.). Boston: Allyn & Bacon.

Bialystok, E. (2002). Acquisition of literacy in bilingual children: A framework for research. *Language Learning, 52*(1), 159–199.

Billow, R. (1975). A cognitive developmental study of metaphor comprehension. *Developmental Psychology, 11,* 415–423.

Blachman, B. (1991). Phonological awareness: Implications for prereading and early reading instruction. In S. Brady & D. Shankweiler (Eds.), *Phonological processes in literacy* (pp. 29–36). Hillsdale, NJ: Erlbaum.

Blackman, B., & James, S. (1985). Metalinguistic abilities and reading achievement in first grade children. In J. Niles & R. Lalid (Eds.), *Issues in literacy: A research perspective* (pp. 280–286). Thirty-Fourth Yearbook of the National Reading Conference.

Bloom, L. (1991). *Language development from two to three.* Cambridge, UK: Cambridge University Press.

Bloom, L., Lahey, M., Hood, L., Lifter, K., & Fiess, K. (1980). Complex sentences: Acquisition of syntactic connectives and the semantic relations they encode. *Journal of Child Language, 7,* 235–261.

Bloom, L., Lifter, K., & Hafitz, J. (1980). Semantics of verbs and the development of verb inflection in child language. *Language, 56,* 386–412.

Bloom, L., Lightbown P., & Hood, L. (1975). Structure and variation in child language. *Monographs of the Society for Research in Child Development, 40.*

Bloom, L., Merkin, S., & Wooten, J. (1982). *Wh*-questions: Linguistic factors that contribute to the sequence of acquisition. *Child Development, 53,* 1084–1092.

Bloom, L., Rocissano, L., & Hood, L. (1976). Adult-child discourse: Developmental interactions between information processing and linguistic interaction. *Cognitive Psychology, 8,* 521–552.

Bloom, P. (1990). Syntactic distinctions in child language. *Journal of Child Language, 17,* 343–356.

Bloom, P., Barss, A., Nicol, J., & Conway, L. (1994). Children's knowledge of binding and coreference: Evidence from spontaneous speech. *Language, 70*(1), 53–71.

Brady, S., & Shankweiler, D. (Eds.). (1991). *Phonological processes in literacy.* Hillsdale, NJ: Erlbaum.

Breinbauer, C., & Maddaleno, M. (2005). *Promoting healthy behaviors in adolescents* (Scientific and Technical Publication No. 594). Pan American Health Organization.

Briggs, A., Austin, R., & Underwood, G. (1984). Phonological coding in good and poor readers. *Reading Research Quarterly, 20,* 54–66.

Brinton, B., & Fujiki, M. (1984). Development of topic manipulation skills in discourse. *Journal of Speech and Hearing Research, 27,* 350–358.

Brinton, B., Fujiki, M., Loeb, D., & Winkler, E. (1986). Development of conversational repair strategies in response to request for clarification. *Journal of Speech and Hearing Research, 39,* 75–82.

Brown, R. (1975). *A first language: The early stages.* Cambridge, MA: Harvard University Press.

Brown, R., & Berko, J. (1960). Word association and the acquisition of grammar. *Child Development, 13,* 1–15.

Bryant, P., Bradley, L., MacLean, M., & Crossland, J. (1989). Nursery rhymes, phonological skills and reading. *Journal of Child Language, 16,* 407–428.

Bryant, P., MacLean, M., & Bradley, L. (1990). Rhyme, language, and children's reading. *Applied Psycholinguistics, 11*(3), 237–252.

Butler, K. (1999). From oracy to literacy: A millennial perspective. *Topics in Language Disorders, 20*(1), 14–32.

Cairns, H. S. (1996). *The acquisition of language* (2nd ed.). Austin, TX: Pro-Ed.

Carlisle, J. F. (2004). Morphological processes that influence learning to read. In C. A. Stone, E. R. Silliman, B. J. Ehren, & K. Apel (Eds.), *Handbook of language and literacy: Development and disorders* (pp. 318–339). New York: Guilford Press.

Catts, H. W. (1991). Early identification of reading disabilities. *Topics in Language Disorders, 12*(1), 1–17.

Catts, H. W. (1996). Defining dyslexia as a developmental language disorder: An expanded view. *Topics in Language Disorders, 16*(2), 14–25.

Catts, H. W., & Kamhi, A. G. (Eds.). (1999). *Language and reading disabilities.* Boston: Allyn & Bacon.

Chall, J. S. (1983). *Stages of reading development.* New York: McGraw-Hill.

Chiappe, P., Siegel, L. S., & Wade-Woolley, L. (2002). Linguistic diversity and the development of reading skills: A longitudinal study. *Scientific Studies of Reading, 6*(4), 369–400.

Chien, Y., & Wexler, K. (1990). Children's knowledge of locality conditions in binding as evidence for the modularity of syntax and pragmatics. *Language Acquisition, 1,* 225–295.

Choi, S. (2000). Caregiver input in English and Korean: Use of nouns in book-reading and toy-play contexts. *Journal of Child Language, 27,* 69–96.

Choi, S., & Gopnik, A. (1995). Early acquisition of verbs in Korean: A cross-linguistic study. *Journal of Child Language, 22,* 497–529.

Chomsky, C. (1969). *The acquisition of syntax in children from 5 to 10.* Cambridge, MA: MIT Press.

Crais, E. R., & Lorch, N. (1994). Oral narratives in school age children. *Topics in Language Disorders, 14*(3), 13–28.

Cuda, R. A., & Nelson, N. (1976, November). *Analysis of teacher speaking rate, syntactic complexity, and hesitation phenomena as a function of grade level.* Paper presented at the Annual Convention of the American Speech-Language-Hearing Association, Houston, TX.

Dale, P. S., & Crain-Thoreson, C. (1993). Pronoun reversals: Who, when, and why? *Journal of Child Language, 20,* 573–589.

de Villiers, J. G., & de Villiers, P. A. (1978). *Language acquisition.* Cambridge, MA: Harvard University Press.

Dever, R. (1978). *TALK: Teaching the American language to kids.* Columbus, OH: Merrill/Macmillan.

De Temple, J., & Snow, C. E. (2003). Learning words from books. In A. van Kleeck, S. A. Stahl, & E. B. Bauer (Eds.), *On reading books to children: Parents and teachers* (pp. 16–36). Mahwah, NJ: Erlbaum.

Dickinson, D., Wolf, M., & Stotsky, S. (1993). Words move: The interwoven development of oral and written language. In J. Berko Gleason (Ed.), *The development of language* (3rd ed., pp. 225–257). Columbus, OH: Merrill/Macmillan.

Dore, J. (1978). Requestive systems in nursery school conversations: Analysis of talk in its social context. In R. Campbell & P. Smith (Eds.), *Recent advances in the psychology of language: Language development and mother-child interaction* (pp. 271–292). New York: Plenum Press.

Drozd, K. F. (1995). Child English pre-sentential negation as a metalinguistic exclamatory sentence negation. *Journal of Child Language, 22*(3), 583–610.

Eisenberg, S., & Cairns, H. S. (1994). The development of infinitives from three to five. *Journal of Child Language, 21,* 713–734.

Elley, W. B. (1989). Vocabulary acquisition from stories. *Reading Research Quarterly, 24,* 174–187.

Ervin, S. (1961). Changes with age in the verbal determinants of word-association. *American Journal of Psychology, 74,* 361–372.

Ervin-Tripp, S. (1970). Discourse agreement: How children answer questions. In J. R. Hayes (Ed.), *Cognition and the development of language* (pp. 79–107). New York: Wiley.

Ervin-Tripp, S. (1980). Lecture, University of Minnesota, May 14, 1980.

Ferreiro, E., & Teberosky, A. (1982). *Literacy before schooling.* Exeter, NH: Heinemann.

Fletcher, J., Shaywitz, S., Shankweiler, D., Katz, L., Liberman, I., Stuebing, K., Francis, D., Fowler, A., & Shaywitz, B. (1994). Cognitive profiles of reading disabilities: Comparison of discrepancy and low achievement definitions. *Journal of Educational Psychology, 86,* 6–23.

Garvey, C. (1975). Requests and responses in children's speech. *Journal of Child Language, 2,* 41–63.

Garvey, C. (1977). The contingent query: A dependent act of communication. In M. Lewis & L. Rosenblum (Eds.), *Interaction, conversation, and the development of language.* New York: Wiley.

Gentner, D. (1982). Why nouns are learned before verbs: Linguistic relativity versus natural partitioning. In S. A. Kuczaj, II (Ed.), *Language development. Vol 2: Language, thought and culture* (pp. 301–334). Hillsdale, NJ: Erlbaum.

Gerber, A. (1981). Problems in the processing and use of language in education. In A. Gerber and D. N. Bryen (Eds.), *Language and learning disabilities* (pp. 75–112). Baltimore: University Park Press.

Gerken, L. (1991). The metrical basis for children's subjectless sentences. *Journal of Memory and Language, 30,* 431–451.

Gillam, R. (1999). Communicative patterns that facilitate language development. www. utexas.edu/ftp/courses/gillam/commpat.html.

Gillam, R., & Johnston, J. (1992). Spoken and written language relationships in language learning impaired and normally achieving school-age children. *Journal of Speech, Language, and Hearing Research, 35,* 1303–1315.

Gleitman, L. R., & Gleitman, H. (1994). A picture is worth a thousand words, but that's the problem: The role of syntax in vocabulary acquisition. In B. Lust, M. Suñer, & J. Whitman (Eds.), *Heads, projections, and learnability* (pp. 291–299). Hillsdale, NJ: Erlbaum.

Goldstein, B. (2000). *Cultural and linguistic diversity resource guide for speech-language pathologists*. San Diego, CA: Singular.

Goldstein, B., & Iglesias, A. (1996). Phonological patterns in normally developing Spanish-speaking 3- and 4-year-olds of Puerto Rican descent. *Journal of Communication Disorders, 29*(5), 367–387.

Golinkoff, R. M., Mervis, C. B., & Hirsh-Pasek, K. (1994). Early object labels: The case for a developmental principles framework. *Journal of Child Language, 21,* 125–155.

Gopnik, M. (1997). *The inheritance and innateness of grammars*. Oxford, UK: Oxford University Press.

Goswami, U., & Bryant, P. E. (1990). *Phonologic skills and learning to read*. Hillsdale, NJ: Erlbaum.

Greene, J. (1996). Psycholinguistic assessment: The clinical base for identification of dyslexia. *Topics in Language Disorders, 16*(2), 45–72.

Greenhalgh, K., & Strong, C. (2001). Literature language features in spoken narratives of children with typical language and children with language impairments. *Language, Speech, and Hearing Services in School, 32,* 114–125.

Grimm, H. (1975, Sept 9). Analysis of short-term dialogues in 5–7 year olds: Encoding of intentions and modifications of speech acts as a function of negative feedback loops. Paper presented at the Third International Child Language Symposium, London.

Haas, A., & Owens, R. (1985, November). *Preschooler's pronoun strategies: You and me make us*. Paper presented at the American Speech-Language-Hearing Association Annual Convention, Washington, DC.

Halliday, M. (1975). *Learning how to mean: Explorations in the development of language*. New York: Edward Arnold.

Halliday, M., & Hasan, R. (1976). *Cohesion in English*. London, UK: Longman.

Harkins, D. A., Koch, P. E., & Michel, G. F. (1994). Listening to maternal story telling affects narrative skill of 5-year-old children. *Journal of Genetic Psychology, 155,* 247–257.

Hatcher, P. J., Hulme, C., & Ellis, A. W. (1994). Ameliorating early reading failure by integrating the teaching of reading and phonological skills: The phonological linkage hypothesis. *Child Development, 65,* 41–57.

Haynes, W. O., & Shulman, B. S. (Eds.). (1998). *Communication development: Foundations, processes, and clinical applications* (pp. 361–386). Baltimore: Williams & Wilkins.

Heath, S. B. (1996). What no bedtime story means: Narrative skills at home and school. In D. Brenneis & R. K. S. Macaulay (Eds.), *The matrix of language* (pp. 12–38). Cumnor Hill: Westview Press.

Henderson, E. H., & Beers, J. W. (Eds.). (1980). *Developmental and cognitive aspects of learning to spell: A reflection of word knowledge*. Newark, DE: International Reading Association.

Henry, M. (1993). Morphological structure: Latin and Greek roots and affixes as upper grade code strategies. *Reading and Writing: An Interdisciplinary Journal, 5,* 227–241.

Hirsh-Pasek, K., & Golinkoff, R. M. (1997). *The origins of grammar: Evidence from early language comprehension*. Cambridge, MA: MIT Press.

Hulit, L. M., & Howard, M. R. (1997). *Born to talk: An introduction to speech and language development*. New York: Macmillan.

Hunt, K. (1965). *Grammatical written at three grade levels* (Research Report no. 3). Champaign, IL: National Council of Teachers of English.

Hyams, N. (1992). A reanalysis of null subject in child language. In J. Weissenborn, H. Goodluck, & T. Roeper (Eds.), *Continuity and change in development* (pp. 249–268). Hillsdale, NJ: Erlbaum.

James, S. (1990). *Normal language acquisition*. Boston: Allyn & Bacon.

Jenkins, J. R., Stein, M. L., & Wysocki, K. (1984). Learning vocabulary through reading. *American Educational Research Journal, 21,* 767–787.

Johnson, C. J., & Anglin, J. M. (1995). Qualitative development in the content and form of children's definitions. *Journal of Speech and Hearing Research, 38,* 612–625.

Jorm, A. F., & Share, D. L. (1983). An invited article: Phonological recoding and reading acquisition. *Applied Psycholinguistics, 4*(2), 103–147.

Jusczyk, P. W. (1992). Developing phonological categories from the speech signal. In C. A. Ferguson, L. Menn, & C. Stoehl-Gammon (Eds.), *Phonological development: Models, research, implications* (pp. 17–64). Timonium, MD: York Press.

Justice, L. M., & Ezell, H. K. (2000). Enhancing children's print and word awareness through home-based parent intervention. *American Journal of Speech-Language Pathology, 9*(3), 257–269.

Justice, L. M., & Schuele, C. M. (2004). Phonological awareness: Description, assessment, and intervention. In J. E. Bernthal & N. W. Bankson (Eds.), *Articulation and Phonological Disorders* (5th ed., pp. 376–411). Boston: Pearson.

Kamhi, A. G., & Catts, H. W. (1991). *Reading disabilities: A developmental language perspective*. Boston: Allyn & Bacon.

Kamhi, A. G., & Hinton, L. N. (2000). Explaining individual differences in spelling ability. In K. G. Butler (Ed.), *Topics in Language Disorders, 20*(3), 37–49.

Kamhi, A. G., & Koenig, L. (1985). Metalinguistic awareness in language disordered children. *Language, Speech and Hearing Services in Schools, 16,* 199–210.

Karmiloff-Smith, A. (1986). Some fundamental aspects of language development after age 5. In P. Fletcher & M. Garman (Eds.), *Language acquisition studies in first language development* (2nd ed., pp. 455–474). New York: Cambridge University Press.

Karmiloff-Smith, A. (1995). *Beyond modularity: A developmental perspective on cognitive science*. Cambridge, MA: MIT Press.

Klima, E., & Bellugi, U. (1966). Syntactic regularities in the speech of children. In J. Lyons & R. Wales (Eds.), *Psycholinguistic papers* (pp. 183–208). Edinburgh, Scotland: Edinburgh University Press.

Kogan, N., & Chadrow, M. (1986). Children's comprehension of metaphor in the pictorial and verbal modality. *International Journal of Behavioral Development, 9,* 285–295.

Konefal, J., & Folks, J. (1984). Linguistic analysis of children's conversational repairs. *Journal of Psycholinguistic Research, 13,* 1–11.

Kuhl, P. K., & Meltzoff, A. N. (1997). Evolution, nativism, and learning in the development of language and speech. In M. Gopnik (Ed.), *The inheritance and innateness of grammars* (pp. 7–44). Oxford, UK: Oxford University Press.

Lahey, M. (1974). The role of prosody and syntactic markers in children's comprehension of spoken sentences. *Journal of Speech and Hearing Research, 17,* 656–668.

Lahey, M., Liebergott, J., Chesnick, M., Menyuk, P., & Adams, J. (1992). Variability in children's use of grammatical morphemes. *Applied Psycholinguistics, 13,* 373–398.

Larson, V. L., & McKinley, N. (1995). *Language disorders in older students, preadolescents and adolescents.* Eau Claire, WI: Thinking Publications.

Larson, V. L., & McKinley, N. L. (1998). Characteristics of adolescents' conversations: A longitudinal study. *Clinical Linguistic and Phonetics, 12,* 183–203.

Larson, V. L., & McKinley, N. L. (2003). *Communication solutions for older students: Assessment and intervention strategies.* Eau Claire, WI: Thinking Publications.

Levin, E., & Rubin, K. (1982). Getting others to do what you want them to: The development of children's requestive strategies. In K. Nelson (Ed.), *Children's language* (Vol. 4). New York: Gardner Press.

Lewis, B. A., Freebairn, L. A., & Taylor, H. G. (2000). Academic outcomes in children with histories of speech sound disorders. *Journal of Communication Disorders, 33*(1), 11–30.

Lewis, B. A., O'Donnell, B., Freebairn, L. A., & Taylor, H. G. (1998). Spoken language and written expression-interplay of delays. *American Journal of Speech-Language Pathology, 7,* 77–84.

Lund, N., & Duchan, J. (1993). *Assessing children's language in naturalistic contexts.* Englewood Cliffs, NJ: Prentice Hall. (Originally published 1983)

MacDonald, G. W., & Cornwall, A. (1995). The relationship between phonological awareness and reading and spelling achievement eleven years later. *Journal of Learning Disabilities, 28,* 523–527.

MacLean, M., Bryant, P., & Bradley, L. (1987). Rhymes, nursery rhymes, and reading in early childhood: Children's reading and the development of phonological awareness [Special issue]. *Merrill-Palmer Quarterly, 33*(3), 255–281.

Masterson, J., & Crede, L. (1999). Learning to spell: implications for assessment and intervention. *Language, Speech, and Hearing Services in Schools, 30,* 243–254.

McBride-Chang, C., & Kail, R. V. (2002). Cross-cultural similarities in the predictors of reading acquisition. *Child Development, 73*(5), 1392–1407.

McGhee-Bidlack, B. (1991). The development of noun definitions. A metalinguistic analysis. *Journal of Child Language, 18,* 417–434.

McGregor, K. C. (2004). Developmental dependencies between lexical semantics and reading. In C. A. Stone, E. R. Silliman, B. J. Ehren, & K. Apel (Eds.), *Handbook of language and literacy: Development and disorders* (pp. 302–317). New York: Guilford Press.

McLaughlin, S. (1998). *Introduction to language development.* San Diego, CA: Singular.

McLean, J., & Snyder-McLean, L. (1999). *How children learn language.* San Diego, CA: Singular.

McNeill, D. (1970). *The acquisition of language.* New York: Harper & Row.

McShane J. (1980). *Learning to talk.* New York: Cambridge University Press.

Menyuk, P. (1969). *Sentences children use.* Cambridge, MA: MIT Press.

Menyuk, P. (1977). *Language and maturation.* Cambridge, MA: MIT Press.

Miller, G., & Gildea, P. (1987). How children learn words. *Scientific American, 257*(3), 94–99.

Miller, J. F. (1981). *Assessing language production in children: Experimental procedures.* Baltimore: University Park Press.

Muter, V., & Diethelm, K. (2001). The contribution of phonological skills and letter knowledge to early reading development in a multilingual population. *Language Learning, 51*(2), 187–220.

Nation, K. (2005). Connections between language and reading. In H. W. Catts & A. G. Kamhi (Eds.), *The connection between lexical and reading disabilities* (pp. 41–54). Mahwah, NJ: Erlbaum.

Nation, K., & Hulme, C. (1997). Phonemic segmentation, not onset-time segmentation, predicts early reading and spelling skills. *Reading Research Quarterly, 32,* 154–167.

Nelson, K. (1973). Structure and strategy in learning to talk. *Monographs of the Society for Research in Child Development, 38.*

Nelson, K., Hampson, J., & Shaw, L. K. (1993). Nouns in early lexicons: Evidence, explanations, and implications. *Journal of Child Language, 20,* 61–84.

Nelson, N. W. (1985). Teacher talk and children listening—Fostering a better match. In C. Simon (Ed.), *Communication skills and classroom success: Assessment of language-learning disabled children* (pp. 65–104). San Diego, CA: College-Hill.

Nelson, N. W. (1986). Individual processing in classroom settings. *Topics in Language Disorders, 6,* 13–27.

Nelson, N. W. (1993). *Childhood language disorders in context: Infancy through adolescence.* New York: Macmillan.

Nelson, N. W. (1998). *Childhood language disorders in context: Infancy through adolescence* (2nd ed.). Boston: Allyn & Bacon.

Ninio, A., & Snow, C. E. (1996). *Pragmatic development: Essays in developmental science.* Boulder, CO: Westview.

Nippold, M. A. (1985). Comprehension of figurative language. *Topics in Language Disorders, 3,* 1–20.

Nippold, M. A. (1988). Figurative language. In M. A. Nippold (Ed.), *Later language development: Ages nine through nineteen* (pp. 179–210). Austin, TX: Pro-Ed.

Nippold, M. A. (1991). Evaluating and enhancing idiom comprehension. *Language, Speech and Hearing Services in Schools, 22*(3), 100–105.

Nippold, M. A. (1998). *Later language development: The school-age and adolescent years* (2nd ed.). Austin, TX: Pro-Ed.

Nippold, M. (2000). Language development during the adolescence years: aspects of pragmatics, syntax, and semantics. *Topics in Language Disorders, 20*(2), 15–28.

Nippold, M. A., Leonard, L., & Kail, R. (1984). Syntactic and conceptual factors in children's understanding of metaphors. *Journal of Speech and Hearing Research, 27,* 197–205.

Nippold, M. A., & Martin, S. T. (1989). Idiom interpretation in isolation versus context: A developmental study with adolescents. *Journal of Speech and Hearing Research, 32,* 59–66.

Nippold, M. A., & Taylor, C. L. (1995). Idiom understanding in youth: Further examination of familiarity and transparency. *Journal of Speech and Hearing Research, 2,* 426–443.

Norris, J. A. (1998). Early sentence transformations and the development of complex syntactic structures. In W. O. Haynes & B. B. Shulman (Eds.), *Communication development: Foundations, processes, and clinical applications* (pp. 263–310). Baltimore: Williams & Wilkins.

O'Connor, R. E., & Bell, K. M. (2004). Teaching students with reading disability to read words. In C. A. Stone, E. R. Silliman, B. J. Ehren, & K. Apel (Eds.). *Handbook of Language and literacy: Development and disorders* (pp. 481–498). New York: Guilford Press.

O'Connor, R. E., Jenkins, J. R., & Slocum, T. A. (1995). Transfer among phonological tasks in kindergarten: Essential instructional content. *Journal of Educational Psychology, 87,* 202–217.

O'Grady, W. (1997). *Syntactic development.* Chicago: University of Chicago Press.

Oller, D. (1978). Infant vocalizations and the development of speech. *Allied Health and Behavior Sciences, 1,* 523–549.

Oshima-Takane, Y., Takane, Y., & Shultz, T. R. (1999). The learning of 1st and 2nd pronouns in English: Network models and analysis. *Journal of Child Language, 26,* 545–575.

Owens, R. (1988). *Language development and communication disorders in children* (2nd ed.). Columbus, OH: Merrill/Macmillan.

Owens, R. E., Jr. (1996). *Language development: An introduction* (3rd ed.). Columbus, OH: Merrill/Macmillan.

Owens, R. E., Jr. (2005). *Language development: An introduction* (6th ed.). Boston: Allyn & Bacon.

Owens, R. E., Jr., Metz, D. E., & Haas, A. (2000). *Introduction to communication disorders: A life span perspective.* Boston: Allyn & Bacon.

Patterson, J. L., & Westby, C. E. (1998). The development of play. In W. O. Haynes & B. B. Shulman (Eds.), *Communication development: Foundations, processes, and clinical applications* (pp. 135–163). Baltimore: Williams & Wilkins.

Peccei, J. S. (1999). *Child language* (2nd ed.). London, UK: Routledge.

Perfetti, C. (1984). Reading acquisition and beyond: Decoding includes cognition. *American Journal of Education, 93,* 40–60.

Piaget, J. (1954). *The construction of reality in the child.* New York: Basic Books.

Ratner, V., & Harris, L. (1994). *Understanding language disorders: The impact on learning.* Eau Claire, WI: Thinking Publications.

Rees, N. (1980). The nature of language. In T. Hixon, L. Shriberg, & J. Saxman (Eds.), *Introduction to communication disorders* (pp. 2–41). Englewood Cliffs, NJ: Prentice Hall.

Rescorla, L. (2002). Language and reading outcomes to age 9 in late-talking toddler. *Journal of Speech, Language, and Hearing Research, 45,* 360–371.

Ricard, M., Girouard, P. C., & Decarie, T. G. (1999). Personal pronouns and perspective taking in toddlers. *Journal of Child Language, 26,* 681–697.

Rispoli, M. (1998). Patterns of pronoun case error. *Journal of Child Language, 25,* 533–554.

Roth, F. P., & Troia, G. A. (2006). Collaborative efforts of promote emergent literacy and efficient word recognition skills. *Topics in Language Disorders, 26*(1), 24–41.

Rubin, H., Patterson, P., & Kantor, M. (1991). Morphological development and writing ability in children and adults. *Language, Speech and Hearing Services in the Schools, 22*(4), 228–236.

Rumelhart, D. (1977). Toward an interactive model of reading. In S. Dornic (Ed.), *Attention and performance, Vol. 6* (pp. 573–606). Hillsdale, NJ: Erlbaum.

Saywitz, K., & Wilkinson, L. C. (1982). Age related differences in metalinguistic awareness. In S. Kuczaj (Ed.), *Language development: Vol. 1. Language, thought and culture* (pp. 249–250). Hillsdale, NJ: Erlbaum.

Scarborough, H. (1990). Very early language deficits in dyslexic children. *Child Development, 61,* 1728–1743.

Scarborough, H., & Dobrich, W. (1990). Development of children with early language delay. *Journal of Speech and Hearing Research, 33,* 7–83.

Schatschneider, C., Fletcher, J. M., Francis, D. J., Carlson, C.D., & Foorman, B. R. (2004). Kindergarten prediction of reading skills: A longitudinal comparative analysis. *Journal of Educational Psychology, 96*(2), 265–282.

Schatschneider, C., & Torgesen, J. K. (2004). Using our current understanding of dyslexia to support early identification and intervention. *Journal of Child Neurology, 19*(10), 759–765.

Schwartz, R. G. (1994). Phonological disorders. In G. H. Shames, E. H. Wiig, & W. A. Secord (Eds.), *Human communication disorders: An introduction* (pp. 250–290). New York: Merrill.

Scott, C. (1984). Adverbial connectivity in conversations of children 6 to 12. *Journal of Child Language, 11,* 423–452.

Scott, C. M. (2004). Syntactic contributions to literacy learning. In C. A. Stone, E. R. Silliman, B. J. Ehren, & K. Apel (Eds.), *Handbook of language and literacy: Development and disorders* (pp. 340–362). New York: Guilford Press.

Scott, C. M., & Erwin, D. L. (1992). Descriptive assessment of writing: process and productions. *Best Practices in School Speech-Language Pathology, 2,* 87–98.

Seymour, H. N., & Roeper, T. (1999). Grammatical acquisition of African American English. In L. B. Leonard & O. L. Taylor (Eds.), *Language acquisition across North America: Cross-cultural and cross-linguistic perspectives* (pp. 109–152). San Diego, CA: Singular.

Share, D. L., & Stanovich, K. E. (1995). Cognitive processes in early reading development: Accommodating individual differences into a model of acquisition. *Issues in Education, 1,* 1–57.

Shaywitz, B. A., Fletcher, J. M., Holahan, J. M., & Shaywitz, S. E. (1992). Discrepancy compared to low achievement definitions of reading disability: Results from the Connecticut longitudinal study. *Journal of Learning Disabilities, 25*(10), 639–648.

Silliman, E. R., & Bahr, R. H., & Peters, M. L. (2006). Spelling patterns in preadolescents with atypical language skills: Phonological, morphological, and orthographic factors. *Developmental Neuropsychology, 29,* 93–123.

Silliman, E. R., & James, S. (1997). Assessing children with language disorders. In D. K. Bernstein & E. Tiegerman-Farber (Eds.), *Language and communication disorders in children* (pp. 197–271). Boston: Allyn & Bacon.

Snow, C., Scarborough, H., & Burns, M. S. (1999). What SLPs need to know about early readings. *Topics in Language Disorders, 20,* 48–58.

Snow, C. E., Perlmann, R., & Nathan, D. (1987). Why routines are different: Toward a multiple-factors model of the relation between input and language acquisition. In K. E. Nelson & A. van Kleeck (Eds.), *Children's language, Vol. 6* (pp. 65–97). Hillsdale, NJ: Erlbaum.

Snowling, M. J. (1991). Developmental reading disorders. *Journal of Child Psychology and Psychiatry, 32,* 49–77.

Snowling, M. J., Hulme, C., Smith, A., & Thomas, J. (1994). The effects of phoneme similarity and list length on children's sound categorization performance. *Journal of Experimental Child Psychology, 58,* 160–180.

Snyder, L. S., & Downey, D. M. (1997). Developmental differences in the relationship between oral language deficits and reading. *Topics in Language Disorders, 17,* 27–40.

Sokolov, J. L., & Snow, C. E. (1994). The changing role of negative evidence in theories of language development. In C. Gallaway & B. J. Richards (Eds.), *Input and interaction in language acquisition* (pp. 38–55). Cambridge, UK: Cambridge University Press.

Stanovich, K. (1980). Toward an interactive-compensatory model of individual differences in the development of reading fluency. *Reading Research Quarterly, 16,* 32–71.

Stanovich, K. E., Cunningham, A. E., & Cramer, B. (1984). Assessing phonological awareness in kindergarten children: Issues of task comparability. *Journal of Experimental Child Psychology, 38,* 175–190.

Stein, N., & Glenn, C. (1979). An analysis of story comprehension in elementary school children. In R. Freedle (Ed.), *New directions in discourse processing* (pp. 53–120). Norwood, NJ: Ablex.

Stein, N., & Glenn, C. (1982). Children's concept of time: The development of a story schema. In W. Friedman (Ed.), *The developmental psychology of time* (pp. 255–282). New York: Academic Press.

Stockman, I. (1999). Semantic development of African American children. In L. B. Leonard & O. L. Taylor (Eds.), *Language acquisition across North America: Cross-cultural and cross-linguistic perspectives* (pp. 61–106). San Diego, CA: Singular.

Stoehl-Gammon, C., & Cooper, J. (1984). Patterns of early lexical and phonological development. *Journal of Child Language, 11,* 247–271.

Strapp, C. M. (1999). Mothers', fathers', and siblings' responses to children's language error: Comparing sources of negative evidence. *Journal of Child Language, 26,* 373–391.

Swanson, H. L., Mink, J., & Bocian, K. M. (1999). Cognitive processing deficits in poor readers with symptoms of reading disabilities and ADHD: More alike than different? *Journal of Educational Psychology, 91*(2), 321–333.

Tardif, T. (1995). Nouns are not *always* learned before verbs, but why? Evidence from Mandarin Chinese. *Proceedings of the Twenty-Sixth Annual Child Language Research Forum, 26,* 224–230.

Tardif, T., Shatz, M., & Naigles, L. (1997). Caregiver speech and children's use of nouns versus verbs: A comparison of English, Italian, and Mandarin. *Journal of Child Language, 24,* 535–565.

Taylor, O. L. (1999). Cultural issues and language acquisition. In O. L. Taylor & L. B. Leonard (Eds.), *Language acquisition across North America* (pp. 21–37). San Diego, CA: Singular.

Taylor, O. L., & Leonard, L. B. (1999). *Language acquisition across North America.* San Diego, CA: Singular.

Temple, C., Nathan, R., Temple, F., & Burris, N. A. (1993). *The beginnings of writing* (3rd ed.). Boston: Allyn & Bacon.

Tiegerman-Farber, E. (1995). *Language and communication intervention in preschool children.* Boston: Allyn & Bacon.

Torgesen, J. K. (1999). Assessment and instruction for phonemic awareness and word recognition skills. In H. W. Catts & A. G. Kamhi (Eds.), *Language and reading disabilities* (pp. 128–153). Boston: Allyn & Bacon.

Torgesen, J. K., Morgan, S., & Davis, C. (1992). Effects of two types of phonological awareness training on word learning in kindergarten. *Journal of Educational Psychology, 84,* 364–370.

Torgesen, J. K., Wagner, R., & Rashotte, C. (1994). Longitudinal studies of phonological processing and reading. *Journal of Learning Disabilities, 27,* 276–286.

Tough, J. (1979). *Talk for teaching and learning.* Portsmouth, NH: Heinemann.

Tunmer, W., & Bowey, J. (1984). Metalinguistic awareness and reading acquisition. In W. Tunmer, C. Pratt, & M. Herriman (Eds.), *Metalinguistic awareness in children: Theory, research and implications* (pp. 144–168). New York: Springer-Verlag.

Tunmer, W., Pratt, C., & Herriman, M. (Eds.). (1984). *Metalinguistic awareness in children: Theory, research and implications.* New York: Springer-Verlag.

Tyack, D., & Gottsleben, R. (1986). Acquisition of complex sentences. *Language, Speech, and Hearing Services in Schools, 17*(3), 160–175.

Tyler, A., & Nagy, W. (1989). The acquisition of English derivational morphology. *Journal of Memory and Language, 28*(6), 648–667.

Valdez-Menchaca, M. C., & Whitehurst, G. J. (1992). Accelerating language development through picture-book reading: a systematic extension to Mexican day care. *Developmental Psychology, 28,* 1106–1114.

Valian, V. (1991). Syntactic subjects in the early speech of American and Italian children. *Cognition, 40,* 21–81.

van Kleeck, A. (1982). The emergence of linguistic awareness: A cognitive framework. *Merrill-Palmer Quarterly, 28,* 237–265.

van Kleeck, A. (1995). Learning about print before learning to read. In K. Butler (Ed.), *Best practices 11. The classroom as an interaction context* (pp. 3–23). Gaithersburg, MD: Aspen.

Vellutino, F. R., & Scanlon, D. (1987). Phonological coding, phonological awareness, and reading ability: Evidence from a longitudinal and experimental study. *Merrill-Palmer Quarterly, 33,* 321–363.

Vellutino, F. R., Scanlon, D., Small, S., & Tanzman, M. (1991). The linguistic bases of reading disability: Converting written to oral language. *Text, 11,* 99–133.

Vosniadou, S., Ortony, A., & Reynolds, R. E. (1984). Children's comprehension of metaphor in the pictorial and verbal modality. *International Journal of Behavioral Development, 9,* 288–295.

Wagner, R. K., Torgesen, J. K., Laughon, P., Simmons, K., & Rashotte, C. A. (1993). Development of young readers' phonological processing abilities. *Journal of Educational Psychology, 85,* 83–103.

Wallach, G. (1984). Who shall be called "learning disabled"? Some new directions. In G. Wallach & K. Butler (Eds.), *Language learning disabilities in school age children* (pp. 1–14). Baltimore: Williams & Wilkins.

Wallach, G., & Butler, K. (1994). *Language learning disabilities in school age children and adolescents.* New York: Macmillan.

Wasik, B. A., & Bond, M. A. (2001). Beyond the pages of a book: interactive book reading and language development in a preschool classroom. *Journal of Educational Psychology, 93,* 243–250.

Wasik, B. H., & Hendrickson, J. S. (2004). Family literacy practices. In C. A. Stone, E. R. Silliman, B. J. Ehren, & K. Apel (Eds.), *Handbook of language and literacy: Development and disorders* (pp. 154–174). New York: Guilford Press.

Wells, G. (1985). *Language development in the preschool years.* New York: Cambridge University Press.

Werker, J., & Tees, R. (1984) Cross-language speech perception: evidence for perceptual reorganization during the first year of life. *Infant Behavior and Development, 7,* 49–64.

Werner, E., & Kresheck, J. (1983). *Structural photographic expressive language test.* Sandwich, IL: Janelle.

Westby, C. E. (1998). Communicative refinement in school age and adolescence. In W. O. Haynes & B. B. Shulman (Eds.), *Communication development: Foundations, processes, and clinical applications* (pp. 311–360). Baltimore: Williams & Wilkins.

White, B. (1975). Critical influences in the origins of competence. *Merrill Palmer Quarterly,* *22,* 243–266.

Whitmire, K. A. (2000). Adolescence as a developmental phase: a tutorial. *Topics in Language Disorders, 20*(2), 1–14.

Wiig, E. H., & Semel, E. M. (1984). *Language assessment and intervention for the learning disabled* (2nd ed.). New York: Merrill/Macmillan.

Windsor, J. (1994). Children's comprehension and production of derivational suffixes. *Journal of Speech and Hearing Research, 37,* 408–417.

Winner, E., Rosentiel, A., & Gardner, H. (1976). The development of metaphoric understanding. *Developmental Psychology, 12,* 189–297.

Witt, B. (1998). Cognition and the cognitive-language relationship. In W. O. Haynes & B. B. Shulman (Eds.), *Communication development: Foundations, processes, and clinical applications* (pp. 101–133). Baltimore: Williams & Wilkins.

World Health Organization (WHO). (2005). *Mental health policy and service guidance package: Child and adolescent mental health policies and plans.* Geneva, Switzerland: WHO Press.

Zeverbergen, A. A., & Whitehurst, G. J. (2003). Dialogic reading: A shared picture book reading intervention for preschoolers. In A. van Kleeck, S. A. Stahl, & E. B. Bauer (Eds.), *On reading books to children: Parents and teachers* (pp. 177–200). Mahwah: NJ: Erlbaum.

Zeverbergen, A. A., & Wilson, G. (1996). *Effects of an interactive reading program on the narrative skills of children in Head Start.* Paper presented at the Head Start's Third National Research Conference, Washington, DC.

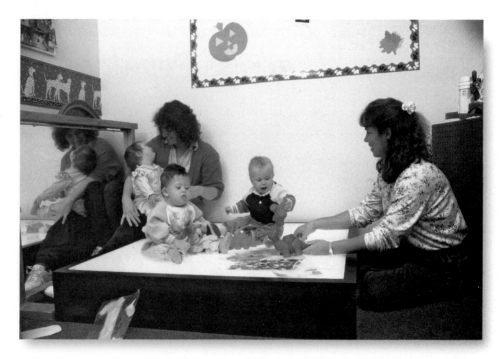

CHAPTER 3

Early Communication Assessment and Intervention

A Dynamic Process

Nancy B. Robinson
San Francisco State University

Michael P. Robb
University of Canterbury, Christchurch, New Zealand

When you finish this chapter, you should be able to

- Identify policy and legislation that defines professional practice for speech-language pathologists in early intervention settings.
- Describe family-centered and culturally competent approaches to early assessment and intervention with infants, toddlers, and families.
- Discuss the roles of early intervention team members and collaborative approaches to assessment and intervention for infants and toddlers.

- Describe infant behaviors that provide indices for assessment and intervention at the prelinguistic and emergent language levels.
- Implement assessment and intervention processes that include selection of appropriate informal and formal methods.
- Discuss current best practices in early language intervention and selection of appropriate strategies for individual children.

In a chapter designed to introduce students to the processes involved in communication assessment and intervention with infants and toddlers, one may question what early communication, speech, and language abilities are found among the youngest of humans. In fact, the term *infant* originates from a Latin term meaning "one unable to speak." The literal interpretation implies a being without communication abilities, a view that was challenged in recent decades, beginning with Chomsky's (1965) proposal that language is an "innate property of the human mind" and that the human enters life in the earliest days with preprogrammed linguistic ability.

Since the development of the nativist proposals articulated by Chomsky, more recent theorists have proposed a more generalized ability in the infant that predisposes the human to the development of spoken language and highly specific prelinguistic skills that lead to interaction with caregivers and the environment (Kent & Hodge, 1991). Parent–child interaction is viewed as the construct that initiates linguistic development (Locke, 1994a). Infants are now assumed to enter the world with a tremendous degree of organization and predilection for language acquisition rather than specific linguistic programming (Paul, 1999).

This chapter focuses on three major areas: early prelinguistic communication; emergent speech and language abilities in the first years of life; and most importantly, assessment and intervention strategies for early intervention specialists, particularly speech-language pathologists, to enhance language development with infants and toddlers at high risk of communication disorders.

Several bodies of research lend support to the efficacy of early intervention to enhance language development, including health and education disciplines of psychology, psychiatry, nursing, medicine, early childhood special education, occupational therapy, physical therapy, speech-language pathology, nutrition, and others. Continuity and predictive relationships between early prelinguistic behaviors in infants and emerging language behaviors in toddlers were found in the last three decades (Bates, Benigni, Bretherton, Camaioni, & Volterra, 1979; Bates, Bretherton, & Snyder, 1988; Lust, 1999; Snow, 1979). Researchers in medicine and psychology also found that parent–child interaction patterns in infancy are related to later developmental outcomes (Brazelton & Als, 1979). The role of the environment in influencing developmental outcomes for young children, particularly language, is further supported in research that investigated long-term outcomes for children in various SES groups (Hart & Risely, 1995; Justice & Ezell, 2001).

Theories of language development during infancy continue to be influenced by many fields—most recently, neurobiology. The late Elizabeth Bates (1999), in her enduring contribution to understanding the nature of language development, summarized research and evidence from neurobiology that challenged the nativist position and illuminated understanding of the critical nature of infant development relative to processes that support and lead to speech, language, and communication behavior in the early years of life. Bates argued that the neurobiological underpinnings of language are based on adaptations of general properties and functions of the brain. She also identified the results of research with adults and infants with focal brain injury that reinforced the notion that the infant's brain is highly plastic, with the ability to permit language learning through alternatives in brain development. According to Bates, research does not support the idea of specific localization in the brain for language functions; however, infants begin life with highly differentiated brain functions, perhaps with certain regions biased toward information processing that are important for language development. The findings reported by Bates and her colleagues strengthened the assumption that the infant's interactions with caregivers in the environment are critical to maximizing language development.

Early intervention professionals are faced with the challenge of identifying young children at risk of communication disorders. Locke (1994b) emphasized the "cascading effect" of even subtle impairments in the ability to process and learn auditory information in young children. The importance of early identification, assessment, and intervention are clearly supported (Calandrella & Wilcox, 2000; Guralnick, 1997).

Recent research has increased our understanding of risk factors that may lead to limitations in communication, speech, and language development in young children and underscored the urgent need for early identification and intervention when brain development is rapid with a high degree of *plasticity*. The goal of this chapter is to introduce to the student a foundation of behaviors that describe the infant's developing linguistic and communication system. The specification of prelinguistic behaviors and stages of development that are now considered predictive of later language development and risk factors for communication disorders is aimed at preparing professionals to better assist these children and families at a critical time in early life.

The chapter is divided into five sections, beginning with U.S. policy guidelines for early communication intervention. The second section of the chapter describes known risk factors that are related to poor developmental outcomes in young children, particularly delays in language development. The third section examines traditional and dynamic approaches to early language assessment and intervention. The fourth section provides an organizational framework for dynamic processes of assessment and intervention and includes suggested methods and tools to implement comprehensive and collaborative intervention for children at risk of communication disorders. Finally, the fifth section applies suggested processes for assessment and intervention to three case studies for demonstration and student discussion.

Due to significant increases in global immigration and migration patterns, the families and children involved in early intervention services are increasingly of diverse cultural and linguistic backgrounds (Parrenas, 2005). Throughout this chapter, practices recommended to support families and children in a multicultural society are included. Further, the chapter is based on the principle that early intervention requires a team approach, with the central member being the family (Bruns & Steeples, 2001; Crais, 1991; Paul, 2007; Polmanteer & Turbiville, 2000; Shelton, Jeppson, & Johnson, 1987). Processes and practices in early communication assessment are applicable for all early intervention professionals and are targeted specifically for the speech-language pathologist (SLP).

U.S. Policy Guidelines for the SLP in Early Intervention

In the United States, the role of the SLP in early intervention was defined more clearly with passage of Public Law (PL) 99-457 in 1986. Subsequent amendments to the Individuals with Disabilities Education Act (IDEA), including the latest reauthorization in 2004, have required early intervention services for children birth to three years of age in Part C (NICHCY, 2007; U.S. Department of Education, 2007). Recent initiatives by the American Speech-Language-Hearing Association (ASHA) focusing on the identification of newborn infants at risk for hearing loss are one example of policies that recognize that the first years of life are critical for language learning (ASHA, 2007a; CDC, 2007).

The policy statement issued by ASHA in 1990 remains current in supporting the role of SLPs in early intervention settings. Reauthorization of IDEA in 1997 strengthened the legal requirements for early intervention and the role of the SLP to assist young families and children. As stated in IDEA 1997:

> Families and their infants and toddlers (birth–36 months) who are at-risk or have developmental disabilities present a broad spectrum of needs that the appropriately certified and/or licensed speech-language pathologist is uniquely qualified to address. These include delays and disabilities in communication, language, and speech, as well as oral-motor and feeding behaviors. Speech-language pathologists, and independent practitioners, assume various roles in addressing these needs of families and their infants.

The earlier ASHA (1989) position statement described the possible roles of SLPs in early intervention to include (1) screening and identification; (2) assessment and evaluation; (3) design, planning, direct delivery, and monitoring of treatment programs; (4) case management; and (5) consultation with and referral to agencies and other professionals. The intention is for the SLP to assume these multiple and changing roles within a community-based, family-centered program as part of an early intervention team. Although brief in content, the position statement embodies considerable thought and broad implications about the way SLPs interact with families and their infants at risk for communicative disorders (Catlett, 1991). More recently, several ASHA documents (2004a, 2004b, 2007c) have identified SLP roles in early intervention with infants and toddlers to include prevention, assessment, and intervention in family-centered and collaborative team contexts.

Children at Risk for Communication/ Language Delays

When genetic heritage and prenatal life are favorable, the infant's roots are securely anchored and normal development should occur (Kopp, 1990). Unfavorable genetic or prenatal factors set the stage for vulnerabilities—that is, the child becomes at risk for developmental delays. Since passage of PL 99-457 in 1986 and subsequent amendments of IDEA, Part C, attention has been directed toward identifying and intervening with the at-risk infant.

There are two basic forms of risk: biological and environmental. *Biological risks* stem from genetic conditions as well as from exposure to *teratogenic* factors (e.g., viral infections, and drug use). *Environmental risks* generally refer to adverse childrearing conditions (e.g., maternal depression, abuse, and environmental toxins).

The following sections describe biological and environmental factors that place infants at risk for communicative disorders. The discussion is not meant to be all inclusive. Many other sources have reviewed well-known biological risks that can be identified early in life, such as Down syndrome, cerebral palsy, cleft lip and palate, and so on. The present review highlights recent information regarding risk factors that are increasingly identified among newborn infants. The risk factors range from minor to significant involvement.

BIOLOGICAL RISKS

Illegal Substances

When considering the perinatal effects of illegal or illicit substances, the basic tenets of maternal–fetal physiology and pharmacology apply (Dattel, 1990). Illicit drugs tend to be of low molecular weight, passing freely between the mother and child within minutes of ingestion. Because of the rapid transfer across the placental barrier, the drug concentration received by the fetus is usually 50 to 100 percent of maternal levels. The effects of drugs on the fetus are also linked to embryological development. For example, most of the body organs and the structures comprising the face and head are formed within the first trimester of pregnancy. Brain development continues throughout pregnancy. So it is not only a matter of which drug and how much of the drug is ingested by the mother but also of when the drug was taken during the pregnancy.

Unfortunately, incidence and prevalence data are difficult to establish. The substance being abused is often illegal; thus, parental disclosure of drug use is rare. In addition, identifying and isolating a specific drug used by a parent is problematic because of the mixture of over-the-counter drugs (e.g., caffeine, alcohol). Estimates of the number of infants exposed in utero to one or more illegal drugs range between 625,000 and 729,000 per year (about 15 to 18 percent) (National Institute on Drug Abuse, 1995). Surveys have shown that between 8 percent and 12 percent of women delivering in hospitals have used illegal drugs at some time during the pregnancy, which suggests that approximately 1 in 10 infants may have been exposed to illicit drugs in utero (Ondersma, Simpson, Brestan, & Ward, 2000).

Cocaine and Methamphetamines. The effects of cocaine (including crack) and methamphetamines (ecstasy, ice, speed) on the central nervous system include increased respiratory and heart rate, restlessness, and excitement. The drugs suppress the mother's appetite, and she is often sleep deprived.

Developmental outcomes of infants exposed to any of these drugs include shorter body length, smaller head circumference, and lower birthweight than infants delivered to drug-free women. If any of these drugs is taken later in the pregnancy, the infant runs a greater risk of being born addicted to the drug and may experience withdrawal symptoms, including cardiovascular problems, seizures, and difficulty sucking, swallowing, and feeding (McElhatton, Bateman, Evans, Pughe, & Thomas, 1999). Because the brain continues to develop throughout pregnancy, it is also possible that the infant may show cognitive impairments (Wouldes, LaGasse, Sheridan, & Lester, 2004). Recent research also indicates that, in addition to having poor developmental outcome, these infants may be more prone to instances of parental abuse during the formative years (Smith, Johnson, Pears, Fisher, & DeGarmo, 2007).

Marijuana. Studies of marijuana use by pregnant women are inconclusive because the drug is often taken in conjunction with other drugs—notably, alcohol and tobacco. Like cigarette smoke, marijuana smoke contains toxins that prevent the baby from obtaining the supply of oxygen that is necessary for intrauterine growth.

Marijuana use during pregnancy is associated with a variety of adverse outcomes, including prematurity, low birthweight, decreased maternal weight gain, complications of pregnancy, difficult labor, congenital abnormalities, increased chance of stillbirth and perinatal mortality, poor neonatal assessment scores, and limited verbal and memory abilities (Fried & Watkinson, 1990). Use of marijuana following birth has also been shown to have an adverse effect on infants who are breastfed (Briggs, Freeman, & Yaffe, 2002).

Howard and Lawrence (1998) found that infants exposed to breastmilk containing the active ingredient in marijuana (delta-9-tetrahydro cannabinol) were lethargic and fed less frequently and for shorter periods of time. The various developmental problems identified in infancy have been shown to extend well into later periods of childhood and adulthood (Goldschmidt, Richardson, Cornelius, & Dan, 2004; Smith, Fried, & Hogan, 2004).

Commonly Used Teratogens

The term *teratogen,* translated literally from its Greek roots, means "monster maker" (*teratos* = monster; *gen* = derived from). The practical application of the term is reserved for substances that produce anomalies when the developing embryo is exposed to them (Shprintzen, 1997). Alcohol, nicotine, and caffeine are teratogenic agents that are capable of interfering with the development of a fetus.

Alcohol.   Alcohol is the most widely used and abused drug in the United States and the United Kingdom, and by most indications, the level of abuse is worsening. In 2001, the number of alcohol-attributed deaths in the United States was a staggering 75,766 (CDC, 2004). The alcohol-related death rate in the United Kingdom increased from 6.9 per 100,000 population in 1991 to 12.9 in 2005 (UK Office for National Statistics, 2006). On average, three of every five women of childbearing age consume alcoholic beverages (ASHA, 1991). Because alcohol can interfere with essentially any developmental process in the embryo, the variation in both the physical and behavior features of the infant can be quite dramatic (Shprintzen, 1997).

Jones and Smith (1974) were the first to describe *fetal alcohol syndrome (FAS),* which results from excessive prenatal exposure to alcohol. FAS is a pattern of altered tissue and organ development that involves cardiovascular problems, craniofacial abnormalities (e.g., cleft lip and/or palate), limb defects, growth deficiency, and poor fine and gross motor coordination (Gerber, 1990). It is still unknown how much alcohol is necessary to produce the symptoms of FAS. Children who demonstrate subtle signs of prenatal alcohol exposure are said to show *fetal alcohol effects (FAE).* FAS appears in 3 per 1,000 live births, and FAE occurs in 10 per 1,000 live births (Shprintzen, 1997). Reported communication problems include delayed language and problems with speech articulation, fluency, voice, and swallowing (ASHA, 1991; Sparks, 1989; Streissguth & Kanter, 1997).

Nicotine.   Nicotine is a stimulant that causes a short-term increase in blood pressure, heart rate, and the flow of blood from the heart. In 2005, 20.3 million women smoked in the United States. More than 14 million of them (28 percent of all women) were of reproductive age, or 18 to 44 years old (CDC, 2006). Approximately 90 percent of the nicotine inhaled from smoking is absorbed into the mother's body (Dattel, 1990).

Smoking during pregnancy—more specifically, the ingestion of nicotine—raises the risk of miscarriage or premature labor. However, the primary danger associated with smoking is low birthweight; this factor explains at least 20 percent of all low-birthweight infants born in the United States. Nicotine depresses the mother's appetite at a time when she should be gaining weight, and smoking reduces the fetus's ability to absorb oxygen. The fetus, being deprived of both nourishment and oxygen, may not grow as it should. Documented effects of nicotine ingestion on the infant include impaired neurological and intellectual development and a higher risk of sudden infant death syndrome (SIDS). A recent report by Key et al. (2007) found that prenatal exposure to tobacco smoke in otherwise healthy babies was linked with significant changes in brain physiology associated with basic perceptual skills that could place the infant at risk for later developmental problems.

Caffeine.   Caffeine is a naturally occurring substance found in the leaves, seeds, and fruits of more than 60 plants (Christian & Brent, 2001). It is found in many foods and beverages and also in prescription and over-the-counter medications. Caffeine acts as a stimulant to the central nervous system. An 8 ounce cup of coffee contains approximately 65 to 120 milligrams of caffeine, and a 12 ounce can of cola contains 45 milligrams. Caffeine is a substance commonly used during pregnancy. At least 80 percent of pregnant women ingest caffeine in some form every day (Dattel, 1990).

Like other chemicals, caffeine freely crosses the placental barrier between mother and child. However, because caffeine is broken down much more slowly than some other substances, its potential influence on the developing child is greater. To date, there has been no definitive evidence to suggest a link between caffeine use and poor developmental outcome in human infants. Recent reports suggest that low to moderate caffeine consumption does not increase the risk for developmental problems (International Food Information Council, 2002). However, mothers may be at an increased risk for miscarriage or fetal death with high caffeine consumption (more than 300 mg/day), particularly in combination with smoking or alcohol, and with extremely high caffeine consumption (more than 800 mg/day) (Bech, Autrup, Nohr, Henriksen, & Olsen, 2005). Some studies have shown that children born to mothers who consumed more than 500 milligrams of caffeine a day were more likely to have a faster heart rate, tremors, and increased breathing rate and to spend more time awake in the days following birth (Eskenazi, 1999). As a general rule, pregnant women are advised to limit their caffeine intake.

Other Health Risks

Two medical conditions that have been shown to impact infants' communication development adversely are middle ear infections and infection with human immunodeficiency virus (HIV), the virus that causes acquired immunodeficiency syndrome (AIDS).

Middle Ear Infections.   The rapid and short onset of signs and symptoms of inflammation in the middle ear is termed *acute otitis media* (Bluestone, 1990). Acute otitis media occurs in almost every child at some time during the first few years of life. Many infants experience multiple episodes of acute otitis media; some spend months with the condition, which is characterized by fluid discharge (or effusion) in both ears (Paradise et al., 1997; Teele, Klein, Chase, Menyuk, & Rosner, 1990). Considerable data show that although otitis media with effusion (OME) produces only a temporary hearing loss, its persistent and recurrent nature produces a fluctuating hearing loss. This hearing loss poses a challenge for young children attempting to acquire speech and language (Gravel & Wallace, 2000). Teele et al. (1990) determined that children who experienced OME during the first three years of life were later found to have lower scores on tests of cognitive ability and on follow-up speech and language tests at 7 years of age. Further, Shriberg, Friel-Patti, Flapsen, and Brown (2000) have suggested that children ages 12 to 18 months who experienced OME with an accompanying mild hearing loss were at a 33 percent risk for developing delayed speech and language by 3 years of age.

HIV/AIDS.   In 1981, the Centers for Disease Control (CDC) reported an outbreak of a rare form of cancer among homosexual men residing in New York and California, known medically as Kaposi's sarcoma. About a year later, the CDC linked the illness to blood and termed the illness *AIDS (acquired immune deficiency syndrome)*. In 1985, the *human immunodeficiency virus (HIV)* was discovered to be the cause of AIDS. HIV has since affected large numbers of heterosexuals, intravenous drug abusers, persons with hemophilia, and other recipients of contaminated blood products (Cohen, 1990).

As of 2005, the total number of AIDS cases reported in the United States to the CDC was 984,155. Adult and adolescent AIDS cases total 943,525, with 761,723 cases in males and 181,802 cases in females. The total number of children under age 13 with AIDS is 9,101. Most infants with HIV contracted the virus by perinatal exposure. The first reports of pediatric AIDS were in 1983, and presently, there are over 2,000 pediatric HIV cases and approximately 270 pediatric AIDS cases in the United States.

The central nervous system is impaired in children with HIV, and recent reports point to communicative impairments as well. McNeilly (2005) states that persons living with HIV are quite likely to develop communication disorders involving language, phonology, voice, or swallowing. In addition, the National Institutes of Health estimate that approximately 75 percent of adults with AIDS experience some degree of hearing impairment, which results from the medications used to combat the virus (Zuniga, 1999).

ENVIRONMENTAL RISKS

Socioeconomic Status

In families experiencing economic hardship, poor living conditions, instability, and/or inadequate alternative child care resources, parenting itself may be disturbed, resulting in a child with an insecure attachment (Lyons-Ruth, Connell, & Grunebaum, 1990; Shaw & Bell, 1993). Attachment difficulties place the child at risk for psychopathology during the school years (Rutter, 1979). Low socioeconomic status also appears to predict lower mental development scores, impoverished language development, placement in special classes, and school failure (Bryant & Ramey, 1987).

Clinical research focused on assisting children from deprived social environments has yielded encouraging results. Specifically, research has shown that universal prekindergarten programs (serving 4-year-olds) and Early Head Start programs (serving infants, toddlers, and their families) contribute to significant gains in children's cognitive and language development (Gormley et al., 2005; Love, Kiskder, Ross, Constantine, & Boller, 2005).

Maternal Influences

In addition to the drug-related maternal influences that place a child at risk for communication delay, there are environmental risks as well. Maternal anxiety can produce a variety of psychological changes and physical changes in heart rate, constriction of blood vessels, and decreases in gastrointestinal motility. Generally, the greater the anxiety, the more severe the response, which ultimately affects the developing fetus (Arimoto & Murashima, 2007).

Childrearing practices also place an infant at risk. It has long been known that high-quality childrearing practices are associated with children having fewer emotional and behavioral problems (Smith, 1994). Alternatively, parental rejection and lack of involvement have been proven damaging to child development, affecting children's cognitive abilities (Lyons-Ruth et al., 1990). Finally, the age of the mother has also been shown to affect the child's subsequent communication development. A recent study by Oxford and Spieker (2006) found poor language development in children of adolescent mothers.

Lead

Lead is a neurotoxic substance that has been shown in numerous research studies to affect brain function and development (Canfield et al., 2003). In the early 1900s, it was recognized that women employed in the lead trades often gave birth to infants who were small, weak, and neurologically damaged (American Academy of Pediatrics, 1987). Lead had crossed the placental barrier, resulting in retarded intrauterine growth and postnatal failure to thrive.

Today, the exact incidence of lead poisoning in the United States is not known, but the incidence in children has declined sharply over the past three decades, due to public education and sustained effort from governmental agencies to publicize the dangers of lead. Even so, lead poisoning continues to be a problem in many areas across the United States, including metropolitan areas and rural communities (CDC, 2005). Children who have been exposed to elevated levels of lead are at increased risk for cognitive and behavioral problems during development.

The biggest potential source of lead is older homes that were painted prior to passage of existing legislation. In these homes, lead-based paint can peel off the walls in flakes and chips or fall on the floors and windowsills as a toxic dust. Among the by-products of older paint, the effectively invisible lead dust is the greatest threat to the health of young children.

In addition to children directly ingesting lead from existing sources, they can be introduced to lead through their mothers. It is now thought that many women of childbearing age who were exposed to lead as children (e.g., in soil and drinking water) have sufficient amounts of the substance accumulated in their bones to threaten the health of their babies many years later (Gonzalez-Cossio et al., 1997). Noted developmental outcomes of lead exposure include lowered IQ, behavioral problems, language learning difficulties, and school failure.

Nutrition and Diet

Meeting the nutritional needs of infants is well recognized as essential for their healthy growth and development (American Academy of Pediatrics, 1993). Proper nutrition during the first year of life plays a vital role in the future growth and development of a child. In addition to meeting nutritional needs, positive feeding experiences can enhance fine motor skills and provide social interaction during infancy (McKinney et al., 2000).

The growth rate during infancy is more rapid than any other time during the life cycle. An infant's birthweight may double by 6 months and triple by 1 year of life. Providing adequate calories, protein, vitamins, and minerals to support optimal growth is essential. Both the American Academy of Pediatrics (1993) and the American Dietetic Association (2001) recommend breastfeeding as the preferred method of feeding during the first year of life.

Malnutrition is the condition that develops when the body does not get the right amounts of vitamins, minerals, and other nutrients it needs to maintain healthy tissues and organ function. About 1 percent of children in the United States suffer from chronic malnutrition, in comparison to 50 percent of children in Southeast Asia. About two-thirds of all the malnourished children in the world are in Asia, and another one-fourth are in Africa (Beers & Berkow, 2004). Worldwide, malnutrition contributes to nearly 7 million child deaths every year (UNICEF, 1998). When it does not kill, poor nutrition can leave children physically impaired (stunted growth), intellectually impaired, and with a weakened immune system.

Table 3.1 summarizes the foregoing discussion, identifying risk factors and predicted developmental outcomes related to each risk factor. The reader should keep in mind that a single risk factor cannot clearly predict a specific outcome, given the mediating effects of the infant's own resiliency and the care-giving environment.

Table 3.1   Selected Risk Factors Related to Adverse Developmental Outcomes

Risk Factor	Possible Outcome
Biological risks	
Cocaine/crack	Low birthweight, shorter body length, smaller head circumference, tremulousness
Methamphetamines, "ice"	Cognitive, social, behavioral differences
Marijuana	Prematurity, low birthweight, congenital abnormalities
Alcohol	Low birthweight, shorter length, fetal alcohol syndrome
Smoking/nicotine	Neurological impairment, respiratory distress
Caffeine	Possible decrease in fetal weight and birth defects
Otitis media	Conductive hearing loss, delayed phonetic development
HIV infection	Central nervous system disorder, death
Environmental influences	
Socioeconomic status	Low mental development, psychopathology
Maternal influences (e.g., stress)	Low mental development
Lead	Mental retardation
Nutrition	Low mental development, learning disorders

Early Language Assessment and Intervention

We now turn to assessment and intervention for very young children with delays in communication and language development. Communication assessment and intervention are inseparable processes, particularly with infants and toddlers and the relatively rapid developmental period that is taking place. The need to assess known risk factors quickly and accurately and to provide effective intervention in support of optimal communication and language development requires a dynamic interaction between assessment and intervention processes. Recently, the term *dynamic assessment* has been applied with somewhat older children at the primary and elementary school–age levels to describe a test–teach–retest approach for specific linguistic targets such as emergent spelling, phonemic awareness, vocabulary, syntax, and concept development.

Butler (1997) described the historic development of assessment practices in speech and language pathology and current trends to sample a child's linguistic skills in real-life contexts, particularly related to reading and writing. She pointed out that the strengths of the approach are based on the collection of assessment data and intervention planning simultaneously. While infants and toddlers do not possess emerging literacy and linguistic skills, their prelinguistic interactions with caregivers provide a context to gather assessment data and to demonstrate intervention strategies in a dynamic process. This section of the chapter includes a comparison of traditional approaches to infant assessment and dynamic approaches that include both assessment and intervention strategies, applied specifically to early language development.

MODELS OF ASSESSMENT: TRADITIONAL AND DYNAMIC APPROACHES

The two most commonly applied models of assessment are developmental models and naturalistic models. *Developmental models* are the traditional approach and rely almost exclusively on age-expected or normative criteria. Developmental assessment tools include age-expected behaviors and represent a *static* form of assessment in which the individual infant is assessed against a given set of age-referenced criteria. Developmental assessment tools can be normative, such as the Bayley Scales of Infant Development (Bayley, 1993), or criterion referenced, such as the Hawaii Early Learning Profile (Furuno et al., 1987).

Wetherby and Prizant (1992) voiced dissatisfaction with many of the available developmental instruments because of their limited scope and difficulty in thoroughly evaluating preverbal communication behaviors. They advocate for a *naturalistic* approach to assessment, which involves viewing the infant's communication skills in commonly occurring settings and contexts such as play and daily routines (Crais, 1995). Far fewer assessment instruments are based on a naturalistic model. Naturalistic approaches and dynamic assessment are closely aligned due to the emphasis on the child's performance in natural contexts and the *process* of determining communication skills. Dynamic assessment can be viewed as a specific application of naturalistic assessment with specific strategies to determine the child's optimal performance when provided with adult support and intervention. A comparative listing of assessment tools that are based on a developmental/traditional model and naturalistic/dynamic approach is given in Table 3.2.

Table 3.2 **Early Language and Communication Assessment Tools for Infants and Toddlers**

Developmental/Traditional Assessment Tools	Naturalistic/Dynamic Assessment Tools
Minnesota Child Development Inventory (Ireton & Thwing, 1974)	Assessing Prelinguistic and Linguistic Behaviors (Olswang et al., 1987)
Preschool Language Sale—3 (Zimmerman, Steiner, & Pond, 1992)	Neonatal Behavioral Assessment Scale, 2nd ed. (Brazelton, 1984)
Battelle Developmental Inventory (Newborg, Stock, & Wnek, 1984)	Assessment of Mother–Child Interaction (Klein & Briggs, 1987)
The Language Development Survey (Rescorla, 1989)	MacArthur Communicative Development Inventories, Infant and Toddler forms (Fenson et al., 1993)
Reynell Developmental Language Scales (Reynell, 1985)	
Bayley Scales of Infant Development (Bayley, 1993)	Parent–Child Interaction Assessment (Comfort & Farran, 1994)
Rossetti Infant-Toddler Language Scale (Rossetti, 1990)	Communication and Symbolic Behavior Scales (Wetherby & Prizant, 1993)
Receptive-Expressive-Emergent Language Scale—2 (Bzoch & League, 1991)	Communication Matrix (Rowland, 2004)
Clinical Linguistic and Auditory Milestones Scale (Capute & Accardo, 1978)	Integrated Developmental Experiences Assessment (Norris, 1992)
Hawaii Early Learning Profile (Furuno et al., 1987)	Assessment, Evaluation, and Programming System (Bricker, 1993)
Sequenced Inventory of Communication Development—Revised (Hedrick, Prather, & Tober, 1984)	Communication Play Protocol (Adamson & Bakeman, 1999)
Early Language Milestone Scale (Coplan, 1993)	Transdisciplinary, Play-Based Assessment (Linder, 1993)
Mullen Scales of Early Learning (Mullen, 1997)	Partners in Play (Ensher, 2007)
Infant/Toddler Checklist for Communication and Language Development (Wetherby & Prizant, 1998)	

Given the rapid sequence and complexity of developmental processes in the first year of life, we agree with Wetherby and Prizant (1992) that developmental assessment models are often too limited in their examination of the infancy period. Naturalistic and dynamic approaches allow much needed flexibility, which is particularly important when confronted with children with special needs. On the other hand, a naturalistic approach may not provide the milestone information necessary to evaluate the child's communication abilities compared to his or her same-age peers.

DYNAMIC ASSESSMENT

The recent emphasis on dynamic assessment in speech and language pathology has relevance for assessment with infants and toddlers and is consistent with emphases in the field of early intervention on processes of communication demonstrated by the child and the social interactive context with caregivers. As Butler (1997) stated, assessment is an essential precursor to intervention and should lead to effective intervention. However, standardized tests measure what a child already knows and are static. In contrast, dynamic assessment provides a sample of the child's performance in the context of interaction with a more knowledgeable partner. Cues and support from the examiner are permitted to determine the extent of the child's emerging language competence and the degree of scaffolding required from adults.

When applied with school-age children with language-learning disabilities, the dynamic assessment process is implemented in a test–intervene–test cycle and attention is paid to the strategies that best support the child to display learning abilities. Swanson (cited in Butler, 1997) asserted that dynamic assessment strategies for children with language learning disabilities contributed to improved information-processing abilities by improving access to previously stored information. While the principles of dynamic assessment appear to have relevance for younger children, Butler cautions that dynamic assessment techniques are more appropriate for use with children with metacognitive abilities.

What similarities are found in dynamic assessment and the dynamic processes recommended for use with infants and toddlers? Butler (1997) outlines the components and purposes of dynamic assessment to evaluate the child's communicative and learning competence in the following areas:

- Address the child's knowledge base.
- Evaluate the child's attention abilities.
- Evaluate the child's encoding of perception and memory, storage, and retrieval.
- Evaluate the child's strategy selection and application.
- Evaluate the child's degree of self-regulation.
- Evaluate the child's analysis of stimuli presented during the assessment process.
- Evaluate the child's ability to modify learning strategies.

DYNAMIC ASSESSMENT APPROACHES
APPLIED TO EARLY INTERVENTION

The principles and procedures of dynamic assessment are generally designed for children with the ability to observe and modify their own learning performance, as stated by Butler (1997). However, the principles of determining the child's true knowledge and degree of scaffolding required to demonstrate emergent abilities are applicable and found in recent assessment practices with infants and toddlers. Key applications include the following:

1. use of parent report to determine the child's performance in natural contexts of daily activities in familiar environments
2. observation of the child and parent or primary caregiver in interactive contexts
3. interview data to determine the child's communication abilities in ideal settings
4. demonstration by the examiner to determine level of scaffolding required for the child to demonstrate emergent abilities

Billeaud (1998) described *serial assessment* of infants and toddlers in natural environments as a method that includes observations of children in (1) routine daily activities, (2) interactions with familiar people, (3) manipulation of objects, and (4) development of play. Videotaping is recommended to allow the SLP to interact freely with the parent and child and to provide documentation for intervention and monitoring of progress. Billeaud further suggested that the assessment process be used as a period of *trial intervention* in the context of play to gather information about the child's typical and preferred means of communication. To extend Billeaud's guidelines, the SLP can further determine the types of strategies that optimally stimulate the child to communicate at higher developmental levels.

There are clear differences between the naturalistic method of assessment recommended by Billeaud and the steps identified to conduct dynamic assessment with older children who comprehend basic language concepts and display some degrees of verbal language. However, there are similarities in the steps used to observe *habitual* or typical communication patterns and to provide appropriate scaffolding to elicit optimal communication behavior.

Play-based assessment is particularly appropriate to conduct a dynamic assessment approach. Using play as the context, the child is assessed in a transdisciplinary or multidisciplinary team. (Differences in the two team models will be discussed in a later section of the chapter.) Play schemes are varied to elicit many aspects of communicative behavior, particularly expressive language. Linder's (1993) model for transdisciplinary play-based assessment allows for the early intervention team to gather assessment data through observation of other professionals interacting with the child and family members. The Communication and Symbolic Behavior Scale (Wetherby & Prizant, 1998) is one tool based on naturalistic assessment procedures and applicable for use in a dynamic assessment approach. Specific activities are constructed in the context of play with the child in order to determine his or her response to natural and novel bids for communication.

The application of a dynamic process of assessment and intervention is particularly appropriate for infants and toddlers at risk for communication delays and disorders. A traditional model of assessment involves several stages, including (1) screening, (2) diagnosis, (3) determination of eligibility for services, and (4) progress evaluation following a period of intervention (Ensher, 1989). Sparks (1989) advised that assessments with infants and toddlers be serial, addressing the child, the family, and their interactions. Assessment tools are developed with this approach in mind for collection of information regarding the child's strengths and weaknesses for purposes of intervention planning. With current policy and practice guidelines leading to a family-centered, dynamic process that incorporates many domains of development and a systems approach to considering family resources, a reconceptualization of communication assessment for infants and toddlers is needed.

Practices and principles described by Billeaud (1998) include the following:

1. Early intervention provides optimal opportunities for infants and toddlers with risk of developmental delays to develop communicative competence for school success.
2. Families are the primary members of the early intervention team and require support to provide optimal environments over the long term.
3. Early intervention for communication delays and disorders requires collaboration and teamwork across a variety of professionals and agencies involved with individual families.
4. Family diversity requires a range of early intervention models and approaches by SLPs and other professionals.
5. Specific knowledge and skills are needed to provide effective early intervention services with infants, toddlers at risk of communication delays and disorders, and their family members.

EFFICACY OF EARLY IDENTIFICATION AND LANGUAGE INTERVENTION

The importance of early identification and early intervention for children at risk for communication disorders is the primary thesis of this chapter. Recent literature is rich with findings that support the rationale for early identification and early intervention.

For example, Oller, Eilers, Neal, and Schwartz (1999) identified the early predictive power of delayed onset of canonical babbling to identify children at risk for delayed speech and language development. While it is well established that delayed onset of babbling is a common characteristic of infants who are deaf or hard of hearing, Oller et al. provided insight regarding the potential role of babbling in language development in other children at risk of delayed development. In their study of 3,400 infants, late onset of canonical babbling (reduplicated sequences of CV units) at 10 months of age was found to be related to smaller productive vocabularies at 18, 24, and 30 months of age compared to the control group. The authors speculated that delayed onset of canonical babbling may assist in predicting apraxia, dysarthria, specific phonological disorders, and perhaps more general speech and language disorders. McCathren, Yoder, and Warren (1999) also reported predictive relationships between a number of specific characteristics of vocalization and later language development (expressive vocabularies) among children with identified developmental delays during infancy and in one-year follow-up when subjects were 17 to 24 months of age.

A further implication of interest related to canonical babbling in infants is that parents tend to respond to this type of babbling as if true speech were produced. As Snow (1979) identified twenty years earlier, parents treat all infant behavior as if meaningful communication occurred. The closer approximation to verbal language creates a setting for critical parent–child interaction at the babbling stage. It follows that delayed onset of canonical babbling may create a situation where parents are less likely to interact verbally with their infants and thus reduce environmental input at a critical language learning point. Thus, while delayed onset of babbling is critical information, it is not the entire picture in the complexities of precursors to potential delays in language development in young children.

Paul (1999) challenged the interpretations presented by Oller et al. (1999), emphasizing the multiple variables that affect language development in infants and toddlers. Further, she questioned the assumption that babbling is a necessary precursor of speech, citing Bleile (1997), who reported only modest and transient delays in speech and language development in children who were tracheostomized and prevented from babbling as infants. Paul cautioned that use of delayed onset of canonical babbling as a clinical indicator of children at risk of delayed speech and language development may result in excessive numbers of false positives, children who are referred needlessly. She argued for a more comprehensive view of risk factors for speech and language delays and early preventative measures that emphasize monitoring of development combined with parent education and language stimulation for young children with late onset of babbling and early vocabularies.

As Robertson and Weismer (1999) pointed out, evidence supporting the efficacy for early language intervention with infants and toddlers is scant. They noted that the "watch and see policy" advocated by Paul (1999) and more active intervention approaches lack clear guidelines in research. Treatment methods studied in infants and toddlers are based on interactive approaches. These authors reported positive increases in a number of linguistic and social skills with late-talking toddlers.

EARLY LANGUAGE INTERVENTION APPROACHES

Iacono (1999) reviewed language intervention with early childhood populations within a framework of early intervention, emphasizing the reciprocal relationship of the wider context of early intervention and language intervention. She described the development of research that demonstrated effectiveness of early intervention as *first-generation research* and referred to *second-generation research* as the more specific questions asked in the later part of the 1990s to determine the effectiveness of certain components of early intervention. Specific areas of second-generation research include parental involvement; program structure, intensity, duration, and timing; location of the intervention; and training of the interventionists. The increasing specificity of effectiveness research in early intervention parallels the development of research in early language intervention, which is becoming increasingly specific regarding the type of intervention strategies implemented with children with communication delays and special needs.

Iacono (1999) provided a comprehensive review of historical developments in early language intervention that has moved from highly structured and didactic to naturalistic and play based. Research in parent–child interaction resulted in current best practice guidelines for team models of early language intervention. Current models have historical foundations in behavioral, psycholinguistic, and sociolinguistic theory and can be understood on a continuum of structure and intrusiveness.

Key features of early language intervention models are highlighted in Table 3.3, with high structure/most intrusive to low structure/least intrusive approaches arranged from left to right. Similarities are found in the use of natural environments and daily routines in all approaches; however, the degree of structure and adult directives varies. Specific features of each model can be compared across several variables,

Table 3.3   **High-Structure/Intrusive to Low-Structure/Nonintrusive Models of Early Language Intervention**

Direct Instruction	Milieu Teaching	Enhanced Milieu Teaching	Responsive Interaction	Conversation-Based Interventions
SLP identifies specific linguistic goals	Child-oriented focus with environmental arrangement	Child-oriented with focus on organizing the environment to increase communication opportunities	Child-oriented with focus on organizing the environment to increase communication opportunities	Intervention is child oriented; child discovers properties of language
Intervention based on incremental steps	Specific language structures are targeted in arranged play	Specific language structures are targeted in arranged play	Generalized child communication gains are targeted	All language domains are interrelated; no specific objectives
Intervention conducted in pull-out settings	Intervention conducted in typical child routines	Intervention in natural environments and typical routines	Intervention in natural environments and typical routines	SLP relies on rich learning environments in natural settings
Drill, practice, and reinforcement methods of teaching to achieve mastery	Adult-directed requests (mand-model) for child response and incidental teaching procedures	Incidental teaching approaches in responsive conversational style	Adult follows child's lead and provides linguistic models in response to child's behavior	Adult–child interaction to achieve reciprocal communication

including (1) directives by adults, (2) plan for intervention, (3) location or contexts, and (4) method of intervention.

Iacono (1999) further compared the key features of each model and discussed outcomes of each model documented in research. The movement toward naturalistic intervention within a context that is familiar for young children is largely supported by current research. Iacono summarized best practices in early language intervention that are found to be effective in supporting language development in children who are developing typically and those with communication delays and disorders. Those practices include the following:

- *Environmental arrangement.* Design of the environment is recommended to be of high interest, with relevant activities and objects that will engage the child. A variety of techniques are recommended to "sabotage" the environment, such as placing materials in view but just out of reach in clear plastic containers and offering choices of materials and activities to engage the child's attention focus.

- *Responsive interaction.* Environments are arranged to engage the child in typical, relevant activities, with adult interaction following the child's lead and building on the establishment of joint attention to expand the child's communication and turn-taking. Specific incidental teaching techniques are used within the context of naturally occurring activities that are the focus of the child's attention. According to Jones and Warren (1991), "Incidental teaching occurs when a child initiates interaction with the teacher in the form of a request, question, comment or other communicative behavior" (p. 49).
- *Prelinguistic milieu intervention.* Modifications of milieu teaching for prelinguistic interventions include the initial uses of requests and comments. Strategies taken from milieu teaching also include following the child's lead, facilitating environmental arrangement, and embedding modeling in routines and social interactions.
- *Augmentative and alternative communication (AAC).* Incorporation of AAC into play-based intervention is recommended to provide opportunities for children at risk of severe communication delays to communicate in meaningful contexts. AAC tools for infants and toddlers may include natural, unaided cues such as gesture cues and sign language or aided methods such as picture cues and voice output communication aids (VOCAs). Strategies to implement AAC may include a range of unaided and aided methods to develop early communicative intent in daily routines and familiar contexts with young children and their caregivers.

THE EFFECTS OF "INPUT"

McCathren, Yoder, and Warren (1995) investigated the role of directives in early language intervention. **Directives** are described as adults' verbal behaviors that communicate to children the expectation that they do, say, or attend to something. These authors identified three types of directives employed: (1) **follow-in directives,** which follow the child's lead; (2) **redirectives,** which initiate a new topic; and (3) **introductions,** or directives given to an unengaged child. The use of directives is a key feature of naturalistic language intervention approaches, including those under the category of milieu and conversational approaches discussed by MacDonald (1985) and by Mahoney and Powell (1984).

Generally, extensive use of directives by the adult is not encouraged in naturalistic language intervention because of the assumption that the child's spontaneous communication will be inhibited. The exception to the caution against heavy use of directives is follow-in directives, which actually follow the child's focus of attention and attempt to expand communication behavior from the foundation of his or her perspective.

The importance of the work by McCathren et al. (1995) is their specific identification of the facilitative effect of follow-in directives on language development in young children. Follow-in directives set the stage for the child to learn salient vocabulary and language concepts and are further reported to affect language development outcomes at later points in time through increased expressive semantic and syntactic development.

Conclusions drawn from this review of the effects of parent interaction on early language development are important because they help to define specific aspects of language that are most effectively facilitated by specific types of directives:

1. Milieu approaches, using follow-in directives, are most effective to facilitate vocabulary and early semantic relations.
2. Directives that are not based on the child's focus of attention are not facilitative of language development.
3. Directives that change the topic (redirectives) or direct the child's attention to new stimuli (introductions) are not positively related to language development outcomes.
4. Although the importance of follow-in directives is established in promoting language development, cultural variation is not accounted for and requires further research.
5. The use of redirectives and introductions has validity in some cases, particularly with children with behavioral problems.

Organizational Framework for Infant Assessment and Intervention

In an earlier version of this chapter, a model to organize assessment and intervention strategies in early communication and language development was proposed, the Communication Assessment Model for Infants (CAMI) (Robinson & Robb, 1997). When evaluated in light of recent literature, the CAMI provides a dynamic process and allows the SLP to move easily between assessment and intervention in working with families and infants and toddlers at risk of language and communication delays. Best practices in early intervention requires that families be at the center of all professional intervention.

The CAMI is organized around six strands: (1) family preferences, (2) developmental processes, (3) individual differences, (4) communicative contexts, (5) early intervention teams, and (6) intervention strategies. Each of these strands includes recent policy and practice in early intervention with infants and toddlers with communication delays and disorders. Together, these strands provide the clinician with a structural plan for observations, data gathering, interviews with family members, and specific test procedures required for comprehensive assessment and intervention planning.

As shown in Figure 3.1, the CAMI establishes a blueprint for the clinician to plan initial assessment questions and select assessment tools for individual children and families. The family preferences strand is always the beginning point, as the information gathered and shared at this level will drive the subsequent assessment and intervention activities. Each strand is distinct yet interdependent, and each has a direct bearing on intervention strategies. Implicit in the CAMI is the flexibility for the SLP to conduct brief assessments of the infant's current status and to immediately implement or demonstrate intervention to support further communication/language development.

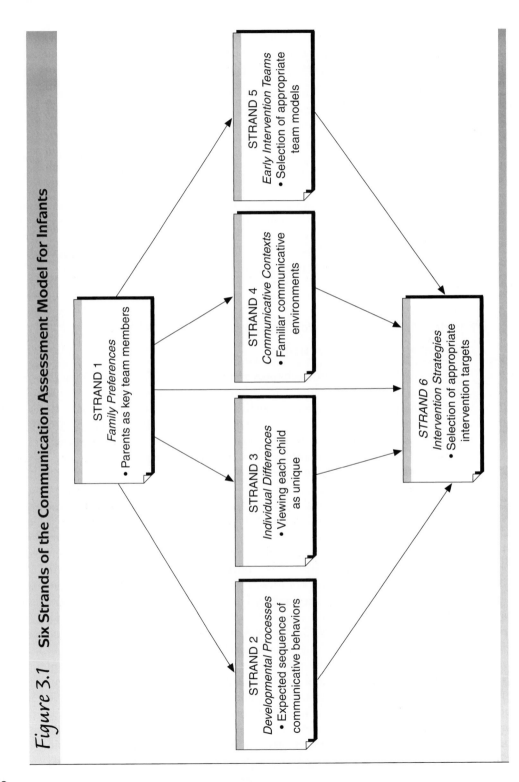

Figure 3.1 **Six Strands of the Communication Assessment Model for Infants**

STRAND 1
Family Preferences
• Parents as key team members

STRAND 2
Developmental Processes
• Expected sequence of communicative behaviors

STRAND 3
Individual Differences
• Viewing each child as unique

STRAND 4
Communicative Contexts
• Familiar communicative environments

STRAND 5
Early Intervention Teams
• Selection of appropriate team models

STRAND 6
Intervention Strategies
• Selection of appropriate intervention targets

STRAND 1: FAMILY PREFERENCES

The field of early intervention is changing rapidly, as professionals move from direct intervention with children to collaborative roles with family members. In many ways, early intervention services are changing with the reorganization of health care. As Cochrane, Farley, and Wilhelm (1990) stated over a decade ago, "The field of early intervention is evolving from discipline specific, child-centered services, to a family oriented context within which professionals from many disciplines address the educational, medical, psychological, and therapeutic needs of handicapped infants and their families" (p. 373). The components of early intervention identified by Cochrane et al. remain current today, as early intervention professionals require competency-based training in family support skills. Specific knowledge and professional responsibilities include communication with families, case management, interdisciplinary teaming, family intervention, and family-centered values and ethics (ASHA, 2004a; Pilkington & Malinowski, 2002).

Given the unique characteristics of families in the United States today, SLPs need to cultivate **cultural competence,** a continuum of knowledge and skills to respond to families of diverse cultural and language backgrounds (ASHA, 2004c, 2005; Goode, 2002; Goode & Jones, 2006; Hanson, Lynch, & Wayman, 1990; NCCC, 2007a; Turnbull & Turnbull, 1990). Diverse cultural groups have differing views that range from seeing the child with a disability as a symbol of good luck to viewing his or her disability as a shameful event caused by wrongdoing in a previous generation. Direct questioning by the professional may be aversive to families from some cultures, and the subject of disability within the family must be approached very gradually. Among native Hawaiians, for example, a "talk story" format of interaction is preferred to build a relationship before focusing on concerns about the child. In addition to the need for sensitivity to cultural styles of interaction, professionals also need to be attuned to individual family styles (e.g., single parents, extended family caregivers, foster families, working parents, and teen parents).

The development of cultural competence is described as a multistage process, beginning with self-awareness and moving toward knowledge and skills to work effectively with families and children of diverse cultures and languages. Goode (2002) and Goode and Jones (2006) have adapted the cultural competence model originally developed by Cross, Bazron, Dennis, and Isaacs (1989) for application in health care systems. The National Center on Cultural Competence (NCCC) provides a number of organizational assessment tools and guidelines for cultural competence in health care services developed by Goode and colleagues; they can be accessed at this web address: www11.georgetown.edu/research/gucchd/nccc.

Cultural competence at the organizational level is defined by Goode and Jones (2006; as adapted from Cross et al., 1989) as follows:

Cultural competence requires that organizations:

- have a congruent, defined set of values and principles, and demonstrate behaviors, attitudes, policies, and structures that enable them to work effectively cross-culturally;
- have the capacity to (1) value diversity, (2) conduct self-assessment, (3) manage the dynamics of difference, (4) acquire and institutionalize cultural knowledge,

and (5) adapt to the diversity and cultural contexts of communities they serve; and

- incorporate the above into all aspects of policymaking, administration, practice, and service delivery and systematically involve consumers, key stakeholders and communities.

Cultural competence is a developmental process that evolves over an extended period of time. Individuals, organizations, and systems are at various levels of awareness, knowledge and skills along the cultural competence continuum. (NCCC, 2007b, p. 3)

In recognition of the cultural competence imperative, ASHA has adopted the NCCC materials and further developed self-assessment tools in cultural competence for the professions of speech-language pathology and audiology (ASHA, 2007b); they can be accessed at www.asha.org/about/leadership-projects/multicultural/self.htm. The tools may be used as checklists, self-assessment, and caseload comparisons to guide the development of culturally competent practices in communication sciences and disorders.

The importance of being sensitive to individual family preferences is clearly important in early communication and language assessment. Because the SLP's initial contact with families begins the assessment and intervention process, the success of that first meeting has implications for the continuing parent–professional relationship and, ultimately, intervention outcomes for the child (Gradel, Thompson, & Sheehan, 1981; Pilkington & Malinowski, 2002). During the initial family contact, the SLP needs to acknowledge that family members play a key role in the team. The initial meeting helps the SLP determine the primary caregiver's main concerns about the child, strengths in parent–child interactions, and appropriate assessment tools.

STRAND 2: DEVELOPMENTAL PROCESSES

Development implies a high degree of continuity and stability in behavior change within and between children across time (Dunst & Rheingrover, 1982). The approach used most often to evaluate the development of a child is to organize the child's changing behavior as a function of stage intervals occurring at a specific chronological age. A **stage model of development** is a description of measurable aspects of behavioral development (Brainerd, 1978). In the typical stage model of development, as shown in Figure 3.2, the sequence of development is based on one behavior serving as the antecedent for the next behavior. The antecedent must occur in order for the ensuing behavior to develop. For the most part, a stage model of development is conceptually similar to the previously described developmental assessment model.

There are at least two primary drawbacks to using a stage model in evaluating a young child. First, an important characteristic of stage models is that the particular stages are assumed to occur in an invariant sequence, yet the determination of stages seems to be quite arbitrary because stage models are constantly being revised. For example, a group of researchers in 1950 may have identified three stages in a child's development of walking; twenty years later, another group of researchers may have

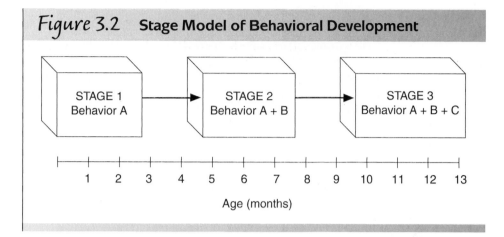

Figure 3.2 **Stage Model of Behavioral Development**

identified five stages. Thus, the more we learn about development, the more stages we seem to require. This is true of Brown's (1973) model of five stages of grammatical morpheme development, which was based on evaluation of only three children. Subsequent work has shown that while children tend to show steady progression in mean length of utterance, their order of grammatical morpheme development is far from being invariant.

The second drawback to using a stage model relates to ascribing an age expectancy to each stage. Chronological age often misrepresents readiness skills and expectant behavior. To post norms based on age is often a matter of convenience and practicality, and deviations should be weighed accordingly, because early- and late-maturing children do not display similar characteristics at the same chronological age. Thus, although a developmental assessment instrument may be useful as a gauge to compare individual children, caution is warranted. One needs to be careful not to adhere too closely to specific age expectations. That is not to say that stages are not important in infant assessment protocols, as stage models play an important role in determining a general guide for the SLP.

We believe that a more appropriate approach to describing a child's ongoing development is through the use of a process model. A **process model of development** allows for overlapping of behavior, as well as for the individual differences displayed by infants. For the most part, a process model of development is conceptually similar to previously discussed dynamic and naturalistic models. Although the advantages of applying a process model to early communication seems clear, surprisingly few commercial instruments are available that adhere to such a philosophy.

Vocal Stages and Processes

A child's early vocal development is usually described with respect to a stage model of development (Stark, 1980; Stoel-Gammon & Cooper, 1984). Several versions of this model have been published, but they differ somewhat in the number of stages recognized, the particular characteristics of each stage, and the age period covered.

Figure 3.3   **Schematic Representation of a Traditional Stage Model of Vocalization Development**

The various stage assignments, according to chronological age, are based on the work of Holmgren et al. (1986), Koopmans van-Beinum and van der Stelt (1986), Oller (1980), Proctor (1989), and Stark (1980). The two-way arrow between reduplicated and variegated babbling stages indicates co-occurring behaviors.

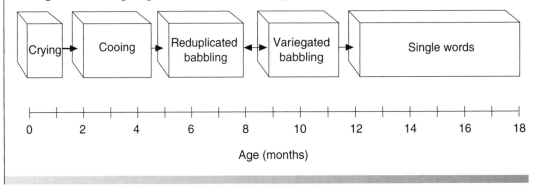

However, most models recognize approximately five major stages, referenced according to chronological age (refer to Figure 3.3):

1. *Reflexive and cry vocalizations.* This is usually thought to occur during the first month of life.
2. *Cooing or gooing.* The basic syllable shapes (V, CV) and consonants /k/ and /g/ are identified between ages 2 and 3 months.
3. *Reduplicated or canonical babbling.* The same CV syllable shape is produced in repetitive strings and occurs by 6 months of age.
4. *Variegated or nonreduplicated babbling.* The variety of sounds and syllable strings produced increases markedly by 8 months of age.
5. *Single-word production.* This occurs around 12 months of age.

Oller et al. (1999) provide a stage model of phonological development based on multiple longitudinal studies conducted since the 1970s. Oller et al. outline the stages of early phonological development as follows:

- *Phonation stage:* quasivowels, glottals
- *Primitive articulation stage:* gooing
- *Expansion stage:* full vowels, raspberries, marginal babbling
- *Canonical stage:* well-formed canonical syllables, reduplicated sequences

Stages of development serve as a useful general framework for organizing early vocalization behaviors (Proctor, 1989). However, because stages are descriptive and somewhat impressionistic, they can become obsolete and their inadequacies more obvious (Shatz, 1983). For example, Mitchell and Kent (1990) challenged the notion that reduplicated babbling precedes nonreduplicated babbling. Upon closer inspection, the researchers found that these two forms of babbling co-occurred. That is, they were not separate stages of vocal development. Faults in the stage model of vocal development have also been found in regard to the single-word stage. Robb, Bauer, and Tyler (1994) found a mixture of identifiable single words, as well as nonwords (e.g., jargon), during the single-word stage. A guideline when using the stage model is to allow for overlap or individual differences from one child to the next.

Gestural Stages and Processes

Stages of gestural development appear to follow a sequence similar to that found in vocal development, as the infant moves from early reflexive activity to intentional control over planned sequences of behavior. Gestural communication proceeds from the infant's first year of life and continues well beyond the emergence of verbal language. Individual differences occur and are expected in the specific gestures used. Furthermore, there seems to be a direct relationship between motor development and the infant's ability to use precise gesturing toward caregivers.

The earliest gestures are found during the first month of life, when the neonate displays engagement and disengagement cues, signaling readiness to interact or to refrain from interaction. Brazelton, Koslowski, and Main (1974) described both subtle and potent forms of engagement and disengagement cues of young infants that let caregivers know how to adjust and respond during daily care and play routines. *Engagement cues* are those that convey to caregivers that the infant welcomes interaction; these nonverbal behaviors include facial brightening, eye widening, smiling, opening of hands, making smooth movements of extremities, head turning toward the caregiver, and reaching toward the caregiver. *Disengagement cues* are signals that the infant is ready for a break from interaction; these behaviors include whimpering, hiccupping, an increased rate of sucking, frowning, yawning, leg kicking, and being immobile. Sensitive and trained caregivers who respond to engagement cues by interacting with the infant and to disengagement cues by giving the baby a break from interaction can assist newborns to express their own communicative behaviors.

During the early months of life, the infant displays increasing mastery over discrete facial expressions and movements of arms, legs, and fingers to express pleasure, anticipation, hunger, and readiness to play. As infants become accustomed to daily caregiving routines, they display to caregivers a range of gestural responses, including lifting legs in diapering routines, grasping adults' hands or facial parts, orienting the whole body toward the parent, and exploring the mother's clothing during feeding.

An infant's reciprocal imitation of facial and hand gestures begins to emerge by 6 months of age (Moore & Meltzoff, 1978). For example, an infant will attempt to restart games such as pattycake and peekaboo by reaching toward the adult's hands or the cloth hiding the adult's face. By 9 months of age, gestures play a key role in the emergence of verbal language, particularly during the period of intentional communication.

Transitions from nonintentional to intentional communication are aided by a range of vocal, gestural, and gaze patterns that differ across individual children. Common patterns are found, however, in the sequence of increased refinement and range of meanings expressed. Infants typically display intentional gesturing during the use of preverbal requests for a specific item or action from the adult. These are called *protoimperatives*. Intentional communication sequences (e.g., giving, showing) that indicate the child's desire to gain adult attention related to a specific object or environmental

Table 3.4   Sequence of Intentional Communication Behavior in Protoimperatives at 9 Months of Age

Communicative Behavior	Example
1. Gaze alternation	Mother and cookie are not in same line of vision. The child looks back and forth from the cookie to the adult, indicating that he expects adult intervention.
2. Repair of failed message	If initial signaling (gaze and/or gesture) fails to result in adult action, child repeats and expands signaling (reaching toward object, looking back at adult, vocalizing loudly).
3. Ritualization of previously instrumental gestures	True reaching toward the object becomes abbreviated grasping motion, and vocalization for the cookie may become insistent "mmmm" sound.

event (protodeclaratives) are also evident at this stage (Bates et al., 1979; Bates, Bretherton, Snyder, Shore, & Volterra, 1980; Crees, 1999; Harding & Golinkoff, 1979; Snyder, Bates, & Bretherton, 1981). Table 3.4 summarizes the sequence of intentional communication behavior in protoimperatives at 9 months of age.

Protoimperative and protodeclarative sequences are observed before the systematic use of pointing in communication. With the development of intentional forms of communication comes the development of *reference,* which is the ability to differentiate one entity from many and to note its presence (Owens, 1992). Reference coincides with the age period of approximately 11 months. Bates et al. (1979) have taken the position that showing and giving gestures are precursors to pointing, as the child learns how to conduct referential communication acts. Bates et al. termed the gestures observed during the intentional period and their rapid ritualization the *gesture complex.* The role of the gesture complex in establishing reference was found to be strongly correlated with the subsequent emergence of verbal naming.

Social Interaction Stages and Processes

As noted in Chapter 2, caregiver–child social routines are important in the development of prelinguistic and early linguistic communication. During the first months of infancy, children take a responsive role in interactions with caregivers; toward the end of the first year, they gain more intentional control. The growth-fostering aspect of social interaction with caregivers is often referred to as *social scaffolding,* providing a context for the development of social, emotional, psychological, and cognitive development (Brazelton & Als, 1979; Brazelton et al., 1974; Bruner, 1983). Through daily caregiving routines, games, and other interactions with caregivers, infants have repeated opportunities to experience the effects of their actions on caregivers and the home environment. The role of the caregiver is a supportive and structural responsibility. The caregiver's ability to make adjustments in timing, verbal stimulation, presentation of objects, changing positions in space, and introducing a variety of activities and experiences contributes to the infant's growing world of referents.

Social interactions develop over the first year of life, expanding from early face-to-face interactions with caregivers to intentional and referential communication in less specific environmental contexts. Key elements in this developmental process include the dyad, the infant's state control, mutuality, reciprocity, synchronicity, and turn taking. The *dyad* refers to the interactive pair of infant and caregiver. Mother–infant dyads are observed most often, but sibling–infant, father–infant, relative–infant, and babysitter–infant are all viable caregiving dyads that may play an important role in fostering the infant's communication development.

Infant state control refers to the neonate's mastery over smooth movement from sleep to wake states. Brazelton and Als (1979) described progressive states, including deep sleep, drowsiness, quiet alert, and crying. Neonates repeatedly cycle through these states during the first month of life, demonstrating increased physiological and neurological maturity. The *quiet alert state* is the optimal state for the infant to interact with caregivers. As the infant matures in state regulation, longer periods of the quiet alert state are observed. Other terms applied to parent–infant communication include *mutuality, reciprocity, synchronicity,* and *turn taking.* These terms, defined in Table 3.5,

Table 3.5   Social Scaffolding Qualities in Caregiver–Infant Interaction

Quality	Definition
Mutuality	Both partners in the interactive dyad are aware and attentive to each other, accepting any contribution to the interaction made by the other partner (Brazelton, Koslowski, & Main, 1974).
Reciprocity	Adaptive modifications are made within the dyad by both partners in response to communicative behavior of the other partner. Reciprocity can be observed in repair strategies by both the mother and child that serve to continue, or repair, the interaction. Infants learn to repair interactions through repeated signaling to reengage caregivers (Brazelton, Koslowski, & Main, 1974).
Synchronicity	Building on sensitivity and awareness of the other partner, synchronous dyads include mutuality and reciprocal interaction. Mutual sensitivity to the emotional and attention state of the other partner is coupled with continuous adjustments in timing and intensity of stimulation (Clark & Siefer, 1983).
Turn taking	A turn is defined as any single communicative act, verbal or nonverbal, that is directed toward another person. Turn taking is considered one of the primary social interaction skills learned in infancy. Parents initially take more turns, but infants later take a more active role in social games and routines. Turns between parents and infants become more balanced as each partner learns to respond contingently to the other (Kaye & Charney, 1981).

refer to qualities of interaction between caregivers and infants that are considered to enhance communication development with young infants over the first year of life.

The supporting role of caregivers is significant to provide multiple opportunities for infants to practice and refine the vocal, gestural, and social communication behaviors. For the SLP and other early intervention professionals, understanding the developmental processes underlying prelinguistic and early linguistic communication is critical to providing appropriate services.

STRAND 3: INDIVIDUAL DIFFERENCES

The third strand of the CAMI involves the notion of individual differences. The possibility that children may follow different paths or strategies in language acquisition was noticed as early as the 1960s, when the prevailing emphasis in the field was on universal aspects of development (c.f. Vihman & Greenlee, 1987). Since then, there have been numerous accounts of variation across subjects in the acquisition of syntax and single-word vocabulary, pragmatic development, and phonological development (Bates, Thal, Whitesall, Fenson, & Oakes, 1989; Stoel-Gammon & Cooper, 1984; Vihman & Greenlee, 1987).

However, individual differences in language acquisition are not limited to vocal/verbal forms of communication. Concomitant aspects of communication development also vary considerably from child to child (DeWeerth, van Geert, & Hoijtink, 1999). Among these aspects are intentional acts (Bates et al., 1988; Harding & Golinkoff, 1979), turn taking (Mahoney & Powell, 1984), and gesturing (Bates et al., 1989).

Given the complexities of communication development and varied opportunities for learning, variability in rate of learning is to be expected. As noted in Chapter 2, we can generally conclude that children exhibit a high degree of variability in the individual competence each brings to communication development. For the SLP, accepting that a child displays individual differences helps in recognizing the uniqueness of a child's development, specifically the approach he or she takes to acquire language. The differing rates and styles of language development increasingly found among typically developing infants support the need to approach developmental assessment of infants and toddlers with language/communication delays with caution. The CAMI acknowledges these differences and incorporates them into the assessment paradigm.

STRAND 4: COMMUNICATIVE CONTEXTS

Language development occurs within familiar contexts (see Chapter 2). Developmentally, children go through a gradual process of *decontextualization,* in which utterances are no longer bound to limited contexts. Snyder, Bates, and Bretherton (1981) have described the process of decontextualization in relation to a child's acquisition of first words and early word combinations. Young children first exhibit utterances that are bound to specific contexts, such as saying "Daddy go" only when Daddy is walking out the front door at home. Later, the same child may generalize such utterances to other people, in other locations, and possibly in picture contexts (i.e., *decontextualization*).

When assessing infants, clinicians need to be aware that familiar routines at home may be the only contexts that elicit vocalizations and communicative intent. Situational variables, such as degree of structure (low/high), environment (familiar/unfamiliar), persons (familiar/unfamiliar), age of communicative partner (adult/peer/younger child), and communicative function (request, comment, showing off, greeting, etc.) influence the communicative and linguistic performance of young children.

For children with language and communication delays, the relationship between familiar context and communicative behavior takes on additional significance. Kennedy, Sheridan, Radlinshi, and Beeghly (1991) recently studied the relationships between play behavior and subsequent language development in a small sample of children with developmental delays. Using play as the context for assessments, symbolic play behavior and early language skills were compared for six children ranging in age from 2 years, 9 months to 3 years, 4 months. Although relationships among language comprehension, expression, and symbolic play schemes were similar to those found in typically developing children of similar language development skills, wide fluctuations in play and language behavior were found. Observed differences in language skills demonstrate that children with language and communication delays may be more sensitive to context, structure of assessment situation, and the demands placed on them (Donahue & Pearl, 1995).

STRAND 5: EARLY INTERVENTION TEAMS

The next strand of the CAMI involves selecting an early intervention team. Three types of team models are identified in the literature and in practice: the multidisciplinary, interdisciplinary, and transdisciplinary models (Campbell, 1987; McCormick & Goldman, 1978). Although clear differences exist among the models in the patterns of interactions with families and the delivery of early intervention services, early intervention professionals actually use variations and combinations of all three team models. The three models can be outlined as follows:

1. *Multidisciplinary model.* Professionals from multiple disciplines work independently to provide services to an individual child and family. For example, in the case of a speech and language delay related to a child born with cleft lip and/or palate, the child's parents may see multiple medical specialists and an audiologist, SLP, genetic counselor, hospital social worker, and other professionals over the course of many months, in relatively separate interactions. Parents and children are involved in a number of different assessments and interventions, as each professional interacts individually with the family.

2. *Interdisciplinary model.* This model involves a greater degree of interaction among disciplines and more coordinated service delivery with families and young children. For example, parents of an infant with health and developmental needs related to prenatal drug exposure and positive HIV status may interact with medical, social work, public health nursing, speech-language pathology, physical therapy, occupational therapy, and psychology professionals. Rather than interact with families individually throughout the identification, assessment, and intervention process, professionals meet together to discuss findings of individual assessment and, most often,

to synthesize individual findings into a single report intended to be comprehensive to family members. Similar to the multidisciplinary model, interdisciplinary services are provided through professionals interacting individually with families and children.

3. *Transdisciplinary model.* The third model of teamwork requires a great deal more communication between team members, as coordinated interactions with families and children with disabilities are the primary goal. Transdisciplinary approaches move beyond single-discipline interactions with families at all levels of identification, assessment, and intervention with young children and their caregivers. For example, a child with early communication and language delays related to combined biological and environmental risks, such as a very low-birthweight infant born to a teenage mother, may have maximum contact with the SLP and minimal contact with other related disciplines. In this case, the SLP relies on the input and consultative roles of professionals from other disciplines, such as the physical therapist, the occupational therapist, the social worker, and others, to provide comprehensive services with the young mother, infant, and other family members involved.

The transdisciplinary model is often considered the preferred model for increasing communication and collaboration among disciplines and for maintaining continuity in services to families (Briggs, 1993). However, individual family and child needs, as well as the particular needs of the program (staffing, location, etc.), may necessitate the use of multidisciplinary and interdisciplinary models at times. For example, children who are identified at birth as having been exposed to drugs require confidentiality to prevent possible stigma. A multidisciplinary model may be required to identify these children; however, a transdisciplinary model may best serve them when planning intervention. Because the transdisciplinary model calls for a primary care provider to maintain contact with the parent and child, the intervention should be more confidential and meaningful to family members.

Collaborative Team Models

The three types of team models just described apply to interactions of team members within teams, or *intrateam* processes. Also critical to the coordination of services for families and young children are the interactions across teams, or *interteam* processes.

Professionals in early intervention services are increasingly urged to develop collaboration across disciplines and service systems to create more effective transitions and services with families. For example, families with high-risk newborns born prematurely are faced with interactions with multiple teams in the hospital, home, and early intervention center. Interactions with each of these teams are made in very rapid succession in the child's early months of life. The importance of coordination and collaboration across teams is defined as best practice in providing family-centered care and links across one team of providers to the next.

Wyly, Allen, Pfalzer, and Wilson (1996) describe collaborative team models within the context of the neonatal intensive care unit with the following key components:

- establishing partnership with family members at the outset
- high-risk infant interventions
- transition information and support to early intervention services

- continuity of care from hospital, home, center-based services
- communication between hospital, home, and center-based team members

As noted in Chapter 9, the role of the speech pathologist has increasingly become one of a consultant and collaborative team member especially in early intervention settings. Billeaud (1998) and Laurel and Westby (1993) identified the primary role of the SLP on the early intervention team as a partner with the family members involved. This fits the broad goal of IDEA, which is to empower the family to enhance the child's development. The natural opportunity available to SLPs is to build partnerships with family members in the assessment, planning, and intervention phases of early intervention.

In addition to having skills to support family members to take part in the team process of assessment and intervention, SLPs also need skills to work as team members with professionals from other disciplines. The degree of contact between the SLP and other disciplines can vary widely, related to the intervention model and setting where services are provided. The role of the SLP and relationship to the family and other professionals will vary widely, from one-time contacts in the assessment process to consultative contacts, intensive short-term services, intermittent assessment, or follow-up. Iacono (1999) described the recent trend for the SLP to change from a direct intervention role to that of consultant to the family and other professional team members involved in the child's early intervention plan, or individualized family support plan.

Briggs (1993) identified the importance of open communication skills to be effective team members and outlined the characteristics of effective teams:

1. There is a mission, purpose, and goals that members understand and accept.
2. Sufficient resources are available.
3. Members have appropriate training, skills, and experience.
4. There is an open communication system that encourages diversity, manages conflict, and seeks feedback.
5. Sufficient time is devoted to examining team norms, values, and beliefs and to fostering the growth of individuals and the team as a whole.
6. An effective problem-solving strategy is utilized.
7. High standards are established internally, and a method for evaluating individual roles, responsibilities, and performance is instituted.
8. A climate of trust and personal, as well as professional support, is established.
9. One leader is identified, or the responsibility is shared appropriately among the members.
10. Organizational support is provided to ensure success of the team process and product.

While recognizing the barriers to becoming an effective team, Briggs identifies the transdisciplinary model as the standard of best practice in early intervention for five key reasons: (1) flexibility in disciplinary boundaries results; (2) role overlap promotes true collaboration; (3) a single coordinator improves efficiency; (4) all members depend on one another rather than one member; (5) family are full members who ultimately make decisions.

Systems theory, an approach that places the early intervention team in the context of the larger ecological system that includes family, child, service providers, program, and policy levels, is a wider context to examine the role of team relationships within and across services and society. Briggs (1997) has defined and discussed a multilayered systems model that includes the family, child, core intervention team, administration, and policy makers related to early intervention programs. She emphasizes the need for SLPs and other early intervention professionals to learn to work across the boundaries of their agencies and the communities within which they function. The interrelatedness of all levels of the system influences the roles and effectiveness of our interventions with families.

STRAND 6: INTERVENTION STRATEGIES

The last strand of the CAMI involves the design of intervention strategies for infants and toddlers. However, intervention begins in the assessment phase and is not the last component in the sequence of the implementation of assessment. Indeed, in a dynamic model of assessment and intervention, the SLP moves between assessment and intervention in an ongoing process to determine a child's communicative strengths and needs and to determine intervention strategies to promote communication and language development.

The selection of intervention strategies is guided by assessment information and individual characteristics of children and families. As the clinician moves through the assessment process, beginning with identification of family concerns, intervention goals may become evident. For example, a parent may identify increased vocalization and talking as intervention targets. Keeping this intervention target in mind, the SLP will gather information regarding developmental processes, individual differences, communicative contexts, and roles of team members, allowing the SLP and parent to refine the initial target and develop collaborative goals. At each stage in the assessment process, linkages to intervention can be developed. The intervention goals are then based on a synthesis of shared information among parents, the SLP, and other team members.

INTERVENTION PLANNING

Bailey (1988) outlined a process of developing collaborative goals and objectives for early intervention personnel and families. An **intervention goal** is a long-term statement that includes an outcome statement for a given timeframe (e.g., six months to one year. An **intervention objective** is a specific, short-term goal that includes (1) the precise behaviors to be accomplished, (2) a description of the context for the behaviors expected of the individual child, and (3) specific criteria to evaluate the attainment of the objective.

The development of precise intervention goals, as recommended in the early 1990s, has been influenced by an increased understanding of the importance of providing early intervention in the context of daily routines with individualized approaches that are tailored to family and child needs. In particular, activity-based interventions provide a framework for developing functional communication and language goals to support parent–child interaction in natural environments and daily routines (Pretti-Frontchzak & Bricker, 2004).

Pilkington and Malinowski (2002) introduced the Everyday Routines, Relationships, Activities, Places, and Partnerships (ERRAPP) model of early intervention, which is based on building a relationship with family members and using "detective work" to determine the intervention approach that best fits the family's and child's needs and offers opportunities for daily interaction. The determination of intervention objectives is based on several sources of information, including (1) developmental characteristics of the infant, (2) family preferences and concerns, and (3) daily routines and activities in which communication may be enhanced and developed. However, the specific nature of the linguistic targets or objectives will vary related to the intervention strategy selected. Direct behavioral intervention strategies may target specific communication behaviors, such as "increased vocalization to request objects," whereas naturalistic approaches may have broader targets, such as "increased imitation of vocalization."

As the student will discover in the case studies presented in the final section of this chapter, individual child characteristics, family preferences, and professional findings influence the selection of intervention approaches. The theoretical bases for early language intervention were discussed in an earlier section of this chapter. This section continues that discussion with specific strategies for intervention.

Two primary types of intervention approaches are used in practice and described in the literature: naturalistic and direct (McCormick, Loeb, & Schiefelbusch, 1997). Differing theories and principles underlie the two types of intervention. *Naturalistic approaches* are based on a developmental, cognitive, and social model, and *direct approaches* are based on a behavioral model incorporating reinforcement principles. Major types and features of naturalistic and direct early language intervention approaches that are consistent with recent research and best practice outlined by Iacono (1999) are described in the following sections.

NATURALISTIC COMMUNICATION INTERVENTION

Naturalistic approaches to language and communication are based on two assumptions: (1) that young children learn to communicate using speech and language in a variety of daily routines and activities with caregivers, and (2) that intervention is best conducted within the context of familiar environments. Based on the work of Hart and Risely (1975), naturalistic approaches to language intervention have their basis in incidental teaching techniques that rely primarily on a time-delay procedure (withholding desired items briefly) in order to elicit further communicative attempts with children with developmental delays.

Since that early research, the many forms and procedures of naturalistic approaches to intervention to support young children with language delays have more commonly been referred to as *milieu approaches*. Other terms that are used to refer to similar methods of embedding language intervention within naturally occurring activities and routines include (1) *transactional teaching*, (2) *pragmatic intervention*, (3) *child-oriented teaching*, (4) *interactive modeling* (Wilcox, Kouri, & Caswell, 1991), (5) *social partnership* (MacDonald & Carroll, 1992), and (6) *enhanced milieu teaching* (Kaiser & Hester, 1995). A more complete review of the past development of naturalistic/milieu intervention approaches was provided by Warren and Gazdag (1990), who defined several common elements, including incidental teaching, social routines, turn taking, and environmental arrangement.

Conversational Approaches

The notion of *balanced* turns between adult and child was incorporated into conversational forms of language intervention by MacDonald and Gillette (1985) and Mahoney and Powell (1984). Turn-taking interventions are planned primarily as play sessions between the parent and child, with the focus on achieving a balanced turn ratio between partners.

MacDonald and Carroll (1992) have more recently proposed a social partnership model that is designed to support parents to learn that communication "develops even from the [child's] simplest actions and sounds." Parents are encouraged to respond to any child behavior that might be communicative, treating each child behavior as one conversational turn. The effects of the social partnership model are reported to increase levels of child imitation, vocalization, and communicative turn taking in the context of interaction with parents.

MacDonald and Carroll (1992) have extended earlier work to support verbal language between children and caregivers to intervention with infants and toddlers. The ECO model has specific applications to children with communication disorders and families in daily routines. The context of play interactions is recommended for assessment and intervention processes with young children and family members. In the ECO approach to intervention, parents are supported to learn that communication "develops even more from the [child's] simplest actions and sounds" and to respond to any child behavior that might be construed as communication. Similar to findings in the work by Yoder, Warren, Kyoungram, and Gazdag (1994), MacDonald and Carroll have reported that parents demonstrated qualitative changes in communication behavior directed toward their children that included actions and words more closely matched to the child's play.

Responsive Interaction

Adults use responsive interactions to follow the child's lead and to comment, request, and expand the child's attention and communication within the context of social interactions and play. Within an environment that is arranged to engage the child in typical, relevant activities, adult interaction follows the child's lead and builds on the establishment of joint attention to expand the child's communication and turn taking.

Milieu Teaching

Milieu approaches are the most well-known methods of naturalistic language intervention and incorporate incidental teaching strategies. The concept and application of incidental teaching has remained central to the application of naturalistic interventions, as SLPs, parents, and other members of the team are required to become skilled in observation and identification of so-called teachable moments with young children. For example, an infant who is reaching toward her bottle provides caregivers the opportunity to hold the bottle momentarily and comment, "Yes, that's Ana's milk!" thus engaging the baby's attention and providing a verbal label for her behavior.

The importance of joint attention between caregiver and child and responsiveness to the child's focus of attention are stressed in naturalistic intervention as the key starting points. Specific incidental teaching techniques are used within the context of naturally occurring activities and focus of the child's attention. According to Jones and Warren (1991), "Incidental teaching occurs when a child initiates interaction with the teacher in the form of a request, question, comment or other communicative behavior" (p. 49).

Enhanced Milieu Teaching

The application of naturalistic intervention approaches was originally demonstrated within the context of early language development in preschool children with developmental delays (Halle, Baer, & Spradlin, 1981). Strategies taken from milieu teaching include following the child's lead, facilitating environmental arrangement, and embedding modeling in routines and social interactions.

Bruner (1983) identified the importance of familiar names and social routines, such as peekaboo, due to their defined structure, repetition, and opportunities for young children to experience anticipation, response, initiation, and conclusion. Bruner described the adult's use of naturally occurring games, interactions, and routines as teaching opportunities with the child as *scaffolding*.

The application of naturalistic or milieu approaches are by nature embedded within daily routines and familiar activities for young children. In application, authors range from carefully planned environments and activities to naturally occurring events; agreement is stated that young children demonstrate increased generalization of language and communication behaviors when familiar routines are used for the context of intervention such as play, mealtimes, bath, and so on (Kaiser & Hester, 1995). Norris and Hoffman (1990) have described specific steps that caregivers can take to structure and respond to child communication through selection of toys, expansion of child behavior, and natural consequences.

Prelinguistic Milieu Intervention (PMT)

Modifications of milieu teaching for prelinguistic interventions with infants and toddlers in stages of prelinguistic communication and emergent language development have been reported in recent years (MacDonald & Carroll, 1992; Norris & Hoffman, 1990; Yoder et al., 1994). Yoder et al. described the application of a modified milieu approach combined with linguistic mapping to teach intentional requesting to young children with Down syndrome. Intervention techniques were implemented in a play setting while adults employed time delay, joint attention, and environmental arrangement to elicit requesting behaviors with young children. In addition, linguistic mapping was employed as adults verbally labeled the child's actions and focus of attention. As children increased intentional requesting (nonverbal gestures to signal requesting), Yoder et al. found that adults also increased verbal labeling (mapping) of the child's actions. The effect of increased child communicative behavior on increased adult responsiveness was described as a transactional effect. As children increased in their intentional communication behaviors, adults increased responsive communication toward the children.

Through the increased modification and demonstration of naturalistic intervention approaches to communication and language intervention with young children, researchers have demonstrated positive effects for the parent–child dyad and the reciprocal communication between child and caregiver, rather than a single focus on the increase in child behavior that was reported in earlier research.

DIRECT COMMUNICATION INTERVENTION

Direct intervention models are based on learning principles, as defined in behavioral psychology. Applications of direct intervention strategies are often incorporated in naturalistic settings with a high degree of structure. The reader is referred to McCormick et al. (1997) for a detailed overview of direct intervention strategies, including modeling, reinforcement, shaping, chaining, fading, and prompting–cueing strategies.

The beginning SLP often feels more comfortable pursuing direct intervention over naturalistic techniques because of the highly structured nature of direct intervention. However, direct intervention approaches are not easily applied with infants and toddlers who have communication and language delays; play-based and naturalistic methods are better aligned with this age group. Drash and Tudor (1990) reported that direct intervention approaches are most effective in developing contingency awareness in infants and toddlers with severe disabilities. Subsequently, early intervention practices within naturally occurring routines were advocated to support generalization of communication and language skills (Pretti-Frontczak & Bricker, 2004).

AAC APPLICATIONS

The development of augumentative and alternative communication (AAC) approaches in early intervention is a natural extension of the best practices to support prelinguistic communication through encouraging all communicative behaviors available to infants and toddlers with disabilities. Cress and Marvin (2003) summarized recent research in the development and implementation of AAC for beginning communicators and emphasized that AAC can be defined as a "progression of communication skills from early [prelinguistic] behaviors to symbolic and technological skills" (p. 254). Expanding the definition of AAC to include a number of aids for children with complex communication needs provides the practitioner with an increased array of tools to build communication behaviors, reciprocal interaction, intentional communication, and transitions to symbolic language.

The communication tools model articulated by Cress (2001, 2002) is particularly applicable for introducing early AAC applications to very young children with complex communication needs. The communication tools model is based on theoretical and applied research in prelinguistic communication development that identifies transitions from preintentional to intentional communication (Acredolo & Goodwyn, 1988; Reichle, Beukelman, & Light, 2002; Thal & Bates, 1988).

Cress (2001, 2002) provided an analysis of prelinguistic communication and emerging language and applies a "tools" model to demonstrate the increasing complexity from single communicative acts to the use of a series of tools to accomplish communication. For example, a child who initiates communication and directly reaches for a desired object is using his or her own body as a communication tool. Cress further outlined increasing complexity in the use of communication tools that include the actual object, communicative messages, and additional communicative behaviors from the child or adult that are all considered tools within a given interaction. Cress advocated gradual transitions from nonsymbolic tools to symbolic tools such as photos, picture icons, and single-message voice output communication aids

(VOCAs) such as a prerecorded message to request more of an activity. The use of graduated and carefully sequenced communication tools in response to the child's interactive communication behaviors (smiles, reaching, vocalizations, picture selection, VOCA activation) supports the transition from preintentional to intentional communication. The communication tools model and applications for broad applications of early AAC use are supported in theory and require additional research to support their efficacy in practice.

Further research and guidelines for applying AAC in early intervention with young children with complex communication needs has focused on the emerging communication and language stage, moving beyond prelinguistic communication. The framework provided by Light et al. (2005) is applicable for developing emerging language and further language development with a focus on expanding the vocabulary repertoire in familiar contexts. Light et al. found that the use of *visual scene displays,* based on familiar contexts for individual children in a dynamic computer system, increased communicative acts and expressive vocabulary among toddlers with physical disabilities and severely limited expressive speech. These researchers advocate for rapid expansion of vocabulary use and concepts in early AAC applications, based on their research to date. As stated by Light et al., the general goal for AAC in early intervention is to maximize language and communication.

Based on additional knowledge of best practices in early intervention, we would also emphasize the importance of maximizing the child's participation in natural environments and inclusive settings. Light et al. identified specific goals within the broader goal for AAC, stated above:

1. Increase participation and build social interaction/turn taking.
2. Express the range of communication functions.
3. Develop the breadth of semantic concepts to support more diverse communication.
4. Build a more complex language structure to support more complex communication.
5. Build phonological awareness and foundations for literacy development.

Incorporation of AAC into play-based intervention is recommended to provide opportunities for children at risk of severe communication delays to communicate in meaningful contexts. Strategies to implement AAC interventions may include formulating precise behavioral objectives and methods as well as following naturalistic procedures to promote the child's use of AAC in communication interactions with peers and adults. The need of children with severe communication disabilities (e.g., cerebral palsy, cognitive disabilities, and autism, to name a few) to have access to communication is becoming increasingly clear, and technological advances provide very young children with alternative means to develop communication and language skills. Prelinguistic communication skills such as imitation, social interaction, symbolic play, and intentional communication have been proven necessary for the successful use of AAC systems and devices (Adamson & Bakeman, 1999; Cress, 2002; Reichle et al., 2002; Romski & Sevcik, 2005). The use of AAC for assessment and intervention with infants and toddlers is a rapidly growing area of research and clinical practice. Continued work in this area will lead to greater understanding of the efficacy for early introduction of AAC tools to enhance communication, language, and literacy. Table 3.6 summarizes examples of AAC tools that support early

Table 3.6   **Examples of AAC Tools in Early Intervention**

	Natural: Unaided	No-/Low-Tech AAC	Low-/High-Tech AAC
Presymbolic: Spontaneous behaviors	Gaze Gesture Vocalization	Cause-effect toys Daily routine objects	Adapted battery-operated toys with switch activation
Presymbolic: Intentional behaviors	Gaze Gesture Vocalization	Cause-effect toys Daily routine objects	Adapted battery-operated toys with switch activation Cause-effect computer programs
Presymbolic: Intentional communication	Gaze Gesture Vocalization	Cause-effect toys Daily routine objects Adapted books Single photos	Adapted battery-operated toys with switch activation Cause-effect computer programs Single-message VOCAs to request, participate in activities
Symbolic: Intentional communication	Gaze Gesture Sign language Verbalization	Photo books Single-picture icons Picture icon activity sequences Adapted toys/books	Adapted battery-operated toys with switch activation Cause-effect computer programs Single-message VOCAs to request, participate in activities Multiple-message VOCAs to combine words, stories Visual scene displays in dynamic computer program

Adapted from Cress (2002) and Light et al. (2005)

presymbolic communication and transitions to symbolic language and communication development.

Applications of Assessment and Intervention Approaches: Three Case Examples

EXAMPLE 1: EARLY INFANCY

The CAMI allows for assessment of infants and toddlers across several periods of development. Case examples are provided in this section to apply the processes of assessment and intervention discussed thus far.

The first case focuses on the period of early infancy. Early infancy is characterized by basic physiological responses to the external world and development of primary relationships with caregivers.

Kwan was born three months prematurely and weighed only 949 grams, placing her within the very-low-birthweight range. Her condition at birth was such that she required breathing assistance with a respirator and feeding with a gavage tube. She remained in the hospital for three months, going home at her term gestational age of nine months. Her weight at discharge had improved, at nearly 1,500 grams. At the time of discharge, Kwan was medically stable, having overcome irregular breathing patterns. She was discharged with a gastrostomy tube for feeding.

Kwan's mother, a twenty-year-old single parent, cared for her with the help of her own mother and sister in the home that the three adults shared. Kwan's mother and her family had immigrated to a large urban area on the U.S. mainland from Taiwan ten years earlier. Kwan's mother and grandmother were referred to the early intervention program through the public health nurse, and a home visit was scheduled for an assessment. Kwan's mother expressed concern because her baby did not seem to make many movements or vocal sounds (except prolonged crying every day between 6:00 and 9:00 P.M.). Kwan's mother reported that she had difficulty handling Kwan, as she cried often and stiffened when picked up out of her crib.

Family Preferences

Because Kwan's mother is young and offers only a small amount of information about her daughter's early development, professionals may mistakenly assume that her limited knowledge in some way contributes to Kwan's fussiness and slow development. However, the characteristics that Kwan brings to the caregiving interaction contribute to her mother's frustration. Further questioning of Kwan's mother and grandmother about their primary concerns for Kwan's development reveal deeply concerned caregivers.

With the help of Kwan's grandmother, Kwan's mother has spent many hours watching her daughter in the hospital and learning how to feed and care for her. The grandmother carries on most of the home chores so that Kwan and her mother can be together. Further, the grandmother and Kwan's mother have different concerns about the baby, and these must be incorporated in the assessment plan. Kwan's mother sincerely wants to learn skills to better handle and soothe her daughter, and the grandmother feels the baby will grow better with formula fed through a bottle rather than a gastrostomy tube. Their concerns and awareness of Kwan will guide assessment and intervention. As the clinician observes and gathers further information about Kwan's early development, Kwan's family members can be encouraged to participate actively as primary informers about Kwan's interactive cues and feeding behaviors at home.

Developmental Processes

Based on information gathered from the brief report provided by Kwan's mother and grandmother, certain questions emerge regarding Kwan's development thus far. Knowing her multiple risks at birth, assessment of Kwan's physiological, sensory, and motor development are needed. The following questions can now be formulated to systematically determine her developmental status and communication development:

1. To what extent does Kwan respond to voices and familiar sounds and voices?
2. What are Kwan's sleep and waking patterns, and how does she transition?
3. What are Kwan's overall muscle tone and movement patterns when she is placed in prone, supine, and feeding positions?
4. What primitive reflexes are observed in Kwan's repertoire at this time?
5. When Kwan is placed in close proximity to her caregivers, what social responses (e.g., brightened gaze, smile, open mouth, arm thrust, foot movement, or other generalized response to caregivers) are observed?
6. What is Kwan's regular intake at each feeding, and how steady is her weight gain?

As these questions indicate, the focus of assessment at this point is to gather further information about critical developmental processes that are typically observed in infants at one month of age. Communication development is clearly not the only concern for Kwan. With her history of very low birthweight, a number of developmental processes are affected.

Developmental tools available include the Minnesota Infant Development Inventory, a subtest of the Minnesota Child Development Inventory (MCDI) (Ireton & Thwing, 1974), and the Hawaii Early Learning Profile (HELP) (Furuno et al., 1987). Both of these tools can be administered through parent report and supplemented with direct observation. Although only limited items assess developmental processes in very young infants, these instruments allow for flexibility and parent report in administration.

Individual Differences

With information regarding the developmental status of Kwan's communication behavior, a more complete picture of Kwan's individual communication patterns emerges.

> Kwan's mother reports that her daughter is beginning to recognize familiar people when she is awake, generally after a feeding and in her swing. Kwan's mother is not sure if her own voice or face are more effective in getting Kwan to gaze in her direction. When observed at home, Kwan did not localize to sounds readily but exhibited a whole-body response when her mother said her name. Her mother reports that Kwan's waking from sleep in midmorning is more gradual than at other times. At other times, Kwan has difficulty waking, sleeping on and off throughout the day, fussing and quickly developing an agitated cry before her mother can get to the room to pick her daughter out of bed. According to the mother, preparation of the gastrostomy tube, formula, and attaching the tube takes more time than Kwan is willing to wait. Her intake of formula is quite good, as the entire 4 ounces are absorbed rapidly through the tube. Kwan does show some reflexive sucking activity near the beginning of feeding, and her family wants to begin bottle feeding. Observations of Kwan's muscle tone and motor development show low muscle tone and weak startle reflexes in response to loud sounds.

Further reports by Kwan's mother and grandmother and direct observation by the SLP will provide a record of sleeping, feeding, and waking times so that they can understand the best times to play with Kwan and support her responsive interactions with her family.

Two different types of assessment tools will be helpful: the Neonatal Behavioral Assessment Scale (NBAS) (Brazelton, 1984) and the Bayley Scales of Infant Development (BSID) (Bayley, 1993). The NBAS requires extensive training to administer and a very clear method to assess sleep, wake, and activity behaviors in very young infants. The BSID, on the other hand, is a standardized test with limited reliability for use with young infants. However, the early items on the BSID will identify Kwan's gaze, reach, and preferred motor positions and will highlight individual differences and strengths. From what is known about her individual preferences thus far, Kwan requires support to adjust to environmental stimulation throughout the day. For example, her intense crying periods in the evening may be a result of increasing stimulation throughout the day that results in potent disengagement cues including body arching, hands at sides, and inconsolable crying.

Communicative Contexts

Kwan's communicative contexts can be determined through her daily caregiving routines. The individual engagement and disengagement behaviors that she displays are intimately tied to the context of the caregiving environment. Observations of parent–child interaction help the clinician and caregiver determine the specific contexts for Kwan's early behavioral signals (i.e., communicative behavior). Tools that are useful at this point in assessment are the Parent-Child Interaction Assessment (Comfort & Farran, 1994) and Assessment of Mother-Child Interaction (Klein & Briggs, 1987). Information from these assessments will enable the SLP and parent to determine optimal methods to respond to Kwan's readiness to engage and interact in prelinguistic "conversations."

Early Intervention Teams

With a baby who is medically at risk, multiple contacts with a range of health care and social service professionals are unavoidable. Thus, a team approach is needed to support Kwan and her family. To minimize the fragmentation the family may experience, a primary care coordinator, or case manager, is recommended. At the hospital level, this person may be the primary care nurse assigned to Kwan's mother or perhaps the SLP or other professional responsible for early assessment and parent education in the neonatal intensive care unit. After the family goes home, the public health nurse often becomes the case manager. At the point when Kwan's family contacts an early intervention program, they will have made several transitions between several different service systems and professionals.

The SLP can build a partnership with Kwan's family by taking a key role in coordinating recommendations from other professionals that affect Kwan's intervention plan. Based on the assessment information gathered thus far, it is clear that concerns about Kwan's motor development, feeding, general health, hearing, vision, and communication will involve at least the following disciplines: speech language pathology, audiology, physical therapy, occupational therapy, nursing, nutrition, pediatrics, and early intervention specialists. In this case, the SLP is the obvious professional to coordinate contacts and recommended interventions with Kwan's family, due to the central nature of her families' concern about Kwan's limited interactions. The team model that most applies in this situation is a combination of transdisciplinary and interdisciplinary approaches, as individual disciplines will continue to have direct involvement with Kwan's family.

Intervention Strategies

Kwan's family identified three primary areas of concern at the outset of the assessment process: difficulty in soothing her when crying, feeding with a bottle, and having a general lack of noncry vocalization. As the SLP and other team members conduct an assessment, these areas of concern can guide assessment and intervention goals. At least three possible goals can be generated for Kwan: (1) develop alternative techniques for Kwan's mother to soothe her daughter, (2) increase Kwan's tolerance for oral feeding, and (3) increase social interaction times between Kwan and her family members.

Several researchers in infant development have provided effective strategies to enhance the infant's self-regulation and tolerance of external stimuli, as shown in Table 3.7. The underlying principle for all the approaches is to continually monitor infant engagement and disengagement cues, adjusting caregiver behaviors in direct response to infant cues. Adjustments of caregiver behavior may include simply taking a break in the interaction, allowing the infant to brace her feet against the caregiver's hand, and providing a small toy for the infant to grasp. Of course, strategies must be individualized for each infant, and the parent and SLP must discover the appropriate techniques through trial and error. Table 3.7 also provides more extensive guidelines that may be applied and modified for individual infants.

Table 3.7   **Communication Intervention Goals, Strategies, and Models for Kwan**

Intervention Goal	Intervention Strategy	Intervention Model
Develop alternative techniques for Kwan's mother to soothe her daughter.	Demonstrate holding, wrapping, and soothing techniques with Kwan and her mother.	Swaddling, self-regulation, and slow movements (Cole, 1996).
Increase Kwan's tolerance for oral feeding.	Provide pacifier or nipple on bottle to increase oral tolerance; gradually increase amounts of formula by mouth.	Consult physician and OT regarding feeding techniques and plan for increasing oral feeding (Ahman & Lipski, 1991).
Increase social interaction times between Kwan and her family members.	Encourage Kwan's mother and grandmother to respond to vocal, visual, and gestural behaviors during Kwan's awake/alert times.	Support parent–child interaction (Hanson & Krentz, 1986; McCollum & Yates, 1994).

EXAMPLE 2: MIDDLE INFANCY

In middle infancy, the child becomes a more active participant in the world around him or her. The child sleeps less, sits upright, and vocalizes often. The following example applies the CAMI components to a child in middle infancy.

> Lucy was referred at age 7 months for an evaluation of her general developmental status, particularly in communication, after her mother reported that "Lucy's muscles are weak and do not allow her to make sounds like my other children." Lucy's mother describes her pregnancy as normal, but Lucy was born in a breech position and diagnosed as having cerebral palsy shortly after birth. An earlier developmental assessment of Lucy performed at 3 months indicated that her cerebral palsy is considered *spastic hemiplegia,* affecting the right side of her body. Reportedly, Lucy is able to sit upright with support. Her mother says she worries about Lucy's speech development, as Lucy makes only a few vocal sounds, including crying and some vowels. Further, Lucy's mother reports that she recently learned about the use of computers with very young children with disabilities and hopes to learn about using technology to support her daughter's communication and development.

Family Preferences

Lucy is the youngest of four siblings. She comes from an extended family consisting of her mother and siblings, her grandmother, and an aunt and uncle, who all reside in the same home. Lucy's mother works outside the home, so Lucy is cared for at home by her aunt and older siblings.

Lucy's siblings and aunt are important to include in the assessment process because of their roles as primary caregivers. Each of Lucy's family members has information about her personality, daily communicative behavior, feeding, fussiness, and overall development. Given these multiple caregivers, the SLP has a unique opportunity to develop teamwork through the use of parent/caregiver interview tools with family members.

Developmental Processes

Information provided thus far by Lucy's mother indicates generalized developmental delays in the areas of gross and fine motor, feeding, and communication. The following questions can be formulated to gather critical information for understanding and planning intervention to support Lucy's progress in developmental and functional skills:

1. What are Lucy's eating patterns and her likes and dislikes of liquid and solid foods?
2. What are Lucy's general muscle tone and independent mobility skills?
3. To what extent does Lucy show intentional communication with caregivers?
4. To what extent does Lucy vocalize and in what contexts?
5. What social and gestural communications does Lucy use with caregivers?
6. In what activities is Lucy most comfortable and observed to communicate?
7. What degree of physical support is needed to help Lucy maintain sitting?
8. What is Lucy's response to her caregivers and objects in her environment?

As discussed, Lucy's extended family plays a critical role in her daily activities and development. Family members may participate to identify Lucy's strengths and needs through a structured interview process and using developmental stages as guidelines for discussion. The Receptive-Expressive Emergent Language Scale (Bzoch & League, 1991) provides an interview guide to determine receptive and expressive milestones, and the results may be scored for normative purposes. Other tools appropriate at this stage of the assessment process include the MacArthur Communicative Development Inventories (Fenson et al., 1993) and the Infant/Toddler Checklist for Communication and Language Development (Wetherby & Prizant, 1998). The Communication Matrix (Rowland, 2004) offers a functional communication assessment profile for children in prelinguistic and emerging language stages. Three formats are available, including a professional version, parent assessment tool, and online format. The online version is available to use at no cost and can be accessed at www.designtolearn.com/pages/matrix.html.

Individual Differences

Having gathered critical information covering the preceding developmental areas, identification of the specific characteristics of Lucy's individual prelinguistic communication patterns can begin. The following information is gained through careful observation and parental information:

> Results of developmental assessment based on family reports and clinical observations show that Lucy has low tolerance for solid foods. She can sit upright with support; however, she has yet to walk on "all fours. " She shows interest in objects presented directly in her line of vision and will reach for them. But when objects are presented away from Lucy's midline, she is less responsive, probably due to her motor and visual limitations. When attempting to have Lucy demonstrate her preference for favorite toys, she turns her head toward noisy toys more often than toward stuffed animals and cuddly toys. She shows a limited degree of persistence to reach toward her favorite toys, demonstrating her ability to show intentional behavior but not consistent communicative intent. She demonstrates differentiated cries for hunger, discomfort, and pain. Aside from crying and other reflexive vocalizations (e.g., burping, sneezing), Lucy occasionally laughs, and she is just beginning to make some vocal sounds, including a grunting "uh" sound and an "aah" sound. She is particularly vocal when lying on her back during diaper changes. She is also generally more attentive toward family members than strangers.

This information leads to forming the hypothesis that Lucy's primary strength is her interest in her environment. Her primary weaknesses are in the areas of motor and verbal development. These weaknesses may prevent Lucy from gaining everyday experiences in the environment that nondisabled children experience without difficulty. Her present oral motor abilities also suggest that normal speech–sound development may be impaired.

Additional questions can now be generated for further assessments and to focus on Lucy's strengths, as well as to further define the range of her motoric and visual limitations:

1. What are Lucy's daily events, and what gestural/vocal behaviors does she display?
2. How does Lucy demonstrate her attentiveness toward familiar people?

3. What are the specific food items that Lucy can and cannot tolerate?
4. What are Lucy's imitation skills, both gesturally and vocally?
5. What specific items/events will Lucy attend to the most and the least?
6. To what degree will Lucy persist to reach for or request favorite toys?
7. To what extent does Lucy demonstrate awareness of cause/effect relationships between her actions and toys or people?

Assessment instruments that will address these specific questions include the Rossetti Infant-Toddler Language Scale (ITLS) (Rossetti, 1990) and the Early Language Milestone Scale (ELM) (Coplan, 1993). The ELM uses parent report, incidental observation, and direct testing to evaluate prelinguistic and emerging linguistic skills, including visual response. Coplan and Gleason (1990) demonstrated that the ELM scale is valid for both normal and at-risk populations. Similar to the ELM scale, the ITLS (Rossetti, 1990) is designed to assess children between the ages of birth and 3 years. It uses both parent report (and interview) and actual testing of children's social interaction, pragmatics, gestural development, play behavior, language comprehension, and language expression.

For Lucy, the developmental ages obtained on both the ELM and ITLS may not be as critical as the degree of effort and attention she displays on the test items. In addition, her functional communication skills can be determined by completion of the Communication Matrix (Rowland, 2004), as can the qualities of her prelinguistic and intentional communication behaviors.

Communicative Contexts

Lucy's prelinguistic behavior appears tied to three different contexts: (1) her family, (2) her daily routines, and (3) her response to toys presented at her midline. Lucy is most attentive when interacting with familiar people. The importance of this context should be stressed, with family members playing the role of primary interactive partners. Daily routines provide opportunities for Lucy to communicate with her caregivers and for her caregivers to communicate in return, choice of favorite objects, turn taking, participation in play with family members, initiation of communication, and gestural and vocal communication. Lucy responds to items and activities presented at her midline, and this will serve as the foundation for presenting new information to her.

Early Intervention Teams

The events at birth that contribute to cerebral palsy seldom result in only one kind of clinical problem. As already noted, Lucy has difficulties in feeding and motor development, as well as a delay in communication development. Other problems associated with cerebral palsy include hearing impairment, mental retardation, and seizure activity. Because the problems associated with cerebral palsy are numerous and complex, intervention involves the integrated efforts of many professionals. Rather than schedule separate evaluations for Lucy's family to see these various professionals, the SLP may wish to use these persons as consultants while maintaining direct contact with the child and family, a transdisciplinary model.

Intervention Strategies

Infants born with special needs, along with their caregivers, require specialized professional support in the early months for optimal communicative interactions. A child with cerebral palsy from birth may have severely limited movement and gesture capabilities, requiring family members to extensively adapt and augment their infant's communicative efforts.

The specific areas that need to be strengthened to support Lucy's prelinguistic and emerging communication skills with her caregivers include (1) fuller use of gaze, gesture, and vocal patterns to maintain interaction with caregivers; (2) increased use of intentional communication to persist in requesting and initiating toward family members; and (3) expanded vocabulary expression in daily routines through objects and photo representation. Due to Lucy's significant risk for limited vocal, verbal, and language development, the use of AAC to make the transition from presymbolic to language communication is critical. Exposure to a gradual sequence of symbolic representation using actual objects, photos, and pictured icons is also recommended. Lucy's receptive and expressive language and intentional communication development will be augmented and encouraged through a gradual transition from actual objects to symbolic communication tools. The use of early AAC strategies can include support for more intentional use of natural gestures, actual objects, photo associations, and VOCAs with single-message output, such as "More" when her favorite activities are halted momentarily.

The intervention goals, strategies, and suggested models shown in Table 3.8 are based on Lucy's developmental needs as well as her reported and observed preferences. Her family members all demonstrate active involvement with Lucy; their preferences for certain intervention strategies will determine what priorities are placed on the goals outlined.

EXAMPLE 3: TRANSITIONS TO TODDLERHOOD

The conclusion of the infancy period and the beginning of toddlerhood is characterized by the emergence of recognizable language. The following example begins the application of recent findings in studies of emerging language to assessment and intervention planning during the period of toddlerhood.

> Josh, age 19 months, was referred for an evaluation of his communication skills based on his parents' report that he is not yet talking. Josh's mother provided the following information: His birth history is reported to be normal, although he was diagnosed to have Down syndrome at birth. His health history is characterized by a "number of ear infections" that "never seem to clear up." His mother stated that "aside from the infections," his health has been "good." Josh's mother also reported that he cannot stand on his own, although he can stand with support. He still drinks fluids from a bottle and is not yet able to tolerate solid foods. Josh communicates with his parents using "only a few sounds" and "lots of gesturing," including gestures for "bye bye" and "eat." When comparing Josh to her older child, Josh's mother said, "Josh is not doing much."

Family Preferences

Josh's family consists of his mother, father, and older brother, age 5. His mother coordinates most of the medical and developmental activities with her children, as their

Table 3.8 **Communication Intervention Strategies for Lucy (Age 7 Months)**

Intervention Goal	Intervention Strategy	Intervention Model
Increase presymbolic gaze, gesture, and vocalization in turn-taking games.	Identify child's attention focus and repeat actions to engage turn taking. Respond to all communication behaviors with matched behavior, adding vocal/verbal model.	Hanen Program (Girolametto, Greenberg, & Manolson, 1986) Social partnership model (MacDonald & Carroll, 1992) Prelinguistic milieu teaching (Yoder & Warren, 1999)
Increase intentional communication using cause/effect toys; objects and photos.	Provide increasing complexity in choices of objects, beginning with one object. Place in field of vision and reach for child and respond to all communicative behaviors to indicate intent. Support graduate transition to two objects before moving to photos with objects.	Communication tools model (Cress, 2002)
Increase expressive vocabulary through objects and photos; VOCA devices; adapted books.	Provide actual photos of child's environment, activities, and toys. Observe and respond to all communicative behaviors as expressive vocabulary and provide verbal model with consequence immediately for the item/activity indicated.	Visual scene displays using dynamic computer programs (Light et al., 2005)

father works full time. However, Josh's father is very much involved in the care of his children and keeps well informed about the special needs of his youngest son. Both parents are very much concerned that they do "everything possible to help Josh."

Josh's parents' initial comments give the impression that they may not perceive his prelinguistic and early linguistic behaviors as strengths. This may alert the SLP that the parents require support and careful guidance to identify every means of communication that Josh exhibits.

Developmental Processes

Having considered the background information, a number of questions can be generated regarding developmental processes present in Josh's communicative behavior. Note that the areas addressed in the preceding description provided by Josh's mother include possible concerns about hearing, motor development, oral motor development, cognitive development, social, and vocal development.

1. Does Josh respond to familiar voices and sounds in his environment?
2. What is Josh's overall muscle tone and body posture in a variety of positions?
3. What are Josh's sucking, swallowing, and chewing patterns?
4. Does Josh demonstrate interest in toys? What types of actions does he perform?
5. How does Josh respond or initiate games with family members?
6. What vocal sounds does Josh make? What changes have been reported in recent months?
7. What are the types and apparent functions of Josh's communicative gestures?

Based on the areas of concern for Josh, several developmental assessment tools may be appropriate to gather initial information with his parents, including the Hawaii Early Learning Profile (HELP) (Furuno et al., 1986), the Sequenced Inventory of Communication Development (SICD) (Hedrick, Prather, & Tobin, 1984), MacArthur Communicative Development Inventories (CDI) (Fenson et al., 1993), the Language Development Survey (LDS) (Rescorla, 1989), and the Infant/Toddler Checklist for Communication and Language Development (Wetherby & Prizant, 1998).

At this point in the assessment, general developmental information is needed. Parent report measures such as the CDI for toddlers may provide the most information about the developmental skills Josh demonstrates. Of the other tools listed, the HELP is a nonstandardized developmental scale, and the SICD is a standardized early assessment that also includes several parent report items for children under 20 months of age. There are several advantages to using a tool such as the CDI for initial assessment and intervention planning with Josh's parents. Recall that Josh's mother reported she does not perceive him to be doing much communicating for his age. Through completion of the CDI with professional support, Josh's parents may be able to identify his specific communication skills and provide the clinician with data for further assessment and initial intervention strategies. Dale (1991) supported the validity of parent report to identify emerging language and communication skills.

The CDI provides two scales, the CDI/Infants and the CDI/Toddlers, to assess preverbal development related to emerging language, including nonverbal gestures, games and routines, actions with objects, imitation of actions, use of early language forms, and the degree of decontextualization present in the young child's language. Dale (1991) reported significant correlations between the CDI/Toddlers and the Bayley Scales of Infant Development (BSID). Miller, Sedey, and Miolo (1995) recently reported strong predictive correlation between CDI vocabulary scores and MLU. Rescorla (1989) conducted multiple studies of the LDS and reported repeatedly high correlations of the LDS with the BSID, the Preschool Language Scale (PLS) (Zimmerman, Steiner, & Pond, 1992), and the Reynell Developmental Language Scales (Reynell, 1985). The LDS was found a reliable predictor of language delay with children at 2 years of age. Although each tool is somewhat different in content and in level of communication and language assessed, all the tools have common elements—in particular, a focus on current and newly emerging communication and language behaviors.

Individual Differences

With specific developmental information, the SLP will learn more of the developmental bases for Josh's delay in language and begin to identify his individual communication patterns. The following information is gained through careful observation and parental information.

> Results of developmental assessment based on parent report and clinical observations show that Josh responds to many environmental sounds and voices of family members. He appears to understand a number of words that refer to names of family members; to familiar items, including his bottle, blanket, teddy bear, and inflated ball with noise makers inside; and to some daily activities, including eating, bathtime, and story time. He enjoys sitting in either parent's lap at bedtime to read stories, although he only looks at the pictures fleetingly. Recently, he has begun to pat the pages of the books. Further observation of his body posture shows that Josh pulls to stand on furniture with his back curved and stomach out. He drops to the floor in sitting and generally sits with legs widespread, with his center of balance on his lower back. Feeding patterns are described as "messy" by his mother, with frequent drooling. Observation of chewing skills shows some vertical munching of soft crackers and forward tongue thrusting when attempting to swallow sips of milk from a small plastic tumbler. Interactions with others are generally described as visual and sometimes vocal responses. Josh's parents feel he tends to use gaze patterns to get attention, followed by pointing when he really wants his bottle. Vocal sounds are described primarily as vowels. Josh uses gestures to indicate "up," "bye bye," "eat," and "no."

This information leads to the hypothesis that Josh's strengths lie in his social responsiveness to members of his family and his understanding of familiar events and daily routines. Concerns about motor development and apparently hypotonic patterns (low muscle tone) involve both large and small body movement and control in space as well as feeding skills and preferences. Consultation with other disciplines, including the physical therapist and occupational therapist, is supported by these observations. Additional questions can now be generated for further assessment, as the first steps of supporting parents to become the primary informants about their own child are accomplished:

1. Which environmental sounds are most likely to get a response from Josh?
2. Does Josh respond to particular voices more than others, and if so, how?
3. What differences are found in Josh's responses when his parents name and point to particular toys and familiar objects versus just naming the same items?
4. How does Josh respond to familiar routines, such as bathtime and mealtime?
5. Does Josh attempt to bring favorite toys to family members and to interact?
6. Does Josh enjoy particular pictures and books in his bedtime story routine?
7. In what positions and with what support is Josh most likely to point and reach?
8. To what extent is Josh able to imitate fine motor gestures?

These questions require more specific information about Josh's individual communicative behaviors. Particularly useful at this point are structured parent report measures that help parents catalog more specific understanding of gestural, vocal, and verbal communication and language. Assessment tools that are useful at this point are the Communication and Symbolic Behavior Scales (CSBS) (Wetherby & Prizant, 1998) and Assessing Prelinguistic and Linguistic Behaviors (APLB) (Olswang, Stoel-Gammon, Coggins, & Carpenter, 1987). The CSBS is a normed measure of communicative means, reciprocity, and social and affective signaling that is based on play activities and interactions with objects. Similarly, the APLB is conducted in an observation format to elicit interactions between the child and adults and assess cognitive antecedents to language, communicative intent, production, and comprehension of language. The use of either tool will yield information that identifies Josh's communicative strengths and needs for intervention.

Communicative Contexts

What are the contexts in which Josh appears to communicate? The work of Bruner (1983) and Snyder et al. (1981) indicates that familiar routines and games are the natural contexts for the expansion and elaboration of early communication forms. Another consideration is the important process of gradual decontextualization in early language. In Josh's case, verbal language has not yet fully emerged, so the clinician might anticipate that his communication behavior is likely to occur in familiar, daily routines with familiar caregivers. Suggested methods to identify communicative contexts include ecological inventories, assessment of play sessions (Kennedy et al., 1991), and direct observations of caregivers and infants.

Early Intervention Teams

To carry out the assessment and initial intervention process for Josh, several other professionals must be involved. Appropriate team members for the completion of Josh's assessment include an audiologist, pediatrician, nurse practitioner, physical therapist, occupational therapist, social worker, and possibly other professionals. The manner of referral and utilization of other disciplines in the assessment process with Josh and his family can be guided by current understanding of best practices in early intervention and, ultimately, the preferences of Josh's parents.

Intervention Strategies

Although Josh's assessment process has been presented as a series of steps leading up to intervention, the process is not actually linear. Intervention may begin at any point in the process, whenever a problem has been identified and Josh's parents and the clinician agree to address it. Some of these points include reports by Josh's mother of her concern about his use of only a few sounds, frequent ear infections, and general pattern of responding rather than initiating games with his family. Further development of family goals around each of these concerns for Josh will provide opportunities for the clinician to assist the parents.

Recommended strategies for each of these concerns are displayed in Table 3.9. General principles to support Josh and his family include enhancing daily routines rather than creating teaching situations; expanding play interactions with Josh; identifying functional communication through Josh's use of gestures, vocalizations, and

Table 3.9 **Communication Intervention Strategies for Josh (Age 19 Months)**

Intervention Goal	Intervention Strategy	Intervention Model
Monitor general health and ear infections.	Consult with pediatrician on regular basis.	Have Josh undergo periodic audiological testing. Use prevention approach for chronic otitis media (Northern & Downs, 2002).
Increase vocalization repertoire in daily routines and games with family members, especially older brother.	Select favorite routine, such as reading books at night, and pause often to give opportunities for Josh to vocalize before turning pages. Imitate and expand his sounds ("aa . . . ba . . . ," "aa . . . da . . . ," "aa . . . ma . . .").	Use conversational teaching (MacDonald, 1985; Mahoney & Powell, 1984; MacDonald & Carroll, 1992). Scaffolding structured intervention (Norris & Hoffman, 1990).
Increase vocal and gestural initiation in games and functional communication.	Before daily activities such as eating, bath time, going in the car, etc. Josh's parents and/or brother should pause and wait for Josh to gesture or vocalize to eat, turn on the bath water, or get picked up to go out to the car.	Enhanced milieu teaching (Kaiser & Hester, 1995). Group intervention (Wilcox, Kouri, & Caswell, 1991).
Increase Josh's social communication with other children and adults.	Involve Josh in playgroup.	

emerging word patterns; and taking a preventative approach to upper respiratory infections.

Summary

The role of early intervention to ameliorate risk factors and to contribute to positive developmental outcomes for the youngest children at risk of communication disorders has become increasingly clear over the past four decades. Federal legislation and resulting policy in the United States provide a foundation to support the requirements for infants, toddlers, and preschool children and their families to have access to appropriate services early in the child's life. The plasticity and resilience of the young child's neurological system is further documented by researchers in the United States and internationally. While public resources to implement known best practice in early intervention are vulnerable to the fluctuating and inequities of the economic conditions in society at large, the critical importance of identifying and serving children who demonstrate biological, environmental, and developmental risk factors is clearly supported.

Recognition of the multiple risk factors that influence early child development and family coping with child-rearing contribute to a systems perspective of early intervention, one that is dynamic and interactive. All parts of that system, including the child, the family, the professionals, and the service system are influenced by the context of today's changing, multicultural society. As one of the early intervention team members, the beginning and practicing SLP plays a critical role in assessing and intervening with children and families at their most critical early experiences. The context of early communication between children and their caregivers provides the setting for environmental influence on the biological make-up of the child, both positive and detrimental. Evidence-based practice in speech-language pathology and related fields demonstrates the power of early language intervention through increased communication opportunities that influence cognitive, social, communicative, and linguistic competence in the young child.

Through the foregoing discussion of the multiple risk factors that face young children and their families, legislation, policy, best practice, assessment, and intervention research, a greater understanding of the complexity and importance of early language intervention emerges. The role of the SLP to improve the communicative environment for young children at risk of communication disorders carries significant responsibilities that include a combination of knowledge, skills, and competence in the following areas:

- cultural competence
- knowledge of developmental systems in children
- collaborative teamwork with related professionals
- knowledge of early intervention and early childhood legislation and policy
- flexibility to adapt to changing child and family needs
- knowledge and practice of family-centered care
- understanding and application of augmentative and alternative communication
- continuing professional development in early intervention
- dynamic assessment methods and tools

This list is not an exhaustive one, as the SLP who participates in early intervention and early childhood settings must often work in community settings that require home-based and center-based services. The ability to transition from one setting to another and to effectively meet the needs of families and children in diverse environments requires a flexible "tool kit" that includes a range of indirect and direct intervention approaches and technology. Increasingly, early intervention research supports the naturalistic approach to implement intervention in play-based settings with young children. However, the art and science of early language intervention requires the ability to structure interactions to meet the developmental needs of the individual child. The SLP, as an early language interventionist, must be able to draw from direct behavioral approaches and child-directed play in order to design the most effective program for each child and family. The challenges facing professionals and families to form partnerships in the act of optimizing communicative and linguistic development for the most vulnerable members of the human community are many. The resources that are available include state-of-the-art assessment and intervention for SLPs willing to embark on the journey of dynamic problem-solving to design effective communication intervention with team members, families, and children.

Study Questions

1. Provide a rationale for early identification and intervention with children at risk for communication disorders that is based on research in developmental neurobiology.
2. Explain the differences between environmental biological risk factors. Provide examples of each.
3. Describe differences in traditional developmental and naturalistic approaches to assessment with infants and toddlers, and identify three types of assessment tools in each category.
4. Identify applications of dynamic assessment for young children at risk for communication disorders.
5. Describe the key components of naturalistic language intervention, and state the rationale for using directives in this context.
6. Describe possible AAC methods in early intervention and their potential application with a 2-year-old boy with complex physical disabilities who does not vocalize or verbalize yet shows appropriate comprehension of vocabulary and basic concepts expected for his age.

References

Abel, E., & Sokol, R. (1986). Fetal alcohol syndrome is now the leading cause of mental retardation. *Lancet, 2,* 1222–1224.

Acredolo, L., & Goodwyn, S. (1988). Symbolic gesturing in normal infants. *Child Development, 59,* 450–466.

Adamson, L. B., & Bakeman, R. (1999). Viewing variations in language development: The Communication Play Protocol. *Augmentative and Alternative Communication, 8,* 2–4.

Ahman, E., & Lipski, K. (1991). Early intervention for technology dependent infants and young children. *Infants and Young Children, 3,* 67–77.

American Academy of Pediatrics. (1987). Statement of childhood lead poisoning. *Pediatrics, 79,* 458–459.

American Academy of Pediatrics & American College of Obstetricians and Gynecologists. (1993). *Guidelines for perinatal care* (4th ed.). Elk Grove, IL: American Academy of Pediatrics.

American Dietetic Association. (2001). Position of the American Dietetic Association: Breaking the barriers to breastfeeding. *Journal of the American Dietetic Association, 10,* 1213–1220.

American Speech-Language-Hearing Association (ASHA). (1989, March). Issues in determining eligibility for language intervention *ASHA, 31,* 113–118.

American Speech-Language-Hearing Association (ASHA). (1990). The roles of speech-language pathologists in service delivery to infants, toddlers, and their families. *ASHA, 32*(suppl. 2), 4.

American Speech-Language-Hearing Association (ASHA). (1991, August). Let's talk: Fetal alcohol syndrome. *ASHA, 32,* 53–54.

American Speech-Language-Hearing Association (ASHA). (2004a). *Preferred practice patterns for the profession of speech-language pathology* [Preferred Practice Patterns]. Retrieved on March 25, 2008, from www.asha.org/policy.

American Speech-Language-Hearing Association (ASHA). (2004b). Knowledge and skills needed by speech-language pathologists providing services to infants and families in the NICU environment. *ASHA Supplement, 24,* 159–165.

American Speech-Language-Hearing Association (ASHA). (2004c). *Knowledge and skills needed by speech-language pathologists and audiologists to provide culturally and linguistically appropriate services* [Knowledge and Skills]. Retrieved on March 25, 2008, on from www.asha.org/policy.

American Speech-Language-Hearing Association (ASHA). (2005). *Cultural competence* [Issues in Ethics]. Retrieved on March 25, 2008, from www.asha.org/policy.

American Speech-Language-Hearing Association (ASHA). (2007a). *Early Hearing Detection & Intervention Action Center.* Retrieved July 24, 2007, from www.asha.org/about/legislation-advocacy/federal/ehdi.

American Speech-Language-Hearing Association (ASHA). (2007b). *Self-assessment for cultural competence.* Retrieved July 23, 2007, from www.asha.org/about/leadership-projects/multicultural/self.htm.

American Speech-Language-Hearing Association (ASHA). (2007c). *Scope of practice in speech-language pathology* [Scope of Practice]. Retrieved on March 25, 2008, from www.asha.org/policy.

Arimoto, A., & Murashima, S. (2007). Child-rearing anxiety and its correlates among Japanese mothers screened at 18-month infant health checkups. *Public Health Nursing, 24*(2), 101–110.

Bailey, D. B. (1988). Considerations in developing family goals. In D. Bailey & R. Simeonsson (Eds.), *Family assessment in early intervention.* Columbus, OH: Merrill/Macmillan.

Bates, E. (1999). Language and the infant brain. *Journal of Communication Disorders, 32,* 195–205.

Bates, E., Benigni, L., Bretherton, I., Camaioni, L., & Volterra, V. (1979). *The emergence of symbols: Cognition and communication in infancy.* New York: Academic Press.

Bates, E., Bretherton, I., & Snyder, L. (1988). *From first words to grammar: Individual differences and dissociable mechanisms.* New York: Cambridge University Press.

Bates, E., Bretherton, I., Snyder, L., Shore, C., & Volterra, V. (1980). Vocal and gestural symbols at 13 months. *Merrill-Palmer Quarterly, 26,* 408–423.

Bates, E., Thal, D., Whitesall, K., Fenson, L., & Oakes, L. (1989). Integrating language and gesture in infancy. *Developmental Psychology, 25,* 197–206.

Bayley, N. (1993). *Bayley Scales of Infant Development.* San Antonio, TX: Psychological Corporation.

Bech, B., Autrup, H., Nohr, E., Henriksen, T., & Olsen, J. (2005). Coffee and fetal death: A cohort study with prospective data. *American Journal of Epidemiology, 162*(10), 983–990.

Beers, M., & Berkow, R. (2004). *Malnutrition: The Merck manual of diagnosis and therapy.* Whitehouse Station, NJ: Merck Research Laboratories.

Billeaud, F. P. (1998). *Communication disorders in infants and toddlers: Assessment and intervention* (2nd ed.). Boston: Butterworth-Heinemann.

Bleile, K. (1997). Where words come from: The origins of expressive language. In R. Paul (Ed.), *Exploring the speech-language connection* (pp. 119–139). Baltimore: Paul H. Brookes.

Bluestone, C. (1990). *Update on otitis media: 1990.* Unpublished manuscript, University of Pittsburgh School of Medicine, Pittsburgh.

Brainerd, C. (1978). The stage question in cognitive developmental theory. *Behavioral and Brain Sciences, 1,* 173–182.

Brazelton, T. (1984). *Neonatal Behavioral Assessment Scale* (2nd ed.). White Plains, NY: March of Dimes Materials and Supplies Division.

Brazelton, T. B., & Als, H. (1979). Four early states in the development of mother–infant interaction. *Psychoanalytic Study of the Child, 34,* 349–369.

Brazelton, T. B., Koslowski, B., & Main, M. (1974). The origins of reciprocity: The early mother–infant interaction. In M. Lewis & L. A. Rosenblum (Eds.), *The effect of an infant upon its caregiver* (pp. 49–76). New York: Wiley.

Bricker, D. (1993). *Assessment, evaluation, and programming system for infants and children. Volume 1: AEPS measurement of birth to three years.* Baltimore: Paul H. Brookes.

Briggs, G. G., Freeman, R. K., & Yaffe, S. J. (2002). *Drugs in pregnancy and lactation* (6th ed.). Philadelphia, PA: Lippincott Williams & Wilkins.

Briggs, M. H. (1993). Team talk: Communication skills for early intervention teams. *Journal of Childhood Communication Disorders, 15,* 33–40.

Briggs, M. H. (1997). A systems model for early intervention teams. *Infants and Young Children, 9,* 66–77.

Brown, R. (1973). *A first language: The early stages.* London, England: George Allen & Unwin Ltd.

Bruner, J. (1983). *Child's talk: Learning to use language.* New York: Norton.

Bruns, D. A., & Steeples, T. (2001). Partners from the beginning: guidelines for encouraging partnerships between and NICU and EI professionals. *Infant-Toddler Intervention, 11*(3–4), 237–247.

Bryant, D., & Ramey, C. (1987). An analysis of the effectiveness of early intervention programs for environmentally at-risk children. In M. Guralnick & F. Bennett (Eds.), *The effectiveness of early intervention for at-risk and handicapped children.* New York: Academic Press.

Butler, K. (1997). Dynamic assessment at the millennium: A transient tutorial for today! *Journal of Children's Communication Development, 19,* 43–54.

Bzoch, K., & League, R. (1991). *Receptive-Expressive Emergent Language Scale (REEL-2).* Austin, TX: Pro-Ed.

Calandrella, A. M., & Wilcox, M. J. (2000, October). Predicting language outcomes for young prelinguistic children with developmental delay. *Journal of Speech, Language, and Hearing Research, 43,* 1061–1071.

Campbell, R. (1987). The integrated programming team: An approach for coordinating professionals of various disciplines in programs for students with severe handicaps. *Journal of the Association for Persons with Severe Handicaps, 12,* 107–116.

Canfield, R., Henderson, C., Cory-Slechta, D., Cox, C., Jusko, T., & Lanphear, B. (2003). Intellectual impairment in children with blood lead concentrations below 10 μg per deciliter. *New England Journal of Medicine, 348,* 1517–1526.

Capute, A., & Accardo, P. J. (1978). Clinical Linguistic and Auditory Milestones Scale. *Clinical Pediatrics, 17,* 847.

Catlett, C. (1991, April). ASHAs early intervention projects. *ASHA, 32,* 50–51.

Centers for Disease Control and Prevention (CDC). (2000). *HIV/AIDS surveillance report, 11*(2). www.cdc.gov/hiv/topics/surveillance/resources/reports/index.htm#surveillance.

Centers for Disease Control and Prevention (CDC). (2004, September 24). Alcohol-attributable deaths and years of potential life lost—United States, 2001, *MMWR Weekly, 53*(37), 866–870.

Centers for Disease Control and Prevention (CDC). (2005, August). *Preventing lead poisoning in young children.* Atlanta, GA: Author.

Centers for Disease Control and Prevention (CDC). (2006). Tobacco use among adults—United States, 2005. *MMWR, 55*(42), 1145–1148.

Centers for Disease Control and Prevention (CDC). (2007). *Early hearing detection & intervention (EHDI) program.* Retrieved July 24, 2007, from www.cdc.gov/ncbddd/ehdi/default.htm.

Chai, A. Y., Zhang, C., & Bisberg, M. (2006). Rethinking natural environment practice: Implications from examining various interpretations and approaches. *Early Childhood Education Journal, 34,* 203–209.

Chasnoff, I. (1987). Parental effects of cocaine. *Contemporary Ob/Gyn, 26,* 1–8.

Chiocca, E. M. (1998). Language development in bilingual children. *Pediatric Nursing, 24,* 43–47.

Chomsky, N. (1965). *Aspects of the theory of syntax.* Cambridge, MA: MIT Press.

Christian, M., & Brent, R. (2001). Teratogen update: Evaluation of the reproductive and developmental risks of caffeine. *Teratology, 64,* 51–78.

Clark, G., & Seifer, R. (1983). Facilitating mother–infant communication: A treatment model for high-risk and developmentally delayed infants. *Infant Mental Health Journal, 4,* 67–82.

Cochrane, C. G., Farley, B. G., & Wilhelm, L. J. (1990). Preparation of physical therapists to work with handicapped infants and their families: Current status. *Physical Therapy, 70,* 372–380.

Cohen, H. (1990). Case management and care coordination for children with HIV infection. In R. Kozlowski, D. Snider, R. Vietze, & H. Wisniewski (Eds.), *Brain in pediatric AIDS.* Basel, Switzerland: Karger.

Cole, J. G. (1996). Intervention strategies for infants with prenatal drug exposure. *Infants and Young Children, 8,* 35–39.

Comfort, M., & Farran, D. C. (1994). Parent–child interaction assessment in family-centered intervention. *Infants and Young Children, 6,* 33–45.

Coplan, J. (1993). *Early Language Milestone Scale* (2nd ed.). Austin, TX: Pro-Ed.

Coplan, J., Contello, K. A., Cunningham, C. K., Weiner, L. B., Dye, T. D., Roberge, L., Wojtowycz, M. A., & Kirkwook, K. (1998). Early language development in children exposed to or infected with human immunodeficiency virus. *Pediatrics, 102,* 8.

Coplan, J., & Gleason, J. (1990). Quantifying language development from birth to 3 years using the Early Language Milestone Scale. *Pediatrics, 86,* 963–971.

Crais, E. (1991). Moving from "parent involvement" to family-centered services. *American Journal of Speech-Language Pathology, 1*(1), 5–8.

Crais, E. (1995). Expanding the repertoire of tools and techniques for assessing the communication skills of infants and toddlers. *American Journal of Speech-Language Pathology, 4,* 47–59.

Crawley, S., & Spiker, D. (1983). Mother–child interactions involving two-year-olds with Down syndrome: A look at individual differences. *Child Development, 54,* 1312–1323.

Crees, C. J. (1999). Transitions from spontaneous to intentional behaviors. *Augmentative and Alternative Communication, 8,* 4–7.

Cress, C. (2001). *A communication "tools" model for AAC intervention with early communicators.* Proceedings of the 24th Annual RESNA Conference, Reno, NV.

Cress, C. (2002). Expanding children's early augmented behaviors to support symbolic development. In J. Reichle, D. Beukelman, & J. Light (Eds.), *Implementing an augmentative communication system: Exemplary strategies for beginning communicators* (pp. 219–272). Baltimore: Paul H. Brookes.

Cress, C., & Marvin, C. (2003). Common questions about AAC services in early intervention. *AAC, 19,* 254–272.

Cross T., Bazron, B., Dennis, K., & Isaacs, M. (1989). *Towards a culturally competent system of care, Volume I.* Washington, DC: Georgetown University Child Development Center, CASSP Technical Assistance Center.

Dale, P. (1995). The value of good distinction. *Journal of Early Intervention, 19,* 102–103.

Dale, R. S. (1991). The validity of a parent report treasures of vocabulary and syntax at 24 months. *Journal of Speech and Hearing Research, 34,* 565–571.

D'Apolito, K. (1998). Substance abuse: Infant and childhood outcomes. *Journal of Pediatric Nursing, 13,* 307–316.

Dattel, B. (1990). Substance abuse in pregnancy. *Summaries in Perinatology, 14,* 179–187.

DeWeerth, C., van Geert P., & Hoijtink, H. (1999). Intraindividual variability in infant behavior. *Developmental Psychology, 35,* 1102–1112.

Donahue, M. L., & Pearl, R. (1995). Conversational interactions of mothers and their preschool children who have been preterm. *Journal of Speech and Hearing Research, 38,* 1117–1125.

Drash, R. W., & Tudor, R. M. (1990). Language and cognitive development: A systematic behavioral program and technology for increasing the language and cognitive skills of developmentally disabled and at-risk preschool children. *Programs in Behavior Modification, 26,* 173–220.

Dunst, C., & Rheingrover, R. (1982). Discontinuity and instability in early development: Implications for assessment. In J. Neisworth (Ed.), *Assessment in special education.* Rockville, MD: Aspen.

Ensher, G. (1989). Newborns at risk. *Topics in Language Disorders, 10,* 80–90.

Ensher, G. (2007). *Partners in play: Assessing infants and toddlers in natural contexts.* Clifton Park, NY: Delmar Cengage Learning.

Eskenazi, B. (1999). Caffeine—Filtering the facts. *New England Journal of Medicine, 341,* 1688–1689.

Fenson, L., Dale., R., Reznick, S., Thal, D., Bates, E., Hartung, J., Pethick, S., & Reilly, J. (1993). *MacArthur Communicative Development Inventories.* San Diego: Singular.

Fried, R., & Watkinson, B. (1990). 36- and 48-month neurobehavioral follow-up of children prenatally exposed to marijuana, cigarettes, and alcohol. *Developmental and Behavioral Pediatrics, 11,* 49–58.

Furuno, S., O'Reilly, K., Inatsuka, T., Hosaka, C., Allman, T., & Zeisloft-Falboy, B. (1987). *Hawaii Early Learning Profile*. Palo Alto, CA: Vort.

Gerber, S. (1990). *Prevention: The etiology of communicative disorders in children*. Englewood Cliffs, NJ: Prentice Hall.

Girolametto, L. (1995). Reflections on the origins of directiveness: Implications for intervention. *Journal of Early Intervention, 19*, 104–106.

Girolametto, L., Greenberg, J., & Manolson, A. (1986). Developing dialogue skills: The Hanen Early Language Parent Program. *Seminars in Speech and Language, 7*, 367–382.

Glascoe, F. P., & Byrne, K. E. (1993). The usefulness of the Developmental Profile-II in developmental screening. *Clinical Pediatrics, 32*, 203–208.

Goldschmidt, L., Richardson, G. A., Cornelius, M. D., & Day, N. L. (2004). Prenatal marijuana and alcohol exposure and academic achievement at age 10. *Neurotoxicology Teratology* 26(4), 521–532.

Gonzalez-Cossio, T., Peterson K. E., Sanin, L., Fishbein S. E., Palazuelos, E., Aro, A., Hernandez-Avila, M., & Hu, H. (1997). Decrease in birth weight in relation to maternal bone lead burden. *Pediatrics, 100*, 856–862.

Goode, T. (2002). *Promoting cultural diversity and cultural competency-self assessment checklist for personnel providing services and supports to children with disabilities and special health care needs*. Washington, DC: National Center for Cultural Competence, Georgetown University Center for Child and Human Development.

Goode, T., & Jones, W. (2006). *Definition of linguistic competence*. Washington, DC: National Census for Cultural Competence, Georgetown University Center for Child and Human Development.

Gormley, W., Gayer, T., Phillips, D., & Dawson, B. (2005). The effects of universal pre-K on cognitive development. *Developmental Psychology, 41*(6), 872–884.

Gradel, K., Thompson, M. S., & Sheehan, R. (1981). Parental and professional agreement in early childhood assessment. *Topics in Early Childhood Special Education, 1*, 31–39.

Gravel, J., & Wallace, I. (2000). Effects of otitis media with effusion on hearing in the first 3 years of life. *Journal of Speech, Language, and Hearing Research, 43*, 631–644.

Guralnick, M. J. (1997). *The effectiveness of early intervention*. Baltimore, MD: Brookes.

Halle, J. W., Baer, D., & Spradlin, J. E. (1981). Teacher's generalized use of delay as a stimulus control procedure to increase language use in handicapped children. *Journal of Applied Behavior Analysis, 14*, 389–411.

Hanson, M. J., & Krentz, M. S. (1986). *Supporting parent–child interactions: A guide for early intervention program personnel*. San Francisco: San Francisco State University, Integrated Special Infant Services Program, Department of Special Education.

Hanson, M. J., Lynch, E. W., & Wayman, K. (1990). Honoring the cultural diversity of the family when gathering data. Topics *in Early Childhood Special Education, 10*, 112–131.

Harding, C., & Golinkoff, R. (1979). The origins of intentional vocalizations in prelinguistic infants. *Precursors of early speech*. New York: Stockton.

Harding, C. G., & Golinkoff, R. M. (1979). The origins of intentional vocalizations in prelinguistic infants. *Child Development, 25*, 140–151.

Hart, B., & Risely, T. (1975). Incidental teaching of language in the preschool. *Journal of Applied Behavioral Analysis, 8*, 411–420.

Hart, B., & Risely, T. (1995). *Meaningful differences in the everyday experiences of young American children*. Baltimore: Paul H. Brookes.

Hedrick, D., Prather, E., & Tobin, A. (1984). *Sequenced Inventory of Communication Development* (Rev.). Los Angeles: Western Psychological Services.

Holmgren, K., Lindblom, B., Aurelius, G., Jaling, B., & Zetterstrom, R. (1986). On the phonetics of infant vocalization. In B. Lindblom & R. Zetterstrom (Eds.), *Precursors of early speech*. New York: Stockton.

Hopkins, K., Grosz, J., & Lieberman, A. (1990). *Working with families and caregivers of children with HIV infection and developmental disability.* Technical report on developmental disabilities and HIV infection. Silver Spring, MD: American Association of University Affiliated Programs.

Howard, C., & Lawrence, R. (1998). Breast-feeding and drug exposure. *Obstetrics and Gynecology Clinics of North America, 25,* 195–217.

Iacono, T. A. (1999). Language intervention in early childhood. *International Journal of Disability, Development and Education, 46,* 383–420.

International Food Information Council. (2002). Caffeine and women's health. Retrieved on March 25, 2008, from http://ific.org/publications/brochures/caffwomenbroch.cfm.

Ireton, H., & Thwing, E. (1974). *Manual for the Minnesota Child Development Inventory.* Minneapolis, MN: Behavior Science Systems.

Jones, H., & Warren, S. (1991). Enhancing engagement in early language teaching. *Teaching Exceptional Children, 23,* 48–50.

Jones, K., & Smith, D. (1974). Outcomes in offspring of chronic alcoholic women. *Lancet, 3,* 1076–1078.

Justice, L. M., & Ezell, H. K. (2001). Word and print awareness in 4-year-old children. *Child Language Teaching and Therapy, 17,* 207–225.

Kaiser, A. B., & Hester, R. R. (1995). Generalized effects of enhanced milieu teaching. *Journal of Speech and Hearing Research, 37,* 1320–1340.

Kaye, K., & Charney, R. (1981). Conversational asymmetry between mothers and children. *Journal of Child Language, 8,* 35–49.

Kennedy, M. D., Sheridan, M. K., Radlinshi, S. H., & Beeghly, M. (1991). Play-language relationships in young children with developmental delays: Implications for assessment. *Journal of Speech and Hearing Research, 34,* 112–122.

Kent, R., & Hodge, M. (1991). The biogenesis of speech: Continuity and process in early speech and language development. In J. Miller (Ed.), *Research on child language disorders.* Austin, TX: Pro-Ed.

Key, A., Ferguson, M., Molfese, D., Peach, K., Lehman, C., & Molfese, V. (2007). Smoking during pregnancy affects speech-processing ability in newborn infants. *Environmental Health Perspectives, 115,* 623–629.

Klein, M. D., & Briggs, M. H. (1987). *Observation of Communicative Interaction.* Los Angeles: University of California, Los Angeles, Mother–Child Communication Project.

Koopmans-van Beinum, F. J., & van der Stelt, J. M. (1986). Early stages in the development of speech movements. In B. Lindblom & R. Zetterstrom (Eds.), *Precursors of Early Speech* (pp. 37–50). New York: Stockton.

Kopp, C. (1990). Risk in infancy: Appraising the research. *Merrill-Palmer Quarterly, 36,* 117–139.

Laurel, M., & Westby, C. (1993). *Teams in early intervention: Speech/language pathology module.* Albuquerque, NM: Center for Family & Community Partnerships.

Light, J., Drager, K., Curran, J., Hayes, E., Kristiansen, L., Lewis, W., May, H., Page, R., Panek, E., Perdergast, S., & White, M. (2005). AAC interventions to maximize language development in young children. Penn State University, Department of Communication Sciences and Disorders. www.aac-rerc.com/pages/news/webcasts.htm.

Linder, T. (1993). *Transdisciplinary, play-based assessment.* Baltimore: Paul H. Brookes.

Locke, J. (1994a). Speech acquisition and mother–child interaction. *American Scientist, 82,* 436–440.

Locke, J. (1994b). Gradual emergence of developmental language disorders. *Journal of Speech and Hearing Research, 37,* 608–616.

Love, J., Kiskder, E., Ross, C., Constantine, J., & Boller, K. (2005). The effectiveness of early Head Start for 3-year-old children and their parents: Lessons for policy and programs. *Developmental Psychology, 41*(6), 885–901.

Lust, B. (1999). Universal grammar: The strong continuity hypothesis in first language acquisition. In W. Ritchie & T. Bhatia (Eds.), *Handbook of child language acquisition* (pp. 111–155). San Diego: Academic Press.

Lyons-Ruth, K., Connell, D., & Grunebaum, H. (1990). Infants at social risk: Maternal depression and family support services as mediators of infant development and security of attachment. *Child Development, 61,* 85–98.

MacDonald, J. (1985). Language through conversation. In S. Warren & A. Rogers-Warren (Eds.), *Teaching functional language.* Austin, TX: Pro-Ed.

MacDonald, J., & Carroll, J. Y. (1992). A social partnership model for assessing early communication development: An intervention model for preconversational children. *Language, Speech, and Hearing Services in Schools, 23,* 113–124.

MacDonald, J., & Gillette, Y. (1985). *Social play: A program for developing a social play habit for communication development.* Columbus, OH: Ohio State University Research Foundation.

Mahoney, G., & Powell, A. (1984). *The transactional intervention program, preliminary teachers' guide.* Unpublished manuscript, School of Education, University of Michigan, Ann Arbor.

Mays, R. M., & Gillon, J. E. (1993). Autism in young children: An update. *Journal of Pediatric Health Care, 7,* 17–23.

McCathren, R. B., Yoder, P. J., & Warren, S. F. (1995). The role of directives in early language intervention. *Journal of Early Intervention, 19,* 91–101.

McCathren, R. B., Yoder, P. J., & Warren, S. F. (1999). The relationship between prelinguistic vocalization and later expressive vocabulary in young children with developmental delay. *Journal of Speech, Language, and Hearing Research, 42*(4), 915–924.

McCollum, J. A., & Yates, T. J. (1994). Dyad as focus triad as means: A family-centered approach to supporting parent–child interactions. *Infants and Young Children, 6,* 54–63.

McCormick, L., & Goldman, R. (1978). The transdisciplinary model: Implications for service delivery and personnel preparation for the severely and profoundly handicapped. *AAESPH Review, 4,* 152–161.

McCormick, L., Loeb, D., & Schiefelbusch, R. (1997). *Supporting children with communication difficulties in inclusive settings: School-based intervention.* Boston: Allyn & Bacon.

McElhatton, P., Bateman, D., Evans, C., Pughe, K., & Thomas, S. (1999). Congenital anomalies after prenatal ecstasy exposure. *Lancet, 354,* 1441–1442.

McGonigel, M., Kaufmann, R., & Johnson, B. (1991). *Guidelines and recommended practices for the individualized family service plan.* Bethesda, MD: Association for the Care of Children's Health.

McKinney, E., Ashwill, J., Murray, S., James, S., Gorrie, T., & Droske, S. (2000). *Maternal–child nursing.* New York: Saunders.

McNeilly, L. (2005). HIV and communication. *Journal of Communication Disorders, 38,* 303–310.

Miller, J. P., Sedey, A. L., & Miolo, G. (1995). Validity of parent report measures of vocabulary development for children with Down syndrome. *Journal of Speech and Hearing Research, 38,* 1037–1044.

Mitchell, R., & Rent, R. (1990). Phonetic variation in multisyllabic babbling. *Journal of Child Language, 17,* 247–266.

Montgomery, J. K., Valdez, F., & Herer, G. R. (1997). Best practice in school speech language assessment: Using early intervention results. *Journal of Children's Communication Development, 19,* 3–11.

Moore, M. K., & Meltzhoff, A. N. (1978). Object permanence, imitation, and language development: Toward a neo-Piagetian perspective. In R. D. Minifie & L. L. Lloyd. (Eds.), *Communicative and cognitive abilities—Early behavioral assessment.* Baltimore: University Park Press.

National Center for Cultural Competence (NCCC). (2007a). Georgetown University Center for Child and Human Development. Retrieved July 23, 2007, from www11.georgetown.edu/research/gucchd/nccc.

National Center for Cultural Competence (NCCC). (2007b). A *guide for advancing family-centered and culturally and linguistically competent care.* Georgetown University Center for Child and Human Development. Retrieved July 23, 2007, from www11.georgetown.edu/research/gucchd/nccc.

National Dissemination Center for Children with Disabilities (NICHCY). (2007). *NICHCY Connections . . . to Resources on IDEA* 2004. Retrieved July 11, 2007, from www.nichcy.org/resources/IDEA2004resources.asp.

National Institute on Drug Abuse. (1995). *Biological mechanisms and perinatal exposure to drugs.* NIDA Research Monograph no. 158.

Newborg, J., Stock, J., & Wnek, I. (1984). *Batelle Developmental Inventory.* Allen, TX: DLM/Teaching Resources.

Norris, D. (1992). Connectionism: A new breed of bottom-up model? In R. G. Reilly & N. E. Sharkey (Eds.), *Connectionist approaches to natural language processing* (pp. 351–371). Hilldale, NJ: Lawrence Erlbaum.

Norris, J. A., & Hoffman, R. (1990). Language intervention within naturalistic environments. *Language, Speech, and Hearing Services in the Schools, 21,* 72–84.

Northern, J. L., & Downs, M. P. (2002). *Hearing in children* (5th ed.). Philadephia: Lippincott, Williams & Wilkins.

Oller, D. K. (1980). The emergence of the sounds of speech in infancy. In G. Yeni-Komshian, J. Kavanagh, & C. Ferguson (Eds.), *Child phonology* (Vol. 1, pp. 93–112). New York: Academic.

Oller, D. K., Eilers, R., Neal, A. R., & Schwartz, H. K. (1999). Precursors to speech in infancy: The prediction of speech and language disorders. *Journal of Communication Disorders, 32,* 223–245.

Olswang, L., Stoel-Gammon, C., Coggins, T., & Carpenter, R. (1987). *Assessing Prelinguistic and Linguistic Behaviors.* Seattle: University of Washington Press.

Ondersma, S., Simpson, S., Brestan, E., & Ward, M. (2000). Prenatal drug exposure and social policy: The search for an appropriate response. *Child Maltreatment, 5*(2), 93–108.

Owens, R. (1992). *Language development: An introduction* (3rd ed.). Columbus, OH: Merrill/Macmillan.

Oxford, M., & Spieker, S. (2006). Preschool language development among children of adolescent mothers. *Journal of Applied Developmental Psychology, 27,* 165–182.

Paradise, J., Rockette, H., Colborn, K., Bernard, B., Smith, C., Kurs-Lasky, M., & Janosky, J. (1997). Otitis media in 2,253 Pittsburgh-area infants: Prevalence and risk factors during the first two years of life. *Pediatrics, 99,* 318–333.

Parrenas, R. S. (2005). *Children of global migration: Transnational families and gendered roles.* Stanford, CA: Stanford University Press.

Paul, R. (1999). Discussion: Early speech perception and production. *Journal of Communication Disorders, 32,* 247–250.

Paul, R. (2007). *Language disorders from infancy through adolescence: Assessment and intervention* (3rd ed.). St. Louis, MO: Mosby.

Pilkington, K. O., & Malinowski, M. (2002). The natural environment II: Uncovering deeper responsibilities within relationship-based services. *Infants and Young Children, 15,* 78–84.

Pine, J. (1992). Maternal style at the early one-word stage: Re-evaluating the stereotype of the directive mother. *First Language, 12,* 169–186.

Polmanteer, K., & Turbiville, V. (2000). Family-responsive individualized family service plans for speech-language pathologists. *Language, Speech, and Hearing Services in Schools, 31,* 4–14.

Pretti-Frontczak, K., & Bricker, D. (2004). *An activity-based approach to early intervention* (3rd ed.). Baltimore: Paul H. Brookes Publishing.

Proctor, A. (1989). Stages of normal vocal development in infancy: A protocol for assessment. *Topics in Language Disorders, 10,* 26–42.

Reichle, J., Beukelman, D., & Light, J. (2002). *Implementing an augmentative communication system: Exemplary strategies for beginning communicators.* Baltimore: Paul H. Brookes.

Reinharten, D. B., Edmondson, R., & Crais, E. R. (1997). Developing assistive technology strategies for infants and toddlers with communication difficulties. *Seminars in Speech and Language, 18,* 283–301.

Rescorla, L. (1989). Language Development Survey. *Journal of Speech and Hearing Disorders, 54,* 587–599.

Reynell, J. (1995). *Reynell Developmental Language Scales.* Los Angeles: Webster Psychological.

Rice, M., Buhr, J., & Nemeth, M. (1990). Fast-mapping word-learning abilities of language-delayed preschoolers. *Journal of Speech and Hearing Research, 55,* 33–42.

Robb, M., Bauer, H., & Tyler, A. (1994). A quantitative analysis of the single-word stage. *First Language, 14,* 37–48.

Roberts, J., Wallace, I., & Henderson, F. (1997). *Otitis media in young children: Medical, developmental, and educational considerations.* Baltimore: Paul H. Brookes.

Robertson, S. B., & Weismer, S. E. (1999). Effects of treatment on linguistic and social skills in toddlers with delayed language development. *Journal of Speech, Language, and Hearing Research, 42,* 1234–1248.

Robinson, N., & Robb, M. (1997). Early communication assessment and intervention: An interactive process. In D. Bernstein & E. Tiegerman (Eds), *Language and communication disorders in children* (4th ed., pp. 155–196). Boston: Allyn & Bacon.

Romski, M. A., & Sevcik, R. A. (2005). Augmentative communication and early intervention: Myths and realities. *Infants & Young Children, 18,* 174–185

Rossetti, L. (1990. *The Rossetti Infant-Toddler Language Scale.* Moline, IL: Lingua Systems.

Rowland, C. (2004). *The Communication Matrix.* Oregon Health Sciences Design to Learn Projects. Retrieved July 25, 2007, from www.designtolearn.com/pages/matrix.html.

Rutter, M. (1979). Protective factors in children's response to stress and disadvantage. In M. Kent & T. Rolf (Eds.), *Social competence in children.* Hanover, NH: University Press of New England.

Sawyer, D., & Butler, K. (1991). Early language intervention: A deterrent to reading disability. *Annals of Dyslexia, 41,* 55–79.

Sevcik, R. A. (1999). Research with young children at risk of speech/language development disorders. *Augmentative and Alternative Communication, 8,* 1–2.

Shatz, M. (1983). On transition, continuity, and coupling: An alternative approach to communicative development. In R. Golinkoff (Ed.), *The transition from prelinguistic to linguistic communication.* Hillsdale, NJ: Erlbaum.

Shaw, D. S., & Bell, R. Q. (1993). Developmental theories of parental contributors to antisocial behaviour, *Journal of Abnormal Child Psychology, 21,* 493–518.

Shelton, T., Jeppson, E., & Johnson, B. (1987). *Family-centered care for children with special health care needs.* Washington. DC: Association for the Care of Children's Health.

Shprintzen, R. (1997). *Genetics, syndromes, and communication disorders.* San Diego, CA: Singular.

Shriberg, L., Friel-Patti, S., Flapsen, P., & Brown, R. (2000). Otits media, fluctuant hearing loss, and speech-language outcomes: A preliminary structural equation model. *Journal of Speech, Language, and hearing Research, 43,* 100–120.

Smith A. M., Fried, P. A., & Hogan, M. J. (2004). Effects of prenatal marijuana on response inhibition: An MRI study of young adults. *Neurotoxicology Teratology, 26*(4), 533–542.

Smith, D., Johnson, A., Pears, K., Fisher, P., & DeGarmo, D. (2007). Child maltreatment and foster care: Unpacking the effects of prenatal and postnatal parental substance use. *Child Maltreatment, 12*(2), 150–160.

Smith, M. (1994). Child-rearing practices associated with better developmental outcomes in preschool-age foster children. *Child Study Journal, 24,* 299–326.

Snow, C. (1979). The role of social interaction and the development of communicative ability. In A. Collins (Ed.), *Children's language and communication.* Hillsdale, NJ: Erlbaum.

Snyder, L., Bates, E., & Bretherton, I. (1981). Content and context in early lexical development. *Journal of Child Language, 8,* 565–582.

Sparks, S. (1989). Assessment and intervention with at-risk infants and toddlers: Guidelines for the speech-language pathologist. *Topics in Language Disorders, 10,* 43–56.

Stark, R. (1980). Stages of speech development in the first year of life. In G. Komishan, J. Kavanagh, & C. Ferguson (Eds.), *Child phonology* (Vol. 1). New York: Academic.

Stoel-Gammon, C., & Cooper, J. (1984). Patterns of early lexical and phonological development. *Journal of Child Language, 11,* 247–271.

Streissguth, A., & Kanter, J. (1997). *The challenge of fetal alcohol syndrome: Overcoming secondary disabilities.* Seattle: University of Washington Press.

Teele, D., Klein, J., Chase, C., Menyuk, R., & Rosner, B. (1990). Otitis media in infancy and intellectual ability, school achievement, speech and language at age 7 years. *Journal of Infectious Diseases, 162,* 685–694.

Thal, D., & Bates, E. (1988). Language and gesture in late talkers. *Journal of Speech and Hearing Research, 31,* 115–123.

Tomblin, J. B., Shonrock, C. M., & Hardy, J. C. (1989). The concurrent validity of the Minnesota Child Development Inventory as a measure of young children's language development. *Journal of Speech and Hearing Disorders, 54,* 101–105.

Turnbull, A., & Turnbull, H. (1990). *Families, professionals, and exceptionality: A special partnership* (2nd ed.). Columbus, OH: Merrill/Macmillan.

UK Office for National Statistics. (2006). Child health. Retrieved on August 25, 2007, from www.statistics.gov.uk/cci/nscl.asp?ID=8456.

UNICEF. (1998). *The state of the world's children.* Oxford, UK: Oxford University Press.

U.S. Department of Education. (2007). Special Education and Rehabilitative Services. IDEA 2004, Part C Regulations, Notice of Proposed Rule Making (NPRM). Retrieved July 23, 2007, from www.ed.gov/policy/speced/guid/idea/part-c/nprm/index.html.

Vihman, M., & Greenlee, M. (1987). Individual differences in phonological development: Ages one and three years. *Journal of Speech and Hearing Research, 30,* 503–521.

Ward, S. (1999). An investigation into the effectiveness of an early intervention method for delayed language development in young children. *International Journal of Language and Communication Disorders, 34,* 243–264.

Warren, S., & Kaiser, A. (1986). Incidental language teaching: A critical review. *Journal of Speech and Hearing Disorders, 51,* 291–299.

Warren, S. R., & Gazdag, G. (1990). Facilitating early language development with milieu intervention procedures. *Journal of Early Intervention, 14,* 62.

Wetherby, A., & Prizant, B. (1992). Profiling young children's communicative competence. In S. Warren & J. Reichle (Eds.), *Causes and effects in communication and language intervention* (pp. 217–253). Baltimore: Paul H. Brookes.

Wetherby, A., & Prizant, B. (1993). Profiling communication and symbolic abilities in young children. *Journal of Childhood Communication Disorders, 15,* 23–32.

Wetherby, A., & Prizant, B. (1998). *Communication and Symbolic Behavior Scale.* Chicago: Riverside.

Wetherby, A., Prizant, B., & Hutchinson, T. (1998). Communication, social/affective, and symbolic profiles of young children with autism and pervasive developmental disorders. *American Journal of Speech-Language Pathology, 7,* 79–91.

Wilcox, M. J., Kouri, T. A., & Caswell, S. B. (1991). Early language intervention: A comparison of classroom and individual treatment. *American Journal of Speech-Language Pathology, 1,* 49–61.

Wing, C. (1990). Defective infant formulas and expressive language delay: A case study. *Language, Speech, and Hearing Services in Schools, 21,* 22–27.

World Health Organization. (2001). *International classification of functioning, disability and health.* Geneva, Switzerland: Author.

Wouldes, T., LaGasse, L., Sheridan, J., & Lester, B. (2004). Maternal methamphetamine use during pregnancy and child outcome: What do we know? *Journal of the New Zealand Medical Association, 117*(1206), 1–10.

Wyly, M., Allen, J., Pfalzer, S. M., & Wilson, J. R. (1996). Providing a seamless service system from hospital to home: The NICU Training Project. *Infants and Young Children, 8,* 77–84.

Yoder, P., & Warren, S. (1999). Prelinguistic communication intervention may be one way to help children with developmental delays learn to talk. *Augmentative and Alternative Communication, 8,* 11–12.

Yoder, P., Warren, S., Kyoungram, K., & Gazdag, G. E. (1994). Facilitating prelinguistic communication skills in young children with developmental delay II: Systematic replication and extension. *Journal of Speech and Hearing Research, 37,* 841–851.

Zimmerman, I., Steiner, V., & Pond, R. (1992). *Preschool Language Scale—3.* San Antonio, TX: Psychological Corporation.

Zuniga, J. (1999, April). Communication disorders and HIV Disease. *International Association of Physicians in Aids Care.* Retrieved on March 26, 2008, from www.thebody.com/content/art12344.html.

CHAPTER 4

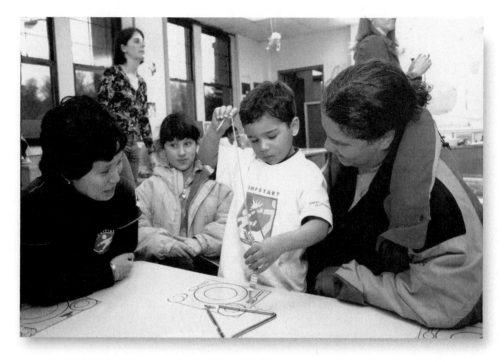

Preschool Language Impairment

Characteristics, Assessment, and Intervention

Liat Seiger-Gardner
Lehman College, City University of New York

Diana Almodovar
Lehman College, City University of New York

When you finish this chapter, you should be able to

- Explain how language form (phonology, syntax, and morphology), content (semantics), and use (pragmatics) are affected in children with language impairment.
- Differentiate between a language delay and a language disorder.
- Identify the hallmark characteristics of children with language impairment and

- current theories accounting for these deficits.
- Distinguish between formal and informal methods for assessing the language of preschool children with language impairment.
- Discuss various treatment methods and strategies for facilitating language abilities in children with language impairment.

Early identification of delayed language development is critical in order to provide early intervention. It is important to determine whether the delay exhibited early on in language development may persist throughout the child's development. A speech-language pathologist needs to be aware of the developmental milestones a child must achieve as well as the course of acquisition of the various areas of language. Linguistic development coupled with nonlinguistic communicative behaviors is key to identifying children in need of speech-language intervention. This chapter will discuss the characteristics of language delay as well as language impairment in preschool-aged children. Methods for formally and informally assessing a child will be reviewed. In addition, methods used to facilitate language development in intervention will be discussed.

Early Language Delay

Most children with language impairments are not identified until the age of 2. In the absence of other significant disabilities (i.e., sensory, motor, or cognitive deficits), the first evidence of a language delay is the late onset of the production of first words and a slow development of vocabulary growth (Leonard, 1998). Toddlers with typical language development acquire their first words between 12 and 18 months of age and produce two-word combinations between 18 and 24 months of age, after they have at least fifty words in their productive lexicon (Nelson, 1973). This stage of development is referred to as the **emerging language stage** (Paul, 1995). Children who fail to meet these linguistic milestones are referred to as **late talkers** (Rescorla, 1989; Rescorla, & Schwartz, 1990). This delay may be due to weak processing skills, articulatory skills, retrieval skills, conceptual skills, or rule-learning skills (Rescorla, 2002).

Delayed phonological development is also a hallmark of late talkers (Paul, 1991; Paul & Jennings, 1992; Rescorla & Ratner, 1996; Roberts, Rescorla, Giroux, & Stevens, 1998). Late talkers are less vocal and verbal compared to their typically developing peers and less accurate in consonantal production. Late talkers exhibit proportionally smaller consonantal and vowel inventories, and their consonantal inventory consists of primarily voiced stops (/d/, /g/, /z/), nasals (/m/, /n/), and glides (/j/, /w/). (See Figure 4.1 for an overview of the age of acquisition of consonants in English.) Late talkers also exhibit a more restricted and less complex array of syllable structures, using predominantly single vowels and consonant–vowel (CV) syllable shapes. Moreover, while meaningful speech increases and the proportion of babbling decreases in typically developing children, in late talkers, the babbling period is extended. These children's babbling is characterized as being less complex.

Lastly, typically developing children, as well as late talkers, use a specific set of strategies to simplify the production of words. These strategies are called **phonological processes** (see Figure 4.2, p. 172). The most prevalent phonological processes are the following:

1. *Consonant-cluster reduction*—reducing the cluster to one consonant; for example, /poon/ for /spoon/ or /tee/ for /tree/
2. *Weak syllable deletion*—omitting the unstressed or weak syllable in multisyllabic words; for example, /nana/ for /banana/ or /ephant/ for /elephant/
3. *Gliding*—replacing the liquids (/l/ and /r/) with glides (/w/ and /j/); for example, /twack/ for /truck/ or /wave/ for /love/
4. *Final consonant deletion*—omitting the final consonant in words; for example, /ca/ for /car/ or /ha/ for /hat/ (Ingram, 1981; Leonard, 1982; Schwartz, Leonard, Folger, & Wilcox, 1980)

While these processes are used by typically developing children until age 4, they usually disappear by age 5. This is not the case for late talkers, however; these processes persist over a longer period of time. In sum, late talkers follow similar patterns (i.e., order of acquisition) of phonological development as their typically developing peers, but phonological development in late talkers continues over a longer period of time (Paul & Jennings, 1992).

Whereas delays in lexical and phonological development are characteristics of late talkers at age 2, morphosyntactic delays are the hallmark of late talkers at age 3 (Rescorla & Roberts, 1997). It is during the second and third years of life that new morphological forms are evident in typically developing children: (1) the appearance of several grammatical morphemes (e.g., present progressive *-ing*, prepositions: *in* and *on*, regular plural *s*) (see Table 4.1, p. 173) and (2) the production of the basic sentence form of subject–verb–object (e.g., *She drinks milk*) and subject–copula–complement (*She is pretty*) (Brown, 1973) (see Table 4.2, p. 174).

One of the most common measures of syntactic development is a developmental index that measures the increase in a child's *mean length of utterance (MLU)* in morphemes. MLU is considered to be a reliable predictor of the complexity of the language of English-speaking children. Researchers have found that late talkers are delayed in syntactic complexity and morphological maturity based on their MLU

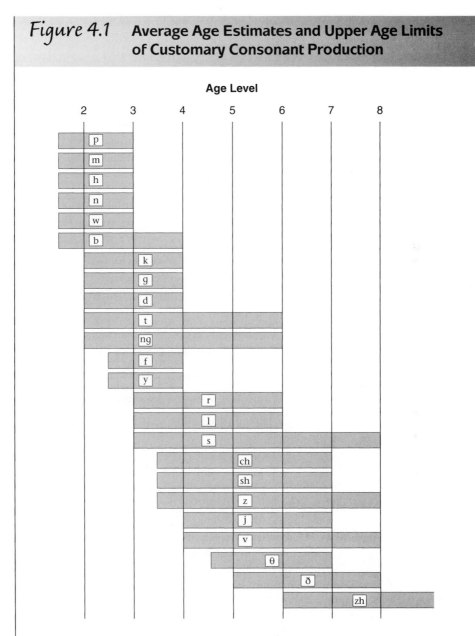

Figure 4.1 Average Age Estimates and Upper Age Limits of Customary Consonant Production

The solid bar corresponding to each sound starts at the median age of customary articulation; it stops at an age level at which 90 percent of all children are customarily producing the sound.

Figure 4.2   **Chronology of Phonological Processes**

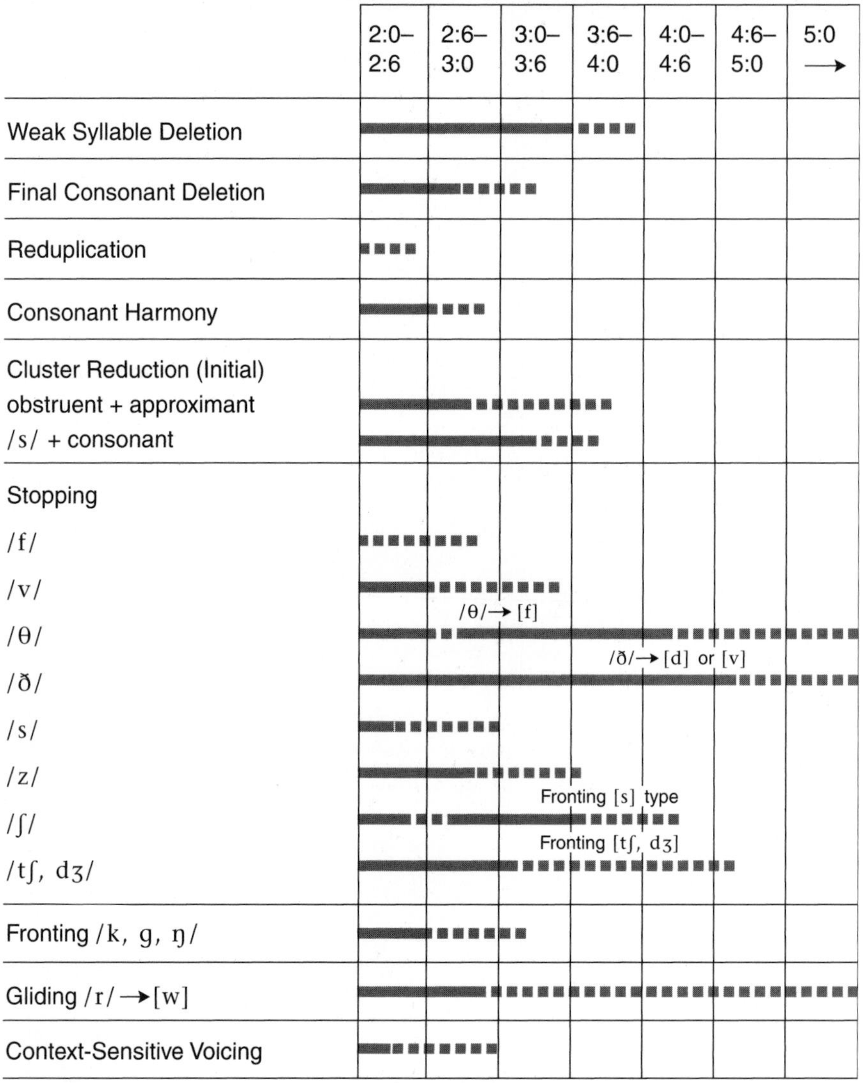

	2:0–2:6	2:6–3:0	3:0–3:6	3:6–4:0	4:0–4:6	4:6–5:0	5:0 →
Weak Syllable Deletion	▬▬▬▬	▬▬▬▬	▬▬▬▬	▪▪▪▪			
Final Consonant Deletion	▬▬▬▬	▬▪▪▪	▪▪▪				
Reduplication	▪▪▪▪						
Consonant Harmony	▬▬▬	▪▪▪					
Cluster Reduction (Initial) obstruent + approximant	▬▬▬▬	▬▬▬	▪▪▪▪▪▪	▪▪			
/s/ + consonant	▬▬▬▬	▬▬▬▬	▪▪▪				
Stopping /f/	▪▪▪▪▪▪	▪▪					
/v/	▬▬	▪▪▪▪▪	▪▪				
/θ/	▬▬▬▬	▬▬	/θ/→ [f]		▪▪▪▪	▪▪▪▪▪	▪▪▪▪
/ð/	▬▬▬▬	▬▬▬▬	▬▬▬▬	▬▬▬▬	/ð/→ [d] or [v] ▪▪	▪▪▪▪	▪▪▪
/s/	▬▪▪	▪▪▪▪					
/z/	▬▬▬	▪▪▪▪	▪				
/ʃ/	▬▬▬	▪▪▬▬▬	Fronting [s] type ▪▪▪	▪▪			
/tʃ, dʒ/	▬▬▬▬	▬▬▬▬	Fronting [tʃ, dʒ] ▪▪▪▪▪▪▪▪	▪▪▪▪			
Fronting /k, g, ŋ/	▬▬▬	▪▪▪▪	▪				
Gliding /r/ →[w]	▬▬▬▬	▪▪▪▪	▪▪▪▪	▪▪▪▪	▪▪▪▪	▪▪▪▪	▪▪
Context-Sensitive Voicing	▬▪▪	▪▪▪▪					

scores (Paul 1993; Paul & Alforde, 1993; Paul & Smith, 1993; Rescorla & Roberts, 1997). Deficits are apparent in both noun and verb morphology (Paul & Alforde, 1993; Rescorla & Roberts, 2002), with the greatest difficulties occurring with nominal morphemes, such as articles (*the, a*) and pronouns (*she, his*), and verbal morphemes, such as the contractible copula (*She's a teacher*) and auxiliary (*He is swimming*). Thus, the acquisition of nominal and verbal morphology in late talkers

Table 4.1 **Stages of Morphosyntactic Development in Typically Developing Children**

Stage	Age (Months)	Morphosyntactic Characteristics	Examples
1	12–26	Single-word utterances and multiword combinations based on word order/semantic-syntactic rules	"Eat cookie" Action + Object "Daddy shoe" Possessor + Possession "Doggie bed" Entity + Locative
2	27–30	Appearance of grammatical morphemes.	"Mommy *is* driving" Present progressive -*ing* and auxiliary *is* "I love dogs" Regular plural -*s*
3	31–34	Simple sentence forms: • Development of noun and verb phrases with the addition of grammatical morphemes, quantifiers, adjectives, and adverbs • Development of different sentence types (declarative, interrogative, imperative, and negative forms)	"Dave eats banana" Subject-verb-object "This *is* Mommy's car" Copula and possessive "Diana has *three* cats" Quantifiers "She has a *blue* cap" Adjectives "She runs *quickly*" Adverbs "I'm eating ice cream" Declarative "What are you eating?" Interrogative "Throw me the ball, *please*" Imperative "I don't want that" Negative forms
4	35–40	Appearance of embedded phrases and subordinate clauses within a sentence Subordinate clauses introduced by conjunction words (*after, although, before, until, while, when*) or relative pronouns (*who, which, whom, that*)	"The woman *in the blue dress* is my teacher" Embedded phrase "The boy, *whom we met last week*, is in my class" Embedded clause
5	41–46	Appearance of conjoined sentences with conjunction words (*and, if, because, when, but, after, before, so*)	"I play the violin, *and* she plays the piano." "She cried *because* she fell down the stairs." "We went to school *after* we ate breakfast." "I like fruit, *but* I don't like vegetables."

From S. A. Raver, *Early Childhood Special Education – 0 to 8 years*, p. 127. Published by Allyn and Bacon, Boston, MA. Copyright © 2009 by Pearson Education. Reprinted by permission of the publisher.

Table 4.2   **Acquisition of Grammatical Morphemes**

Morpheme	Example	Age of Mastery (in Months)
Present progressive -*ing* (no auxiliary verb)	*Mommy driving.*	19–28
In	*Ball in cup.*	27–30
On	*Doggie on sofa.*	27–30
Regular plural -*s*	*Kitties eat my ice cream.*	27–33
Irregular past	*came, fell, broke, sat, went*	25–46
Possessive *'s*	*Mommy's balloon broke.*	26–40
Uncontractible copula (verb *to be* as main verb)	*He is my teacher.*	27–39
Articles	*I see a kitty.* *I throw the ball to Daddy.*	28–46
Regular past -*ed*	*Mommy pulled the wagon.*	26–48
Regular third-person -*s*	*Kathy hits.*	26–46
Irregular third-person form	*She does like me.* *He has the ball.*	28–50
Uncontractible auxiliary	*He is wearing a hat.*	29–48
Contractible copula	*Daddy's big* (for *Daddy is big*).	29–49
Contractible auxiliary	*Daddy's drinking juice* (for *Daddy is drinking juice*).	30–50

From R. Owens, *Language Development: An Introduction* (6th ed.), 2005. Published by Allyn and Bacon, Boston, MA. Copyright © 2006 by Pearson Education. Adapted with permission of the publisher.

is protracted, although it follows a pattern similar to that of typically developing peers.

Chronic morphosyntactic deficits at the sentence level are also apparent in the narratives of 4-year-old late talkers (Paul & Smith, 1993). Four-year-olds who were identified as late talkers at age 2 performed significantly more poorly on all measures of narrative skills (i.e., cohesion, semantic content, lexical diversity, and syntax) compared to their typically developing peers. The late talkers' narratives reflected their difficulties in encoding, organizing, and linking schemes, as well as in retrieving precise and diverse words from their lexicons. The ability to narrate a story requires a child to be able to convey ideas and sequence events in a cohesive manner, to use context-related vocabulary, to understand cause-effect relationships, and to structure the story in a way that will help the listener understand it. The difficulties late talkers exhibit in language content (semantics), form (phonology, morphology, and syntax), and use (pragmatics) are evidenced in their narratives and known to be good predictors of later academic skills.

DIFFERENTIAL DIAGNOSIS: LATE TALKERS VERSUS LATE BLOOMERS

Some toddlers with slow expressive vocabulary growth (i.e., late talkers) catch up to their typically developing peers in expressive language skills by age 3 or 4 (Paul, 1996; Recorla & Lee, 2000; Rescorla, Mirak, & Singh, 2000; Whitehurst & Fischel, 1994). Some refer to these children as *late bloomers* (Thal & Tobias, 1992; Thal, Tabias, & Morrison, 1991). Late bloomers, although slow in developing their productive lexicon in the first 2 years of life, make progress in expressive vocabulary development after their second birthday and by their third birthday look very similar to their typically developing peers (Rescorla et al., 2000). However, many toddlers with expressive language delays never really catch up to their peers and continue to show persistent language delays even after the age of 3. These children are often identified at age 4 as having specific language impairment (SLI).

The question is, How can we distinguish transient language difficulties (i.e., late bloomers) from persistent language impairments (i.e., late talkers)? What clinical markers may distinguish late talkers from late bloomers?

Two markers were identified as potential predictors of persisting language delays:

1. *A delay in the development of the receptive lexicon* (Thal, Reilly, Seibert, Jeffries, & Fenson, 2004; Thal & Tobias, 1992; Thal et al., 1991). Comprehension at 13 months of age has been shown to predict the development of receptive vocabulary and grammatical complexity (i.e., MLU) at 28 months of age in typically developing children (Bates, Bretherton, & Snyder, 1988). Comprehension is suggested to play an important role throughout the second year of life in both receptive and expressive language acquisition (Watt, Wetherby, & Shumway, 2006).

2. *A delay in the use of conventional gestures (e.g., pointing, showing) and symbolic gestures (e.g., panting like a dog, sniffing to indicate a flower)* (Thal & Tobias, 1992; Thal et al., 1991). Typically developing children use conventional and symbolic gestures before they use words to communicate with others (Acredolo & Goodwyn, 1988; Caselli, 1990; see Capone & McGregor, 2004, for a full review) (see Table 4.3). The use of gestures early in the second year of life has been shown to correlate highly with the development of receptive language at age 3 (Watt et al., 2006) and with total vocal production at 20 months (Capirci, Iverson, Pizzuto, & Volterra, 1996). Late bloomers were found to use more communicative gestures compared to their typically developing peers in order to compensate for their lack of words. In contrast, late talkers failed to show an increase in communicative gestures as a compensation for their verbal delay (Thal & Tobias, 1992). Thus, compensatory use of communicative gestures is a positive prognostic sign for later typical language development.

Can children who are slow in developing their expressive lexicon recover? Data from longitudinal studies suggest a recovery rate of about 50 percent per year from age 2 to age 5 (Rescorla, Dahlsgaard, & Roberts, 2000). Approximately 50 percent of the late talkers identified between the ages of 2 years and 2 years, 7 months exhibited MLU scores within normal range by age 3 (Rescorla & Roberts, 1997). Of the 50 percent that were still delayed at age 3, half exhibited within normal range MLUs at age 4 (Rescorla et al., 2000). At age 5, half of the late talkers that still exhibited language

Table 4.3 **Timeline of Gesture Development**

10–13 Months	12–13 Months	15–16 Months	18–20 Months	2–5 Years	School Age
Showing Giving Pointing Ritualized request	Representational gestures, play schemes	Gesture or vocal preference	Spoken word preference, gesture-plus-spoken combinations	Speech-gesture integration, beat gestures emerge	Mismatched gesture-plus-spoken combinations
POINT predicts first words	First words emerge		Significant increase in words (types, tokens)	Gesture scaffolds spoken expression and comprehension	Mismatches indexes the transitional knowledge state
Other prelinguistic behaviors include: Eye contact, joint attention, and turn taking	Gesture serves a complementary function to spoken forms		Increased pointing in combination with spoken words Transition to empty-handed play schemes	Transition from BPO to IO gestures Iconic and beat gestures accompany longer utterances	Gesture aids in the transition to concept acquisition

Note: BPO = body part as object; IO = imaginary object

From "Gesture Development: A Review for Clinical and Research Practices," by N. Capone and K. McGregor, 2004, *Journal of Speech, Language, and Hearing Research, 47*, pp. 173–186.

delays at age 4 recovered; hence, 75 to 85 percent of the late talkers identified at age 2 recovered and scored within normal range at age 5 (Paul, 1996; Rescorla, 2002).

LATE TALKERS VERSUS CHILDREN WITH SLI

It was recently suggested that late talkers and children with SLI are the same children at different ages (Rescorla, 2000, 2002; Rescorla & Roberts, 2002). Preschoolers with SLI, like late talkers, are identified by a process of exclusion. They typically have performance IQs within normal limits, normal hearing acuity, no behavioral or emotional disorders, and no gross neurological deficits. However, they present with significant deficits in language production and/or comprehension (Leonard, 1998). Thus, children who present with language impairment that is secondary to another condition, such as autism, mental retardation, or hearing loss, are usually not diagnosed as being late talkers or as having SLI (Leonard 1998; Whitehurst & Fischel, 1994).

Moreover, one of the hallmarks of preschool children with SLI is a morphosyntactic deficit—specifically, a deficit in verb morphology (Bedore & Leonard, 1998; Rice & Wexler, 1996; Rice, Wexler, & Cleave, 1995). Similarly, late talkers identified at age 2 were reported to acquire fewer tense-marking morphemes by age 4 compared to their language-matched typically developing peers (Paul & Alforde, 1993).

Rescorla and Roberts (2002) suggested that diagnostic caution led to the distinction between children with SLI and late talkers. It seemed as though both clinicians and researchers were reluctant to label a young child with mild (or expressive-only) language delay as having SLI. However, both disorders are suggested to fall on a continuum from:

1. preschoolers with SLI whose delays continue into school-age years (severe impairment), to
2. preschoolers with SLI who seem to recover by age 5 (moderate impairment), to
3. late talkers with continuing delay (moderate to severe delay in receptive expressive skills), to
4. late bloomers (mild expressive delay), to
5. typically developing children (average to above average language abilities).

It has been suggested that the term *late talkers* be used to describe children who are delayed in acquiring language and who are between the ages of 2 and 4 and that the term *SLI* be used to describe children who exhibit persisting language impairments at age 4 or older (Rescorla & Lee, 2000).

Characteristics of Preschool Language Impairment

As mentioned earlier, children with SLI typically have performance IQs within normal limits, normal hearing sensitivity, no behavioral or emotional disorders, and no gross neurological deficits in the presence of significant language deficits (Leonard, 1998). The language deficits can be manifested in the expression of language or in the expression *and* comprehension of language, and they can affect one or more areas of language (i.e., form—phonology, syntax, morphology; content—semantics; and use—pragmatics).

SLI affects about 7 percent of children (Leonard, 1998). It often runs in families and is suggested to have a genetic component (Newbury, Bishop, & Monaco, 2005), although a clear inheritance pattern or specific genes are yet to be identified. Although the disorder is defined as one that shows no evidence of frank neurological impairment (e.g., brain lesions, seizures), subtle irregularities in brain structure suggest neurological involvement in the disorder. Atypical left–right perisylvian area configurations, with a larger than usual right perisylvian area that equals or exceeds the size of the left perisylvian area, has been associated with SLI (Leonard, 1998).

Children with SLI form a heterogeneous group. To address the heterogeneity, several subgroups of SLI have been identified based on their linguistic profiles:

1. *Children who exhibit a lexical-syntactic deficit*—These children exhibit no problems with articulation but reveal morphosyntactic difficulties that can be manifested in both language comprehension and expression.
2. *Children who exhibit verbal apraxia*—These children exhibit phonological deficits that are manifested mainly in their expressive language.
3. *Children who exhibit phonologic programming deficit*—These children exhibit articulation and phonological deficits and difficulties in expressive language.
4. *Children who exhibit phonological-syntactic deficit*—These children exhibit articulation, phonological, and morphosyntactic deficits. Their deficits can be manifested in both domains of language comprehension and production.
5. *Children who demonstrate difficulties with word meaning (semantics) and/or with language usage in discourse (pragmatic skills)* (Conti-Ramsden & Botting, 1999; Conti-Ramsden, Crutchley, & Botting, 1997).

Classifying children with SLI into subgroups based on their linguistic profiles is advantageous for clinical purposes. Identifying the specific linguistic profile of a child allows the clinician to form a more focused remediate program that centers on the specific areas of deficit.

LIMITATIONS IN LANGUAGE CONTENT: SEMANTICS

Children with SLI exhibit a slower rate of lexical acquisition (Rice, Buhr, & Nemeth, 1990; Windfuhr, Faragher, & Conti-Ramsden, 2002) and have a less diverse and more restricted receptive and expressive lexicon (Watkins, Kelly, Harbers, & Hollis, 1995). Several explanations have been offered for their limited lexicon. One suggests the cause is lexical gaps, or the absence of a word/concept from the child's lexicon. In this case, the child produces a word he or she knows that captures some features of the item to be named (e.g., *bird* for *ostrich*). Another suggested cause is fragile semantic representations, in which the semantic representations of words/concepts in the child's lexicon are not well elaborated; the child has limited concept knowledge. In this case, the child would produce a word usually from the same semantic category (e.g., *horse* for *zebra*) (McGregor, Friedman, Reilly, & Newman, 2002; McGregor, Newman, Reilly, & Capone, 2002).

The semantic difficulties of preschoolers with SLI are apparent in these areas:

1. *Speech errors*—The most frequently produced speech errors by children with SLI are semantic in nature (e.g., saying *dog* for *horse*; *clown* for *circus*; *fish* for *shark*).

2. *Low performance on lexical comprehension tests* (Lahey & Edwards, 1999; McGregor, 1997) *and tasks focusing on multiple levels of noun hierarchy*—These tasks examine children's comprehension of work meaning on various semantic levels. For example, it examines a child's knowledge of general categories (superordinate), such as *furniture,* basic lexical items under this category (coordinate), such as *chair,* and a more specific label (subordinate), such as *rocking chair* (McGregor & Waxman, 1998).

3. *Word-finding difficulties*—These children have difficulties generating a specific word for any given situation (Rapin & Wilson, 1978). These difficulties are manifested in single-word naming tasks as well as in discourse (German & Simon, 1991). The language of children with word-finding difficulties is characterized by repetitions, substitutions, reformulations, and pauses and by the use of nonspecific words (e.g., *stuff, thing*) (Faust, Dimitrovsky, & Davidi, 1997; German, 1987; McGregor & Leonard, 1989).

4. *Difficulty fast mapping new words* (Dollaghan, 1987; Gray, 2003, 2004; Rice et al., 1990)—*Fast mapping* is the process by which children represent and store new lexical items in their mental lexicon after only few exposures (Carey & Bartlett, 1978; Dollaghan, 1985). This ability is suggested to contribute to the rapid acceleration in lexical development that occurs at approximately 18 months of age (e.g., Golinkoff, Hirsh-Pasek, Bailey, & Wenger, 1992). Children with SLI reveal difficulties in fast mapping (Alt & Plante, 2006; Gray, 2006); they require many more exposures to learn a new lexical label compared to their typically developing peers (Gray, 2004; Rice, Oetting, Marquis, Bode, & Pae, 1994; Riches, Tomasello, & Conti-Ramsden, 2005).

5. *Difficulty learning new words in contexts that provide limited support*—This occurs in contexts that involve fast mapping (Rice, Buhr, & Oetting, 1992; Rice et al., 1994) as well as in contexts where more explicit instructions regarding relevant words and their meanings are provided to children (Gray, 2003, 2004; Nash & Donaldson, 2005).

6. *Difficulty in the acquisition of relational word meanings (e.g., spatial, temporal, quantitative, and dimensional words)*—Relational words play a major role in expressing a number of grammatical relationships and are prevalent in the language of the school curriculum (Edmonston & Litchfield Thane, 1992). Preschoolers with SLI exhibit difficulties understanding and using relational words that mark spatial relations (*on, in, above, behind*), temporal relations (*tomorrow, before, after*), kinship relations (*grandmother, sister, daughter*), causal relations (*because, why*), sequential relations (*first, next, finally*), and physical relations (*hard/soft, wide/narrow, shallow/deep*).

7. *Difficulty in verb learning*—Verb learning poses more of a challenge compared to noun or concept learning in that it requires the child to associate the word (verb) with the physical action, which is short lived and transitory. The verb lexicon of children with SLI is characterized as limited and less diverse, with a heavy reliance on general all purpose (GAP) verbs (e.g., *go, make, do, look*) (Conti-Ramsden & Jones, 1997; Rice & Bode, 1993; Thordardottir & Weismer, 2001). Difficulty with verb tensing was recognized as a clinical marker of preschool children with SLI (Conti-Ramsden, 2003; Hadley & Short, 2005; Rice & Wexler, 1996).

LIMITATIONS IN LANGUAGE FORM: PHONOLOGY

The Acquisition of Phonemes

Children with SLI show many of the same phonological characteristics as younger children with typically developing language. Children with SLI are late in acquiring their consonant inventory but follow the same pattern of acquisition as typically developing children. The sounds acquired early by typically developing children (e.g., /n/, /m/, /b/, /w/) are also those acquired by children with SLI. However, the sounds acquired later (e.g., /s/, /v/) continue to be difficult for children with SLI even into the school-age years.

The phonological difficulties of preschool children with SLI are apparent in tasks that require the repetition of nonsense words and the recall of lists of real words. These difficulties have been suggested to reflect imprecise phonological representations, limited phonological storage capacity, or rapid decay of phonological traces in phonological working memory (Gathercole & Baddeley, 1990; Montgomery, 1995).

Phonological Working Memory

The phonological working memory of preschool children with SLI can be assessed using a variety of conventional short-term memory measures, such as standardized digit span and word span tasks. The informal nonword repetition task (Dollaghan & Campbell, 1998; Gathercole & Baddeley, 1990, 1995) has been proven an especially sensitive index of phonological working memory in preschool and young school-age children with and without SLI. In this task, children are asked to repeat individual nonwords varying in length from one to four or five syllables. The task involves the perception and temporary storage of an unfamiliar sequence of phonemes, the construction of a new phonological representation, and the production of a novel articulatory sequence. A deficit in phonological working memory is indicated by markedly poor repetition of the longer multisyllabic nonwords. Edwards and Lahey (1998) found that preschoolers with SLI made more errors of syllable structure and produced a higher percentage of phoneme deletions than did their typically developing peers. The researchers interpreted these children's performance as resulting from difficulty forming a finely detailed phonological representation. It was suggested that the phonological representations of children with SLI are more holistic, resembling those of younger children with typical language development (Maillart, Schelstraete, & Hupert, 2004).

Nonword repetition has been used in many investigations (e.g., Dollaghan & Campbell, 1998; Gathercole & Baddeley, 1990, 1995; Gathercole, Willis, Baddeley, & Emslie, 1994; Marton & Schwartz, 2003; Weismer et al., 2000) to identify impairments in the phonological working memory of children with SLI. Poor performance on this task was even suggested as a clinical marker for SLI. One of the drawbacks of the nonword repetition task is the absence of normative data. Speech-language pathologists using this task need to compare the performance of a child with SLI to the performance of a typically developing child to identify a deficit in phonological working memory.

Phonological Awareness

Montgomery (2002) emphasized the importance of speech-language pathologists promoting better phonological working memory skills in children with SLI to facilitate their phonological encoding and storage abilities. Practicing phonological awareness skills can improve phonological working memory abilities.

Phonological awareness refers to the explicit awareness that words in the language are composed of syllables and phonemes (i.e., consonants and vowels) (Catts, 1991) and that words can rhyme or begin with the same sound. Preschoolers can demonstrate phonological awareness by tapping syllables (i.e., segmenting multisyllabic words into their syllable components), recognizing and producing rhymes, segmenting words into their phoneme components, blending and manipulating sounds within words, and understanding letter–sound correspondence. Phonological awareness plays an important role in the acquisition of print literacy.

Children with SLI exhibit difficulties in activities that involve phonological awareness (Fazio, 1997). Mann and Liberman (1984) suggested that having children listen to nursery rhymes might prove beneficial in facilitating their phonological working memory. Nursery rhymes and other activities that promote phonological awareness teach children how to attend to and discover the internal phonological structures of words and require them to phonologically encode and store the phonemic sequence in phonological working memory.

LIMITATIONS IN LANGUAGE FORM: MORPHOLOGY

Children with typical language development start to acquire grammatical morphemes as early as 27 to 30 months of age (Brown Stage II of morphosyntactic development) (See Tables 4.1 and 4.2). However, grammatical morphology presents a major challenge for children with specific language impairment (SLI). These children exhibit extraordinary difficulty in producing nominal morphology (e.g., noun plural -*s* inflection) and verb morphology (e.g., third-person singular -*s*, regular past tense -*ed*, auxiliary *be* forms), with the latter being most challenging (Bedore & Leonard, 1998; Norbury, Bishop, & Briscoe, 2001; Rice et al., 1995). When compared to language or age-matched peers, children with SLI produce verb and noun morphological markers less consistently and use them less frequently in obligatory contexts (e.g., sentence completion tasks) and in spontaneous speech (Leonard, Eyer, Bedore, & Grela, 1997; Rice & Wexler, 1996; Rice et al., 1995).

The cause for the grammatical deficit is unclear and debatable. Three theories have been offered to account for the grammatical deficit in SLI: (1) the input-processing theory, which is also known as the surface hypothesis (Leonard, 1998); (2) the grammar-specific theory (van der Lely & Christian, 2000; van der Lely, Rosen, & McClelland, 1998); and (3) the extended optional infinitive theory (Rice, 2000, Rice & Wexler, 1996; Rice et al., 1995).

The *input-processing theory* suggests children with SLI have a general processing capacity limitation or reduced speed of processing and specific difficulty with the perception and production of surface features of specific morphemes. These morphemes—such as the third-person singular -*s* and past-tense -*ed* inflections, possessive '*s*, articles, and the copula and auxiliary *be* forms—are characterized by short duration and low perceptual saliency. Children with SLI not only have difficulty perceiving these morphemes but also have difficulty conceptualizing their grammatical functions.

The *grammar-specific theory* suggests a deficit that is localized in the grammatical system or the representations of grammatical morphemes. This suggests that within the heterogeneous group of SLI, there is a subgroup of children, referred to as G-SLI, that presents a grammar-specific deficit (van der Lely, 1998). These children show persisting grammatical impairment in language comprehension and production in the absence of severe phonological, pragmatic, or nonverbal cognitive deficits.

Finally, the *extended optional infinitive theory* suggests that children with SLI follow the same developmental pattern of morphological acquisition as their typically developing peers. Like typically developing children, children with SLI have partial knowledge of finiteness, thus treating tense marking as optional (Norbury et al., 2001). However, whereas the grammatical representations of finiteness in typically developing children are fully developed by the age of 4 years, 6 months, the development of finiteness in children with SLI extends over a longer time period (Rice et al., 1995; Rice & Wexler, 1996). This theory has focused specifically on verb phrase morphology and identified it as a clinical marker for SLI.

Regardless of theory, the deficits in morphology apparent in preschoolers with SLI are characterized by the limited use of grammatical morphemes or their omission. Children with SLI are likely to omit the auxiliaries, which are the *be* verb forms (i.e., *am, is,* and *are*), or the present progressive *-ing* form when producing a sentence in the present tense. Thus, sentences such as *I going to swim in the pool* (omitting the auxiliary) and *I'm play with the cars now* (omitting the present progressive) occur frequently in the productions of children with SLI. In addition, children with SLI exhibit many grammatical errors. They are likely to misuse the *be* verb form, as in the sentence *She were going to the store* (misuse of auxiliary *be* form) or in the sentence *The boy and the girl is not happy* (misuse of copula *be* form).

Another area of difficulty for children with SLI is the production of pronouns. A pronoun is a word that can be substituted for a noun or noun phrase in a sentence. For example, in the sentence *The girl was watching her dog when it bit the neighbor's child*, the pronoun *her* replaces the words *the girl* and the pronoun *it* replaces the words *the dog*. The development of pronoun use begins around age 2; the use of subjective pronouns (e.g., *he, she, they*) develops first followed by objective pronouns (e.g., *him, her, them*), possessive pronouns (e.g., *his, her, their*), and finally, around age 5, reflexive pronouns (e.g., *himself, herself, themselves*) (Owens, 2005).

The lengthy development of pronouns in typically developing children reflects the complex interaction of form, content, and use. Pronouns are grammatical markers that make semantic distinctions based on gender, person, and number. They also serve as conversational devices, providing cohesion between old and new information. New information is initially identified as is and then is referred to by a pronoun.

The complexity involved in the acquisition of pronouns is evident in the difficulty children with SLI exhibit in mastering the pronominal system and especially the pronoun case. This difficulty is revealed in the misuse of pronouns. For example, in the sentence *There was a boy making cookies with her sister*, the objective pronoun is misused based on gender marking. A common mistake made by children with SLI is replacing the pronoun *I* with *me*, as in the sentence *Me play with the doll*. Research on the acquisition of pronouns in children with SLI is limited. Some research suggests that the difficulty children with SLI have with subjective pronouns may be accounted for by the surface theory. In general, research suggests that children with SLI follow a typical but delayed pattern of pronoun development (Moore, 1995, 2001).

LIMITATIONS IN LANGUAGE FORM: SYNTAX

The limitations children with SLI exhibit in syntactic structure are manifested in the reduced length and complexity of the syntactic forms they use. These children produce shorter sentences (Scott & Windsor, 2000), do not elaborate on the noun and verb phrases within sentences, and, when attempting to produce complex sentences, often do so by adding a simple conjunction, such as *and*. Children with SLI fail to use prepositional phrases, as in *The house around the corner is my parents*, and verb-embedded phrases, as in *She fought with courage* and *The girl in the red jeans is nice* (Gillam & Johnston, 1992; Schuele & Dykes, 2005; Schuele & Nicholls, 2000; Schuele & Tolbert, 2001).

LIMITATIONS IN LANGUAGE USE: PRAGMATICS

During the preschool years, typically developing children acquire many conversational skills and improve at responding to their conversational partners. They are capable of engaging in short dialogues with a few turns. Their presupposition skill is developing, revealing the ability to adjust the language style to the conversational partner. These children are also capable of self-monitoring and self-correcting of errors produced during conversation, and they can provide clarifications for misunderstandings.

Children with SLI exhibit delays in the development of conversational skills. They exhibit difficulties initiating and sustaining conversation beyond a few turns, and difficulties in auditory comprehension and short-term memory impede their ability to maintain the flow of conversation. Because these children are less likely to respond to other children's conversational initiations or interaction attempts (Hadley & Rice, 1991), they engage in fewer peer interactions (Hadley & Rice, 1991; Rice, Sell, & Hadley, 1991) and their participation in social interactions is often limited. Due to their social–pragmatic difficulties, children with SLI are less likely to be selected by their typically developing peers as conversational partners.

Other conversational skills that are impaired in children with SLI and impede their ability to socialize with others include presupposition and clarifying misunderstandings. *Presupposition* is the ability to adjust the speech style and language to the listener's age, social status, and language ability. Children with SLI exhibit limited presupposition skill (Leonard, 1998). They also have difficulty asking for clarification and providing it to others when experiencing a communication breakdown (Brinton & Fujiki, 1982; Brinton, Fujiki, Winkler, & Loeb, 1986; Fujiki, Brinton, & Sonnenberg, 1990). Due to their language deficits, children with SLI have difficulty resolving conflicts in a verbal manner, which makes them either withdraw or become aggressive (Leonard, 1998).

EXECUTIVE FUNCTIONS AND LANGUAGE

Language may not be the only domain affected in children with SLI. Some may have deficits in *executive functions*, which are the abilities that allow (1) attending to and shifting attention from one task to another, (2) screening irrelevant information, and (3) organizing information in working memory (Im-Bolter, Johnson, & Pascual-Leone, 2006). Several studies have shown that children with SLI have difficulties inhibiting irrelevant information while focusing on target stimuli (Hanauer & Brooks, 2005; Marton & Schwartz, 2003). Another related mechanism that may be deficient in children with SLI is **attention** (Stevens, Sanders, & Neville, 2006). Children with SLI may not have difficulties inhibiting irrelevant information but rather attending to or focusing on salient or relevant information. After all, approximately two-thirds of preschoolers with attention-deficit hyperactivity disorders also exhibit language disorders. Deficits in working memory were also documented in children with SLI (Archibald & Gathercole, 2006; Marton & Schwartz, 2003; Marton, Schwartz, Farkas, & Katsnelsor, 2006; Montgomery, 2003), revealing low performance compared to typically developing peers on working memory tasks that require processing and storing information simultaneously.

Whether deficiencies in these executive functions or mechanisms cause the language impairment or co-occur with it is unclear. However, speech-language pathologists need to be aware of the possibility that other nonlinguistic functions (e.g., attention, working memory, and inhibition) may be deficient in children with SLI and thus may need to be addressed directly or indirectly in therapy. For example, a speech-language pathologist treating a child with SLI who also exhibits an attention deficit needs to consider these attentional demands when selecting the tasks and materials to address the child's language deficits. Similarly, a child with deficits in verbal working memory may need visual scaffolding and many repetitions to process and store new linguistic information. Deficits in executive functions become more salient as the child transitions from preschool into the school-age years, when linguistic and cognitive demands increase.

Assessment of Preschool Language Impairment

Early identification of children with difficulties in language form, content, or use is vital. A full language evaluation, performed by a certified speech-language pathologist (SLP), should be the method of choice when early signs of language impairment are present. The purpose of a language evaluation is twofold: identification and diagnosis.

It is important to initially identify or rule out the existence of language impairment. During this identification process, the child's language abilities are compared to norms gathered from typically developing children of the same chronological age. This process is used to determine the eligibility of the child for speech and language services. Following the identification process, the speech-language pathologist diagnoses the child in order to understand the nature of his or her language problem. The SLP confirms the presence of a language disorder and determines whether it is primary, as in SLI, or secondary, resulting from other deficits (e.g., cognitive deficit, autism, hearing loss, etc.). During the diagnosis, the SLP gathers information about the child's strengths and weaknesses, his or her needs, the family's concerns and priorities, and the resources available to the child and parents. It is vital, especially in the case of a young child, to involve the caregivers in the evaluation process. It is also important to gather information from multiple sources, such as teachers, pediatricians, and other professionals working with the child, as well as family members that frequently interact with the child and can provide information about his or her abilities. This information will eventually guide intervention and ensure that intervention will be carried out effectively.

Evaluation of a child's language and communication skills can be done through the use of standardized tests (also called *norm-referenced measures*), through the use of criterion-referenced measures, and through the use of performance assessment procedures, which are procedures that evaluate the preschooler's knowledge, abilities, and achievements in a more naturalistic manner.

STANDARDIZED TESTS

A standardized test ranks the child's performance on the test against that of typically developing children in the same age group. *Norms,* which are measures of the average performance of children in a specific age group, are used to compare a child's score to that of his or her age-matched, typically developing peers. Using norms allows the speech-language pathologist to determine whether a child's score falls within the age-expected range or below it, suggesting the presence of language impairment. Having the scores from standardized tests is usually necessary to determine a child's eligibility for services. These tests are standardized with regard to scoring and testing procedures; the speech-language pathologists administering the tests are expected to follow the exact instructions for administration and scoring to get proper results.

Most standardized tests consist of a set of subtests that are designed to measure various aspects of receptive and expressive language in one or more areas of language (i.e., phonology, syntax, morphology, semantics, and pragmatics). Subtests that require the child to manipulate objects or point to pictures usually measure receptive language skills, whereas subtests that require the child to imitate, complete, or formulate sentences or provide descriptions usually measure expressive language skills.

Although the use of standardized tests is the most common method for evaluating a child's language abilities and is mandated by the state boards of education as well as other agencies to determine children's eligibility for speech and language services, these tests have several drawbacks. For instance, standardized tests are limited in the content and scope of what is being tested, usually dedicating only a few items to each linguistic form. They provide a cursory overview of the child's linguistic abilities, not an in-depth evaluation, which minimizes the potential of using the results to determine intervention goals. Furthermore, most of the standardized tests used by SLPs to evaluate children do not evaluate language use, social communicative skills, and play skills. The fact that the tests are standardized removes them from a meaningful and communicative context. Table 4.4 provides a sample of standardized measures used to evaluate preschool language development.

CRITERION-REFERENCED MEASURES

Criterion-referenced measures are nonstandardized tools that measure the child's linguistic abilities in terms of absolute level of mastery. In contrast to performance on a

Table 4.4   **Most Commonly Used Standardized Tests and Criterion-Referenced Measures for Preschool Language Evaluation**

Standardized Tests	Clinical Evaluation of Language Fundamentals–Preschool–CELF-P (Wiig, Semel, & Secord, 2004)
	Preschool Language Scales—PLS (Zimmerman, Steiner, & Pond, 2002)
	Test of Language Development Primary—TOLD:P (Newcomer & Hammill, 1997)
	Test of Auditory Comprehension of Language—TACL (Carrow-Woolfolk, 1999)
	Peabody Picture Vocabulary Test—PPVT (Dunn & Dunn, 1997)
	Expressive One-Word Picture Vocabulary Test—EOWPVT (Gardner, 2000)
Criterion-Referenced Measures	Assessment of Phonological Processes, Revised (Hodson, 1986)
	Multilevel Informal Language Inventory (Goldsworthy, 1982)
	Preschool Language Assessment Instrument (Blank, Rose, & Berlin, 1978)
	Sequenced Inventory of Communication Development—SICD (Hedrick, Prather, & Tobin, 1984)
	Wiig Criterion Referenced Inventory of Language (Wiig, 1990)

standardized test, a child's performance on a criterion-referenced test is not compared to that of his or her age-matched peers to determine whether he or she differs significantly from the norm. Criterion-referenced measures provide more in-depth information about the child's performance in specific domains and as such provide more appropriate information for intervention planning and formulating goals.

Whereas in a standardized test, the SLP evaluates the child's performance *quantitatively*, computing a score that is compared to that of age-matched peers, in a criterion-referenced measure, the SLP evaluates the child's responses *qualitatively*, looking for any missing forms that can be targeted in therapy. The results of a child's performance on criterion-referenced measures are presented as pass/fail scores, percentages correct, and performance rates. These results indicate the child's level of mastery of a specific linguistic form and thus can be used to develop goals for therapy. For example, if a 5-year-old preschooler with language impairment produced the auxiliary -*be* form only 40 percent of the time, the speech-language pathologist would target this form as a goal in therapy with the expectation to reach a mastery level of 90 percent production. Table 4.4 provides a sample of criterion-referenced measures most often used by SLPs to assess preschool language development.

PERFORMANCE ASSESSMENT PROCEDURES

Performance assessment procedures are methods by which the speech-language pathologist can evaluate a preschooler's linguistic knowledge, abilities, and achievements in a more naturalistic manner. **Language sampling** is one of the most common procedures used by SLPs to assess a child's strengths and weaknesses in all language areas: (1) syntax and morphosyntax (e.g., calculating MLU, examining the length and complexity of utterances), (2) phonology (e.g., phonetic inventory, syllable structure complexity, and phonological processes), (3) semantics (e.g., vocabulary size), and (4) pragmatics (e.g., conversational skills, the use of gestures, maintenance of eye contact). Language sampling can also be used to establish treatment goals and to monitor progress in therapy or assess the effects of intervention by comparing the language samples before and after intervention.

Language sampling is performed while the child is engaged in free play with the SLP or the child's caregiver, or it can be carried out in more structured situations using predictable contexts (i.e., scripts), which employ familiar toys with which the child can play. Ideally, language sampling should be done in a number of situations— for instance, at school, in the clinic, and at home. However, when only one session of direct observation is possible, it is important to arrange a setting that will allow for collecting the best and most representative language sample possible. Following language sample collection, the SLP transcribes and analyzes the sample for the presence or absence of specific linguistic forms.

When language sampling is used to assess a child's language skills and formulate treatment goals, it is important to ensure that the language sample is representative of the child's productive language capabilities. Often, a child may not verbalize much at the beginning of the session, taking a while to warm up to the speech-language pathologist or to the new setting. Thus, the first ten to fifteen minutes of the language sampling may not be representative of the child's productive language capabilities and may need to be discarded from the analysis. A representative language sample should consist of at least 100 utterances.

To elicit more language and more complex linguistic structures, the speech-language pathologist should limit the number of questions asked (Miller, 1981). Questions increase the number of ellipses, responses that contain omissions of words or information that can reduce the mean MLU, one of the most common measures of morphosyntactic development in the preschool years. For example, an adult asks a child, "Look at the picture. What's Tigger doing?" The child may respond, "Bouncing." This response is technically correct; however, it does not allow the full grammatical form "He is bouncing." Thus, it reduces the MLU. When questions are used during language sampling, they should be open-ended questions instead of yes/no questions, which tend to elicit single-word responses. Every question should be followed by the request to "Tell me more about it," which is helpful in eliciting more language.

The assessment of **narratives** is another commonly used procedure in the evaluation of language abilities of preschool and school-age children with SLI (Paul &

Smith, 1993). In a narrative, all language components come together to form a cohesive, well-formulated, meaningful story. The analysis of narratives provides information about the child's morphological and syntactic abilities (Scott & Windsor, 2000), the child's ability to use cohesive devices (e.g., *because, after, if*) to relate meanings across sentences (Hesketh, 2004; Liles, 1985a, 1985b, 1987; Liles, Duffy, Merritt, & Purcell, 1995), and the child's ability to organize and sequence story content in a meaningful way (Liles et al., 1995; Merritt & Liles, 1989; Scott & Windsor, 2000).

Like language sampling, the analysis of narratives provides a lot of information about a child's language. Although much of this information can also be gathered from having a conversation with a child or from taking a language sample, some preschoolers with language impairments may have more difficulties engaging in conversation. The relative structure provided by a narrative may facilitate the child's production and provide the speech-language pathologist with a more representative sample (Wagner, Nettelbladt, Sahlen, & Nilholm, 2000).

Narratives can be elicited from children using sequencing cards or wordless books or by having children describe routine events and personal experiences. Two procedures are often used to elicit narratives from children: story generation and story retelling. In *story generation,* the child is instructed to compose a story by himself or herself from sequencing cards or wordless books. In *story retelling*, the child is asked to listen to a story narrated by the speech-language pathologist and then to tell the story back to the SLP. Both procedures require the child to produce a story that will be composed of well-formed, well-organized, coherent sentences. However, the procedures differ in that story generation requires the child to self-conceptualize the story plot, whereas story retelling requires the child to understand the plot narrated by the speech-language pathologist and then narrate the story as the SLP told it (Merritt & Liles, 1989).

Miller and colleagues (2005) raised several issues that a speech-language pathologist should consider when collecting a narrative from a child. The SLP needs to make sure that the narrative task is age appropriate; children younger than 4 years of age should not be expected to produce reliable narratives. When using story retelling, it is important to select stories that children have ample experience with and to provide them with very clear instructions. The speech-language pathologist also needs to be aware of cultural differences when selecting stories (Miller et al., 2005).

Two types of narrative scoring systems are used by SLPs to evaluate the narrative skills of children: Applebee's six levels of narrative development and story grammar categories (Miller et al., 2005). Applebee's six levels of narrative development categorize children's stories into six developmental stages that span from age 2 to age 7 (see Table 4.5, p. 190). This scoring system can be used to evaluate fictional stories and stories depicting personal experiences but not script narratives.

The story grammar scoring system identifies the elements that must be present for a complete story: title, introduction, main characters, supporting characters, conflict, cohesion, resolution, conclusion, and listener awareness (see Table 4.6). According to this system, a narrative can fall into one of three categories: (1) *proficient,* meaning that the child demonstrates proficient use of all the elements of the story; (2) *emerging,* meaning that the child demonstrates emerging or inconsistent use of the story grammar

Table 4.5 Applebee's Six Levels of Narrative Development

Narrative Stage	Age of Emergence	Description
Heaps	2 years	Few links from one sentence to another.
Sequences	2–3 years	Superficial but arbitrary sequence in time, no causal links between events.
Primitive narratives	3–4 years	Concrete core, surrounded by a set of complementary attributes that amplify and clarify it.
Unfocused chains	4–4 years, 6 months	Incidents leading directly from one to another, but attributes that link them shift.
Focused chains	5 years	The center is a main character who experience a series of events, but nothing abstract to indicate a true concept.
True narratives	5–7 years	Stories begin to have a theme or moral.

From *Language Sample Analysis II: The Wisconsin Guide–Revised,* by J. F. Miller, S. Long, N. McKinley, S. Thormann, M. A. Jones, & A. Nockerts, 2005, Milwaukee, WI: Wisconsin Department of Public Instruction.

elements and requires prompts from the speech-language pathologist; or (3) *immature or minimal*, meaning that the child demonstrates immature use of the story grammar elements by leaving out some elements or revealing no awareness of the category. A score of 5 is assigned to any element in which the child demonstrates proficient use; a score of 3 is assigned to any element in which the child demonstrates emerging use; and a score of 1 is assigned to any element in which the child demonstrates minimal or no use. A score of 50 is the maximum a child can receive in this analysis.

Another type of assessment that can be used to assess the language skills of a preschooler is **transdisciplinary play-based assessment** (Linder, 2005). This type is advantageous in that it allows the assessment of not only language and communication skills but also social-emotional, cognitive, and sensory-motor abilities. As suggested by its name, the assessment is implemented by a team that includes the child's parents and professionals from various disciplines (i.e., speech-language pathologists, occupational therapists, physical therapists, psychologists, etc.). The context of the assessment is play activities that vary depending on the child and the areas being evaluated.

Transdisciplinary play-based assessment is a natural and dynamic process that follows the child's attentional needs. It is less stressful and demanding compared to other assessment tools (e.g., standardized tests), which is helpful when assessing the language abilities of children exhibiting language impairments secondary to other disorders, such as autism spectrum disorder (ASD) and mental retardation (MR), as well as children from bilingual homes. Information gathered during play-based assessment is very useful in developing treatment goals and assessing treatment

Table 4.6   **Story Grammar Categories**

Characteristic	Proficient	Emerging	Minimal/Immature
Title	Title stated without prompt.	Title stated after prompt or student attempts to give title but can't recall it.	Launches into story; no attempt to state title.
Introduction to story	Setting and story theme stated.	Setting or theme stated.	Launches into story with no attempt to provide setting or story theme.
Main character(s)	Main character(s) introduced to listener by name and relationship to others; physical description or personality traits provided.	Main character(s) referred to by name, relationship, or description. Minimal character information provided.	Main character(s) predominantly referred to by pronouns. No attempt to refer to character(s) by name, relationship, or description.
Supporting character(s)	Same as main character(s).	Same as main character(s).	Same as main character(s).
Referencing	Consistent use of specific referents; cues into listener's awareness of who is talked about.	Inconsistent use of specific referents. Nonverbal clarifiers used. Able to clarify when asked by the listener.	Use of excessive pronouns. No verbal clarifiers/cues. Unaware that the listener is confused. May not be able to respond to listener's request for clarification.
Conflict	Includes rationale for character's behavior. Provides the relationship connecting event and actions.	Vague or incomplete rationale for the character's behavior. Makes statements reflecting confusion regarding the story conflict, e.g., "I don't know why it happened." Provides a series of unconnected events.	Story is missing critical events. No rationale for character's behaviors. No attempt to provide a relationship connecting events and actions.
Cohesion	Events follow a logical order. Critical events are included and minor events ignored. Smooth transitions provided between events.	Events follow a logical order. Both critical and minor events are given equal importance. Inconsistent provisions of transitions between events.	Events are provided in random order. Minimal or no connection between events. Transitions between events are lacking.

Characteristic	Proficient	Emerging	Minimal/Immature
Resolution	Clear resolution regarding character, conflicts, and events.	Some resolution provided for characters, conflicts, and events.	No resolution provided.
Conclusion	Smooth transition to conclusion. Might provide insight into the character's feelings or effects of the ending.	Abruptly states, "The end—that's all."	Stops talking and the listener may need to ask if that is the end.
Listener awareness	Provides listener(s) with appropriate or adequate background information throughout the story. Provides connected information between characters, settings, and events.	Relies on the listener(s) to provide verbal or nonverbal cues for clarification. Excessive use of rising intonation.	Presupposes shared listener knowledge. Fails to recognize nonverbal or verbal cues indicating a lack of understanding.
Total (50 possible points)	Number___ × 5= _____	Number___ × 5= _____	Number___ × 5= _____

From *Rubric for Completing a Story Grammar Analysis,* by M. A. Jones and C. Lodholz, 1999, Madison, WI: Madison Metropolitan School District.

progress, especially in the areas of pragmatics and discourse, which standardized measures usually neglect.

Although this chapter is dedicated to the assessment and treatment of primary language impairments in preschoolers, the assessment methods just discussed and the treatment procedures discussed in the next section can also be used to treat the language impairments of children exhibiting language impairments secondary to other disorders, such as ASD, MR, attention-deficit hyperactivity disorder (ADHD), and others.

Intervention for Preschool Language Impairment

The development of treatment programs for preschool-age children with SLI is a complex process that depends much on the severity of the impairment. Preschool-age children exhibiting language impairment may have difficulties in more than one area of language, may have difficulties attending to an activity for extended periods of time, and may have additional social-communicative difficulties that need to be addressed when constructing a remediation plan. In addition, other developmental skills necessary for impending academic demands (e.g., phonological awareness skills) may need to be targeted. When developing a treatment program, the speech-language pathologist must keep in mind the facilitative techniques and treatment programs available to target specific areas of language.

FACILITATIVE TECHNIQUES

To better understand how to treat various language deficits, it is necessary to understand the terminology used to describe intervention strategies. These facilitative techniques are employed with a variety of populations and are not limited to children with SLI. In addition, these techniques can be modified for children from toddlerhood through the school-age years.

Modeling is a technique in which the targeted linguistic form or behavior is presented to the child by the speech-language pathologist (Leonard, 1975). Modeling a particular form for the child allows him or her to hear the appropriate target in a naturalistic context. This technique can be used in a variety of ways. For example, while playing with a child, the SLP can hold a toy doll and act out the action of jumping. An example of a verbal model for the present progressive -*ing* form would be "The boy is jumping!" The correct sentence form is provided for a child while the visual cue of the act of jumping is provided.

Modeling can be carried a step further in a more conversational context by using techniques called **expansion** and **recasting.** Both are used when a child incorrectly produces a particular linguistic form; the SLP then reinforces the interaction by repeating the child's utterance but with the grammatical and semantically appropriate forms (Camarata, Nelson, & Camarata, 1994; Nelson, Camarata, Welsh, Butkowsky, & Camarata, 1996). The difference between the two techniques is that in recasting, the SLP can change the type of utterance—for example, from a statement to a question—or change the voice or mood in which the utterance is being produced.

The following exchange demonstrates the use of modeling, expansion, and recasting:

SLP: Look at the boy. The boy is jumping! (Modeling)

Child: Boy jump.

SLP: Yes, the boy is jumping. (Expansion)

Child: Jumping.

SLP: The boy is jumping, right? (Recasting)

Enhanced milieu teaching is a method of intervention that employs language facilitating techniques in a naturalistic, conversation-like context (Kaiser, 2000; Kaiser & Hester, 1994). This form of intervention focuses on four types of teaching strategies:

1. *Modeling*—Linguistic models are provided by the SLP or caregiver.
2. *Mand-model procedure*—The SLP mands (explicitly directs, "Tell me what this

is") or provides the child with a choice ("Is the ball red or blue?"). A model is provided by the therapist or caregiver.

3. *Time delay procedure*—Anticipating a child's needs or desires, the SLP intentionally waits until the child initiates a request for a toy or assistance with an activity.

4. *Incidental teaching procedure*—This is similar to facilitative play, in which toys are strategically placed to elicit specific linguistic or communicative forms. Modeling, manding, and time delay are employed to encourage language use.

Often contrasted to the more naturalistic modeling techniques are forms of **elicitation** or **imitative techniques** (Connell, 1987; Haley, Camarata, & Nelson, 1994; Nelson et al., 1996). Nelson et al. (1996) described their procedure for eliciting a response from a child as follows: (1) the child receives a visual prompt, such as a picture or a toy, that provides him or her with an incentive to verbalize; (2) a verbal model is provided, such as "The boy is running;" (3) the child is specifically asked to imitate the target, such as "Say 'The boy is running;'" and finally, (4) the child's response is reinforced by verbal praise or a token.

Studies that contrasted this technique with more naturalistic, conversation-based techniques found that techniques such as recasting, which serve as a more indirect method of eliciting language, have more favorable outcomes. Children appear to produce more spontaneous language and generalize faster in more naturalistic-based approaches (Haley et al., 1994; Nelson et al., 1996). These approaches do not typically require children to respond and are based on the premise that children will be bombarded with the correct linguistic form and will independently produce it when they are ready to.

Most studies comparing naturalistic and imitative techniques have demonstrated improvement over time (Connell & Stone, 1994). However, there are differences in how children's language skills improve. Imitative techniques result in more frequent and an overall faster rate of use of target forms compared to basic modeling procedures (Kouri, 2005). In a treatment efficacy study examining social skills in children with SLI (Haley et al., 1994), improvement was noted for all participating children regardless of the intervention type: imitation based or conversation based (i.e., modeling, conversational recasting, expansion). The central difference noted was the greater amount of spontaneous language and active participation from the children in the conversation-based group. These children appeared more engaged and generally happier during the intervention. In contrast, the children receiving the imitative intervention were quieter and more passive throughout the sessions.

Despite the criticism of imitative techniques, they should be incorporated into the intervention process for several reasons. Doing so does not appear to limit a child's vocalizations or hinder his or her progress. To the contrary, the effectiveness of this strategy is supported by empirical evidence. Researchers who have supported naturalistic-based interventions have also stressed the significance of imitative approaches (Fey, Long, & Finestack, 2003). Using these approaches allows the SLP to ensure that the child is attending to an activity by repeating the target forms and lets him or her practice producing forms that may be phonologically difficult. Fey et al. (2003) argued that using imitation methods does not mean that language can be acquired solely in this manner but that this approach is an important part of the intervention process. Children acquire language and generalize new information better with naturalistic forms of intervention, but imitative elicitation is an integral part of increasing their awareness to linguistic targets.

TREATMENT PROGRAMS

The facilitative techniques reviewed in the previous section can be incorporated into a session in a variety of ways. Some of the methods of incorporation involve indirect language facilitation, as seen in more naturalistic and play-based interventions, whereas others involve more direct instructions, in which the target is explicitly taught and elicited. The following play-based activities can be used in children with minimal language skills and can be modified for those with more productive and receptive language skills:

1. *Facilitative play/indirect language stimulation:* Language is facilitated by using toys or objects that draw the child's interest. Toys can be manipulated throughout the session to facilitate language and establish joint attention and play skills. This method is child guided in that the child's skill level will dictate how objects and toys will be used during the session. For example, for a child who has a limited attention span, limited eye contact, or limited productive language, the toy can be placed in front of him or her. The SLP will typically wait until the child's attention is drawn to the object or the child initiates eye contact, signaling interest in play. To facilitate requesting, a desired item is placed out of reach and when the child points or reaches for the object, a verbal model of a request is provided. To increase joint attention during play, parallel play is often used. In parallel play the SLP plays alongside the child while imitating his or her actions. Additionally, the SLP can provide verbal models describing the child's actions (parallel talk) or models describing his or her own actions (self talk).

2. *Scripted play:* During a scripted play routine, the child and the SLP enact a play routine based on common scripts the child may already be familiar with. These can range from daily routines, such as a morning routine (waking up, brushing teeth, eating breakfast, etc.), to special occasion scripts, such as planning a birthday party. Scripted play can be used to work on a variety of linguistic areas, including increasing vocabulary and grammatical morphology (e.g., verb tensing), as well as higher-level executive functions, such as planning (e.g., "Let's make a list of what we'll need for our party"), attention, and recall of events.

3. *Focused stimulation:* This approach bombards the child with the target form in a variety of contexts. The therapy session employs materials that will encourage spontaneous productions of target forms following the SLP's repeated models. For example, when targeting word-initial bilabial stops (i.e., /p/ or /b/), the modeled repertoire may sound like this:

> *SLP:* Let's *b*low *b*ubbles. Look at the *b*ig *b*ubble. I'm going to pop the *b*ig *b*ubble. Do you want to *b*low a *b*ubble?

In this example, bilabial stops are provided to the child in several ways and the environment and activity are set up in a way that will encourage his or her production.

ADDITIONAL CONSIDERATIONS

While monitoring the progress of intervention during a single session or over the course of several sessions, these elements should be considered to establish goals and assess progress:

1. *Frequency of presentation*—Children with language impairment frequently require repetition to acquire new target forms (Childers & Tomasello, 2002). A particular form may need to be repeated several times and in various contexts before it is fully acquired. The necessary frequency of presentation may vary from child to child and should be monitored accordingly. Although a child may appear to demonstrate some improvement on a goal within a single session, true mastery typically is achieved over the course of several sessions (Riches et al., 2005).

2. *Spacing of presentation of target items*—Children with SLI perform best when appropriate time is allowed between presentations of target items. These children may require more time to process and formulate their thoughts than typically developing children.

3. *Prompts/cues required to achieve a target*—In addition to verbal instruction or modeling, children with SLI may require additional cueing. Cues can be provided visually (e.g., through a picture/toy, with or without the SLP pointing directly to it), verbally (e.g., using verbal prompts, "Look at my mouth"), or through tactile cues (e.g., hand-over-hand assistance). As a child begins to demonstrate improvement over the course of a session, the cues are faded (i.e., reduced in frequency).

PRE-ACADEMIC SKILLS

In addition to targeting form, content, and use when planning intervention goals, the SLP needs to keep in mind the academic demands the child will encounter upon entering school. Many preschoolers with SLI are at risk for pervasive language-based learning problems during the school years; thus, it is important to address pre-academic skills early on. Significant areas include preliteracy skills and early reading comprehension skills.

As noted earlier, phonological awareness is a precursor for later reading ability. Phonological awareness refers to the knowledge that words are constructed of smaller units (syllables and phonemes) and that the addition, deletion, or substitution of a phoneme can cause a change in meaning. The following phonological awareness activities can be used with a preschooler with SLI (Catts, 1991):

1. *Rhyming*—Rhyming can be targeted through a word play game of creating rhymes and identifying rhymes in songs or nursery rhymes.
2. *Syllable tapping*—The child is asked to tap out and identify the number of syllables in a word.
3. *Sound manipulation*—The child plays games that require him or her to add, subtract, or substitute a sound in order to create a new word.
4. *Blending*—The child can blend individual sounds/syllables to create new words.

Another method for increasing pre-academic skills is joint storybook reading (Fey, Catts, & Larrivee, 1995). As the SLP and child engage in a book reading activity, the

SLP uses some of the language facilitation techniques mentioned previously to enhance language comprehension and production. The SLP can encourage language production by using *wh-* questions, which require the child to provide detailed descriptions about the story plot. The SLP should select age- and language-appropriate books; a book for a 4-year-old may not be entirely appropriate if the child is having difficulty comprehending at that level. This method is advantageous in that it can easily be carried out by a caregiver at home.

Summary

Preschool children with SLI are a heterogeneous population that can have deficits in one or more of the five areas of language (i.e., phonology, morphology, syntax, semantics, and pragmatics). Early identification of language impairment can be challenging, as some children who appear delayed during the toddler years catch up to their peers by age 4. For children who continue to present language deficits, identification and treatment are necessary, as these difficulties can persist and affect later academic success.

To assess language impairment, both formal (standardized tests) and informal (language sample, narratives) measures can be used to provide a complete picture of a child's language level. Once a child has been identified as having language impairment, several intervention methods can be employed to facilitate language skills. These methods include naturalistic, conversation-based techniques, such as modeling, expansion, and recasting, along with more direct methods, such as eliciting imitations of target forms. Ultimately, the goal of the SLP is to correctly identify the child's language deficits and provide appropriate treatment to ensure his or her success in communication and later academic development.

Case Study **Preschool Language Impairment**

Mark was 4 years, 2 months old when first referred for a speech and language evaluation to address his unintelligible speech. Mark's mother reported that the prenatal and birth history were unremarkable and that Mark's developmental milestones were attained within normal age ranges. She reported that Mark said his first words around 12 months of age and used short sentences around 2½ years of age.

The speech-language pathologist informally assessed Mark's language performance by collecting a language sample of 100 utterances. Analysis of Mark's language sample revealed that his mean length of utterance (MLU) was 3.68, which falls within the normal range (3.46–5.34) for his age. However, morphological analysis revealed inconsistent use of several grammatical morphemes that should have been mastered by Mark's age: present progressive (-*ing*), plural (-*s*), possessive ('*s*), uncontractible copula (*is, was*), prepositions (*in, on*), articles (*a, the*), and contractible copula and auxiliary (*that's, they're*). Mark's sentences were judged to be simple and short, containing few adjectives and adverbs and no embedded phrases or clauses, and he used no compound sentences.

Approximately 25 percent of Mark's utterances were unintelligible. Phonological analysis revealed the use of the following phonological processes: consonant cluster reduction, final consonant deletion, fronting, and gliding. Semantic analysis revealed an impoverished lexicon with limited use of different word classes (i.e., adverbs, adjectives, and verbs) and a small nominal vocabulary. Mark often used nonspecific words (e.g., *this, that, over there*) to describe objects, actions, and locations, which was characteristic of his limited lexicon and word-finding deficit. Mark's pragmatic skills appeared to be typical for his age. He demonstrated eye contact, turn taking, joint attention, and joint action. He enjoyed playing with the SLP and was able to attend to the activities for the 45-minute session.

Formal assessment revealed significant deficits in both receptive and expressive language abilities. The CELF Preschool was administered to evaluate Mark's language skills. He scored one standard deviation below the age-expected mean on the receptive portion of the CELF and two standard deviations below the age-expected mean on the expressive portion of the CELF.

The SLP recommended that Mark receive speech and language services twice a week that would focus on increasing speech intelligibility and improving receptive and expressive language skills. More specifically, the SLP recommended targeting correct and consistent use of grammatical morphemes, expansion of vocabulary size and decrease usage of nonspecific words, increased complexity and length of sentences, and decreased use of phonological processes.

Study Questions

1. What two clinical markers can help differentiate between late bloomers and late talkers?
2. Describe some of the limitations children with SLI exhibit in language form, content, and use.
3. Collect narrative samples from a preschooler once using story generation and then again using story retelling. Analyze the samples using the story grammar scoring system, and compare and contrast the results from the two procedures.
4. Describe some of the facilitative treatment techniques used with preschoolers exhibiting SLI.

References

Acredolo, L., & Goodwyn, S. (1988). Symbolic gesturing in normal infants. *Human Development, 28*, 40–49.

Alt, M., & Plante, E. (2006). Factors that influence lexical and semantic fast mapping of young children with specific language impairment. *Journal of Speech, Language, and Hearing Research, 49,* 941–954.

Archibald, L. M. D., & Gathercole, S. E. (2006). Short-term and working memory in specific language impairment. *International Journal of Language and Communication Disorders, 41,* 675–693.

Bates, E., Bretherton, I., & Snyder, L. (1988). *From first words to grammar: Individual differences and dissociable mechanisms.* Cambridge, MA: Cambridge University Press.

Bedore, L., & Leonard, L. (1998). Specific language impairment and grammatical morphology: A discriminant function analysis. *Journal of Speech, Language, and Hearing Research, 41,* 1185–1192.

Blank, M., Rose, S. A., & Berlin, L. J. (1978). *Preschool Language Assessment Instrument.* Austin: Pro-Ed.

Brinton, B., & Fujiki, M. (1982). A comparison of request response sequences in the discourse of normal and language disordered children. *Journal of Speech and Hearing Disorders, 47,* 57–62.

Brinton, B., Fujiki, M., Winkler, E., & Loeb, D. (1986). Responses to requests for clarification in linguistically normal and language-impaired children. *Journal of Speech and Hearing Disorders, 51,* 370–378.

Brown, R. (1973). *A first language: The early stages.* Cambridge, MA: Harvard University Press.

Camarata, S., Nelson, K., & Camarata, M. (1994). Comparison of conversational-recasting and imitative procedures for training grammatical structures in children with specific language impairment. *Journal of Speech and Hearing Research, 37,* 1414–1423.

Capirci, O., Iverson, J., Pizzuto, E., & Volterra, V. (1996). Gestures and words during the transition to two word speech. *Journal of Child Language, 23,* 645–673.

Capone, N., & McGregor, K. (2004). Gesture development: A review for clinical and research practices. *Journal of Speech, Language, and Hearing Research, 47,* 173–186.

Carey, S., & Bartlett, E. (1978). Acquiring a new single word. *Papers and Reports on Child Language Development, 15,* 17–29.

Carrow-Woolfolk, E. (1999). *CASL: Comprehensive Assessment of Spoken Language.* Circle Pines, MN: American Guidance Service.

Caselli, M. (1990). Communicative gestures and first words. In V. Volterra & J. Erting (Eds.), *From gesture to sign in hearing and deaf children* (pp. 56–67). New York: Springer-Verlag.

Catts, H. W. (1991). Facilitating phonological awareness: Role of speech-language pathologists. *Language, Speech, and Hearing Services in Schools, 22,* 196–203.

Childers, J., & Tomasello, M. (2002). Two-year-olds learn novel nouns, verbs, and conventional actions from massed or distributed exposures. *Developmental Psychology, 38,* 967–978.

Connell, P. (1987). An effect of modeling and imitation teaching procedures on children with and without specific language impairment. *Journal of Speech and Hearing Research, 30,* 105–113.

Connell, P., & Stone, C. (1992). Morpheme learning of children with specific language impairment under controlled instructional conditions. *Journal of Speech and Hearing Research, 35,* 844–852.

Conti-Ramsden, G. (2003). Processing and linguistic markers in young children with specific language impairment (SLI). *Journal of Speech, Language, and Hearing Research, 46,* 1029–1037.

Conti-Ramsden, G., & Botting, N. (1999). Classification of children with specific language impairment: Longitudinal considerations. *Journal of Speech, Language, and Hearing Research, 42,* 1195–1204.

Conti-Ramsden, G., & Jones, M. (1997). Verb use in specific language impairment. *Journal of Speech, Language, and Hearing Research, 40,* 1298–1313.

Conti-Ramsden, G., Crutchley, A., & Botting, N. (1997). The extent to which psychometric tests differentiate subgroups of children with SLI. *Journal of Speech, Language, and Hearing Research, 40,* 765–777.

Dollaghan, C. (1985). "Fast mapping" in preschool children. *Journal of Speech and Hearing Research, 28,* 449–454.

Dollaghan, C. (1987). Fast mapping in normal and language-impaired children. *Journal of Speech and Hearing Disorders, 52*(3), 218–222.

Dollaghan, C., & Campbell, T. F. (1998). Nonword repetition and child language impairment. *Journal of Speech, Language, and Hearing Research, 41,* 1136–1146.

Dunn, L., & Dunn, L. (1997). *Peabody Picture Vocabulary Test—Third Edition.* Circle Pines, MN: American Guidance Service.

Edmonston, N. K., & Litchfield Thane, N. (1992). Children's use of comprehension strategies in response to relational words: Implications for assessment. *American Journal of Speech-Language Pathology, 1,* 30–35.

Edwards, J., & Lahey, M. (1998). Nonword repetitions of children with specific language impairment: Exploration of some explanations for their inaccuracies. *Applied Psycholinguistics, 19*(2), 279–309.

Faust, M., Dimitrovsky, L., & Davidi, S. (1997). Naming difficulties in language-disabled children: Preliminary findings with the application of the tip-of-the-tongue paradigm. *Journal of Speech, Language, and Hearing Research, 40,* 1037–1047.

Fazio, B. B. (1997). Learning a new poem: Memory for connected speech and phonological awareness in low-income children with and without specific language impairment. *Journal of Speech, Language, and Hearing Research, 40,* 1285–1297.

Fey, M., Catts, H., & Larivee, L. (1995). Preparing preschoolers for the academic and social challenges of school. In M. Fey, J. Windsor, S. Warren (Eds.), *Language intervention: Preschool through the elementary years.* Baltimore, MD: Paul H. Brookes.

Fey, M., Long, S., & Finestack, L. (2003). Ten principles of grammar facilitation for children with specific language impairment. *American Journal of Speech-Language Pathology, 12,* 3–15.

Fujiki, M., Brinton, B., & Sonnenberg, E. A. (1990). Repair of overlapping speech in the conversations of specifically language-impaired and normally developing children. *Applied Psycholinguistics, 11,* 201–215.

Gardner, M. (2000). *Expressive One-Word Picture Vocabulary Test—Revised.* Circle Pines, MN: American Guidance Services.

Gathercole, S., & Baddeley, A. (1990). Phonological memory deficits in language disordered children: Is there a causal connection? *Journal of Memory and Language, 29,* 336–360.

Gathercole, S. E., & Baddeley, A. D. (1995). Short-term memory may yet be deficient in children with language impairments: A comment on van der Lely & Howard (1993). *Journal of Speech, Language, and Hearing Sciences, 38,* 463–472.

Gathercole, S. E., Willis, C. S., Baddeley, A. D., & Emslie, H. (1994). The Children's Test of Nonword Repetition: A test of phonological working memory. *Memory, 2*(2), 103–127.

German, D. J. (1987). Spontaneous language profiles of children with word-finding problems. *Language, Speech, and Hearing Services in Schools, 18,* 217–230.

German, D. J., & Simon, E. (1991). Analysis of children's word-finding skills in discourse. *Journal of Speech and Hearing Research, 34,* 309–316.

Gillam, R. B., & Johnston, J. R. (1992). Spoken and written language relationships in language/learning impaired and normally achieving school-aged children. *Journal of Speech and Hearing Research, 35,* 1303–1315.

Goldsworthy, C. (1982). *Multilevel Informal Language Inventory.* San Antonio: Harcourt Brace Jovanovich.

Golinkoff, R. M., Hirsh-Pasek, K., Bailey, L. M., & Wenger, N. R. (1992). Young children and adults use lexical principles to learn new nouns. *Developmental Psychology, 28,* 99–108.

Gray, S. (2003). Word learning by preschoolers with specific language impairment: What predicts success. *Journal of Speech, Language, and Hearing Research, 46,* 56–67.

Gray, S. (2004). Word learning by preschoolers with specific language impairment: Predictors and poor learners. *Journal of Speech, Language, and Hearing Research, 47,* 1117–1132.

Gray, S. (2005). Word learning by preschoolers with specific language impairment: Affect of phonological or semantic cues. *Journal of Speech, Language, and Hearing Research, 48,* 1452–1467.

Gray, S. (2006). The relationship between phonological memory, receptive vocabulary, and fast mapping in young children with specific language impairment. *Journal of Speech, Language, and Hearing Research, 49,* 955–969.

Hadley, P. A., & Rice, M. L. (1991). Conversational responsiveness of speech-and language-impaired preschoolers. *Journal of Speech and Hearing Research, 34,* 1308–1317.

Hadley, P. A., & Short, H. (2005). The onset of tense marking in children at risk for specific language impairment. *Journal of Speech, Language, and Hearing Research, 48,* 1344–1362.

Haley, K., Camarata, S., & Nelson, K. (1994). Social valence in children with specific language impairment during imitation-based and conversation-based language intervention. *Journal of Speech and Hearing Research, 37,* 378–388.

Hanauer, J. B., & Brooks, P. J. (2005). Contributions of response set and semantic relatedness to cross-modal stroop-like picture-word interference in children and adults. *Journal of Experimental Child Psychology, 90,* 21–47.

Hedrick, P., Prather, E., & Tobin, R. (1984). *Sequenced Inventory of Communication Development, Revised.* Los Angeles, CA: Western Psychological Services.

Hesketh, A. (2004). Grammatical performance of children with language disorder on structured elicitation and narrative tasks. *Clinical Linguistics and Phonetics, 18,* 161–182.

Hodson, B. (1986). *The assessment of phonological processes-Revised.* Austin: Pro-Ed.

Im-Bolter, N., Johnson, J., & Pascual-Leone, J. (2006). Processing limitations in children with specific language impairment: The role of executive function. *Child Development, 77,* 1822–1841.

Ingram, D. (1981). *Procedures for the phonological analysis of children's language.* Baltimore, MD: University Park Press.

Jones, M. A., & Lodholz, C. (1999). *Rubric for completing a story grammar analysis.* Madison, WI: Madison Metropolitan School District.

Kaiser, A. (2000). Teaching functional communication skills. In M. E. Snell & F. Brown (Eds.), *Instruction of students with severe disabilities* (5th ed., pp. 453–492). Upper Saddle River, NJ: Merrill/Prentice Hall.

Kaiser, A., & Hester, P. (1994). Generalized effects of enhanced milieu teaching. *Journal of Speech and Hearing Research, 37,* 1320–1340.

Kouri, T. A. (2005). Lexical training through modeling and elicitation procedures with late talkers who have specific language impairment and developmental delays. *Journal of Speech, Language, and Hearing Research, 48,* 157–171.

Lahey, M., & Edwards, J. (1999). Naming errors of children with specific language impairment. *Journal of Speech, Language, and Hearing Research, 42,* 195–205.

Leonard, L. (1975). Modeling as a clinical procedure in language training. *Language, Speech, and Hearing Services in Schools, 6,* 72–85.

Leonard, L. (1982). Phonological deficits in children with developmental language impairment. *Brain and Language, 16,* 73–86.

Leonard, L. (1998). *Children with specific language impairment.* Cambridge, MA: MIT Press.

Leonard, L., Eyer, J., Bedore, L., & Grela, B. (1997). Three accounts of the grammatical morpheme difficulties of English-speaking children with specific language impairment. *Journal of Speech and Hearing Research, 40,* 741–753.

Liles, B. Z. (1985a). Narrative ability in normal and language disordered children. *Journal of Speech and Hearing Research, 28,* 123–133.

Liles, B. Z. (1985b). Production and comprehension of narrative discourse in normal and language disordered children. *Journal of Communication Disorders, 18,* 409–427.

Liles, B. Z. (1987). Episode organization and cohesive conjunctives in narratives of children with and without language disorders. *Journal of Speech and Hearing Research, 30,* 185–196.

Liles, B. Z., Duffy, R. J., Merritt, D. D., & Purcell, S. L. (1995). Measurement of narrative discourse ability in children with language disorders. *Journal of Speech and Hearing Research, 38,* 415–425.

Linder, T. W. (2005). *Transdisciplinary play-based assessment: A functional approach to working with young children* (Rev. ed.). Baltimore, MD: Paul H. Brookes.

Maillart, C., Schelstraete, M., & Hupert, M. (2004). Phonological representations in children with SLI: A study of French. *Journal of Speech Language and Hearing Research, 47,* 187–198.

Mann, V., & Liberman, I. (1984). Phonological awareness and verbal short-term memory: Can they presage early reading problems? *Journal of Learning Disabilities, 17,* 592–599.

Marton, K., & Schwartz, G. R. (2003). Working memory capacity and language processes in children with specific language impairment. *Journal of Speech Language and Hearing Research, 46,* 1138–1153.

Marton, K., Schwartz, G. R., Farkas, L., & Katsnelsor, V. (2006). Effect of sentence length and complexity on working memory performance in Hungarian children with specific language impairment (SLI): A cross-linguistic comparison. *International Journal of Language and Communication Disorders, 41,* 653–673.

McGregor, K. K. (1997). The nature of word-finding errors of preschoolers with and without word finding deficits. *Journal of Speech and Hearing Research, 40,* 1232–1244.

McGregor, K. K., Friedman, R. M., Reilly, R. M., & Newman, R. M. (2002). Semantic representation and naming in young children. *Journal of Speech, Language, and Hearing Research, 45,* 332–346.

McGregor, K. K., & Leonard, L. B. (1989). Facilitating word-finding skills of language-impaired children. *Journal of Speech and Hearing Disorders, 54,* 141–147.

McGregor, K. K., Newman, R. M., Reilly, R. M., & Capone, N. C. (2002). Semantic representation and naming in children with specific language impairment. *Journal of Speech, Language, and Hearing Research, 45,* 998–1014.

McGregor, K. K., & Waxman, S. R. (1998). Object naming at multiple hierarchical levels: A comparison of preschoolers with and without word-finding deficits. *Journal of Child Language, 25,* 419–430.

Merritt, D. D., & Liles, B. Z. (1989). Narrative analysis: Clinical applications of story generation and story retelling. *Journal of Speech and Hearing Disorders, 54,* 429–438.

Miller, J. (1981). *Assessing language production in children.* Baltimore, MD: University Park Press.

Miller, J. F., Long, S., McKinley, N. Thormann, S., Jones, M. A., & Nockerts, A. (2005). *Language sample analysis II: The Wisconsin guide* (Rev. ed.). Milwaukee, WI: Wisconsin Department of Public Instruction.

Montgomery, J. W. (1995). Sentence comprehension in children with specific language impairment: The role of phonological working memory. *Journal of Speech, Language, and Hearing Research, 38,* 187–199.

Montgomery, J. W. (2002). Understanding the language difficulties of children with specific language impairments: Does verbal working memory matter? *American Journal of Speech Language Pathology, 11,* 77–91.

Montgomery, J. W. (2003). Working memory and comprehension in children with specific language impairment: What we know so far. *Journal of Communication Disorders, 36,* 221–231.

Moore, M. E. (1995). Error analysis of pronouns by normal and language-impaired children. *Journal of Communication Disorders, 28,* 57–72.

Moore, M. E. (2001). Third person pronoun errors by children with and without language impairment. *Journal of Communication Disorders, 34,* 207–228.

Nash, M., & Donaldson, M. L. (2005). Word learning in children with vocabulary deficits. *Journal of Speech, Language, and Hearing Research, 48,* 439–458.

Nelson, K. (1973). Structure and strategy in learning to talk. *Monographs of the Society for Research in Child Development, 38*(1–2), 1–135.

Nelson, K., Camarata, S., Welsh, J., Butkowsky, L., & Camarata, M. (1996). Effects of imitative and conversational recasting treatment on the acquisition of grammar in children with specific language impairment and younger language-normal children. *Journal of Speech, Language, and Hearing Research, 39,* 850–859.

Newbury, D. F., Bishop, D. M. V., & Monaco, A. P. (2005). Genetic influences on language impairment and phonological short-term memory. *Trends in Cognitive Sciences, 9,* 528–534.

Newcomer, P., & Hammill, D. (1997). *Test of Language Development 3: Primary.* Austin, TX: Pro-Ed.

Norbury, C. F., Bishop, D. V. M., & Briscoe, J. (2001). Production of English finite verb morphology: A comparison of SLI and mild-moderate hearing impairment. *Journal of Speech Language and Hearing Research, 44,* 165–178.

Owens, R. (2005). *Language development: An introduction* (6th ed.). Boston: Allyn & Bacon.

Paul, R. (1991). Profiles of toddlers with slow expressive language growth. *Topics in Language Disorders, 11,* 1–13.

Paul, R. (1993). Patterns of development in late talkers: Preschool years. *Journal of Childhood Communication Disorders, 15,* 7–14.

Paul, R. (1995). *Language disorders from infancy through adolescence: Assessment and intervention.* St. Louis, MO: Mosby-Year Book.

Paul, R. (1996). Clinical implications of the natural history of slow expressive language development. *American Journal of Speech-Language Pathology, 5,* 5–21.

Paul, R., & Alforde, S., (1993). Grammatical morpheme acquisition in 4-year-olds with normal, impaired, and late developing language. *Journal of Speech and Hearing Research, 36,* 1271–1275.

Paul, R., & Jennings, P. (1992). Phonological behavior in toddlers with slow expressive language development. *Journal of Speech and Hearing Research, 35,* 99–107.

Paul, R., & Smith, R. L. (1993). Narrative skills in 4-year-olds with normal, impaired, and late-developing language. *Journal of Speech and Hearing Research, 36,* 592–598.

Rapin, I., & Wilson, B. (1978). Children with developmental language disability. Neurological aspects and assessment. In M. Wyke (Ed.), *Developmental dysphasia* (pp. 13–41). New York: Academic Press.

Rescorla, L. (1989). The language development survey: A screening tool for delayed language in toddlers. *Journal of Speech and Hearing Disorders, 54,* 587–599.

Rescorla, L. (2000). Do late talkers turn out to have reading difficulties a decade later? *Annals of Dyslexia, 50,* 87–102.

Rescorla, L. (2002). Language and reading outcomes to age 9 in late-talking toddlers. *Journal of Speech, Language, and Hearing Research, 45,* 360–371.

Rescorla, L., Dahslgaard, K., & Roberts, J. (2000). Late-talking toddlers: MLU and IPSyn outcomes at 3;0 and 4;0. *Journal of Child Language, 27,* 643–664.

Rescorla, L., & Lee, E. C. (2000). Language impairments in young children. In T. Layton, E. Crais, & L. Watson (Eds.), *Handbook of early language impairment in children, Vol. I: Nature* (pp. 1–38). New York: Delmar.

Rescorla, L., Mirak, J., & Singh, L. (2000). Vocabulary growth in late talkers: Lexical development from 2;0 to 3;0. *Journal of Child Language, 27,* 293–311.

Rescorla, L., & Ratner, N. B. (1996). Phonetic profiles of typically developing and language-delayed toddlers. *Journal of Speech and Hearing Research, 39,* 153–165.

Rescorla, L., & Roberts, J. (1997). Late-talkers at 2: Outcomes at age 3. *Journal of Speech and Hearing Research, 40,* 556–566.

Rescorla, L., & Roberts, J. (2002). Nominal versus verbal morpheme use in late talkers at ages 3 and 4. *Journal of Speech, Language, and Hearing Research, 45,* 1219–1231.

Rescorla, L., & Schwartz, E. (1990). Outcome of toddlers with expressive language delay. *Applied Psycholinguistics, 11,* 393–407.

Rice, M. L. (2000). Grammatical symptoms of specific language impairment. In D. V. M. Bishop & L. B. Leonard (Eds.), *Speech and language impairments in children: Causes, characteristics, intervention and outcome.* Hove, UK: Psychology Press.

Rice, M. L., & Bode, J. V. (1993). Gaps in the verb lexicons of children with specific language impairment. *First Language, 13,* 113–131.

Rice, M. L., Buhr, J., & Nemeth, J. (1990). Fast mapping word learning abilities of language delayed preschoolers. *Journal of Speech and Hearing Disorders, 55,* 33–42.

Rice, M. L., Buhr, J. A., & Oetting, J. B. (1992). Specific-language-impaired children's quick incidental learning of new words: The effect of a pause. *Journal of Speech, Language and Hearing Research, 35,* 1040–1048.

Rice, M. L., Oetting, J. B., Marquis, J., Bode, J., & Pae, S. (1994). Frequency of input on word comprehension of children with specific language impairment. *Journal of Speech and Hearing Research, 37,* 106–122.

Rice, M. L., Sell, M. A., & Hadley, P. A. (1991). Social interactions of speech and language impaired children. *Journal of Speech and Hearing Research, 34,* 1299–1307.

Rice, M. L., & Wexler, K. (1996). Toward tense as a clinical marker of specific language impairment in English-speaking children. *Journal of Speech and Hearing Research, 39,* 1239–1257.

Rice, M. L., Wexler, K., & Cleave, P. L. (1995). Specific language impairment as a period of extended optional infinitive. *Journal of Speech and Hearing Research, 38,* 850–863.

Riches, N. G., Tomasello, M., & Conti-Ramsden, G. (2005). Verbal learning in children with SLI: Frequency and spacing effects. *Journal of Speech, Language and Hearing Research, 48,* 1397–1411.

Roberts, J., Rescorla, L., Giroux, J., & Stevens, L. (1998). Phonological skills of children with specific expressive language impairment (SLI-E): Outcome at age 3. *Journal of Speech, Language, and Hearing Research, 41,* 374–384.

Schuele, C. M., & Dykes, J. (2005). A longitudinal study of complex syntax development in a child with specific language impairment. *Clinical Linguistics and Phonetics, 19,* 295–318.

Schuele, C. M., & Nicholls, L. M. (2000). Relative clauses: Evidence of continued linguistic vulnerability in children with specific language impairment. *Clinical Linguistics and Phonetics, 14,* 563–585.

Schuele, C. M., & Tolbert, L. (2001). Omissions of obligatory relative markers in children with specific language impairment. *Clinical Linguistics and Phonetics, 15,* 257–274.

Schwartz, R. G., Leonard, L. B., Folger, M. K., & Wilcox, M. J. (1980). Early phonological behavior in normal-speaking and language disordered children: Evidence for a synergistic view of linguistic disorders. *Journal of Speech and Hearing Disorders, 45,* 357–377.

Scott, C. M., & Windsor, J. (2000). General language performance measures in spoken and written narrative and expository discourse of school-age children with language learning disabilities. *Journal of Speech, Language, and Hearing Research, 43,* 324–339.

Stevens, C., Sanders, L., & Neville, H. (2006). Neurophysiological evidence for selective auditory attention deficits in children with specific language impairment. *Brain Research, 1111,* 143–152.

Thal, D. J., Reilly, J., Seibert, L., Jeffries, R., & Fenson, J. (2004). Language development in children at risk for language impairment: Cross-population comparisons. *Brain and Language, 88,* 167–179.

Thal, D. J., & Tobias, S. (1992). Communicative gestures in children with delayed onset of oral expressive vocabulary. *Journal of Speech and Hearing Research, 35,* 1281–1289.

Thal, D. J., Tobias, S., & Morrison, D. (1991). Language and gesture in late talkers: A 1-year follow-up. *Journal of Speech and Hearing Research, 34,* 604–612.

Thordardottir, E. T., & Weismer, E. S. (2001). High frequency verbs and verb diversity in the spontaneous speech of school-age children with specific language impairment. *International Journal of Language and Communication Disorders, 36,* 221–244.

van der Lely, H. K. J. (1998). SLI in children: Movement, economy and deficits in the computational syntactic system. *Language Acquisition, 72,* 161–192.

van der Lely, H. K. J., & Christian, V. (2000). Lexical word formation in children with grammatical SLI: A grammar-specific versus an input-processing deficit? *Cognition, 75,* 33–63.

van der Lely, H. K. J., Rosen, S., & McClelland, A. (1998). Evidence for a grammar-specific deficit in children. *Current Biology, 8,* 1253–1258.

Wagner, C. R., Nettelbladt, U., Sahlen, B., & Nilholm, C. (2000). Conversation versus narration in pre-school children with language impairment. *International Journal of Language and Communication Disorders, 35,* 83–93.

Watkins, R. V., Kelly, D. J., Harbers, H. M., & Hollis, W. (1995). Measuring children's lexical diversity: Differentiating typical and atypical learners. *Journal of Speech and Hearing Research, 39,* 1349–1355.

Watt, N., Wetherby, A., & Shumway, S. (2006). Prelinguistic predictors of language outcome at 3 years of age. *Journal of Speech, Language, and Hearing Research, 49,* 1224–1237.

Weismer, S. E., Tomblin, J. B., Zhang, X., Buckwalter, P., Chynoweth, J. G., & Jones, M. (2000). Nonword repetition performance in school-age children with and without language impairment. *Journal of Speech, Language, and Hearing Research, 43,* 865–878.

Whitehurst, G., & Fischel, J. (1994). Practitioner review: Early developmental language delay: What, if anything, should the clinician do about it? *Journal of Child Psychology and Psychiatry, 35,* 613–648.

Wiig, E. (1990). *Wiig Criterion Referenced Inventory of Language.* San Antonio, TX: The Psychological Corporation.

Wiig, E. H., Semel, E. M., & Secord, W. (2004). *CELF-Preschool: Clinical Evaluation of Language Fundamentals—Preschool.* San Antonio, TX: The Psychological Corporation.

Windfuhr, K., Faragher, B., & Conti-Ramsden, G. (2002). Lexical learning skills in young children with specific language impairment (SLI). *International Journal of Language and Communication Disorders, 37,* 415–432.

Zimmerman, I. L., Steiner, V. G., & Pond, R. E. (2002). *Preschool Language Scale: 4.* San Antonio, TX: Psychological Corp.

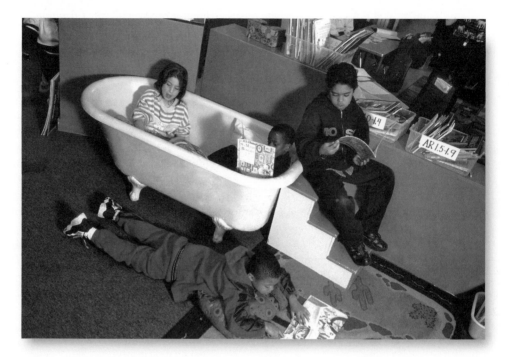

CHAPTER 5

Understanding the Nature and Scope of Language Learning Disability

Characteristics, Frameworks, and Connections

Cheryl Smith Gabig

Lehman College, City University of New York

When you finish this chapter, you should be able to

- Identify the four subgroups of children who may demonstrate academic language difficulty and could be considered as having a language learning disability.
- Distinguish four separate types of reading disability.
- Explain the difference between response-to-intervention (RtI) and use of an IQ-achievement discrepancy in the identification of children with language learning disability.
- Identify the oral language and cognitive characteristics of children with language learning disability.
- Discuss the reciprocal relationship between phonological processing and reading/spelling.

The relationship between spoken and written language is a fairly recent area of scholarly inquiry. For many years, spoken and written language were considered two separate skills, distinct from each other, and attributed to separate cognitive functions and modalities. The individual's competence or disability in oral language was viewed as unrelated to the skill or disability seen in the written domain.

In 1971, a research conference sponsored by the National Institute of Child Health and Human Development (NICHD), one of the divisions within the National Institutes of Health (NIH), explored the relationship between speech and learning to read. The aim of the conference was to understand reading as a cognitive process and to begin to formulate a psychological theory of how the mind interprets print for meaning. The conference proceedings were published in a text called *Language by Ear and by Eye* (Kavanagh & Mattingly, 1972) which emphasized the processes of speaking and listening as integral to the process of reading. As stated by Mattingly, "Speaking and listening are primary linguistic activities; reading is a secondary and rather special sort of activity that relies critically upon the reader's awareness of these primary activities"(1972, p. 133).

This important conference opened a floodgate of focused research on the relationship between spoken and written language, why some individuals have difficulty acquiring written language, and how to teach children and adults who do not or cannot read or produce a written form of language. The connection between ability in oral language and reading and writing skill is now accepted by cognitive scientists, psychologists, neuropsychologists, speech-language pathologists, and many educators.

The purpose of this chapter is to discuss those children who fail to make the connection between oral and written language forms: children with a language learning disability (LLD). Many children struggle with reading, writing, and spelling, yet they display different characteristics and can be grouped into several subtypes. For example, some children show poor auditory (listening) comprehension in the classroom during academic language tasks in addition to having poor reading, spelling, and written language skills. Other children have advanced oral language skills yet show deficits specific to reading and spelling.

Two important questions must be considered in defining LLD. The first is, does the diagnostic category apply only to children who have difficulty in both spoken (i.e., listening and speaking) and written (i.e., reading, writing, and spelling) language, or can children show deficits limited to the written language domain and thereby qualify for inclusion in the classification of LLD? The second question is, should nonverbal intelligence play a factor in identifying children as LLD?

This latter question has significant implications in light of the history of the use of an IQ–achievement discrepancy over the past thirty years to implement federal policy for identifying children with *specific learning disability*. Use of a discrepancy-based identification method has been a major influence of educational policy in the identification of specific learning disabilities in schools. This method has been criticized on theoretical grounds for its tendency to either over- or underidentify children with language impairment who are struggling with reading, spelling, and academic language in the classroom (Aram, Morris, & Hall, 1992; Cole, Mills, & Kelly, 1994; Fletcher, Coulter, Reschly, & Vaughn, 2004). Moreover, the use of an IQ–achievement discrepancy does not predict specific cognitive and language differences in low-achieving children or children with a reading disability nor does it predict how children will respond to remediation (Lyon, 1989; Siegel, 1989; Siegel & Himel, 1998).

This chapter begins with a discussion of the types of children who demonstrate academic learning difficulty, each with separate characteristic criteria. Then the discussion examines the educational policies and federal legislation that have shaped the definition and identification of a learning disability. Since oral language is the foundation for competence in academic language and literacy, the oral language and metalinguistic characteristics of children who demonstrate difficulty with these applied language areas is provided. Finally, the connection between oral and academic language is discussed as a framework for understanding the oral–written language continuum: communicating by language in both its spoken and written forms.

Definition of Language Learning Disability

Language learning disability (LLD) is a broad term used to describe a heterogeneous group of children who have difficulty with aspects of language and communication that interfere with academic performance in the classroom. The language and communication difficulty is manifested in academic areas such as reading, spelling, and writing and in the discourse demands of the classroom.

As noted, individuals with LLD are a mixed group who demonstrate considerable variation in language performance during listening, speaking, reading, spelling, and writing. There is no current consensus on a definition of LLD in the literature nor is there an agreed upon set of diagnostic criteria for classifying individuals as LLD. Rather, a number of subgroups of children who demonstrate academic language difficulty are frequently included within the LLD classification.

SPECIFIC LANGUAGE IMPAIRMENT

The most prevailing subgroup of children considered LLD are those who meet the standard clinical classifications of developmental language impairment (LI) based on impairments in the oral language system, corresponding intact nonverbal cognitive ability, and difficulty in learning to read, write, and spell. These children are typically identified as *specific language impaired (SLI)* because they demonstrate a deficit specific to the linguistic system (i.e., less than 85 standard score) yet show nonverbal abilities within the average range (i.e., greater than 85 standard score).

Various clinical markers evident in the language behavior of children with this classification have been identified, including difficulty with grammatical processing, especially tense marking (Leonard, 1998; Rice, 2003). For example, children with SLI often fail to mark the third-person present tense using the morpheme *-s* (*sit/sits*) or the past-tense morpheme *-ed* (*jump/jumped*). In addition to using verb tense as a marker for SLI, researchers have noted other markers, including deficits in phonological processing, as evidenced by poor performance on a task on nonword repetition (Bishop, North, & Dolan, 1996; Gathercole & Baddeley, 1990), and phonological memory, as evidenced by impaired ability in sentence imitation (Conti-Ramsden, Botting, & Faragher, 2001).

The presence of SLI during the preschool years places a child at risk for difficulty in learning to read (Aram & Nation, 1980; Catts, 1986, 1993; Menyuk et al., 1991; Scarborough & Dobrich, 1990). Moreover, those with persistent expressive language problems at 5½ years showed poor reading outcome at 8½ years (Bishop & Adams, 1990; Catts, Fey, Tomblin, & Zhang, 2002). However, as a group, not all children with SLI during the preschool years go on to develop reading difficulty in first or second grade. There is some controversy about which aspects of language functioning and disability during the preschool or kindergarten years predict poor reading outcomes in first or second grade. Some investigators note that children with language impairment in syntax or semantics are more likely to develop reading problems than children who demonstrate problems with articulation or phonology (Bishop & Adams, 1990; Menyuk et al., 1991; Shriberg & Kwiatiwski, 1988).

In addition to specific deficits in aspects of language, two areas of cognitive linguistic functioning, phonological awareness and rapid automatic naming, have been associated with written word recognition in typically developing children and children with reading disability (Liberman, Shankweiler, Fischer, & Carter, 1974; Vellutino & Scanlon, 1987, 1991; Wagner & Torgesen, 1987; Wolf, 1984). Catts (1993) examined receptive and expressive language abilities, phonological awareness, and rapid automatic naming in a group of kindergartners (N = 41) who demonstrated a language impairment (LI) on standardized testing and another group (N = 15) who met only the criteria for an articulation impairment (AI). Reading achievement was assessed in first and second grade for word identification and decoding and speed and accuracy of word recognition and for reading comprehension in second grade. Results indicated that children with SLI in kindergarten were more likely to have reading problems in first and second grade but that variability in reading achievement was related to certain speech and language abilities. Articulation ability in kindergarten was not related to reading achievement in either first or second grade. Children who had been identified as having only articulation impairment (AI group) performed similarly to the typically developing control group of children assessed for reading achievement. Standardized assessments of receptive and expressive language abilities, as well as measures of phonological awareness and rapid automatic naming in kindergarten, were related to reading achievement in first and second grade. However, measures of phonological awareness and rapid automatic naming were the best predictors of word identification and decoding ability in first and second grade.

Since difficulty with written word recognition while reading is associated with *dyslexia,* a specific type of reading disability, Catts and colleagues (2005) examined the hypothesis that SLI and development dyslexia are related or overlapping conditions by examining the prevalence of dyslexia in the second, fourth, and eighth grades among children identified with SLI in kindergarten. The researchers identified two groups of children in kindergarten. One group was identified as SLI by meeting the following criteria: performance of less than 1.25 standard deviations (SDs) on two language composite scores, a nonverbal IQ greater than 1 SD, and no sensory or neurological impairment. A second large group of children was identified as being without language impairment. The children were assessed in the second, fourth, and eighth grades for word recognition and word decoding abilities using subtests from the Woodcock Reading Mastery Tests–Revised (Woodcock, 1987). At each grade level, the presence of a specific reading disability (dyslexia) was assessed by applying a strict definitional criteria for *dyslexia:* a full-scale IQ–achievement discrepancy and low achievement in word recognition. Although one-third (33 percent) of the children with SLI had poor word recognition in the second, fourth, and eighth grades, only approximately 20 percent of them met the strict criteria of low achievement plus a full-scale IQ–achievement discrepancy. These results were interpreted to demonstrate a limited overlap between SLI and dyslexia, although the significance of oral language deficits and reading disability was still noted.

Much of the current research on the nature of language learning disabilities in children has included children who meet the SLI criteria in defining the targeted group under study, especially the criteria of normal nonverbal performance in the average range (i.e., standard score greater than 85) and documented language impairment on a standardized assessment of language ability (Masterson, 1993; Scott & Windsor, 2000; Silliman, Bahr, & Peters, 2006). A problem with the prevailing view of limiting the identification of children with academic learning difficulties who meet the nonverbal intelligence criteria of greater than 85 as LLD is the notion of cognitive referencing (i.e., an IQ–achievement discrepancy) inherent in the identification method.

The criteria for diagnosis of SLI are based on the original research of Stark and Tallal (1981), who attempted to create a definition of SLI that included inclusionary and exclusionary criteria for the purpose of distinguishing a group of children with similar characteristics for research. (For a full discussion of the criteria used in defining SLI, refer to Chapter 4 in the text.) In the original research, the most significant exclusionary criterion adopted by Stark and Tallal was the use of a nonverbal performance IQ (standard score) of greater than or equal to 85, well above the standard score of 70 used as the cutoff for a diagnosis of mental retardation or learning impairment. The reasoning behind this decision was that the nonverbal performance score reflected a measure of inherent intelligence that would not be influenced by depressed verbal ability and therefore was a better referent point for possible discrepancy.

The validity of cognitive referencing was recently challenged in a study that used measures of nonverbal intelligence and oral language ability to identify three groups of children: (1) one group that met the standard definition of SLI (i.e., nonverbal IQ greater than 85 and composite language skills less than 1.25 SDs below age); (2) one group with a general delay in both cognitive and language ability (i.e., nonverbal IQ less than 85 and composite language skills less than 1.25 SDs for age); and (3) a group with no impairment in nonverbal ability or language (Tomblin & Zhang, 1999). Both language-impaired groups differed considerably from their typically developing peers on language measures, and some differences between the two language-impaired groups were also noted. For the most part, the two language-impaired groups performed similarly on language measures, with the exception of sentence comprehension (grammatical understanding); the general delay group of children showed a more severe deficit in this area than the SLI group. Tomblin and Zhang (1999) noted that deficits in this area of language processing were not unique to one group. The two groups were closely parallel, although the children with the general language and cognitive delays showed more severe deficits. The practice of using an IQ–achievement discrepancy as a criteria for identifying children as language impaired or SLI (or LLD) has not been supported (Plante, 1998; Tager-Flusberg & Cooper, 1999).

NONSPECIFIC LANGUAGE IMPAIRMENT

A second group of children with a more generalized developmental delay across both language and cognitive functioning may also be identified as LLD because of significant difficulties in classroom reading and language performance. This second group has been referred to as *nonspecific language impairment (NSLI)* because the developmental disability is not specific to the linguistic system but is also evident in the nonverbal domain of function (Catts, Hogan, & Fey, 2003). Children with NSLI do not meet the criteria for inclusion in the SLI category because their nonverbal IQ falls below a standard score of 85 nor are they considered for classification as mental retardation or learning impairment because their overall IQ is above 70. Moreover, these children do not demonstrate the behavioral and adaptive problems associated with a diagnosis of mental retardation using criteria outlined in the *Diagnostic and Statistical Manual of Mental Disorders (DSM-IV-TR)* (APA, 2000).

Children with NSLI have significant difficulty with oral language and demonstrate much poorer outcomes in reading achievement than children with SLI (Bishop & Adams, 1990; Catts et al., 2003). Children with NSLI manifest more severe and global deficits across language components than children who meet the criteria for SLI and have lower nonverbal IQ scores, yet they are not mentally retarded. It has been argued that children who meet the characteristics for NSLI should qualify for inclusion in the LLD classification because of their significant difficulty with academic language functioning in the classroom.

STAGE V ORAL LANGUAGE DEVELOPMENT

According to Brown (1973), specific aspects of syntactic development and the acquisition of grammatical morphology by children can be conceptualized in developmental stages as a guide to language learning. Stage V corresponds to a minimum mean length of utterance of 4.0 and is characterized by the competent use of the majority of early grammatical morphemes and the basic sentence types, including complex sentences.

The LLD classification has also been applied when children have acquired basic competency in oral language, as defined as beyond Brown's Stage V in vocabulary and sentence development, but have significant difficulty in acquiring and using higher levels of language (Paul, 2001). The construct of LLD applied in this perspective has been reserved for children who demonstrate a well-developed level of everyday oral language competence, as demonstrated by the use of grammatical morphemes and full sentences containing conjunctions or conjoined and embedded clauses. Yet these children have difficulty with aspects of language functioning in the classroom, such as full participation in discourse, reading comprehension, written language, and spelling.

CHILDREN WITH READING DISABILITY

Finally, there are two types of children with reading disability (RD) that have language deficits and should be included in the LLD classification. The first group demonstrates a phonological-based reading disability. The *phonological core deficit hypothesis* (Stanovich, 1986, 1988) suggests that deficits in phonological processing impair word recognition and decoding of unfamiliar words during reading and cause subsequent deficits in reading comprehension and vocabulary. The phonological core deficit is primarily seen in children with dyslexia (Lyon, Shaywitz, & Shaywitz, 2003). There is some controversy about whether dyslexia belongs in the LLD classification, since the difficulty is theoretically confined to "cracking the code" in reading and spelling and does not involve a lack of competence in the primary oral language system. Some have argued that dyslexia should be included as a subgroup along the continuum of LLD, since deficits in phonological processing cause deficits in word recognition and spelling (Paul, 2001; Snowling, 1996).

A second group of children with a specific deficit in reading comprehension has been shown to have corresponding oral language difficulties, even though none of the children had been previously diagnosed with oral language impairment (Nation, Clarke, Marshall, & Durand, 2004). All of the children had fluent and accurate word reading skills and adequate phonological processing ability yet demonstrated difficulty understanding what they read. Assessment of oral language skills showed deficits across a broad range of language areas, including aspects of morphosyntax and semantics and higher aspects of language processing, but showed adequate phonological processing ability. Similar to children with SLI, all the children with poor reading comprehension had nonverbal cognitive ability in the average range (i.e., standard score greater than 85); however, they differed from children with SLI in that their performances on phoneme awareness and nonword repetition tasks were not impaired. It has been suggested that children with specific reading comprehension deficits and overlapping oral language impairment may be a specific subtype of LLD (Nation et al., 2004).

Definition and Identification: Educational Policies

Understanding of the construct of LLD has evolved over the past thirty years as part of the broader learning disability movement in education and professional practice. *Learning disability (LD)* is a concept with a relatively complex history in both federal policy in special education and as an area of applied research, including clinical research on individual differences in learning and performance. Of particular interest are the definition and identification of learning disability, as federal legislation has guided policy and practice in three critical areas: (1) the definition and criteria used in the identification of children having learning disabilities; (2) the recent mandate for research-based alternatives to identify children, including the practice of response to intervention (RtI); and (3) the delivery of teaching and intervention services by highly qualified personnel using scientific or evidenced-based practice.

Federal mandates and policies regarding the identification and provision of specialized services for children with learning difficulties were defined in legislation passed more than thirty years ago. The term *specific learning disability* was first used in federal legislation in 1975, when the U.S. Congress passed the historically significant Education for All Handicapped Children Act, Public Law (PL) 94-142. This legislation officially recognized learning disability as a category eligible for federal funding and applied special education services. The law was implemented in 1977 using a definition of learning disabilities developed by the National Advisory Committee on Handicapped Children (U.S. Office of Education, 1968) for the purpose of identifying children with specific learning disabilities. A major focus within education was the identification of students as LD using common definitions and procedures. Children who were struggling in the classroom were evaluated using criteria derived from the federal definition of LD, which included aspects of discrepancy, heterogeneity, and exclusion.

In 1977, the U.S. Office of Education (USOE) defined a *specific learning disability* as

> a disorder in one or more of the basic psychological processes involved in understanding or in using language, spoken or written, which may manifest itself in an imperfect ability to listen, think, speak, read, write, spell, or to do mathematical calculations. The term includes such conditions as perceptual handicaps, brain injury, manual brain dysfunction, dyslexia, and developmental aphasia. The term does not include children who have learning problems which are primarily the result of visual, hearing, or motor handicaps of mental retardation, or emotional disturbance, or of environmental, cultural, or economic disadvantage.

Federal regulation has interpreted this definition as requiring the application of a discrepancy formula in identifying students for classification as LD. A *discrepancy* is indicated by a difference between aptitude and achievement or between IQ and academic achievement test scores in learning areas such as reading, mathematics, oral language ability, and spelling. *Heterogeneity* is represented by the multiple domains of learning that can qualify a student as LD: listening, speaking, reading, writing, mathematical calculations, and spelling. Finally, the *exclusionary* component is represented by the part of the USOE definition that states that LD cannot be attributed to sensory or motor handicaps, learning impairment, emotional disturbance, or inadequate socioeconomic, linguistic, or educational opportunities.

A significant aspect of the 1977 USOE definition of learning disability is the specification of spoken or written language affecting adequate speaking, listening, reading, writing, spelling, or reasoning. The majority of children identified and classified as learning disability have specific difficulty in reading, writing, and spelling (Lyon, 1995). Despite including language difficulty as an essential component of the definition, reading problems in children have often been seen as a separate and distinct disability. The classification of reading disability was used to distinguish children with significant reading difficulties from those with speech and language impairment.

The 1977 USOE definition is still the definition of learning disability used by the federal government. However, other definitions have been developed over the years, including the influential 1990 definition of the National Joint Committee on Learning Disabilities (NJCLD) (ASHA, 1991), a consensus group made up of organizations representing professional interests and parental advocacy associations, including the American Speech-Language-Hearing Association. According to that definition,

> learning disabilities is a general term that refers to a heterogeneous group of disorders manifested by significant difficulties in the acquisition and use of listening, speaking, reading, writing, reasoning, or mathematical abilities. These disorders are intrinsic to the individual, presumed to be due to central nervous system dysfunction, and may occur across the life span. Problems in self-regulatory behaviors, social perception, and social interaction may exist with learning disabilities but do not by themselves constitute a learning disability. Although learning disabilities may occur concomitantly with other handicapping conditions (for example, sensory impairment, learning impairment, or serious emotional disturbance), or with extrinsic influences (such as cultural differences, insufficient or inappropriate instruction), they are not the result of those conditions or influences. (ASHA, 1991)

This definition was revisited by the NJCLD in 1997 (ASHA, 1998) to recommend operational procedures for ongoing assessment and intervention for children from preschool through secondary school. Five important constructs were identified:

1. Learning disabilities are heterogeneous both within and across individuals.
2. Learning disabilities are manifested by significant difficulties in the acquisition and use of listening, speaking, reading, writing, reasoning, or mathematical skills, even with effective instruction and opportunity to learn.
3. The disorder is intrinsic to the individual and occurs across the life span.
4. Learning disabilities may co-occur with other disabilities but are not the result of those conditions.
5. Learning disabilities are not the result of extrinsic factors, such as cultural differences and insufficient opportunity to learn. Although learning difficulties can result form insufficient opportunity to learn or inappropriate education, they should not be confused with learning disabilities.

SIGNIFICANT EDUCATIONAL REFORM: IDENTIFICATION OF CHILDREN UNDER IDEA AND NCLB

The most recent educational reform efforts are the 2004 reauthorization of the Individuals with Disabilities Education Act (IDEA 2004) and passage of the No Child Left Behind Act (NCLB) in 2001. Both were meant to have an immediate impact on the identification and eligibility of students for special education and to reduce the number of minority children classified as LD. (See Chapter 11 for further discussion of this point.) Fundamental to NCLB is the Reading First initiative, which emphasizes scientifically based reading instruction founded on research and recognized by leading experts in reading (Snow, Burns, & Griffin, 1998).

The reauthorization of IDEA in 2004 was keyed to NCLB. For many years, the majority of students identified as LD and eligible for special education services were those with reading difficulties (Lyon et al., 2001). Both IDEA 2004 and NCLB focus on the notion of instructional accountability and the use of scientific standards of reading instruction for all children. Both of these legislative acts were strongly influenced by a series of consensus reports that suggested schools should implement evidenced-based reading instruction and ensure access to the general educational curriculum, thus reducing the number of students identified as LD and removed from the classroom for special education. Of particular concern was the overrepresentation of minority students in special education. (See Fletcher et al. [2004] for a discussion of IDEA and NCLB.)

Both NCLB and IDEA 2004 prescribe the prevention of reading problems through early intervention, assessment of progress, and accountability for results (Fletcher et al., 2004). Significant requirements include following a more proactive course of evidenced-based instructional approaches and tightening eligibility criteria for the identification of students with LD. Children who are struggling in the classroom may be assessed and served according to a model of response to intervention (RtI) and not subject to the previous "wait-to-fail" policies of many states and schools (Torgesen, 2002). To ensure appropriate instruction for children with learning disabilities, assessment must be directly related to instruction. State and local education agencies should use the child's RtI in determining eligibility. The child may undergo a series of specialized classroom-based assessment and intervention measures administered by qualified professionals before being referred for possible special education assessment for federal classification, placement, and program planning. Classroom teaching of content and intervention practices also must be evidence based, such that valid and reliable scientific research informs practice.

The other significant change resulting from IDEA 2004 concerned the discrepancy formula (i.e., the discrepancy between achievement and aptitude) often used by state and local education agencies to make eligibility decisions. IDEA 2004 stipulated that proving an achievement–aptitude gap is not required to classify a student as having a learning disability. However, the bill does not mandate the replacement of IQ–discrepancy with RtI, and the use of a discrepancy formula for identification is left up to the individual states. Recent research has shown that IQ is ineffective in identifying LD, and its use has been highly criticized as unreliable and lacking scientific evidence (Bradley, Danielson, & Hallahan, 2002; Lyon 1989).

NEW CHALLENGES: UNDERSTANDING LEARNING DISABILITY IN THE CONTEXT OF THE CLASSROOM AND CLINIC

A major outcome of the 2004 reauthorization of IDEA has been the loosening of the federal regulatory definition of LD to allow states not to use the IQ–achievement discrepancy formula as part of the process of identification of LD and to use response to instruction (RtI) criteria instead. Alternative approaches to the identification of LD in students have been proposed by LD researchers and special education consensus groups, including the President's Commission on Excellence in Special Education (USOE, 2002).

As noted by Fletcher et al. (2003), proposed alternatives to the identification of children with LD share three essential components: (1) the need to specify low achievement, (2) the identification of exclusionary factors, and (3) the use of RtI. The role of the speech-language pathologist (SLP) in the identification of students as having LLD must embrace each of these components: (1) the child demonstrates deficient achievement, (2) the child does not adequately respond to consistently presented evidenced-based intervention practices, and (3) the child does not have evidence of any exclusionary criteria that could cause the lack of learning or achievement.

The roles, responsibilities, and practices of the SLP have expanded considerably in the past six years into the domain of literacy development for all children; this includes the prevention of oral and written language difficulties and the assessment and intervention of language learning disabilities (ASHA, 2001). A major goal for SLPs is to develop collaborative partnerships with regular and special education teachers to meet the mandates of literacy education for all children under NCLB and IDEA.

According to Silliman and colleagues (2004), SLPs have three challenges as they move toward more visibility and collaboration in the classroom. The first is to be informed about how educational policies at the state and federal levels are implemented in the local educational setting. The second challenge is to implement research-based practices in literacy-related instruction, assessment, classroom accommodation, and intervention for both at-risk children and children with LLD. Finally, SLPs must develop a thorough understanding of the fundamental relationship between oral and written language and how oral language competence influences and supports literacy, not only during the early stages of literacy development but throughout the acquisition and integration of the advanced literacy knowledge and skills needed to function successfully in the larger society.

Oral Language and Metalinguistic Characteristics of Language Learning Disability

Children with LLD typically have difficulty with learning to read, write, and spell, although they also may have problems in other areas, such as mathematics, or the use of higher-level oral language needed for academic proficiency. The foundation for academic performance in all of these areas is oral language competence. This means that basic skills in all aspects of the oral language system are well developed and available to the individual as he or she engages in literacy learning in academic events. Sometimes, deficits in the oral language system are obvious; for instance, the child may demonstrate difficulties in pronouncing words or producing grammatical sentences. Research has shown that many of the children who struggle with reading and spelling have oral language impairments that include difficulties in phonological processing, speech articulation, vocabulary, syntax, and narrative development (Catts, Fey, Zhang, & Tomblin, 1999). Other times, the difficulties in the oral language system are quite subtle and not readily observed except in specific decontextualized (e.g., clinical) assessment of language processing.

CHILDREN WITH A HISTORY OF PRESCHOOL SPEECH-LANGUAGE IMPAIRMENT

There is ample evidence that children with a preschool history of speech and language impairment are at risk for later academic difficulties even if the speech and language difficulty has presumably been resolved. In a landmark study published in 1984, children originally identified as speech and language impaired during the preschool years were more likely to demonstrate academic and social problems ten years later and to be identified as needing special education services (Aram, Ekelman, & Nation, 1984). The children having the most difficulty with academic performance ten years later were those who demonstrated the poorest language abilities and decreased diadochokinetic speech rate during the preschool years (Aram et al., 1984).

Children with a preschool history of speech and language impairment are also considerably at risk for developing a reading disability, and research has confirmed the relationship between oral language impairment and reading disabilities. However, not all children with this clinical history have poor reading outcomes (Bishop & Adams, 1990; Catts, 1993). Some children seem to resolve their early speech-language difficulties; others do not, however, and the unresolved primary oral language deficit influences their reading outcome. A follow-up study of adolescent children at 15 years of age who had an earlier diagnosis of language impairment but were not classified as such at 8 years of age showed subtle oral language problems and significant reading difficulties when assessed in middle adolescence (Stothard, Snowling, Bishop, & Chipcase, 1998). Researchers have called the presumed recovery of early language difficulty "illusory" and noted that oral and written language problems often recur in individuals who seem to have resolved them (Scarborough & Dobrich, 1990).

METALINGUISTIC AWARENESS AND PHONOLOGICAL PROCESSING

The term *metalinguistic awareness* refers to the explicit recognition of the formal features of one's language—for example, the number of words in a sentence, the number of syllables within a word, and the separate phonemes that make up individual words. Metalinguistic awareness is usually assessed by asking the child to make an out-of-context linguistic judgment, such as "How many words are in the sentence *The boy ran down the street?*" or "How many sounds do you hear in the word *split?*"

The development of metalinguistic ability in children is a metacognitive skill that emerges toward the end of the preschool period and is characterized by a cognitive shift in intellectual functioning when a child can begin to treat language as an object of thought. For example, the child may begin to notice how words are related in rhyming games or how words sound the same in an alliteration game, such as "Silly Suzy sat still." This ability to reflect on language has been attributed to emergence of the Piagetian stage of concrete operations that begins to develop between 5 and 7 years of age (Fowler, 1991; Van Kleek, 1984).

Phonological awareness is a specific type of metalinguistic awareness that involves the explicit recognition of the sound structure of speech (Liberman et al., 1974; Vellutino & Scanlon, 1987; Wagner & Torgesen, 1987). Children's development of phonological awareness progresses from larger units in words to smaller units of sounds within words (Fox & Routh, 1975; Stanovich, Cunningham, & Cramer, 1984). For example, children begin first to isolate and segment words in sentences and then syllables within words. This is followed by phonological awareness of rhyme and finally discrete phoneme awareness and isolation of individual sounds within words (Liberman et al., 1974; Lundberg, Frost, & Peterson, 1988).

Research over the past twenty years has shown that phonological awareness of the discrete sounds in words and the ability to manipulate sounds in words is directly related to the development of word recognition and decoding ability in reading (Bradley & Bryant, 1983; Liberman & Shankweiler, 1985; Pennington & Lefly, 2001; Stanovich, 1986) and is essential for accuracy in spelling (Ball, 1993; Ehri, 2000; Fischer, Shankweiler, & Liberman, 1985; Treiman, 1984). To acquire efficiency in word recognition ability and proficiency in spelling, an individual must be explicitly aware of the individual speech sounds within words. The term *explicit* is used to mean the active, conscious awareness of discrete speech sounds, not letter names. Phonological awareness is a metacognitive process and is not the same as phonics. *Phonics* is a lower-level, paired-associate skill that links letters and sounds (Clark & Uhry, 1995).

Phonological awareness is significantly impaired in children with reading disorders (Catts et al., 2002; Kamhi, Lee, & Nelson, 1985; Vellutino & Scanlon, 1987, 1991). The causal role of deficits in phonological awareness and reading disabilities is evident in studies that have demonstrated a link between low phonological awareness in preschool and kindergarten and reading difficulty in first or second grade (Catts et al., 1999; Pennington & Lefly, 2001).

Children with a history of speech and language impairment show a delay in the overall development of phonological awareness. Kamhi and associates (1985) examined metalinguistic awareness of words, syllables, and sounds in fifteen language-disordered children, fifteen typically developing children matched for mental age, and fifteen chronologically age–matched children. Results indicated that 5- and 6-year-old children with language disorders lacked metalinguistic awareness of words, syllables, and sounds and did not perform as well as younger mental age–matched children, placing them at risk for difficulty in learning to read, write, and spell.

Webster and Plante (1992) examined phonological awareness in twenty-two children between 6 years, 5 months and 8 years, 6 months, all of whom had persistent moderate to severe expressive phonological impairment. Researchers compared their performance on five tasks of word and phoneme segmentation to that of a group of mental age–matched typically developing children. The segmentation tasks required the children to listen to a sentence, a real word, or a pseudoword and to represent using blocks the number of words in the sentence, syllables in the word, or phoneme segments in a real or a pseudoword. Results showed that the children with persistent phonological impairment and low speech intelligibility performed more poorly on all segmentation tasks at the word, syllable, and phoneme levels and that phonological awareness was correlated with speech production independent of mental age and educational experience.

Poor metalinguistic awareness has also been demonstrated in other aspects of language. Children with language disorders have shown a lack of syntactic awareness (Nation & Snowling, 2000) and morphological awareness (Carlisle, 1987; Rubin, Patterson, & Kantor, 1991). Carlisle (1987) demonstrated that students in the ninth grade diagnosed with a specific learning disability in reading and spelling had difficulty completing an orally presented metalinguistic task that involved producing a derived form and performed like typically developing younger students (e.g., "Warm. He chose the jacket for its ____ ").

SPEECH ARTICULATION AND PHONOLOGICAL DISORDERS IN LANGUAGE LEARNING DISABILITY

Children who have difficulties with both oral and written language (e.g., reading, spelling) are referred to as having a *language learning disability* (LLD). Articulation problems and expressive phonological difficulty are frequently observed in children with LLD. The phonological deficit may be obvious in that the child demonstrates speech sound production errors during articulation of well-known words, or it may be more subtle in that phonological difficulty is not observed unless assessment entails more phonologically complex tasks involving repetition of multisyllabic words and nonwords. Moreover, children with expressive phonological disorders in kindergarten and first grade are more likely to demonstrate poor phonological awareness and poor reading outcomes at the end of first grade (Larrivee & Catts, 1999).

Some investigators have indicated that the presence of isolated speech sound disorders in a young child does not by itself guarantee that he or she will develop a reading or spelling disability (Lewis, Freebairn, & Taylor, 2000). However, recent evidence suggests that when language impairment and phonological processing difficulty occur with a speech sound disorder, the child is at increased risk for reading disability. This set of comorbid features should be viewed as a clinical marker of a subtype of phonologically impaired children who are likely to be classified as LLD (Rvachew, 2007).

Persistent phonological problems can be seen in children with reading impairment. In a study of children between 12 and 16 years classified by psychoeducational achievement and IQ–discrepancy criteria for reading disability (RD), significantly more errors across three tasks of phonological processing were made by the RD group than the age-matched, typically developing group (Catts, 1986). Subjects completed three phonological tasks involving multisyllabic or phonetically complex words, nonwords, and phrases. For example, during the naming task, subjects were shown pictures of objects represented by multisyllabic words, such as *thermometer* and *rhinoceros*, and asked to name the objects. In the word repetition task, forty-five multisyllabic words with complex phonetic sequences, such as *specific* and *aluminum*, were spoken by the examiner and then repeated by the subject. Finally, the complex phrase repetition task required each subject to repeat twenty-two short phrases, such as *brown bread and blue pants*. Children with an RD made significantly more errors on all three complex speech articulation tasks than typically developing children. A positive correlation was found between the overall total errors on the three tasks of phonological processing and reading level in the children with an RD. It was concluded that children with RD have an underlying phonological processing deficit that may affect both their spoken and written language performance.

MORPHOLOGIC AND SYNTACTIC DEFICITS IN CHILDREN WITH LANGUAGE LEARNING DISABILITY

Structural aspects of language are areas of difficulty for children with language-based learning problems. Children with LLD produce more errors in word morphology in their oral and written language (Carlisle, 1987; Rubin et al., 1991) and often demonstrate difficulty with the comprehension and production of more complex sentence structures (Paul, 1990; Roth & Spekman, 1989; Wiig, 1982). The term *word morphology* refers to the structures of words, including free morphemes and root word vocabulary, and bound morphemes reflected in the use of grammatical inflections and derivational morpheme endings. In both LLD children and adults with literacy problems, errors have been noted on both grammatical inflections and derivational morphological endings in spoken and written language (Rubin et al., 1991). For example, grammatical morpheme errors were noted in the reading and writing of words such as *speaking/speaker* and *talk/talked*.

One question is whether these individuals lack implicit, internalized knowledge of the rules for applying morphemes to the ends of words. Rubin and associates (1991) conducted an oral language task in which children and adults were given a nonsense word within a stimulus sentence and asked to supply the word with the appropriate morphological ending. The researchers found that both LLD and typically developing second-grade students had not mastered the rules for adding morphological endings, although the children with LLD performed significantly worse than their typically developing peers. Surprisingly, the adults with literacy problems performed similarly to the typically developing second-graders, which was an unexpected finding, given that the adults had had many more years of education and exposure to language. Furthermore, on an explicit task of morphological knowledge in which the three groups (i.e., typically developing children, children with LLD, and adults with literacy problems) were asked to write a word with the correct morphological ending during a dictated sentences task, performance by the children with LLD and adults with literacy problems was consistent with their performance on the oral language elicitation task. Rubin and associates (1991) concluded that individuals with LLD lack both implicit and explicit levels of morphological knowledge and that these deficits are not resolved with maturation or increased exposure to written language.

Children with LLD also demonstrate difficulty learning and using derivational morphology in their spoken and written language (Carlisle, 1987; Templeton, 1989; Templeton & Scarborough-Franks, 1985). The term *derivational morphology* refers to prefixes and suffixes that are combined with root words to form words with new meanings. For example, use of the prefix *un-* with a root word such as *happy* (*unhappy*) or *do* (*undo*) conveys a negative element or opposite meaning or, if applied to a verb, the reversal of the action. Derivational morphemes used as suffixes at the ends of root words most often change the part of speech of the root word and express the additional meaning contained within the morpheme itself. For example, the morpheme *-tion* changes a verb to a noun, as in *transport/ transportation* and *subtract/subtraction,* and conveys the additional meaning of a thing or object.

Carlisle (1987) found that typically developing children between the fourth and eighth grades developed knowledge and skill with words containing derivational morphemes by being exposed to vocabulary during the reading of more advanced texts. Because children with LLD have low levels of reading ability, they have less exposure to derived forms in print and often lack the metalinguistic awareness and phonological processing ability needed to analyze the structures of words for spoken and written tasks (Moats & Smith, 1992).

In addition to deficits in morphology, children with LLD also demonstrate deficits in processing sentences and abstracting the rules for sentence structure in their spoken and written language (Idol-Maestas, 1980; Wiig, 1982). Research has demonstrated that the mean length of utterance (MLU) used by children with reading disabilities is at or beyond stage V of language development (Brown, 1973), a stage of complex sentence development (Wiig, 1982). Utterance length, as measured by MLU, was significantly lower for second-, fourth-, and sixth-grade children with RD than age-matched typically developing children. Moreover, examination of the structural integrity of the children's utterances indicated more grammatical errors across sentence types (Idol-Maestas, 1980).

In a longitudinal investigation of the relationship between oral language ability and reading difficulty in young children, Catts et al. (1999) found that 56 percent of poor readers in the second grade had shown previous deficits in the language domain of grammar when evaluated in kindergarten. These researchers tested over 600 children's oral language ability in kindergarten and then followed them into second grade and assessed their reading ability. The group was divided into good and poor readers, and the oral language measures taken in kindergarten were examined for the unique contribution the language area made to reading achievement in second grade. While in kindergarten, the children's oral language competence in grammar was assessed using three subtests of a standardized measure of language ability, the Test of Language Development–Primary (TOLD-P; Newcomer & Hammill, 1988), including the subtests of grammatical understanding, grammatical completion, and sentence imitation. Performance on all three subtests was combined to form a composite grammar score. Children with reading impairment in second grade had significantly lower mean composite scores than children with reading ability. The fundamental relationship between oral language competence and literacy achievement was underscored by this research.

DISCOURSE AND NARRATIVE DEFICITS IN LANGUAGE LEARNING DISABILITY

Discourse is a broad term that includes a variety of oral forms, including conversation, story narrative, and exposition. Of these three forms, conversation and story narrative have been the most investigated in children with LLD.

The ability to engage in conversation is rooted in the ability of the *speaker* to construct utterances based on shared information or a common ground of shared knowledge with the *listener* (Horton & Gerrig, 2005). There is some evidence that school-age children with LLD are delayed in developing the metalinguistic or metacognitive understanding of the importance of the speaker in message construction in conversation and instead place more of the weight of the conversation on the listener (Meline & Brackin, 1987). When asked to make a judgment in response to an inadequate message of request in a story, children with LLD performed more like typically developing younger children in blaming the listener for the inadequate message, rather than the speaker. Age-matched typically developing children were more likely to correctly judge the speaker as the one to blame for the inadequate message.

Similarly, school-age children with language disorders have difficulty understanding the perspective of the listener. Brinton, Fujiki, and Sonnenberg (1988) demonstrated that school-age children with language disorders had difficulty responding to requests for clarification of a message in conversation and were less able to adjust their message to listener feedback. In addition to difficulty with speaker–listener perspective, children with LLD have difficulty accessing or joining an ongoing interaction with same-age peers, and once engaged in the interaction, they have fewer utterances and less collaboration and are addressed less than the typically developing children in the interaction (Brinton, Fujiki, & Spencer, 1997). Difficulty with the structure and function of conversation puts the child with LLD at a disadvantage for academic and social interaction in the classroom with both peers and teachers.

Another area of discourse that is often impaired in children with LLD is the comprehension and production of a story narrative. Story narrative ability relies on the use of an internalized *story grammar* that includes both content schema and a macrostructure of the story called a *story text grammar* (Mandler & Johnson, 1977). The *content schema* of a story refers to the framework of story elements, including the setting, the goal, the complications, and the resolution. The content schema helps the child process the story as it unfolds and acts as a cognitive scaffold to support both the understanding of the story elements and the temporal and causal relations among them. The text *macrostructure* refers to the larger organization of meaning across utterances and is characterized by the cohesive ties between and among sentences and parts of the text. For example, the use of pronouns, conjunctions, and transition words and phrases link ideas within and across sentences and back through the story text to aid in comprehension.

Liles (1985) investigated narrative comprehension and production ability by school-age children with language disability and found that those with LLD had poorer overall story comprehension and less adequate use of cohesive devices and narrative organization when retelling a story to a naïve listener. Other researchers have also shown that children with LLD produce simpler narratives using fewer cohesive devices and less complex syntax. They also make fewer inferences and more syntactic, semantic, and morphological errors during story retelling tasks (Merritt & Liles, 1987; Norbury & Bishop, 2003; Roth & Spekman, 1989). Decreased competence in story narrative has profound implications for the child or adolescent with LLD in the academic setting. An internalized, well-formed cognitive framework for story narrative is needed to facilitate reading comprehension for story texts (Just & Carpenter, 1987) and written language production for story narratives (Perera, 1984).

WORD RETRIEVAL DEFICITS IN LANGUAGE LEARNING DISABILITY

Rourke (1994) noted that some children with LLD demonstrate specific deficits in word retrieval and oral formulation. He suggested that difficulty in word finding may be an isolated deficit in the retrieval of words in memory and that the problem may constrain verbal expression, even though other areas of cognitive/linguistic functioning remain intact. Rourke speculated that this profile may be a specific subtype of language learning disability called *word-finding disorder (WFD)*. The question is whether WFD exists in the absence of other difficulties in language and learning.

Wolf (1984, 1999) noted that naming and reading deficits frequently co-occur in children with developmental dyslexia, placing them at increased risk for poor reading outcomes. Wolf (1999; Wolf & Bowers, 2000) developed the *double-deficit hypothesis* to conceptualize subtypes of reading disability that result from a possible breakdown in one or both core systems involved in the reading process: phonological processing and naming speed. Other researchers (German, 1982, 1987; Kail & Leonard, 1986) have noted the presence of word-finding deficits in children with language impairment. Word-finding difficulty in children with language impairment can be explained as either a problem with the storage or retrieval of words from memory. A storage-deficit hypothesis suggests that word-finding difficulty reflects inadequate or degraded phonological representations of vocabulary in memory. A retrieval-deficit hypothesis suggests that the difficulty results from a breakdown in the retrieval process itself.

German (1987) examined the word-finding behaviors and language productivity of children diagnosed with language impairment in their connected speech. *Connected speech* refers to spontaneous use of language phrases, sentences, and discourse. As a group, children with language impairment who had difficulty in a confrontational naming task also demonstrated word repetitions, reformulations, and substitutions in their spontaneous connected speech. Furthermore, the study identified two spontaneous language profiles of children with word-finding difficulty. One profile showed an overall reduction of oral language productivity characterized by limited story length, while the other showed adequate story generation similar in length to that of the normative group. The two groups differed on word-finding characteristics during connected speech. The low-productivity group had fewer word-finding behaviors in their spontaneous speech, while the adequate-productivity group showed more of the characteristics classified as word finding in their spontaneous connected speech. German (1987) noted that children with either of these language profiles will have difficulty in academic requirements for longer discourse, either in terms of limited output (profile 1) or existing word-finding behaviors during connected speech (profile 2).

Relationship between Oral and Academic Language

The classroom environment is a distinct context with unique language-processing demands, as evident in the oral language used during instruction and the written language used in textbooks. A student's ability to acquire the content of the general education curriculum depends on his or her ability to navigate the language of the classroom and develop proficiency in academic language (Wilkinson & Silliman, in press). Of particular concern is the student's acquisition of literacy skills, including the functional abilities to read and write and the more advanced applications involved in understanding the complex language and abstract content found in textbooks and in developing skills for inductive and deductive reasoning.

These varying levels of literacy are referred to as *basic, critical,* and *dynamic literacy,* and each has its own functional skill level. The three levels develop sequentially, and ability in each is dependent on competencies acquired in the preceding level or levels (Westby, 2002).

ORAL AND WRITTEN LANGUAGE COMPREHENSION: SIMILARITIES AND DIFFERENCES

Language comprehension, both spoken and written, is a complex cognitive process that involves both lower levels of cognitive processing in perception and higher levels of cognitive processing in accessing and retrieving stored language in long-term memory. At a basic level, spoken language comprehension requires the individual to perceive and discriminate phonemes in the spoken words, to organize and map phonological sequences to stored representations in the lexicon (vocabulary), and to apply syntactic, grammatical, and semantic rules so the meaning can be derived and the message comprehended. Similarly, basic comprehension of a written message requires the individual to perceive and discriminate letters shapes, to transform them into phonemes and create a phonological sequence for mapping, and to retrieve similar representations stored in memory during the processes of word recognition and text construction in reading. Each type of comprehension interacts with the lexicon, where information about individual words is stored, including the phonological, semantic, and syntactic parameters of the word. Over time, as an individual gains experience in reading and manipulating print, additional information is coded for the word in the form of a visual representation of its spelling pattern (Adams, 1992).

In this view, listening comprehension is the basis for reading comprehension, since one must understand a language in its spoken form to be able to read and adequately understand its written form (Cain & Oakhill, 2007). Although the basic psychological processes are similar for spoken and reading comprehension, reading comprehension is said to be "piggy-backed' onto oral listening comprehension in that it derives stored information about oral language experiences from vocabulary, sentence structure, and discourse. Comprehension of the increasingly more literate oral language found in the academic discourse and language register of the classroom continues to support the reading comprehension demands of academic textbooks (Cain & Oakhill, 2007).

Nonetheless, competence in listening comprehension does not guarantee competence in reading comprehension (Oakhill & Cain, 2007). Developing a more advanced level of language comprehension, whether spoken or written, means being able to construct a mental model of the situation at hand, whether experienced in the classroom or described in a written text (Cain & Oakhill, 2007). Comprehending longer texts requires additional cognitive and linguistic processing skills in that information contained in different parts of a text needs to be integrated in order to create an overall meaningful representation.

Research has identified a number of ways in which written and spoken language comprehension differ. The first is that the vocabulary and syntax used in written language are frequently more sophisticated or unfamiliar to the reader; sentences are often complex and contain vocabulary that is not used in everyday social interactions. For example, consider the following sentence from a child's written narrative (Cosgrove, 1977):

> Being the poor fisherman that he was, he couldn't afford to buy another wooden leg so he *fashioned* one out of an old *mop handle*, thinking that it would just have to do.

Unusual vocabulary includes the phrase *mop handle* and the use of *fashioned* as a verb, and complex syntax is noted by the use of dependent clauses and conjunctions. This type of sentence is not usually heard in everyday spoken language. The same essential content would most likely be stated in several more simple sentences, and the vocabulary would be more colloquial.

Another way in which spoken and written language differ is that written language is *decontextualized;* that is, it is set apart from the here and now, the immediate time and place. This means the reader must project his or her mental image to the distant context of the text. In addition, written language comprehension often requires the integration and organization of varying levels of language across a longer discourse frame, such as a narrative or expository text, which does not frequently occur with spoken language comprehension (Denny, 1991).

THE ROLE OF PHONOLOGICAL PROCESSING IN READING AND SPELLING

Awareness of the phonemic structures of words is a causal factor in reading outcomes in first- and second-grade children (Catts et al., 1999; Pennington & Lefly,

2001), and as will be discussed later, is impaired in children and adults with reading disability (RD). Frequently, the term *phonological awareness* is used interchangeably with *phonological processing,* although scientists distinguish the two terms. The term *phonological awareness* is more often associated with ability at the level of the phoneme and syllable: the explicit recognition and manipulation of the individual syllables and phonemic segments in words (Ball, 1993; Ball & Blachman, 1991; Gillon, 2004). *Phonological processing* is a broader term that refers to the use of phonological information for the purpose of encoding analyzed phonological data in long-term memory. One must develop a memory trace of a word—a phonological representation—that is used in the recognition of spoken and written words. Phonological processing also includes the cognitive process of retrieving a word's phonological representation during naming and spelling (Gillon, 2004; Wagner & Torgesen, 1987). In this view, phonological awareness is a subset of the broader construct of phonological processing.

Critical to understanding the roles of phonological awareness and phonological processing in reading and spelling is the notion of the development and expansion of *phonological representations* in long-term memory. Phonological representations in memory begin to develop holistically in infancy, as the infant and young child recognize more and more spoken words in context (Gillon, 2004). Over time, phonological representations of words become more finely segmented into discrete phonemes that are stored for rapid recognition and comprehension without the need of situational context. For example, the mature phonological representation of the word *train* that is stored in memory contains the discrete phonemes /t/ /r/ /e/ /n/. Activation of this stored sequence is needed for both accurate listening comprehension and spoken word production and is critical during reading and spelling of the word (Gillon, 2004).

A reciprocal relationship exists between phonological awareness and the development of literacy in both reading and spelling. Internalized word representations become more fine tuned as the child begins to associate spoken and written forms of a word (Ehri, 2000). As the child reads more words, his or her memory for spelling patterns improves (Ehri & Wilce, 1979) and is integrated with stored phonological information. Similarly, learning to spell influences word recognition while reading (Ehri & Wilce, 1980, 1987) and is integrated with stored phonological information. A spelling pattern, called an *orthographic representation,* is associated with the sound structure of the word in memory. In this way, spelling and reading are aided by knowledge of the alphabetic principle (i.e., that letters represent speech sounds), phonological processing of the word structure, and the stored visual representation or spelling pattern of the word.

READING

Reading is a process by which meaning is derived from print. It involves two basic neuropsychological processes: word recognition and comprehension. Although intricately related, there is evidence that skill in word recognition is necessary but not sufficient for ability in reading comprehension. Individuals may demonstrate adequate and fluent word recognition yet have poor reading comprehension, which is referred to as a *specific comprehension deficit* (Cain & Oakhill, 2007).

Word recognition is the process that transforms or decodes unfamiliar words seen in print to speech or that automatically recognizes familiar printed words in their spoken forms. The decoding aspect of word recognition is critically tied to the alphabetic principle, which acknowledges that the letters of the alphabet represents phonemes in spoken words, and to the development of phonological awareness, which is the nonverbal cognitive awareness that words are made up of linguistic units at the level of the phoneme and syllable (Liberman et al., 1974). Phonological processing ability in kindergarten has been identified as the single best predictor of reading ability, particularly word recognition and decoding, at the end of first grade (Share, Jorm, Maclean, & Matthews, 1984).

Comprehension is the complex cognitive process that assigns meanings to words, phrases, sentences, and texts. During reading, meaning is processed and assigned from varying levels of language and integrated into a coherent text structure. To comprehend written text, the reader must construct a meaning-based representation of the state or event described in print.

Constructing a meaningful representation requires being able to read the words on the page. It follows that problems with reading comprehension are frequently associated with problems with word recognition. Research has shown a significant correlation between word recognition and reading comprehension ability in typically developing children and children diagnosed with dyslexia (Perfetti, 1985; Stanovich, 1986). Additionally, reading comprehension involves tracking and assimilating messages from across a long written text and using existing knowledge, inference, and devices of writing and storytelling to derive meaning (Cain, 2003; Cain & Oakhill, 1996, 2007; Cain, Oakhill, Barnes, & Bryant, 2001). Facility with each of these aspects of written text and language processing contributes to a level of dynamic literacy needed by members of a technologically advanced society (Westby, 2002).

Developmental Changes in Reading

Reading researchers have noted that in the early elementary grades, from kindergarten to third grade, children develop skill and automaticity in word recognition, allowing for increased reading accuracy, fluency, and rate. These three fundamental aspects of word recognition—accuracy, fluency, and rate—are essential as the child navigates new academic language and content featured in texts. From fourth through eighth grade, reading becomes the avenue for learning new knowledge, acquiring a robust vocabulary, and gaining experience with complex syntax, as children encounter more complex and unfamiliar language in textbooks, newspapers, and literature (Chall, 1983; Chall, Jacobs, & Baldwin, 1990). In high school, functional reading requires a wide study of the social, physical, and biological sciences as well classic and contemporary literature. There is also an increased focus on the study of the morphological structure of words through analysis of word parts, including prefixes, suffixes, and roots.

Reading research has focused on the psychological process of reading and consistently highlighted the role of oral language competence as a foundation for reading and literacy. Chall (1983) identified six stages of reading development in the typical child but cautions that the age ranges applied are approximations:

- *Stage 0: Prereading Stage (Birth to 5–6 years).* This stage is referred to as the *emergent literacy* stage and is characterized by the development of basic concepts about literacy activities within a society, such as the purpose of reading, the relationships between pictures and print, beginning awareness of the alphabet, and development of metalinguistic ability to rhyme, segment syllables, and sounds within words.
- *Stage 1: Decoding: (5–7 years).* During this stage, the child acquires rules of phoneme–grapheme correspondence and solidifies the concept of the *alphabetic principle.* In this stage, children develop the ability to attend to the specific graphic elements within words, rather than treat words as whole units.
- *Stage 2: Further Consolidation (7–9 years).* Confidence in decoding skills is consolidated during this stage, as the child uses the knowledge gained in the previous stage to recognize patterns and redundancies within print and thus gains speed and fluency in reading.
- *Stage 3: Reading to Learn (9–14 years).* Decoding skills are fully automatic at this stage, and the child now uses reading to learn. Specific subject reading is introduced (e.g., science and social studies), and the child is able to focus on the comprehension of longer texts and vocabulary development through reading.
- *Stage 4: Multiple Viewpoints (14–18 years).* During this stage, the child is more cognitively able to consider multiple perspectives on a topic or issue. There is a continued emphasis on reading to learn through content-area reading and literature.
- *Stage 5: Constructive Reading (18 years and beyond).* This stage of reading development involves the individual's construction of knowledge from the ideas of others. The individual becomes a more critical reader and applies higher-level cognitive processes, such as inductive/deductive reasoning, during the reading process.

Reading Disability

Individuals with a reading disability (RD) have difficulty in word recognition, reading comprehension, or both. As noted previously, reading comprehension has its foundation in oral listening comprehension.

This view underlies a reading theory called the *simple view of reading* (Gough & Tummer, 1986; Hoover & Gough, 1990), which states that reading comprehension is the result of two components: word recognition and listening comprehension. In other words, an individual's overall reading comprehension ability can be predicted from scores on a word recognition task and a listening comprehension task. Using the simple view of reading model, researchers have identified four subtypes of reading disability based on the individual's word recognition ability and skill in listening comprehension (Catts et al., 2003). These four subtypes are described Table 5.1.

The first subtype, *dyslexia,* is a specific reading disability that is characterized by difficulties in word recognition and spelling but adequate oral listening comprehension.

Table 5.1 **Subtypes of Reading Disability Based on Word Recognition and Listening Comprehension**

	Word Recognition	Listening Comprehension
Dyslexia	Poor	Good
Mixed	Poor	Poor
Specific comprehension	Good	Poor
Nonspecific	Good	Good

Based on Catts, Hogan, & Fey, 2003.

The disorder is linked to deficits in phonological processing that are evident in difficulty with word decoding, word recognition, spelling, and subsequent poor vocabulary development. Current definitions of dyslexia emphasize the primary deficit in word recognition and spelling ability, as demonstrated by the following definition of dyslexia developed by members of a committee of the International Dyslexia Association (Lyon et al., 2003):

> Dyslexia is a specific learning disability that is neurological in origin. It is characterized by difficulties with accurate and/or fluent word recognition and by poor spelling and decoding abilities. These difficulties typically result from a deficit in the phonological component of language that is often unexpected in relation to other cognitive abilities and the provision of effective classroom instruction. Secondary consequences may include problems in reading comprehension and reduced reading experience that can impede growth of vocabulary and background knowledge. (p. 2)

The second subtype is called a *mixed reading disability* because it demonstrates deficits in both word recognition and listening comprehension. Individuals in this group are thought to have both an oral language disability and a written language disability, manifested by difficulty with word recognition and reading comprehension. This subgroup has also been identified with the term *language learning disability (LLD)* to emphasize the oral and written language disorder and to classify it separately from pure dyslexia, a primary learning disability affecting word recognition and spelling. However, individuals in both the LLD subtype and the dyslexia subtype have difficulty with phonemic awareness and the phonological processing of words (Fletcher et al., 1994; Gillon, 2004).

Children in the third subtype, a *specific comprehension deficit,* showed a primary deficit in oral language comprehension, even though their word recognition ability was adequate. These individuals do not demonstrate significant difficulty in decoding words or reading text fluently; rather, their difficulty is seen in the comprehension of larger discourse units in both oral and written contexts (Cain & Oakhill, 2007; Catts et al., 2005). There is converging evidence that children who demonstrate reading comprehension deficits also demonstrate inadequate comprehension of longer discourse units in spoken language, such as story narrative. This indicates a specific disability in constructing the meaning of longer oral and written discourse. This subtype of reading disability is often seen in older children beyond the early primary grades and is most associated with problems in inferencing, semantic and syntactic processing, and working memory (Cain et al., 2001).

Finally, the fourth subtype of reading disability, which is called *nonspecific,* includes children who have adequate word recognition and listening comprehension ability yet struggle to read. Other psychological and social factors may be associated with this subtype of reading disability, including motivational factors or attention deficit (Catts et al., 2003).

SPELLING

Spelling is a complex cognitive-linguistic process that encompasses both the storage and retrieval of phonologic, orthographic, and semantic information about words. Spelling is related to word recognition because it involves knowledge of the alphabetic principle and phonological processing of phoneme/letter correspondences. Spelling is distinct from reading, however, in that the segmenting and sequencing of syllables and letter patterns involves multiple cognitive-processing demands (Ehri, 2000).

There are two competing theories of the cognitive processes involved in spelling. One is the *dual-route theory* of spelling, which suggests there are two separate pathways in the neurobiological network, one phonologic and one orthographic, that are linked but also can be accessed separately in the spelling or reading of a word (Ellis, 1993; Frith, 1980). According to this theory, each entry in the lexicon has a phonological representation and an orthographic representation, each stored as a separate module. Information about the sound structure of a word is stored in the phonological module, while information about the letter sequences of a word is stored in the visual-orthographic module. The visual-orthographic module contains spelling patterns for words that have been memorized. The two storage modules are linked to the meaning of a word and can communicate with each other, yet each module can be accessed independently during spelling and reading. Spelling of a word can be accomplished in either of two ways: (1) by directly retrieving the visual-orthographic representation of the word in memory and converting it to a written form via the grapheme output buffer or (2) by accessing the phonological representation of the word through its pronunciation and converting its sound structure to print via the link between the phoneme and grapheme output buffers. Figure 5.1 represents the dual-route theory of spelling (based on Ellis, 1993).

In contrast, the *connectionist theory* of spelling suggests that both the visual-orthographic spelling and the phonological representation of a word are activated simultaneously in skilled readers and spellers (Adams, 1992; Ehri & Wilce, 1980; Seidenberg & McClelland, 1989). Through exposure to print, readers and spellers are able to process spelling patterns of words and associate their meanings with their pronunciations, creating what Ehri (1987, 2000) describes as an amalgam or fused connection among the multiple layers of information about a word. According to

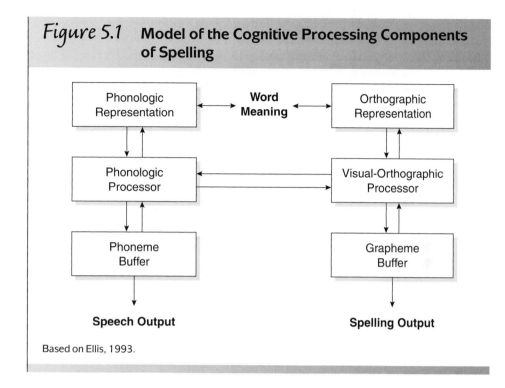

Figure 5.1   **Model of the Cognitive Processing Components of Spelling**

Based on Ellis, 1993.

this theory, it is critical that an association is made between the visual spelling of a word and its auditory phonemic components, especially since words vary in the transparency of their phonemic components (Treiman & Bourassa, 2001). Thus, the influence of repetition and previous experience with spelling patterns is a central feature of the theory of connectionism.

Developmental Changes in Spelling

The developmental changes in children's knowledge and representations of the orthographic patterns of words have been well documented in the research literature (Ehri, 1987; Henderson, 1990). Like reading development, spelling development can be explained with a stage theory. Doing so is useful in conceptualizing the knowledge and skill acquired by children as they become more familiar with print and the spelling patterns of words. There is evidence that children use several different strategies and linguistic processes as they become mature spellers (Treiman & Bourassa, 2000).

Spelling development moves through fairly predictable stages as the child continues to acquire knowledge of orthographic patterns and spellings of words, syllables, and grammatical/derivational morphemes. The following four stages of spelling development were proposed by Moats (1995):

- *Stage 1: Precommunicative Writing.* This stage is marked by the young child's early attempts at writing. There is no evidence that the child understands the concept of a word. Rather, word boundaries and spacing are missing, and whole phrases such as *thank-you* are frequently represented by a combination of letters and nonletter scribbles.

- *Stage 2: Semiphonetic Stage.* In this stage, the child has a rudimentary understanding that letters correspond to speech sounds, although the entire word may not be represented. Instead, the child will choose a few consonants to denote syllables and words, as in this example reported by Bissex (1980) from her 5-year-old son: *RUDF* ("Are you deaf?").

- *Stage 3: Phonetic Spelling.* The child in this stage uses a variety of letters and has learned letter–sound correspondence patterns to represent all speech sounds within words. Spelling is characterized as *surface phonetic* because the child does not understand and represent the morphophonemic structure of the word; rather, the letters chosen in spelling are often related to speech articulation. For example, when producing the letter name *Y*, the child lip-rounds and produces a /w/ speech sound. Consequently, a child in this stage may use the letter *Y* to spell words such as *YL* ("will") and *YAR* ("where") (cf. Moats, 1995).

- *Stage 4: Transitional Spelling: Within-Word Patterns and Beyond.* This stage marks additional learning and consolidation of knowledge of the underlying morphophonemic structures of words. The child grasps that speech sounds are often represented by groups of letters, such as the digraphs *-ch* and *-sh,* and that each syllable represented in print contains a vowel. As reading skill and fluency continue to develop, the child has increased exposure and experience with vocabulary and spelling. Knowledge of standard spellings of grammatical morphemes, such as the use of *-ed* at the end of a word to signal the past-tense morpheme and the plural *-s,* is learned and internalized by children between the second and third grades (Bailet, 1990). In addition, common homophones are recognized and spelled correctly, such as *to, two,* and *too,* and early developing derivational morphemes are used consistently. The initial spellings of prefixes and suffixes include those that do not change the spelling of the root word or the phonological aspects of the word during pronunciation—for example, *-un* in *unhappy, -ment* in *enjoyment,* and *-ful* in *respectful.* By fourth grade, children have a greater understanding of the relationship between root words and are better able to apply more advanced derivational morpheme suffixes that alter the spelling of the root and the pronunciation of the derived form (*televise/television; circle/circular,* etc.).

These stages should be considered as only a guide. Many children exhibit more than one stage of spelling as they acquire more linguistic knowledge and cognitive strategies, and some children never achieve the more advanced levels of spelling.

Spelling Disability

Spelling deficits are common among children with RD (Carpenter, 1983; Moats, 1996) and LLD (Gerber & Hall, 1987, 1989; Silliman et al., 2006), and spelling frequently remains problematic into late adolescence and adulthood for individuals with dyslexia, even if their word recognition and decoding skills are adequate (Bruck,

1993; Gerber, Schneiders, Paradise, & Reiff, 1990; Guyer, Banks, & Guyer, 1993; Moats, 1996).

For many years, research has focused on the spelling errors made by children and adolescents with RD to investigate whether their spelling is phonetically less accurate than that of normally progressing younger children and to determine whether persistent error patterns can be distinguished in the spelling of children with RD (Bruck, 1988; Carslisle, 1987; Moats, 1983). The results of research on group differences revealed that children with spelling disability and RD produced spellings that were typical of younger children in earlier stages of development and that their error types were not qualitatively different. These findings led investigators to conclude that spelling disability is best characterized as a developmental delay in spelling acquisition.

Moats (1996) argued that this developmental-delay hypothesis masks the linguistic problems evident in children with RD and spelling disability. She noted that many of the spelling errors made by children with dyslexia stem from a subtle disorder in phonological processing that is manifested in the spellings of words with less perceptually salient (i.e., undistinctive) phonological features—for example, words that have obscured sounds during co-articulation within syllables, such as the vocalic /r/ in *work,* which might be spelled as *wok.* Moats (1993; 1996) found that older adolescent students with a history of speech articulation delay in the production of the liquid phonemes /l/ and /r/ made a higher proportion of spelling errors on words containing these sounds, providing evidence for a subtle phonological processing deficit and a degraded phonological representation in memory. A liquid is a phoneme produced with minimal obstruction of the air stream in the mouth, but not enough to cause friction. Acoustically, they are similar to vowels and are classified as containing features of both consonants and vowels.

The majority of research on spelling patterns and disability has focused on typically developing children and children with dyslexia or a reading disability. Few studies have investigated the spelling errors of children diagnosed with LLD. Silliman, Bahr, and Peters (2006) examined the spelling performance of eight children (mean age 7 years, 5 months) who met strict inclusion criteria into the LLD group and two comparison groups of children: one spelling age–matched group (SA) and one chronological age–matched group (CA). The criteria for inclusion in the LLD group included (1) eligibility for special education services in speech-language; (2) nonverbal intelligence within the normal range; (3) a score below the expected age-level criterion on the Clinical Evaluation of Language Fundamentals Screening Test–Third Revision (CELF-3, ST-3; Semel, Wiig, & Secord, 1996); and (4) a score 1 SD below the mean score for chronological age ($M = 100$) on the reading subtest of the Wide Range Achievement Test: Revison 3 (WRAT-3; Wilkinson, 1993) and/or the Test of Written Spelling—Fourth Edition (TWS-4; Larsen, Hammill, & Moats, 1999). Children were given an experimental spelling measure, the Phonological, Orthographic, and Morphological Assessment of Spelling (POMAS), a spelling test involving thirty real words that was designed to reflect increasing levels of spelling development and complexity of phonological, morphologic, and orthographic structure (Silliman et al., 2006).

Qualitative analyses of children's spellings were scored for phonological accuracy, orthographic legality, and visual accuracy. Qualitative error analysis of spellings for the three groups of children showed that the LLD group continued to demonstrate phonological errors in their spellings, similar to findings of spelling error patterns in children with RD (Cassar, Treiman, Curry Pollo, & Kessler, 2005; Moats, 1993, 1996). Children with LLD more often omitted spellings of less perceptually salient phonemes within words, such as the vocalic -*r* (e.g., *cules/curls*) and consonant clusters within words (e.g., *foud/found*). In addition, these children more often omitted grammatical features in words such as plural markers, verb tenses, and derivational morphemes. The specific pattern of spelling errors seen in children with LLD is similar to that seen in children with RD and dyslexia (Carlisle, 1987; Moats, 1996). Similarly, omission of inflectional morphemes is also seen in the oral language profiles of younger children diagnosed with SLI (Rice, 2003), suggesting that specific linguistic problems go unresolved and are later manifested in written/spelling form.

Summary

Children with language learning disability are a heterogeneous group that present with varying characteristics and degrees of severity of deficit within and across the functional language systems of listening, speaking, reading, and writing/spelling. As noted, the concept of language learning disability is not fully understood and its definition, identification, and intervention practices are still emerging in the scientific and educational communities. Children with a language learning disability demonstrate deficits with the oral-written language continuum, communicating with language in both its spoken and written form. Several types of children are known to demonstrate language-learning difficulties in the classroom, including children with a history of developmental speech and language problems noted during the preschool years; children with generalized language and cognitive delays; children with specific reading disability in either word decoding, characteristic of dyslexia, or with deficits in reading comprehension; and children with advanced oral language skills who struggle with the academic language demands of the classroom.

A language learning disability may manifest itself differently in similar children, in that varying patterns and levels of difficulty may be seen within and across aspects of language functioning. Understanding the concept of a language learning disability and the interrelationships of the functional language systems means answering the following questions:

1. Do variations in symptoms and behavioral expressions of language deficits indicate specific subtypes of LLD?
2. Do different patterns of language processing and deficits suggest a particular configuration of academic achievement (i.e., well developed word recognition and spelling ability compared to poor oral and/or written discourse ability)?

3. Do developmental variations in the expression of language difficulties in listening, speaking, reading, and writing/spelling dictate the use of specific and targeted intervention practices that can predict a child's response to intervention and long-term behavioral outcomes?

These are only a few of the questions that can be asked as we continue to learn about the concept of a *language learning disability.*

Children who do not have intact language development and processing across the language continuum do not have the necessary foundation to support the development of academic language and literacy. Future research should focus on the developmental interactions among the language systems and the recognition and identification of the early signs of disability. Doing so will help us to develop a more comprehensive model of language learning disability and its effect on children, academic achievement, and society.

Case Study   Meghan

Meghan is an 8-year, 10-month-old girl in third grade in a parochial school. She was initially identified during her preschool years as having a significant articulation and phonological disorder characterized by rapid, unintelligible speech and the presence of a number of phonological processes such as final consonant deletion, cluster reduction, and stopping. From 2½ to 4 years of age, Meghan received speech intervention focusing on articulation training, phonological processes, and speech rate reduction at a hospital-based outpatient program. Meghan entered a small private preschool program at the age of 4 years and speech intervention for articulation and phonological processes continued through her kindergarten year at a private parochial school. By 7 years of age, speech articulation and the use of developmental phonological processes had improved significantly, although speech rate continued to be problematic and sometimes interfered with her speech intelligibility. However, she was able to monitor her rate and would modify and slow her rate when reminded by her parents, teachers, or therapists. In first grade, assessment of oral language competence using the Test of Language Development-P (TOLD-P) indicated no language impairment; Meghan scored within the average range for overall language quotient and for all subtests. Meghan's improved speech articulation and intelligibility was considered a great success. She was doing well in school and in conference with her parents, so it was decided that Meghan should be dismissed from weekly speech intervention yet continue to be monitored for school-related oral language or speech articulation problems. Two years later, at the beginning of third grade, Meghan's mother contacted the speech and language clinic at Lehman College to request a re-evaluation of Meghan's speech and language. She indicated that Meghan was not doing well in school, specifically in the areas of reading and spelling. Although Meghan appeared to not have any difficulty in first grade with learning to read, difficulty was now noted in third grade in completing assignments, reading unfamiliar words, reading comprehension, and spelling. Meghan was seen for an evaluation of oral language, phonological processing, reading, and spelling. Oral language ability was found to be within normal limits for her age but deficits were found in her phonological processing, reading, and spelling. The following standard scores were obtained:

Comprehensive Test of Phonological Processing (CTOPP)
Phonological Processing Composite: 85 (standard score); 16th percentile
Phonological Memory Composite: 88 (standard score); 21st percentile
Rapid Naming Composite: 85 (standard score); 16th percentile

Woodcock Reading Mastery Test (WRMT)
Total Reading Cluster: 85 (standard score); 16th percentile
Basic Skills Cluster: 88 (standard score); 20th percentile
Subtests:
    Word Identification: 87 (standard score); 19th percentile
    Word Attack: 93 (standard score); 31st percentile
    Passage Comprehension: 85 (standard score); 16th percentile

Test of Written Spelling (TOWS)
77 (standard score); 6th percentile
Spelling Errors:

Target Word	Meghan's Spelling	Error analysis
spring	sping	consonant cluster reduction
storm	stom	omission of vocalic -r
myself	mysef	omission of glide /l/, consonant cluster reduction
people	popel	orthographic vowel error and consonant -le
hardly	hardley	orthographic
able	adall	orthographic letter reversal (d/b), consonant -le
everyone	everone	syllable deletion
uncle	encl	vowel, orthographic consonant -le

Impression
Meghan continues to demonstrate phonological deficits, but now the difficulty is expressed in her reading, spelling, and phonological processing. Her initial gains in speech articulation and phonology are now viewed as an *illusory recovery* (Scarborough & Dobrich, 1990), meaning that although her oral speech production had improved, the phonological problems remain, although in a different form. Her spelling errors show many phonological processing errors including cluster reduction, syllable deletion, and omission of liquid phonemes /l/ and /r/, noted by researchers investigating spelling patterns in children with RD and LLD (Moats, 1996; Silliman et al., 2006). Meghan demonstrates poor phonological processing as evidenced by below average scores on phonological awareness and phonological memory composites. Reading is poor for word identification (e.g., sight word vocabulary), a by-product of overall reduced reading ability. As noted by Stanovich (1986), reading difficulty inhibits the acquisition and mapping of more sight words into one's orthographic representation and storage of words creating the "Matthew effect" where the "rich get richer and the poor get poorer." Meghan has good decoding ability as evidenced by her standard score of 93 on the Word Attack subtest of

the WRMT, but she is not applying this knowledge during reading of unfamiliar words. The combined effect is reducing her overall reading comprehension. Meghan's history of significant phonological deficits during the preschool years and extending past the age of 5 years into early elementary school placed her at an increased risk for having a language learning disability, now evident in third grade.

Study Questions

1. Compare and contrast the cognitive and linguistic characteristics of four types of children who may be classified as language learning disabled.
2. How did NCLB and the IDEA reauthorization change how children with academic language difficulty are identified in the schools as having a specific learning disability? Why is this change significant?
3. What are the similarities and differences between spoken and written language comprehension?
4. Define phonological processing within a framework of metalinguistic awareness. What is the role of phonological processing in learning to read and spell?
5. Describe the linguistic spelling patterns and deficits seen in children who are language learning disabled. Are these similar to or different from spelling patterns seen in children who are reading disabled?

References

Adams, M. J. (1992). *Beginning to read: Thinking and learning about print.* Cambridge, MA: MIT Press.

American Psychiatric Association (APA). (2000). *Diagnostic and statistical manual of mental disorders* (text revision) (*DSM-IV-TR*). Washington, DC: Author.

American Speech-Language-Hearing Association (ASHA). (1991). *Learning disabilities: Issues on definition.* Retrieved April, 2008 from www.asha.org/policy.

American Speech-Language-Hearing Association. (1998). *Operationalizing the NJCLD definition of learning disabilities for ongoing assessment in schools* [Relevant Paper]. Available from www.asha.org/policy.

American Speech-Language-Hearing Association (ASHA). (2001). *Roles and responsibilities of speech-language pathologists with respect to reading and writing in children and adolescents.* Position statement, Executive Summary of Guidelines, Technical Report. Rockville, MD: Author.

Aram, D., & Nation, J. (1980). Preschool language disorders and subsequent language and academic difficulties. *Journal of Communication Disorders, 13,* 159–170.

Aram, D. M., Ekelman, B. L., & Nation, J. E. (1984). Preschoolers with language disorders: Ten years later. *Journal of Speech and Hearing Research, 27,* 232–244.

Aram, D. M., Morris, R., & Hall, N. E. (1992). The validity of discrepancy criteria for identifying children with developmental language disorders. *Journal of Learning Disabilities, 25,* 549–554.

Ball, E. W. (1993). Phonological awareness: What's important and to whom. *Reading and Writing: An Interdisciplinary Journal, 5,* 141–159.

Ball, E. W., & Blachman, B. A. (1991). Does phoneme awareness training in kindergarten make a difference in early word recognition and developmental spelling? *Reading Research Quarterly, 26,* 49–66.

Bailet, L. L. (1990). Spelling rule usage among students with learning disabilities and normally achieving students. *Journal of Learning Disabilities, 23,* 121–128.

Berninger, V. W. (2000). Development of language by hand and its connections with language by ear, mouth, and eye. *Topics in Language Disorders, 20,* 65–84.

Bishop, D.V., North, T., & Dolan, C. (1996). Nonword repetition as a behavioral marker for inherited language impairment: Evidence from a twin study. *Journal of Child Psychology and Psychiatry, 37,* 391–403.

Bishop, D. V. M., & Adams, C. (1990). A prospective study of the relationship between specific language impairment, phonological disorders, and reading retardation. *Journal of Child Psychology and Psychiatry, 31,* 1027–1050.

Bradley, L., & Bryant, P. (1983). Categorizing sounds and learning to read: A causal connection. *Nature, 301,* 419–421.

Bradley, R., Danielson, L., & Hallahan, D. (Eds.). (2002). *Identification of learning disabilities: Research to practice.* Mahwah, NJ: Lawrence Erlbaum.

Brinton, B., Fujiki, M., & Sonnenberg, E. (1988). Responses to requests for clarification by linguistically normal and language impaired children in conversation. *Journal of Speech and Hearing Disorders, 53,* 383–391.

Brinton, B., Fujiki, M., & Spencer, J. C. (1997). The ability of children with specific language impairment to access and participate in an ongoing interaction. *Journal of Speech, Language, and Hearing Research, 40,* 1011–1025.

Brown, R. (1973). *A first language: The early stages.* Cambridge, MA: Harvard University Press.

Bruck, M. (1988). The word recognition and spelling of dyslexic children. *Reading Research Quarterly, 23,* 51–69.

Bruck, M. (1993). Component spelling skills of college students with childhood diagnoses of reading disability. *Learning Disability Quarterly, 16,* 171–184.

Cain, K. (2003). Text comprehension and its relation to coherence and cohesion in children's fictional narratives. *British Journal of Developmental Psychology, 21,* 335–351.

Cain, K., & Oakhill, J. (1996). The nature of the relationship between comprehension skill and the ability to tell a story. *British Journal of Developmental Psychology, 14,* 187–201.

Cain, K., & Oakhill, J. (2007). *Children's comprehension problems in oral and written language: A cognitive perspective.* New York: Guilford Press.

Cain, K., & Oakhill, J. V. (2007). Reading comprehension difficulties: Correlates, causes, and consequences. In K. Cain & J. V. Oakhill (Eds.), *Children's comprehension problems in oral and written language: A cognitive perspective.* New York: Guilford Press.

Cain, K., Oakhill, J. V., Barnes, M. A., & Bryant, P. E. (2001). Comprehension skill, inference-making ability, and the relation to knowledge. *Memory and Cognition, 29,* 850–859.

Carlisle, J. F. (1987). The use of morphological knowledge in spelling derived forms by learning-disabled and normal students. *Annals of Dyslexia, 37,* 90–108.

Carpenter, D. (1983). Spelling errors profiles of able and disabled readers. *Journal of Learning Disabilities, 16,* 102–104.

Cassar, M., Treiman, L., Curry Pollo, T., & Kessler, B. (2005). How do the spellings of children with dyslexia compare with those of nondyslexic children? *Reading and Writing: An Interdisciplinary Journal, 18,* 27–49.

Catts, H. W. (1986). Speech production/phonological deficits in reading-disordered children. *Journal of Learning Disabilities, 19,* 504–508.

Catts, H. W. (1993). The relationship between speech-language impairments and reading disabilities. *Journal of Speech and Hearing Research, 36,* 948–958.

Catts, H. W., Adlof, S. M., Hogan, T. P., & Weismer, S. E. (2005). Are specific language impairment and dyslexia distinct disorders? *Journal of Speech, Language, and Hearing Research, 48,* 1378–1396.

Catts, H. W., Fey, M. E., Tomblin, J. B., & Zhang, X. (2002). A longitudinal investigation of reading outcomes in children with language impairments. *Journal of Speech, Language, and Hearing Research, 45,* 1142–1157.

Catts, H. W., Fey, M. E., Zhang, X., & Tomblin, J. B. (1999). Language basis of reading and reading disabilities: Evidence from a longitudinal investigation. *Scientific Studies of Reading, 3,* 331–361.

Catts, H. W., Hogan, T. P., & Fey, M. E. (2003). Subgrouping poor readers on the basis of individual differences in reading-related abilities. *Journal of Learning Disabilities, 36,* 151–164.

Chall, J. S. (1983). *Learning to read: The great debate.* New York: McGraw-Hill.

Chall, J. S., Jacobs, V. A., & Baldwin, L. E. (1990). *The reading crisis: Why poor children fall behind.* Cambridge, MA: Harvard University Press.

Clark, D. B., & Uhry, J. K. (1995). *Dyslexia: Theory and practice of remedial instruction.* Baltimore, MD: York Press.

Cole, K. N., Mills, P. E., & Kelley, D. (1994). Agreement of the assessment profiles used in cognitive referencing. *Language, Speech, and Hearing Services in Schools, 25,* 25–31.

Conti-Ramsden, G., Botting, N., & Faragher, B. (2001). Psycholinguistic markers for specific language impairment (SLI). *Journal of Child Psychology and Psychiatry, 42,* 741–748.

Cosgrove, S. (1977). *Cap'n Smudge.* Danbury, CT: Grolier.

Denny, J. P. (1991). Rational thought in oral culture and literate decontextualization. In D. Olsen & N. Torrance (Eds.), *Literacy and orality.* Cambridge: Cambridge University Press.

Ehri, L. (1987). Learning to read and spell words. *Journal of Reading Behavior, 19,* 5–31.

Ehri, L. (2000). Learning to read and learning to spell: Two sides of a coin. *Topics in Language Disorders, 20,* 19–36.

Ehri, L. C., & Wilce, L. S. (1979). The mnemonic value of orthography among beginning readers. *Journal of Educational Psychology, 71,* 26–40.

Ehri, L. C., & Wilce, L. S. (1980). The influence of orthography on readers' conceptualization of the phonemic structure of words. *Applied Psycholinguistics, 1,* 371–385.

Ehri, L. C., & Wilce, L. S. (1987). Does learning to spell help beginners learn to read words? *Reading Research Quarterly, 22,* 47–65.

Ellis, A. W. (1993). *Reading, writing, and dyslexia: A cognitive analysis* (2nd ed.). Hove, England: Lawrence Erlbaum.

Fischer, F. W., Shankweiler, D., & Liberman, I. Y. (1985). Spelling proficiency and sensitivity to word structure. *Journal of Memory and Language, 24,* 423–441.

Fletcher, J. M., Coulter, W. A., Reschly, D. J., & Vaughn, S. (2004). Alternative approaches to the definition and identification of learning disabilities: Some questions and answers. *Annals of Dyslexia, 54,* 304–331.

Fletcher, J. M., Lyon, G. R., Fuchs, L. S., & Barnes, M. A. (2007). *Learning disabilities: From identification to intervention.* New York: Guilford Press.

Fletcher, J. M., Morris, R. D., & Lyon, G. R. (2003). Classification and definition of learning disabilities: An integrative perspective. In H. L. Swanson, K. R. Harris, & S. Graham (Eds.), *Handbook of learning disabilities.* New York: Guilford Press.

Fowler, A. E. (1991). How early phonological development might set the stage for phoneme awareness. In S. A. Brady & D. P. Shankweiler (Eds.), *Phonological processes in literacy.* Hillsdale, NJ: Lawrence Erlbaum.

Fox, B., & Routh, D. K. (1975). Analyzing spoken language into words, syllables, and phonemes: A developmental study. *Journal of Psycholinguistic Research, 4,* 331–342.

Frith, U. (1980). *Cognitive processes in spelling.* New York: Academic Press.

Gathercole, S. E., & Baddeley, A. D. (1990). Phonological memory deficits in language disordered children: Is there a causal connection. *Journal of Memory and Language, 29,* 336–360.

Gerber, M., & Hall, R. (1987). Information processing approaches to studying spelling deficiencies. *Journal of Learning Disabilities, 20,* 34–42.

Gerber, M., & Hall, R. (1989). Cognitive-behavioral training in spelling for learning handicapped students. *Learning Disability Quarterly, 12,* 159–171.

Gerber, P., Schneiders, C., Paradise, L., & Reiff, H. (1990). Persisting problems of adults with learning disabilities: Self-reported comparisons from their school-age and adult years. *Journal of Learning Disabilities, 23,* 570–573.

German, D. J. (1982). Word-finding substitutions in children with learning disabilities. *Language, Speech, and Hearing Services in Schools, 13,* 223–230.

German, D. J. (1987). Spontaneous language profiles of children with word-finding problems. *Language, Speech, and Hearing Services in Schools, 18,* 217–230.

Gillon, G. (2004). *Phonological awareness: From research to practice.* New York: Guilford Press.

Gough, P. B., & Tummer, W. E. (1986). Decoding, reading, and reading disability. *Remedial and Special Education, 7,* 6–10.

Guyer, B. P., Banks, S. R., & Guyer, K. E. (1993). Spelling improvement for college students who are dyslexic. *Annals of Dyslexia, 43,* 186–193.

Henderson, E. (1990). *Teaching spelling.* Boston: Houghton Mifflin.

Hoover, W. A., & Gough, P. B. (1990). The simple view of reading. *Reading and Writing: An Interdisciplinary Journal, 2,* 127–160.

Horton, W. S., & Gerrig, R. J. (2005). Conversational common ground and memory processes in language production. *Discourse Processes, 40,* 1–35.

Idol-Maestas, L. (1980). Oral language responses of children with reading difficulties. *Journal of Speech Education, 14,* 386–404.

Just, M. A., & Carpenter, P. A. (1987). *The psychology of reading and language comprehension.* Boston: Allyn & Bacon.

Kail, R., & Leonard, L. (1986). Word-finding abilities in language-impaired children. *ASHA Monograph, 25,* 1–36.

Kamhi, A. G., Lee, R. F., & Nelson, L. K. (1985). Word, syllable, and sound awareness in language-disordered children. *Journal of Speech and Hearing Disorders, 50,* 207–212.

Kavanagh, J. F., & Mattingly, I. G. (Eds.). (1972). *Language by ear and by eye*. Cambridge, MA: MIT Press.

Larrivee, L. S., & Catts, H. W. (1999). Early reading achievement in children with expressive phonological disorders. *American Journal of Speech-Language Pathology, 18,* 118–128.

Larsen, S. C., Hammill, D. D., & Moats, L. C. (1999). *Test of written spelling* (4th ed.). Austin, TX: Pro-Ed.

Leonard, L. B. (1998). *Children with specific language impairments*. Cambridge, MA: MIT Press.

Lewis, B. A., Freebairn, L. A., & Taylor, H. G. (2000). Follow-up of children with early expressive phonology disorders. *Journal of Learning Disabilities, 33,* 433–444.

Liberman, I. Y., & Shankweiler, D. (1985). Phonology and the problems of learning to read and write. *Remedial and Special Education, 6,* 8–17.

Liberman, I. Y., Shankweiler, D., Fischer, F. W., & Carter, B. (1974). Explicit syllable and phoneme segmentation in the young child. *Journal of Experimental Child Psychology, 18,* 201–212.

Liles, B. Z. (1985). Cohesion in the narratives of normal and language-disordered children. *Journal of Speech and Hearing Research, 28,* 123–133.

Lundberg, I., Frost, J., & Petersen, O. P. (1988). Effects of an intensive program for stimulating phonological awareness skills in preschool children. *Reading Research Quarterly, 23,* 263–284.

Lyon, G. R. (1989). IQ is irrelevant to the definition of learning disabilities: A position in search of logic and data. *Journal of Learning Disabilities, 22,* 504–512.

Lyon, G. R., Fletcher, J. M., Shaywitz, B. A., Torgesen, J. K., Woods, F. B., et al. (2001). Rethinking learning disabilities. In C. E. Finn, Jr., A. J. Rotherham, & C. R. Hokanson, Jr. (Eds.), *Rethinking special education for a new century*. Washington, DC: Thomas B. Fordham Foundation and Progressive Policy Institute.

Lyon, G. R., Shaywitz, S. E., & Shaywitz, B. A. (2003). A definition of dyslexia. *Annals of Dyslexia, 53,* 1–14.

Mandler, J. M., & Johnson, N. A. (1977). Remembrance of things parsed: Story structure and recall. *Cognitive Psychology, 9,* 111–151.

Masterson, J. J. (1993). The performance of children with language-learning disabilities on two types of cognitive tasks. *Journal of Speech, Language, Hearing Research, 36,* 1026–1036.

Mattingly, I. G. (1972). Reading: The linguistic process and linguistic awareness. In J. K. Kavanagh & I. G. Mattingly (Eds.), *Language by ear and by eye*. Cambridge, MA: MIT Press.

Meline, T., & Brackin, S. (1987). Language-impaired children's awareness of inadequate messages. *Journal of Speech and Hearing Disorders, 52,* 263–270.

Menyuk, P., Chesnick, M., Liebergott, J., Korngold, B., D'Agostino, R., & Belanger, A. (1991). Predicting reading problems in at-risk children. *Journal of Speech and Hearing Research, 34,* 893–903.

Merritt, D. D., & Liles, B. Z. (1987). Story grammar ability in children with and without language disorder: Story generation, story retelling, and story comprehension. *Journal of Speech and Hearing Research, 30,* 539–552.

Moats, L. C. (1983). A comparison of the spelling errors of older dyslexics and second-grade normal children. *Annals of Dyslexia, 33,* 121–139.

Moats, L. C. (1993). Spelling error analysis: Beyond the phonetic/dysphonetic dichotomy. *Annals of Dyslexia, 43,* 174–185.

Moats, L. C. (1995). *Spelling: Development disability and instruction.* Baltimore, MD: York Press.

Moats, L. C. (1996). Phonological spelling errors in the writing of dyslexic adolescents. *Reading and Writing: An Interdisciplinary Journal, 8,* 105–119.

Moats, L. C., & Smith, C. (1992). Derivational morphology: Why it should be included in language assessment and instruction. *Language, Speech, and Hearing Services in Schools, 23,* 312–319.

Nation, K., Clarke, P., Marshall, C. M., & Durand, M. (2004). Hidden language impairments in children: Parallels between poor reading comprehension and specific language impairment? *Journal of Speech, Language, and Hearing Research, 47,* 199–211.

Nation, K., & Snowling, M. J. (2000). Factors influencing syntactic awareness skills in normal readers and poor comprehenders. *Applied Psycholinguistics, 21,* 229–241.

Newcomer, P. L., & Hammill, D. D. (1997). *Test of Language Development–Primary (TOLD–P).* Austin, TX: Pro-Ed.

Norbury, C. F., & Bishop, D. V. M. (2003). Narrative skills in children with communication impairments. *International Journal of Language and Communication Impairments, 38,* 287–313.

Oakhill, J., & Cain, K. (2007). Introduction to comprehension development. In K. Cain & J. V. Oakhill (Eds.), *Children's comprehension problems in oral and written language: A cognitive perspective.* New York: Guilford Press.

Paul, R. (1990). Comprehension strategies: Interactions between world knowledge and the development of sentence comprehension. *Topics in Language Disorders, 10*(3), 63–75.

Paul, R. (2001). *Language disorders from infancy through adolescence: Assessment and intervention.* St. Louis, MO: Mosby.

Pennington, B. F., & Lefly, D. L. (2001). Early reading development in children at family risk for dyslexia. *Child Development, 72,* 816–833.

Perera, K. (1984). *Children's writing and reading.* London, England: Blackwell.

Perfetti, C. A. (1985). *Reading ability.* New York: Oxford University Press.

Plante, E. (1998). Criteria for SLI: The Stark and Tallal legacy and beyond. *Journal of Speech, Language, and Hearing Research, 41,* 951–957.

Rice, M. L. (2003). A unified model of specific and general language delay: Grammatical tense as a clinical marker of unexpected variation. In Y. Levy & J. Schaeffer (Eds.), *Language competence across populations: Toward a definition of specific language impairment.* Mahwah, NJ: Lawrence Erlbaum.

Roth, F. P., & Spekman, N. J. (1989). The oral syntactic proficiency of learning disabled students: A spontaneous story sampling analysis. *Journal of Speech and Hearing Research, 32,* 67–77.

Rourke, B. P. (1994). Neuropsychological assessment of children with learning disabilities: Measurement issues. In G. Reid Lyon (Ed.), *Frames of reference for the assessment of learning disabilities: New views on measurement issues.* Baltimore, MD: Paul H. Brookes.

Rubin, H., Patterson, P. A., & Kantor, M. (1991). Morphological development and writing ability in children an adults. *Language, Speech, and Hearing Services in Schools, 22,* 228–235.

Rvachew, S. (2007). Phonological processing and reading in children with speech sound disorders. *American Journal of Speech-Language Pathology, 16,* 260–270.

Scarborough, H. S., & Dobrich, W. (1990). The development of children with early language delay. *Journal of Speech and Hearing Research, 33,* 70–83.

Scott, C. M., & Windsor, J. (2000). General language performance measures in spoken and written narrative and expository discourse in school-age children with language learning disabilities. *Journal of Speech, Language, and Hearing Research, 43,* 324–339.

Seidenberg, M., & McClelland, J. (1989). A distributed, developmental model of word recognition and naming. *Psychological Review, 96,* 523–568.

Semel, E., Wiig, E. H., & Secord, W. A. (1993). *Clinical Evaluation of Language Fundamentals Screening Test–Third Revision* (CELF-3, ST). San Antonio, TX: Harcourt Assessment.

Share, D. L., Jorm, A. F., Maclean, R., & Matthews, R. (1984). Sources of individual differences in reading acquisition. *Journal of Educational Psychology, 76,* 1309–1324.

Shriberg, L., & Kwiatiwski, J. (1988). A follow-up study of children with phonologic disorders of unknown origin. *Journal of Speech and Hearing Disorders, 53,* 144–156.

Siegel, L. S. (1989). IQ is irrelevant to the definition of learning disabilities. *Journal of Learning Disabilities, 22,* 469–486.

Siegel, L. S., & Himel, N. (1998). Socioeconomic status, age, and the classification of dyslexics and poor readers: The dangers of using IQ scores in the definition of reading disability. *Dyslexia, 4,* 90–104.

Silliman, E. R., Bahr, R. H., & Peters, M. L. (2006). Spelling patterns in preadolescents with atypical language skills: Phonological, morphological, and orthographic factors. *Developmental Neuropsychology, 29,* 93–123.

Silliman, E. R., Wilkinson, L. C., & Brea-Spahn, M. R. (2004). Policy and practice imperatives for language and literacy learning: Who will be left behind? In C. A. Stone, E. R. Silliman, B. R. Ehren, & K. Apel (Eds.), *Handbook of language & literacy: Development and disorders.* New York: Guilford Press.

Snow, C. E., Burns, M. S., & Griffin, P. (1998). *Preventing reading difficulties in young children.* Washington, DC: National Academy Press.

Snowling, M. J. (1996). Developmental dyslexia. In M. Snowling & J. Stackhouse (Eds.), *Dyslexia, speech, and language: A practitioners handbook.* London, England: Whurr.

Stanovich, K. E. (1986). Matthew effects in reading: Some consequences of individual differences in the acquisition of reading. *Reading Research Quarterly, 21,* 360–406.

Stanovich, K. E. (1988). Explaining the differences between the dyslexic and the garden-variety poor reader: The phonological-core variable-difference model. *Journal of Learning Disabilities, 21,* 590–604.

Stanovich, K. E., Cunningham, A., & Cramer, B. (1984). Assessing phonological awareness in kindergarten children: Issues of task comparability. *Journal of Experimental Child Psychology, 38,* 175–190.

Stark, R., & Tallal, P. (1981). Selection of children with specific language deficits. *Journal of Speech and Hearing Disorders, 46,* 114–122.

Stothard, S. E., Snowling, M. J., Bishop, D. V. M., & Chipcase, B. B. (1998). Language-impaired preschoolers: A follow-up to adolescence. *Journal of Speech-Language-Hearing Research, 41,* 407–418.

Templeton, S. (1989). Tacit and explicit knowledge of derivational morphology: Foundations for a unified approach to spelling and vocabulary development in their intermediate grades and beyond. *Reading Psychology, 10,* 233–253.

Templeton, S., & Scarborough-Franks, L. (1985). Spelling's the thing: Knowledge of derivational morphology in orthography and phonology among older students. *Applied Psycholinguistics, 6,* 379–389.

Tager-Flusberg, H., & Cooper, J. (1999). Present and future possibilities for defining a phenotype for specific language impairment. *Journal of Speech, Language, and Hearing Research, 42,* 1275–1278.

Tomblin, J. B., & Zhang, X. (1999). Language patterns and etiology in children with specific language impairments. In H. Tager-Flusberg (Ed.), *Neurological disorders* (pp. 362–381). Cambridge, MA: MIT Press.

Torgesen, J. K. (2002). The prevention of reading difficulties. *Journal of School Psychology, 40,* 7–26.

Treiman, R. (1984). Individual differences among children in spelling and reading styles. *Journal of Experimental Child Psychology, 37,* 463–477.

Treiman, R., & Bourassa, D. C. (2000). The development of spelling skill. *Topics in Language Disorders, 20,* 1–18.

Treiman, R., Cassar, M., & Zukowski, A. (1994). What types of linguistic information do children use in spelling? The case of flaps. *Child Development, 65,* 1130–1329.

U.S. Office of Education. (1968). *First Annual Report of the National Advisory Committee on Handicapped Children.* Washington, DC: U.S. Department of Health, Education, and Welfare.

U.S. Office of Education (1977). *Education of handicapped children.* Implementation of Part B of the Education for Handicapped Act. Federal Register. Part II. Washington, DC: U.S. Department of Health, Education, and Welfare.

U.S. Office of Education (2002). *A new era: Revitalizing special education for children and their families.* Report of the PCESE. Washington, DC: U.S. Department of Education.

Van Kleek, A. (1984). Assessment and intervention: Does "meta" matter? In G. P. Wallach & K. G. Butler (Eds.), *Language learning disabilities in school age children.* Baltimore, MD: Williams & Wilkins.

Vellutino, F. R., & Scanlon, D. M. (1987). Phonological coding, phonological awareness, and reading ability: Evidence from longitudinal and experimental study. *Merrill Palmer Quarterly, 33,* 321–363.

Vellutino, F. R., & Scanlon, D. M. (1991). The preeminence of phonologically based skills in learning to read. In S. A. Brady & D. P. Shankweiler (Eds.), *Phonological processes in literacy.* Mahwah, NJ: Lawrence Erlbaum.

Wagner, R. K., & Torgesen, J. K. (1987). The nature of phonological processing and its causal role in the acquisition of reading skills. *Psychological Bulletin, 101,* 192–212.

Webster, P. E., & Plante, A. S. (1992). Effects of phonological impairment on word, syllable, and phoneme segmentation and reading. *Language, Speech, and Hearing Services in Schools, 23,* 176–182.

Westby, C. (2002). Beyond decoding: Critical and dynamic literacy for students with dyslexia, language learning disabilities (LLD), or attention deficit-hyperactivity disorder (ADHD). In K. Butler & E. R. Silliman (Eds.), *Speaking, reading, and writing in children with language learning disabilities.* Mahwah, NJ: Lawrence Erlbaum.

Wiig, E. (1982). Language disabilities in school-age children and youth. In G. Shames & E. Wiig (Eds.), *Human communication disorders: An introduction* (2nd ed.). Columbus, OH: Merrill.

Wilkinson, G. S. (1993). *Wide Range Achievement Test–Revision 3* (WRAT–3). Wilmington, DE: Jastak Association.

Wolf, M. (1984). Naming, reading, and the dyslexias: A longitudinal overview. *Annals of Dyslexia, 34,* 87–116.

Wolf, M. (1999). Rapid serial naming and the double-deficit hypothesis. *Annals of Dyslexia, 49,* 1–28.

Wolf, M., & Bowers, P. (2000). The question of naming-speed deficits in developmental reading disability: An introduction to the double-deficit hypothesis. *Journal of Learning Disabilities, 33,* 322–324.

Woodcock, R. W. (1987). *Woodcock Reading Mastery Tests–Revised.* Circle Pines, MN: American Guidance Services.

CHAPTER 6

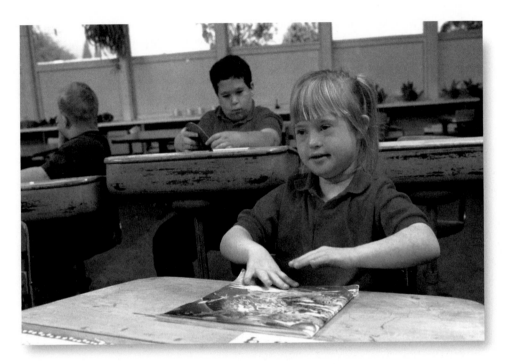

Mental Retardation/
Intellectual Disability

Robert E. Owens, Jr.
State University of New York at Geneseo

When you finish this chapter, you should be able to

- Discuss how we characterize or define the mentally retarded population.
- List the cognitive and linguistic characteristics of the mentally retarded population.
- Discuss intervention techniques that are suggested by the learning characteristics of the mentally retarded population.

- Describe the developmental intervention approach, and how it is used.
- Describe behaviors that should be targeted, and techniques that should be used in intervention by the speech-language pathologist.

> I wanted to make this book all about pop music, but my Dad says people will be more interested in my adventures. But I must write a bit about pop. (Hunt, 1967, p. 89)

In *The World of Nigel Hunt*, the author expresses the interests of many other teenagers. This particular adolescent has mental retardation. He was born with Down syndrome, a genetic disorder that is one of hundreds of identifiable causes of or factors related to mental retardation. Yet Nigel is more like his typically developing peers than he is unlike them.

It is difficult to characterize people with mental retardation because they are so diverse. This heterogeneous population includes individuals who are totally dependent and those who are nearly independent in their daily living. We can say, however, that in general, they develop more slowly or at a more delayed rate than the typically developing population. In other ways, people with mental retardation are different from the typically developing population. These characteristics can be seen in several aspects of the development of individuals with mental retardation, including language.

This chapter will explore a definition of mental retardation, sometimes called *intellectual disability*, and discuss the implications for communication and language development. The chapter will also characterize the special language problems of this population and suggest intervention techniques and programs that might be helpful for the speech-language pathologist.

Before we begin, I should share my biases with you. First, and research supports my contention, it is best to begin intervention and schooling as early as possible. The benefits of early intervention for the child and family are well documented. Second, language and communication intervention should be functional in nature, which means it should target communication use and include a child's caregivers as communication facilitators.

Training should occur in the environments in which language will be used: home, school, and day care. Both topics will be discussed more later in the chapter. For now, let's examine what mental retardation is and is not.

A Definition of Mental Retardation/Intellectual Disability

The American Association on Mental Retardation (AAMR), the primary organization for professionals working with the mentally retarded population, defines *mental retardation (MR)* as a "significantly subaverage general intellectual functioning, existing concurrently with related limitations in two or more adaptive skill areas [and] manifest[ed] before age 18" (AAMR, 1992). To understand this definition fully, we must look at its various components.

Significantly subaverage is generally defined as an IQ of 68 or lower, but this upper limit is not inflexible. In the entire population, the mean, or average, IQ is 100, but the range of normality extends from 86 to 116. This range contains two-thirds of the population. In other words, two-thirds of the population is considered to have average intelligence. An IQ of 68 is significantly below average.

Intellectual functioning refers to the results of a culture-free standardized test of general intelligence. The generally accepted measurement of intelligence is IQ, which is a ratio of mental age to chronological age. If the mental age is 10 years and the chronological age is 10 years, the relationship is 10/10 or 1, which is interpreted as an IQ of 100. In contrast, a mental age of 5 and a chronological age of 10 yields 5/10 or 0.5, which is an IQ of 50.

Testing should be pluralistic and culture free. A test based solely on language abilities would be unfair to many second-language learners and to many children with learning disabilities. Intelligence testing should also assess nonlinguistic abilities, such as problem solving, sensorimotor development, and social skills. Again, culturally biased tests would be prejudicial to many minorities. I know of a Southeast Asian immigrant who was unfairly classified as mentally retarded based on the results of an English receptive vocabulary test.

Adaptive skills vary for different ages. During infancy and the preschool years, adaptive skills include sensorimotor, speech and language, self-help, and interactional development. In middle childhood and early adolescence, the emphasis shifts to academic and reasoning skill development and to group and interpersonal relationships. Late-adolescent and adult adaptive skill development relates to vocational and social responsibility. Although adaptive behavior frequently correlates very positively with intelligence, this is not always true.

The period *prior to age 18* is considered by many to be the **developmental period.** For those with MR, development may be slow, arrested, or incomplete. The developmental rate decreases as all humans reach their late teens. Thus, young adults with MR may experience only moderate developmental change after age 18, although they will function at a mental age below 18 years.

The AAMR (1992) definition includes only those individuals who meet all the criteria. Children who have learning disabilities are not included because most possess normal intelligence, and elderly patients who have aphasia do not qualify because their disorder did not manifest itself during the developmental period. Although individuals with both types of disorders might function within the retarded range on some tasks, they cannot be classified as mentally retarded. Figure 6.1 illustrates the AAMR definition.

The AAMR (1992) definition does not specify causes or etiologies but emphasizes the current functioning level of the individual. In other words, it is not assumed that Down syndrome is synonymous with mental retardation. In part, the definition reflects a belief that functioning levels can be modified or changed—that the individual with MR is a developmental being.

Currently, there is a debate in the professional literature about what to call the disability just described. Other disabilities have also undergone name changes. For instance, autism is now called *autism spectrum disorder*. The new name proposed for mental retardation is *intellectual disability*. The fine points of the discussion underlying this change are beyond the scope of this chapter. I will use the older term and occasionally the new one, mainly for variety.

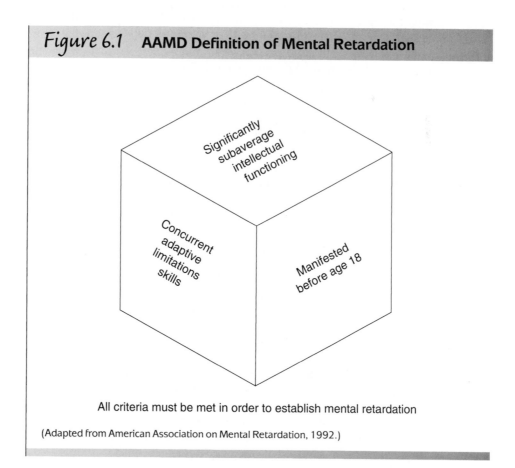

Figure 6.1 **AAMD Definition of Mental Retardation**

Significantly subaverage intellectual functioning

Concurrent adaptive limitations skills

Manifested before age 18

All criteria must be met in order to establish mental retardation

(Adapted from American Association on Mental Retardation, 1992.)

Prevalence and Levels of Functioning

The exact number of individuals with MR in the United States is unknown. Estimates vary from 1 to 3 percent of the population, or approximately 3.5 to 10 million individuals. To place these figures in perspective, mental retardation is approximately fifteen times more prevalent than blindness. Most of the approximately 130,000 individuals with retardation born in the United States each year are only mildly retarded.

There are four categories of mental retardation, all based on IQ: mild, moderate, severe, and profound. The characteristics of each category are listed in Table 6.1.

The distribution of mental retardation within the population is not uniform. The population of individuals with severe and profound retardation reflects the general population in terms of family socioeconomic status and race and ethnicity. Among those with mild and moderate retardation, there are greater percentages of poor and minority individuals as well as a greater percentage of individuals with a family history of retardation.

The disproportionately higher percentage of MR among poor and minority populations may reflect the environmental effects of poverty. In American culture, many individuals from racial and ethnic minorities are found in the lower socioeconomic levels because of poor education and a lack of social mobility. Lack of proper nutrition and poor health may also contribute to delayed development among the poor. In addition, because parents with mild mental retardation are most likely to find themselves among the poor, genetic influences may play a role. Adults with MR

Table 6.1 Categories of Mental Retardation

Category	IQ Range	% of MR Population	Characteristics
Mild	52–68	89	Usually absorbed into the community, where they work and live independently
Moderate	36–51	6	Capable of learning self-care skills and working within a sheltered environment; live semi-independently, with relatives, or in a community residence
Severe	20–35	3½	Capable of learning some self-care skills and are not totally dependent; often exhibit physical disabilities and deficits in speech and language
Profound	Below 20	1½	Capable of learning some basic living skills but require continual care and supervision; often exhibit severe physical and/or sensory problems

Adapted from American Association on Mental Retardation, 1992.

are more likely than nonretarded adults to produce offspring with depressed cognitive functioning. This factor does not occur within the severely and profoundly retarded population, because very few of these individuals produce offspring.

Causes of Mental Retardation/ Intellectual Disability

AAMR groups the causes of MR into two large categories: biological and social-environmental (AAMR, 1992). These categories are not mutually exclusive, and biological factors may be magnified or lessened by social and environmental factors. In addition, mental retardation may co-occur with other disabilities, such as autism spectrum disorder, hearing loss, and cerebral palsy, to name a few. I worked with a young man with both Down syndrome, a genetically related form of MR, and learning disability. The most challenging individual with whom I have worked was a child with profound MR, deafness, blindness, and cerebral palsy. Multiple disabilities increase as IQ decreases. Known causes of mental retardation are listed in Table 6.2.

Table 6.2 Known Causes of Mental Retardation

Type	Examples	Characteristics
Biological		
Genetic and chromosomal	Down syndrome (Trisomy 21)	Broad head and characteristic facial features, small stature, mental retardation
	Klinefelter syndrome (sex-linked, XXY)	Feminine roundness to body, small testes, possible mental retardation
	Cri-du-chat syndrome	Catlike cry, microcephaly, mental retardation
Infectious processes	Maternal rubella	Cardiac defects, cataracts, hearing loss, microcephaly, possible mental retardation
	Congenital syphilis	Deafness, vision problems, possible epilepsy or cerebral palsy, mental retardation
Toxins and chemical agents	Fetal alcohol syndrome	Persistently deficient growth, low brain weight, facial abnormalities, cardiac defects, mental retardation
	Lead poisoning	Central nervous system and kidney damage, hyperactivity
Nutrition and metabolism	Phenylketonuria (PKU)	Reduced pigmentation, motor coordination problems, convulsions, microcephaly, mental retardation
	Tay-Sachs disease	Progressive deterioration of nervous system and vision, mental retardation, death in preschool years
	Inadequate diet	Small stature, possible mental retardation

(continued)

Table 6.2 **Continued**

Type	Example	Characteristics
Gestational disorders	Hydrocephalus	Enlarged head caused by increased volume of cerebrospinal fluid, visual defects, epilepsy, mental retardation
	Cerebral malformation	Absence or underdevelopment of cerebral cortex and resultant mental retardation
	Craniofacial anomalies	Malformed skull and associated mental retardation
Complications of pregnancy and delivery	Extreme immaturity or preterm infant	Low birthweight, higher prevalence of central nervous system disorders
	Exceptionally large baby	Possible birth injury to central nervous system
	Maternal nutritional disorders	Low birthweight, higher prevalence of central nervous system disorders
Gross brain diseases	Tumors and tuberous sclerosis	Tumors in heart, seizures, tuberous "bumps" on nose and cheeks, mental retardation
	Huntington disease	Degenerative neurological functioning evidenced in progressive dementia and cerebral palsy
Social-Environmental		
Psychosocial disadvantage	Subnormal intellectual functioning in immediate family and/or impoverished environment	Functional retardation
Sensory deprivation	Maternal deprivation Prolonged isolation	Functional retardation and failure to thrive

Adapted from American Association on Mental Retardation, 1992.

Biological causes are a factor for more than half of the individuals with MR and include many factors. Included in biological causes are genetic and chromosonal factors; congenital factors, such as metabolic disorders and malformations of the skull and brain; and illness or toxin-related factors, such as maternal rubella and lead poisoning. The relationship between severity of retardation and biological factors is very strong.

Social-environmental factors are not as easy to identify as biological factors and involve many interactive variables. Poor housing and hygiene, as well as inadequate medical care and nutrition, may contribute. Lack of prenatal care and infant stimulation may affect the developing child more directly.

Advances in human genetics have demonstrated that over 750 genetic disorders are associated with mental retardation and may account for 30 to 50 percent of all children with MR (Opitz, 1996; Stromme & Hagberg, 2000). In the future, the incidence figures for all chromosomal causes of MR may change because of the availability of prenatal chromosomal screening. Parents may elect to terminate the pregnancy of an affected fetus.

Although many of the genetic/chromosomal syndromes occur rarely, others, such as Down syndrome and fragile X syndrome, are relatively common. Let's examine some of the more common genetic causes.

DOWN SYNDROME (DS)

Down syndrome (DS), or trisomy 21, is the most common *chromosomal* cause of mental retardation. It results when all or part of an extra twenty-first chromosome is contributed by one parent at conception. The U.S. Centers for Disease Control (CDC, 2006) estimates the incidence of DS to be 1 per 733 live births, which means over 5,400 infants are born with DS in the United States each year. DS is usually identified at birth based on an infant's physical features and then confirmed by chromosome testing.

Characterized by a combination of differences in body structure and development and in impairment of cognitive ability, DS is most often associated with moderate retardation. Some but not all of the physical features of DS also appear in people with a standard set of chromosomes. The most obvious physical traits include almond-shaped eyes, caused by an eyelid fold in the inner corner of the eyes, along with shorter stature and poor muscle tone.

Older parental age increases the likelihood of conceiving a baby with DS. Although the risk increases with maternal age, 80 percent of newborns with DS are conceived by women under 35, reflecting the primary childbearing years.

FRAGILE X SYNDROME (FXS)

Fragile X syndrome (FXS) is the most common inherited cause of intellectual disability and the most common cause of mental retardation after Down syndrome. A weakness in the female, or X, chromosome found in all humans is related to mental retardation and possibly to other learning disorders. Fragile X is a recessive trait most prevalent in males because they carry only one X chromosome. FXS occurs in 1 of every 1,350 live male births and 1 of every 2,033 live female births in the United States (Love & Webb, 1986). Most males with FXS also have MR, whereas only about one-third of females with the trait are so affected (Caron, 1994).

In one study of twenty-four boys with full FXS mutation, the average IQ score was 49.8 (range 25–90) (Alanay et al., 2007). Four, or 17 percent, had IQs above 70. Other co-occurring disorders in some boys were attention-deficit hyperactivity disorder (ADHD), pervasive developmental disorder (including autism), seizures, and psychiatric disorders. The co-occurrence of these disorders in people with FXS is higher than in the general population. The most severe cognitive delays in young children with both FXS and autism compared with those with only FXS continue into adolescence and young adulthood (Lewis et al., 2006). One study found a significant delay in both expressive and receptive language skills with FXS, especially in males, even those whose IQs were within normal limits (Caron, 1994).

KLINEFELTER SYNDROME

Klinefelter syndrome (KS) is a relatively common sex-linked genetic syndrome caused by an extra X chromosome in males, resulting in an XXY. It occurs in 1 of every 500 to 1,000 live births in the United States. In most cases, physical, neurological, and behavioral characteristics are mild, and KS is not usually associated with moderate or severe MR. Often, however, KS is associated with significant language learning impairment and problems in executive dysfunction. A study of a small group adolescents and adults with KS reported mild maladaptive behaviors and learning disabilities (Geschwind & Dykens, 2004).

Associated Neurological Disorders

There is a higher incidence of neurological disorders among the mentally retarded population, especially that segment that is severely and profoundly affected. Cerebral palsy and/or epilepsy are also found in greater percentages of the mentally retarded population than in the nonretarded population. These differences are especially evident among those with severe and profound retardation. Among those with cerebral palsy (CP), approximately half have IQs lower than 70. This may reflect the co-occurrence of the two disorders or the difficulty of testing with standard procedures when there is neuromuscular interference. Nonetheless, it seems safe to conclude that a substantial proportion of people with CP also exhibit MR.

Although epilepsy affects less than 1 percent of the general population, the percentage increases with decreased intelligence. Up to 65 percent of those with profound MR exhibit seizure activity. Related neurological disorders further complicate learning tasks for persons with MR. The co-occurrence of neurological disorders with MR is an indication of the underlying organic cause for the more severe forms of retardation.

Cognitive Functioning

Although volumes have been published on the cognitive abilities of individuals with MR, researchers do not fully understand the cognitive and learning processes of this population (Cegelka & Prehm, 1982). First, because the complex nature of the cognitive process necessitates research that targets very limited aspects of cognitive ability, there are no definitive studies of the entire process of cognitive functioning among either the retarded or the nonretarded population. Second, in many studies, the cognitive functioning level of subjects with MR is poorly defined, making it difficult to draw conclusions across studies. Finally, it is difficult to extrapolate from a study conducted in a limited experimental setting to the daily environments of individuals.

In general, individuals in the mentally retarded population develop many cognitive skills in a developmental sequence similar to that of the nonmentally retarded population. There are variances, however, that indicate fundamental processing differences. Some of these similarities and differences can be identified in learning processes and in memory. **Learning** is a change in behavior that results from rehearsal of the behavior to be learned. Cognitive abilities important for processing information and learning include attention, discrimination, organization, memory, and transfer. Figure 6.2 demonstrates this process schematically.

ATTENTION

Attention includes awareness of a learning situation and active cognitive processing. As noted in Figure 6.2, people do not attend to all stimuli; if they did, their brains would quickly become overburdened.

Research on attention has examined the orientation and reaction times of individuals with MR. **Orientation** is the ability to sustain attention over time. In general, individuals with mild retardation exhibit equal or slightly greater ability to sustain attention and to orient compared to their mental age–matched, typically developing peers.

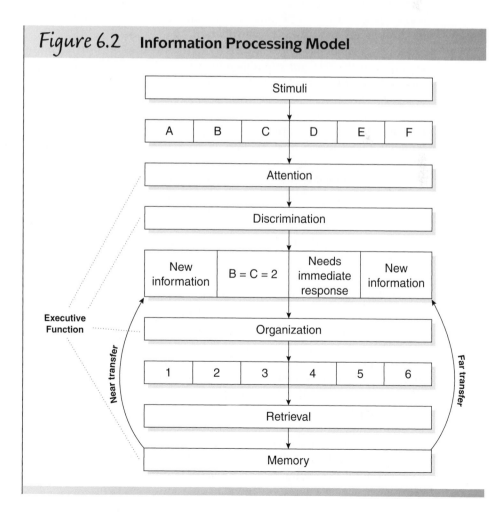

Figure 6.2 **Information Processing Model**

Reaction time refers to the amount of time required for an individual to respond to a stimulus. In Figure 6.2, the subject responds to stimulus E immediately. Individuals with mild mental retardation react similarly to mental age–matched, typically developing peers. In part, reaction time is a function of the individual's ability to select the relevant dimensions of a task before responding. Individuals with MR appear to have deficits in their abilities to scan and attend selectively.

In general, persons with MR seem able to attend as well as their mental age–matched, typically developing peers. They may be less able, however, to select the relevant information from a field. Therefore, new or relevant features of a task need to be highlighted to call attention to them (Meador, 1984).

DISCRIMINATION

Discrimination is the ability to identify differing stimuli from a field of similar stimuli, such as finding a circle among ovals. In a more complicated task, the subject might be asked to find only the small yellow circles among a sample of competing colors, shapes, and sizes. In Figure 6.2, stimuli B and C are found to be similar. In contrast, stimuli A and F are new information.

In general, individuals with MR exhibit difficulties identifying and maintaining attention to the relevant stimulus dimensions. As a group, persons with mild and moderate retardation attend to fewer dimensions of a task than do the nonretarded, and these dimensions are not necessarily the salient or important ones. This deficiency reduces an individual's ability to compare new information with stored information from previous learning, making learning more difficult. In addition, persons with MR take a longer time and need more practice to understand the dimensions of a task. Once a task is understood or learned, however, individuals with MR can perform as well as their mental age–matched, typically developing peers.

In general, individuals with MR who have higher functioning abilities can learn discrimination tasks more rapidly than those who have lower functioning abilities (Ellis et al., 1982). There are substantial individual differences among persons with severe and profound retardation, however, and some subjects learn tasks as well as those with mild retardation (Nugent & Mosley, 1987).

ORGANIZATION OF INPUT MATERIAL

The organization of incoming sensory information is very important for later retrieval. This organization can be demonstrated when someone tries to recall the name of an object. Frequently, the names of related objects also come to mind. Therefore, the individual may name the washing machine *dryer* or *refrigerator* but rarely *spoon* or *window*. As shown in Figure 6.2, information is organized, or "chunked," by category for easy retrieval. Stimuli B and C are placed in storage bin 2.

Although nonretarded persons and those with mild MR exhibit similar developmental trends in the grouping of information, individuals with MR exhibit difficulty developing categorizing strategies for organizing newly learned material. Because it is much more difficult to remember unrelated bits of information, any organizational deficit will hinder later recall and quickly overload memory capacity.

Every reader can recognize that it is easier to recall a ten-word sentence than ten un-related words. If storage capacity is fixed, more efficient processing will require in-creasingly better organization, in turn leaving more room for new input.

Individuals with mild and moderate MR do not seem to rely on mediation or as-sociative learning strategies or use them as efficiently as do the nonretarded. In *mediating strategies,* a word or symbol forms a link between two inputs. For exam-ple, a person's name might relate past experiences with feelings, lifestyles, or opin-ions. In *associative strategies*, one word or symbol aids in recall of another. Common examples are *Salt and* _____, *Black and* _____, and so on. Mildly retarded individuals can use associative strategies if the two symbols are easily asso-ciated and nonabstract.

Two processes, simultaneous synthesis and sequential (or successive) synthesis, are used for coding input and for planning behavior. In *simultaneous synthesis,* which takes place in the occipital-parietal region of the brain, separate elements are organ-ized into groups so that all members of the group can be retrieved simultaneously. For example, various examples of dogs are coded for the *dog* category. In sentence cod-ing, the overall meaning, rather than the individual syntactic and phonological units, is processed. *Sequential,* or *successive, coding* is related to language form and takes place in the frontal-temporal region of the brain. Linguistic information is coded in linear fashion. Obviously, these coding processes are influenced by sensory input, memory, and other intellectual processes.

Nonretarded persons and those with mild MR exhibit both simultaneous and successive coding, although the two groups may employ the coding process differ-ently. As a group, for example, persons with Down syndrome perform more poorly than either individuals who are brain damaged or other mental age–matched indi-viduals with MR on successive processing tasks. This deficiency may be an under-lying cause for auditory memory and expressive language problems of the DS population and may indicate a structural difference in the processing portions of the brain (Ellis, Deacon, & Wooldridge, 1985; Lincoln, Courchesne, Kilman, & Galambos, 1985).

In general, individuals with MR demonstrate some organizing difficulties and thus benefit from having preorganized input. Organizational deficits can hinder recall and generalization, both essential for learning.

MEMORY

The ability to retrieve needed information that was previously learned is necessary for recall, or **memory.** Individuals with mild and moderate MR seem to be able to retain information within long-term memory as well as nonretarded individuals, although their overall recall is slower (Merrill, 1985). Organizational deficits, however, may re-sult in an overreliance on rote memory by persons with mild MR. In contrast, indi-viduals with profound MR exhibit significant forgetting of learned behavior within only a short interval.

Deficiencies in short-term memory, which is used in discrimination, are more ev-ident in the retarded population. Individuals with MR may experience difficulty with short-term storage due to a lack of associational strategies, as mentioned previously

(Gutowski & Chechile, 1987). Short-term memory is particularly affected by the rapid rate of forgetting found in the MR population, especially forgetting within the first ten seconds. Increased encoding time does not normalize the rate of forgetting, indicating both encoding and storage deficits (Ellis et al., 1985).

Information is retained and/or transferred to long-term memory through rehearsal or repetition. It has been reported that persons with MR do not rehearse information spontaneously even when given increased time to do so (Reid, 1980; Turner & Bray, 1985).

The type of information and the stimulus mode greatly affect memory. For example, there appears to be little difference in spatial location memory for children and adults without MR and adults with MR, even those with IQs as low as 30 (Ellis, Woodley-Zanthos, & Dulaney, 1989). In contrast, adults with MR perform much less well on free-recall tasks of auditory information.

Auditory memory deficits are particularly evident in people with DS (Marcell & Weeks, 1988). Auditory working memory, which is the ability to remember briefly what has been heard even when it is no longer present, is a passive retention strategy related to immediate recall of linguistic stimuli and seems to be most efficient with the fast rates found in conversation. Among individuals with DS, however, this echo may decay more rapidly or at a rate at which the slower processing of those with DS cannot access it. In general, persons with MR demonstrate poorer recall than mental age–matched, typically developing peers. Not all areas are affected equally, and there is some indication that memory for spatial location is a strength that can be used to enhance learning in auditory memory tasks (Nigro & Roak, 1987).

TRANSFER

Transfer, or generalization, is the ability to apply previously learned material in the solving of similar but novel problems. Although persons with mild MR can be taught cognitive processing strategies, attempts to generalize these strategies have been less successful. The learning of individuals with more severe retardation is characterized by even weaker transfer (Ellis et al., 1982; Reid, 1980). Learning enhances performance but not generalization.

Near transfer involves only minimal differences between learned information and a novel problem, whereas **far transfer** involves substantial changes. In Figure 6.2, stimulus A is considered to be similar enough to stored information to qualify for near transfer. Stimulus F is less similar and thus represents far transfer. Persons with MR have difficulty with both near and far transfer, which appears to be a function not of the similarity of the old and new tasks but of the level of awareness required for a person to detect such similarities.

Understanding the task is essential for transfer. Individuals with MR benefit from training in all components of a task and in applying these components to new task settings (Burger, Blackman, Clark, & Reis, 1982). However, explicit training does not appear to be necessary for all individuals with MR. Like their nonretarded peers, persons with mild MR can gain knowledge to increase transfer solely through observing the task (Burger, Blackman, & Clark, 1981).

The generalization deficits of individuals with MR may reflect the selection and organization deficits and subsequent memory problems noted previously. Generalization can be facilitated, however, if the client is helped in analyzing the similarities between old and new tasks.

People who are mentally retarded seem to develop cognitively in a manner similar to those who are not retarded but at a slower rate. Overall, the mental development of adults, as measured in individuals, continues well into midlife, albeit at a slower rate for adults with MR than for typical adults (Berry, Groeneweg, Gibson, & Brown, 1984). Some cognitive processing differences exist, however, especially in organization and memory. It is important to remember that these differences alone do not explain mental retardation and may represent the cause, the result, or a concurrent problem (Leonard, 1987).

For persons with mild MR, IQ or cognitive processing alone is not a particularly powerful predictor of life adjustment. Many individuals with MR exhibit integrated problem-solving abilities daily. For example, they make decisions regarding daily schedule, personal hygiene, nutrition, and employment. Individuals with MR who are independent or receive early intervention services are even more flexible problem solvers, because they have developed internal models of the mechanics of addressing problems (Levine & Langness, 1985).

Language and Communication Skills

The language behavior of people with MR is frequently one of the most problematic areas of adaptive behavior and may be the most important characteristic of this population. For example, in a longitudinal study of the development of boys (ages 12 to 36 months) with fragile X syndrome, motor skills appeared least delayed, whereas communication skills appeared most delayed (Roberts, Hatton, & Bailey, 2001). Ultimately, language behavior will determine an individual's ability to function independently in the outside world. Although mental age–matched, typically developing individuals and those with MR may be similar in many cognitive functions, individuals with MR often exhibit difficulty with symbolic functions, including language (Kamhi, 1981). Although children with FXS have moderate to severe delays in communication development, in speech and in all areas of language, those with both FXS and co-occurring autism spectrum disorder tend to have even more severe language impairment (Philofsky, Hepburn, Hayes, Hagerman, & Rogers, 2004; Roberts, Mirrett, & Burchinal, 2001).

The exact relationship between cognition and language for humans is unknown. The relationship may be inconsistent. Cognition might influence language at some phases of development, and language might influence cognition during other phases (Miller, Chapman, & MacKenzie, 1981). Among individuals with MR, several patterns emerge and may vary with age, severity of retardation, and task. The most frequent patterns are as follow (Miller et al., 1981):

1. Comprehension and cognition are at similar levels, but production is below that of cognition.
2. Both comprehension and production are below the level of cognition.
3. Both comprehension and production are at the level of cognition.

Although boys with FXS with and without autism spectrum disorder do not differ from each other in language comprehension, both groups perform lower than typically developing boys. Boys with DS score even lower in language comprehension than boys with FXS (Price, Roberts, Vandergrift, & Martin, 2007).

As many as half the people with MR may display the third pattern. It is important to note, however, that the relationship between cognition and language is not stable over time for any individual (Cole, Dale, & Mills, 1992).

Studies of the language development of people with MR have a number of limitations (Kamhi & Masterson, 1989). First, the MR population is not homogeneous, which means it is difficult to make generalizations. Second, results may vary with the assessment instruments used. Third, attempts to match subjects by mental or even language age may be inappropriate, given the lack of knowledge of the relationship between cognition and language.

The major characteristics of the language of people with MR are listed in Table 6.3, which is based on summarized group data. Individuals and specific subgroups, especially those with more severe impairment, may exhibit different behavior. Some individuals with profound retardation will not use expressive language beyond single symbols, if at all.

PARAMETERS OF LANGUAGE

Five parameters of language are generally recognized: pragmatics, semantics, syntax, morphology, and phonology. All five parameters have been examined in research studies of the language of persons with MR.

Pragmatics

Pragmatic functions first become evident with the development of gestures. At this point, children begin to express primitive intentions, such as signaling notice, attracting attention, and making demands. Both typically developing children and those with mild and moderate MR accompanying Down syndrome exhibit gestures at the same level of cognitive development (Greenwald & Leonard, 1979). Both groups of children use gestures to enlist help or to gain an object and use declarative gestures to gain attention.

Gestures may be classified as *contact,* such as touching an object or a person, or as *distal,* such as pointing. More mature distal gestures are associated with a wider range and greater frequency of communication functions across both those with MR and those who are developing typically (McLean, Brady, McLean, & Behrens, 1999).

For children with severe MR, gestures appear later in their cognitive development than they do for children with milder forms of MR (Lobato, Barrera, & Feldman, 1981). The gestures of individuals with profound MR primarily function to regulate the behavior of others and are often performed in isolation with little vocalization (Ogletree, Wetherby, & Westling, 1992). Among children with DS, word comprehension and gestural production appear to be closely correlated, suggesting that a strong gestural repertoire influences comprehension (Caselli et al., 1998).

In general, the language of typically developing children and those with MR fulfills the functions expressed earlier in gestures. The distribution of most functions is

Table 6.3 Language Characteristics of Children with Mental Retardation

Pragmatics	Gestural and intentional developmental patterns similar to those of children developing normally
	Delayed gestural requesting
	May take less dominant conversational role
	No difference in clarification skills from mental age–matched peers developing typically
Semantics	More concrete word meanings
	Slow vocabulary growth
	More limited use of a variety of semantic units
	Children with Down syndrome able to learn word meanings from exposure in context as well as mental age–matched peers developing typically
Syntax/morphology	Length–complexity relationship similar to that of preschoolers developing typically
	Same sequence of general sentence development as children developing typically
	Shorter, less-complex sentences, with fewer subject elaborations or relative clauses than mental age–matched peers developing typically
	Sentence word order takes precedence over word relationships
	Reliance on less mature forms, though capable of more advanced
	Same order of morpheme development as preschoolers developing typically
Phonology	Phonological rules similar to those of preschoolers developing typically but reliance on less mature forms, though capable of more advanced ones
Comprehension	Poorer receptive language skills, especially children with Down syndrome, than mental age–matched peers developing typically
	Poorer sentence recall than mental age–matched peers
	More reliance on context to extract meaning

Based on Abbeduto, Davies, Solesby, & Furman (1991); Abbeduto, Short-Meyerson, Benson, & Dolish (1997); Bender & Carlson (1982); Chapman, Kay-Raining Bird, & Schwartz (1990); Chapman, Schwartz, & Kay-Raining Bird (1988); Kernan (1990); Klink, Gerstman, Raphael, Schlanger, & Newsome (1986); Lobato, Barrera, & Feldman (1981); McLeavey, Toomey, & Dempsey (1982); Merrill & Bilsky (1990); Mervis (1988); Moran, Money, & Leonard (1984); Mundy, Kasari, Sigman, & Ruskin (1995); Owens & MacDonald (1982); Prater (1982); Rondal, Ghiotto, Bredart, & Bachelet (1988); Rosin, Swift, Bless, & Vetter (1988); Shriberg & Widder (1990).

similar for both groups of children when matched for language development level (Owens & MacDonald, 1982). Both groups of children are able to answer and ask questions spontaneously, to reply to the comments of others, to make spontaneous declarations and demands, to name or label entities, and to imitate and practice language spontaneously.

Imitation of others and self-repetition may develop differently for individuals with Down syndrome (Owens & MacDonald, 1982; Sokolov, 1992). In general, imitation decreases for typically developing children as they begin to learn syntax. The rate of decrease is significantly less for children with DS. This difference may indicate a continued reliance on outmoded learning strategies by children with MR. Typically developing children may discard inefficient strategies more readily.

At the single-word or early multiword stage, typically developing children begin to demonstrate *presuppositional skills*. They presuppose that their communication partners are aware of redundant or old information in a situation and therefore label only aspects of a situation that are undergoing change or provide new information. For example, the child may not name the cup on the high chair each morning but may label with the word *cup* a new cup recently received from Grandma. Toddlers with mild MR also exhibit this behavior.

Presuppositional skills may be a forerunner of several perspective-taking behaviors used in everyday communication, such as the ability to assume the communication partner's perceptual viewpoint in interpretation of terms such as *here* and *there* and to assess a partner's knowledge or emotional state. In one study, children with mild and moderate MR and younger typically developing second-graders matched for cognitive abilities exhibited similar perspective-taking behaviors (Bender & Carlson, 1982).

Although individuals with MR reportedly are delayed in role taking and referential communication, these differences are not found when subjects are matched for social maturity (Blacher, 1982). *Referential communication* refers to a target referent by distinguishing it from others, such as "the girl with the white dress" and "big doggie." Children with MR are less able to distinguish referents for their listeners than are their mental age–matched peers who are developing typically (Brownell & Whitely, 1992). These referential skills can be taught, however.

Individuals who are mentally retarded seem as adept as their mental age–matched, typically developing peers in selecting the appropriate referent or subject of discussion within context, but they are less skilled in requesting clarification of information when the context is unclear (Abbeduto, Davies, Solesby, & Furman, 1991). This conclusion seems odd, given the abilities of individuals with MR to request clarification (Abbeduto & Rosenberg, 1980) and to use the context and linguistic memory for referent identification (Abbeduto & Rosenberg, 1980; Abbeduto, Short-Meyerson, Benson, Dolish, & Weissman, 1998). Possibly, the requirements of conversation are such that the individual with MR cannot integrate these skills when needed. An inability to seek such clarification may be critical, given a report that individuals with Down syndrome have difficulty understanding sentences without a supporting extralinguistic context (Kernan, 1990).

The requirements of the conversational context may also account for the amount of verbal perseveratives found in the speech of adults with MR (Rein & Kernan,

1989). *Verbal perseveration* is excessive talking on a topic even when inappropriate or previously addressed in the conversation. Such behavior may be used by individuals with MR to maintain the interaction or "buy time" until they can produce a more appropriate response. The use of verbal perseveratives varies within the retarded population. For example, males with fragile X syndrome have been shown to produce more perseverative, repetitive, inappropriate, and off-topic utterances than males with Down syndrome (Sudhalter, Cohen, Silverman, & Wolf-Schein, 1990; Wolf-Schein et al., 1987).

Although boys with FXS and those with DS both make more off-topic responses than typically developing boys, those with FXS make more off-topic comments than children with other forms of MR or autism spectrum disorder (Sudhalter & Belser, 2001). Boys with FXS use more perseverative and overly repetitious speech than girls with FXS, although the difference is not based solely on gender but is affected by the communication context (Roberts, Martin et al., 2007). In general, more perseveration occurs in conversation than in narratives (Murphy & Abbeduto, 2007).

All of the preceding skills are interrelated in the conversational context. In a conversation, roles and topics change, and each partner must try to assess how much information his or her partner needs. In general, individuals with MR are less able to judge the nonverbal emotions of their communication partners than are mental age–matched, typically developing peers and thus are less able to respond appropriately (Marcell & Jett, 1985).

The conversational role of persons with MR seems to be one of nondominance. Children with MR are more likely to keep greater interpersonal distance, a possible reflection of their perception of having little personal control. Likewise, adults with MR rarely exert dominance in a conversation, even when the communication partner is a child, although they possess the communication skills to do so. This subservient conversational behavior is more pronounced in institutionalized populations and can be noted in the case study at the end of the chapter.

Semantics

Every auditory event has a sensory or sign impression and an abstract or symbolic representation, such as a word for that event. The sign is meaningful but nonlinguistic, such as the sound of a horn signaling an automobile. In contrast, the abstract representation, or word, is linguistic in nature. Children with MR and mental age–matched, typically developing preschoolers have similar recall for signal information, but children with MR have significantly poorer recognition and recall of symbolic representations (Lamberts, 1981). Word storage and linkage to meanings may be a deficit.

As a group, individuals with MR exhibit poorer semantic skills. Comprehension deficits are evidenced by the poorer receptive language skills than their mental age–matched, typically developing peers. There are many variations among individuals, however, which may reflect type and severity of mental retardation, the language task, or the environment (Abbeduto, Furman, & Davies, 1989). During conversation, boys with FXS produce fewer different words than do typically developing boys matched for nonverbal mental age (Roberts, Hennon et al., 2007).

The word meanings of people with MR seem more concrete than those of non-retarded people. For example, *cold* may be defined in relation to temperature but not to the psychological aspects, as in *a cold personality*. There appears to be no difference in the quality of definition, however, as measured by the Stanford-Binet intelligence test (Papania, 1954).

Word meanings are established in a two-step process that includes (1) a quick, general determination of meaning from the context (a process called *fast mapping*) and (2) a slower evolution of meaning from use. Children with DS are as skilled as mental age–matched peers who are developing typically in inferring novel word meanings. Children with DS are also equally skilled at producing words correctly thereafter (Chapman, Kay-Raining Bird, & Schwartz, 1990).

As might be expected, figurative and idiomatic language pose particular difficulties. Context is extremely important in aiding comprehension for individuals with DS (Ezell & Goldstein, 1991).

Syntax

In general, the overall sequence of development of syntax is similar for children with mild MR and those developing typically; however, the rate of development is slower among those with MR. Both sentence length and complexity increase with development. In addition, the same sentence types appear and are used in the same order for both groups. There is a general trend from simple declarative to negative sentences and then from interrogative to negative interrogative sentences. Within interrogatives, the order of development is also similar, with *what* and *where* types developing initially and *when, why,* and *how* appearing last.

Even at equivalent mental age levels, however, individuals with MR appear to use shorter, less complex sentences than their typically developing peers (McLeavey, Toomey, & Dempsey, 1982; Roberts, Hennon et al., 2007). These characteristics are evident in the case study at the end of this chapter. Individuals with mild MR use fewer complex structures, such as subject elaborations and relative clauses. Boys with FXS use less complex noun phrases, verb phrases, and sentence structure than typically developing boys but use a similar number of questions and negations. This suggests that the language difficulties in boys with FXS reflect an overall expressive language impairment and not a specific syntactic or vocabulary delay (Roberts, Hennon et al., 2007).

These deficiencies may reflect poorer linguistic rule generalization. Poor rule generalization does not imply an inability to learn language rules, although persons with MR seem to rely more on sequential placement than on grammatical rules. In other words, sentence word order takes precedence over the relationships between different word classes. The result is a less flexible linguistic structure, although still a rule-oriented approach to language (McLeavey et al., 1982). Even individuals with severe MR are capable of using linguistic rules. Taken together, these findings suggest that although persons with MR learn and use linguistic rules, they rely more on primitive word order rules than do their typically developing language peers. Advanced syntactic forms are learned but used less frequently.

One measure of sentence complexity for initial sentence development is *mean length of utterance (MLU)*. For children both with DS and those who are developing typically, MLU correlates strongly with chronological age and predicts the complexity and diversity of sentence development (Rondal, Ghiotto, Bredart, & Bachelet,

1988). MLU appears to be a good measure of complexity. For both groups, the average MLU is 3.5 morphemes.

Finally, individuals with MR exhibit poorer recall of sentences than their mental age–matched, typically developing peers (Merrill & Bilsky, 1990). Sentence recall involves reproduction of the memory and then encoding of the text. Because individuals with MR make frequent word substitution errors, performance may break down in the second stage (Bilsky, Walker, & Sakales, 1983). Poor sentence recall indicates a breakdown in syntactic-semantic analysis (Merrill & Mar, 1987). Although individuals with DS seem to have recall patterns similar to those of nonretarded individuals, they have greater difficulty when there is no supporting extralinguistic context (Kernan, 1990). Males with FXS appear to have more difficulty with auditory sequential memory and auditory reception in general than males with DS (Hagerman, Kemper, & Hudson, 1985). This poorer performance may reflect either poorer quality mental representations or an inability to encode and recall holistic, integrated semantic information (Merrill & Mar, 1987).

Sentence recall and context utilization for individuals with MR can be enhanced when the semantic relatedness of the words in a sentence is increased (Merrill & Jackson, 1992). For example, the sentence *The hunter shot the rabbit* has more relatedness across the words (hunters shoot) than *The photographer chased the rabbit* (photographers take photos) and is thus easier to recall. Poor reading recall, on the other hand, may be related to failure to use this important textual information for organization (Luftig & Johnson, 1982).

Morphology

In developmental studies, the same order of morphological acquisition has been reported for both the retarded and nonretarded populations. The pattern of development seems to be delayed, even beyond what one might expect for mental age, but not significantly different for people with MR.

Both individuals with mild MR accompanying Down syndrome and mental age–matched, typically developing individuals display all features of verbs and noun inflections, such as plural *-s* and past tense *-ed*, although individuals with Down syndrome use these features less frequently.

Phonology

Infants with profound MR vocalize less when gesturing than do typically developing infants, and their vocalizations often lack consonants (Ogletree et al., 1992). Infants with DS and less severe retardation babble in a fashion similar to that of chronologically age–matched, typically developing infants (Steffens, Oller, Lynch, & Urbano, 1992). Over time, both groups of children produce more mature vowels and more well-formed syllables and fewer quasi-vowel sounds and partial syllables.

The articulation and phonologic characteristics of people with MR can be summarized as follows (Shriberg & Widder, 1990):

- Articulation errors are more common than in the nonretarded population.
- The most frequent error is the deletion of consonants.

- Errors are likely to be inconsistent.
- Patterns are similar to those of nonretarded children or children with a functional delay.
- Individuals with Down syndrome have perceptually and acoustically distinct prosody (i.e., spoken rhythm and intonation).

The types of errors and level of mental retardation do not seem to be related, although a majority of institutionalized individuals and those with severe MR exhibit articulation disorders.

In general, preschoolers with MR use the same phonological learning processes, such as weak syllable deletion (*elphant* for *elephant*), as typically developing preschoolers but with greater frequency (Klink, Gerstman, Raphael, Schlanger, & Newsome, 1986; Moran, Money, & Leonard, 1984). Although there is much individual variability, the most common phonological processes exhibited by people with MR are reduction of consonant clusters (*top* for *stop*) and deletion of the final consonant (*ca* for *cat*) (Bleile & Schwartz, 1984; Klink et al., 1986; Oller & Seibert, 1988; Sommers, Patterson, & Wildgren, 1988; Van Borsel, 1988). Boys with FXS make errors similar to those of younger typically developing preschoolers, but those with DS have more significant phonological differences than might be expected by delayed development alone (Roberts et al., 2005).

Although the phonological processes of children with MR are the same as those of younger, typically developing children, those with MR may use them even when they are capable of producing the deleted or modified sound (Prater, 1982). It is possible, therefore, that these processes serve a different purpose. For example, consonant deletions may reflect cognitive processing limitations in the motor assembly stage of speech production (Shriberg & Widder, 1990).

Oral language skills correlate closely with reading skills. *Phonological awareness*—rhyming, syllabication, phoneme recognition and identification—is a corequisite of reading. Children with DS develop phonological awareness skills in a manner similar to typically developing children (Cupples & Iacono, 2000).

Several studies have indicated that the language abilities of individuals with MR are delayed beyond expectations based on mental age alone, although the course of development is similar to that for nonretarded persons. This language delay, particularly common among individuals with Down syndrome (Mahoney, Glover, & Finger, 1981), becomes evident soon after language acquisition begins, as the level of vocabulary development begins to lag behind cognitive development (Cardosa-Martins, Mervis, & Mervis, 1985).

Individuals with DS continue to develop language well into adolescence and early adulthood. In general, these individuals produce shorter utterances with fewer words and fewer different words than mental age–matched, typically developing peers (Chapman, Seung, Schwartz, & Kay-Raining Bird, 1998). Down syndrome is only one of hundreds of possible conditions related to mental retardation. Others may exhibit distinct patterns of speech, language, and communication (Alvares & Downing, 1998). This variability only strengthens the need for thorough assessment of individual language ability.

Differences in mental age and language may reflect symbol-processing deficiencies within the MR population. Therefore, in language therapy, it seems prudent to target the underlying process when these deficiencies are evident.

ENVIRONMENTAL INFLUENCES ON LANGUAGE

Individuals with MR are generally found in two types of environments: home centered and residential. Residential settings can be further divided into large institutions and smaller group settings or community residences. In general, individuals who live in large institutions have fewer adaptive skills and are more dependent, although these effects can be reduced with adequate staff training. Institutionalization can affect some aspects of language more than others, especially pragmatics and semantics. The adult described in the case study at the end of this chapter exhibits few conversational initiations. Her verbal behavior is mostly responsive.

Parent–Child Interaction

Although home placement is beneficial for children, some features of the language learning home environment of children with MR may account for their language impairment. The importance of early mother–child interaction has been increasingly recognized as critical to the established repertoire of communication skills of typically developing preverbal infants. The infant's communication skills develop within the interaction of mother and child (Owens, 2008).

The development of communication in children, especially those with more severe MR, depends in part on the responsiveness of adults to all forms of communicative behavior. Although it is difficult to predict the performance of any group of children over time, prelinguistic or early linguistic children with DS have better productive language later if they experience frequent optimal parental responding (Yoder & Warren, 2004).

The stress that accompanies the birth of an infant with a disability may alter the dynamics of family relations. Because the interactional process is one of mutual adaptation by the two partners, a child with MR may alter the mother's behavior differently than will a typically developing infant. The situation is made more acute for the mother and family by a lack of information on and assistance with development, by possible feelings of grief and guilt, and by fear of an unknown future.

Developmental delays of early social behaviors in babies with DS are likely to affect patterns of interaction with caregivers. At 8 weeks, infants with DS are less communicative and lively than typically developing babies. Although at 8 weeks, their mothers' behaviors do not differ from those of mothers of typically developing babies, there are significant differences in the mothers' behaviors at 20 weeks (Slonims & McConachie, 2006). And while the social behaviors of babies with DS improve over time, the differences between mothers seem to remain. Still, parents of children with Down syndrome show prosodic characteristics more typical of infant-directed speech than do parents of children with other types of MR (Fidler, 2003).

All mothers act according to their expectations of their infants' behavior and attempt to keep their infants within these expectations. In general, more active and less irritable infants receive optimum maternal responsiveness. Infants with DS and early medical disorders exhibit rather inactive behavior. It might be expected, therefore, that the mothers of these children will be less responsive than mothers of nondisordered infants and that the lack of maternal responsiveness might result in the infants' withdrawal. Further research is needed in this area.

Predictable and responsive infants participate more in the parent–infant interactional environment. At-risk infants are less predictable and less responsive (Affleck, Allen, McGrade, & McQueeney, 1982). Nevertheless, research does not support the conclusion that mothers of infants with MR are more restrictive of the infants' activities and less responsive. In fact, these mothers interpret more of their children's behaviors as communicative than do mothers of typically developing children (Yoder & Feagans, 1988). For example, parents of children with MR describe their children as using a wide range of behaviors to communicate, including facial expressions, body movements, vocalizations, gestures, word approximations and words, formal and made-up signs, and object and picture symbols (Stephenson & Dowrick, 2005). It is the mother's attribution of meaning to the child's behavior, not just the behavior itself, that affects the mother's responses (Harding, 1984).

Mothers of preschool children with DS and mental age–matched, typically developing children both use directive speech to support and encourage their children's play (Tannock, 1988). As a group, mothers of children with DS exert more verbal control, whereas mothers of typically developing children are more likely to watch quietly (Tannock, 1988). In teaching situations, both groups of mothers have been found equally directive (Davis, Stroud, & Green, 1988). The patterns of directives used by mothers of children with DS and typically developing children are similar over time, although the mothers of children with DS demonstrate more reluctance to change to more mature patterns such as indirect requests ("Can you . . . ?"), possibly out of fear of being misunderstood (Maurer & Sherrod, 1987).

The mothers of children with DS talk to their children more (Berger & Cunningham, 1983). They initiate more topics, repeat more utterances, and take more turns (Maurer & Sherrod, 1987). Although children with DS are more passive and do not respond as frequently, mothers of children with DS and those of typically developing children are equally responsive when their children do verbalize. In studies of the mothers of children with MR and chronological age–matched, typically developing peers, the mothers of the former have been found to use more primitive forms of speech. Mothers of children with DS alter their linguistic input appropriately for the language level of their children. Research has found only small differences between the mothers of children with DS and mothers of typically developing children in both verbal and nonverbal behaviors (Cardosa-Martins & Mervis, 1990). For example, although mothers of children with DS use more comments and replies and fewer whole and partial repetitions than mothers of mental age–matched, typically developing children, these behaviors are the same patterns of language used by their children and may reflect the age differences of the two groups of children.

Maternal changes accompany children's changing abilities (Petersen & Sherrod, 1982). With both children with MR and typical development and those with language delay, mothers use language more prominently in interactions as their children's language progresses. Requests for nonverbal behavior decrease, and language-seeking utterances and verbal feedback increase. Language-seeking utterances consist of questions, including requests for elaboration, labeling, and imitation. Both negative and positive feedback increase with children's increasing language abilities, as mothers become more discriminating and more demanding.

Nevertheless, differences exist. In general, mothers of children with MR dominate the parent–child interaction more than mothers of chronological age–matched, typically developing children. They are more directive, initiate interactions more frequently, imitate more, and incorporate fewer of their children's topics than do the other mothers (Eheart, 1982; A. Miller & Newhoff, 1978; Petersen & Sherrod, 1982). In turn, children with MR respond less frequently to their mothers' initiations (Eheart, 1982) and initiate communication only half as often as typically developing children.

Staff–Client Interaction

In general, a lack of appropriate verbal interactions seems to exist within large residential settings. Much of the communication of the institutional staff involves issuing directives. Such behavior is unlikely to elicit much verbal interchange. Clients are least responsive following staff directives, the most frequent staff verbal behavior. In contrast, the least frequent behavior, staff-initiated conversation, elicits the most verbal client responses. When clients do verbalize, staff are as likely to ignore the behavior as to respond with a verbal comment or reply. The most frequent staff behavior is a nonverbal agreement in the form of a head nod. Although residing in a large institutional setting is likely to have its greatest effect on pragmatics, individuals who reside in smaller community residences are more likely to develop pragmatic skills (McLean et al., 1999; Van Der Gagg, 1989).

Professionals must shoulder some of the blame for the less dominant role that individuals with MR take in conversations (Peter, 2000). The language used by professionals tends to objectify these individuals. Many aspects of the lives of individuals with MR are defined by others. Professional staff expect control in part through their use of directives and questions, two speech acts found infrequently among individuals with MR (Domingo, Barrow, & Amato, 1998). Persons with MR are often treated as members of a category, rather than as individuals, and are labeled with terms that demean or note their abnormality (Danforth & Navarro, 1998). In part, these conditions are fueling the debate over use of the term *mental retardation* versus *intellectual disability.*

Individuals with MR receive better linguistic input and more conversational opportunities within a home or small-group environment. The mother–child data are mixed, however, suggesting that although mothers adapt form and content to the linguistic competence of their children, they also provide primarily a responsive verbal environment. Thus, children with MR initiate less communication than their typically developing peers.

We cannot assume, however, that differences indicate a cause for language delay. The differences in speech and language of the mother may be in response to the child's language problems, rather than their cause. Even if mothers of children with MR did provide linguistic form, content, and use styles similar to those of mothers of typically developing children, it might not be appropriate for the special language learning needs of their children with MR. For example, although parents interpret many behaviors as communicative, they still need support from professionals to encourage presymbolic communication–appropriate behaviors and speech as well as alternative and augmentative communication use at home (Stephenson & Dowrick, 2005).

Language and Communication Intervention

Many of the language and communication intervention techniques discussed in this text for use with other children with language impairment can also be used with individuals with MR. Some intervention methods, however, seem particularly appropriate for this population. Current knowledge of the cognitive functioning and language processes of the many people with MR, although limited, suggests some principles and techniques for intervention. In addition, growing knowledge of the relative strengths and weaknesses associated with some common syndromes suggests other avenues of intervention.

These topics will be discussed globally before specifically addressing various aspects of language assessment and intervention, although the breadth of this topic will allow for only general discussion. Also, the discussion will be based on evidence-based practice (EBP), consisting of a combination of efficacy research, best practices, and clinical experience.

PRINCIPLES OF ASSESSMENT AND INTERVENTION

The reported characteristics of the mentally retarded population suggest some guiding principles for speech-language pathologists (SLPs). Of necessity, these principles will be general. These principles are summarized in Table 6.4. An SLP must remember, however, that each person with MR is an individual and that individual differences—such as age, level of cognitive functioning, previous training, residential environment, and learning style—will alter the methods actually used.

Principles Related to Information Processing

The information processing of people with MR, discussed previously, should be considered when designing intervention strategies. Although these processes offer some

---

Table 6.4   **Principles for Intervention with Clients Who Are Mentally Retarded**

1. Highlight new or relevant material.
2. Preorganize information.
3. Train rehearsal strategies.
4. Use overlearning and repetition.
5. Train in the natural environment.
6. Begin as early as possible.
7. Follow developmental guidelines.

guidance, an SLP must consider the skills the client brings to the task and those skills required for successful learning of the communication target. For example, to require too much in the form of new learning or transfer often hinders the client's ability to be successful. Some structured training is usually necessary for initial learning, and repetition of initial procedures may aid further learning of the targeted skill. It may even facilitate learning if the material is presented in the same order until a certain criterion of performance is reached. Transfer can be facilitated by keeping the training situation as close to the everyday environment as possible. The clever SLP will use objects, persons, and events from this environment for training or, better still, train in the everyday environment.

Highlight New or Relevant Material. Individuals with MR are capable of attending well when they understand to what they should attend. New information, materials, and methods should be highlighted so the client does not miss them or assume they are unimportant. For example, new pictures on a communication board might be drawn in a different color or placed in a special area of the board. Stimuli that require certain responses or language features that govern language use should also be highlighted. For example, words such as *yesterday* and *last week* signal use of past tense. The waiter's utterance "What may I get for you?" signals a requesting response.

Attending need not be targeted directly for intervention. Improved attending has been reported as a result of augmentative communication training for institutionalized children and adults with severe MR (Abrahamsen, Romski, & Sevcik, 1989). Generalization is enhanced by a related principle: *Train scanning of a task for relevant or similar stimuli.* Generalization is often difficult for individuals with MR, because they are unsure of which stimuli are relevant. Signs of similarity can be trained by an SLP along with the training target.

Preorganize Information. An SLP can aid learning by pregrouping information to facilitate organization and storage and later recall. In general, persons with MR are able to retain information better if it is organized first and the learning task is explained by the teacher. Individuals with mild MR have better recall if material is grouped spatially, rather than presented singly (Harris, 1982). For example, an individual who is experiencing difficulty recalling four digits, such as 6–3–8–5, may do better if the digits are grouped in pairs to form 63 and 85. Such grouping does not seem to aid the recall of nonretarded individuals, possibly because they already employ this strategy. In similar fashion, sentences can be grouped into logical phrases to aid memory.

Organizational strategies, such as physical arrangement, grouping, and consistent ordering, can also be used to aid learning. In addition, instructions and procedures should be clear, logically sequenced, and involve as many senses as possible (Pruess, Vadasy, & Fewell, 1987).

Train Rehearsal Strategies. Individuals with mild and moderate mental MR can improve their memory abilities through the training of rehearsal strategies, something they seem not to do on their own (Burger, Blackman, & Tan, 1980; Reid, 1980).

Rehearsal aids the transfer of learned material to long-term storage. This may be especially true for visual information, such as communicative signs and gestures, the learning of which enhances associated word recall (Bowler, 1991).

Use Overlearning and Repetition.   Although rehearsal and extra training facilitate learning and recall, they do not seem to directly enhance transfer (Day & Hall, 1988). Individuals who receive extra training, however, subsequently need less assistance with transfer.

Principles Related to Various Syndromes

Some genetically based syndromes show etiology-related behaviors, especially Down syndrome, fragile X syndrome, Prader-Willi syndrome, and Williams syndrome. Although the exact mechanisms by which a syndrome increases the likelihood of a certain behavior are unknown, data on related behaviors suggest strengths and weaknesses that may be used effectively in intervention with some children. As a rule, these strengths and weaknesses become more evident as children become older. It must be added that researchers know only the basics of cognitive, linguistic, and adaptive strengths and weaknesses, and this information exists only for a small number of the genetic causes of MR. Much more research is needed, especially research in support of evidence-based practice (EBP) or the best methods to intervene.

Children with Down syndrome, the most common and most familiar genetic cause of MR, differ in their behaviors from children with other types of MR. Children with DS display relative strengths in visual short-term memory and weakness in auditory short-term memory. Furthermore, babies and toddlers with DS show a tendency for remembering hand movements and other visual gestures comparable to that of typically developing children (Harris, Bellugi, Bates, Jones, & Rossen, 1997). In contrast, most children with DS have weak skills in expressive language, grammar, and articulation, with most showing expressive syntax well below their mental age (Chapman et al., 1998).

In contrast, children with Williams syndrome, a relatively rare genetic disorder (approximately in 1 out of 7,500 births) caused by a deletion on chromosome 7, show a relative strength in auditory short-term memory (Mervis, Morris, Bertrand, & Robinson, 1999) and in expressive language skills. However, only about 5 percent have chronological age–appropriate performance (Bishop, 1999; Mervis et al., 1999). Language skills and auditory processing are considered to be relative strengths, nonetheless. Even so, many children with Williams syndrome perform poorly on tasks involving visuospatial skills (Dykens, Rosner, & Ly, 2001).

Not every person with a specific genetic disorder necessarily shows the characteristic behavior or behaviors of that disorder. For example, even though those with Down syndrome as a group show extreme difficulties in language relative to their mental age, there are some striking exceptions. Consider Francoise, a 32-year-old woman with an overall IQ of 64, who reportedly often used 10- to 15-word sentences with many relative clauses (Rondal, 1995).

Although some behaviors seem unique to a single syndrome, particular behaviors are more commonly shared by two or more genetic syndromes (Hodapp, 1997). For example, both boys with fragile X syndrome and children with *cri-du-chat* syndrome exhibit hyperactivity. *Cri-du-chat* syndrome is a genetic disorder in which genetic material is missing from chromosome 5.

Because children with a particular genetic disorder are predisposed to display a particular strength or weakness, parents and teachers may unintentionally reinforce such propensities by encouraging what the child is able to do more successfully while avoiding interactions that focus on his or her weaker areas (Hodapp, Des-Jardin, & Ricci, 2003). SLPs in early intervention programs face the dilemma of whether to teach to a child's strengths, remediate weaknesses, or do both. In general, it seems wise to use a child's strengths as the vehicle for teaching to weaker areas of development.

An SLP must be mindful of individual learning styles as well as those of certain identifiable groups of children. For example, accommodations must be made in intervention for the special learning needs of boys with FXS. In short, when working with these boys, an SLP can take advantage of their more visual learning style while stressing listening and comprehension. Intervention sessions must accommodate these boys' short attention span, difficulty with transitions to new activities and topics, other sensory deficits, and low tolerance of stress (Mirrett, Roberts, & Price, 2003). Intervention suggestions are presented in Table 6.5.

Historically, professionals in early intervention have considered the cause of a child's mental retardation to be unimportant in making decisions about intervention (Hodapp & Dykens, 1994). This seems short sighted. Because etiology-related strengths and weaknesses of children with genetically based causes of MR gradually emerge with age and through interaction with environmental input, SLPs can best provide more focused and more effective interventions by considering the strengths and weaknesses that will likely emerge (Hodapp et al., 2003). Of course, these decisions must be based on sound diagnostic data, but strengths and weakness reported in the professional literature for different genetic causes of mental retardation provide clues that may potentially inform these assessments. Only through thorough assessment, however, can an SLP adequately describe the behavior of an individual child.

Principles Related to Functional Language

Functional language intervention is a philosophical approach to teaching communication skills in the environment in which they occur, using natural stimuli, child-based content, and a child's caregivers as facilitators. By teaching in an environment in which the communication occurs or is highly likely to occur, an SLP facilitates use within that context and increases the likelihood of transfer to it. For example, in four in home studies using *responsivity education/prelinguistic milieu teaching* (RE/PMT), a type of functional intervention, nonverbal and minimally verbal children with developmental disabilities made advances in intentional expressive communication (Fey et al., 2007; Yoder & Warren, 1998, 2001a, 2002). RE/PMT targets children's gestures, vocalizations, and coordinated eye gazes. Parents are taught to respond to a child's vocalization with a vocal imitation (*baba* following *baba*) or when the reference is to a specific entity with compliance and/or a linguistic expression of the child's intended message. For example, if the child

Table 6.5 Strengths and Weaknesses Associated with Selected Genetic Syndromes

Syndrome	Strengths	Weaknesses	Intervention Strategies
Down syndrome	Visual short-term memory	Auditory short-term memory	Visual cues
			Picture/photo activity schedules
			Color-coded pictures
			Picture communication to compliment or supplement oral language
			Real objects, materials, actual labels and wrappers
	Simultaneous processing	Sequential processing	Semantic/meaning-based language
	Visual gestures	Grammar	Sign language or gestures to compliment or supplement oral language
		Expressive language	
		Articulation	
Williams syndrome	Language skills	Visual-spatial construction	Use of language expansions and parallel talk
	Linguistic affect		
	Auditory short-term memory	Perceptual-motor	Auditory cues
	Music	Difficulty with loud noises	Music activities, singing/rhyming songs and toys with soft sounds
Fragile X syndrome	Simultaneous processing	Sequential processing	Semantic/meaning-based language
		Language	Language through movement and object manipulation
		Visuospatial	Object-reference tasks
	Repetitive tasks	Extreme reaction to change and loud noise	Quiet, calm space
			Visually and verbally warning of change
			Picture/photo activity schedules
			Routines, repetition
		Low attention	Object manipulation
	Integrated, practical, experiental learning across tasks	Hyperactivity	Teaching within movement-based, practical tasks where a task accomplished
	One-on-one interaction	Large-group interaction	Own space
			Avoid large group

Adapted from Hodapp, DesJardin, & Ricci, 2003. Additional information from Hodapp, Dykens, Ort, Zelinsky, & Leckman, 1991; Owens, 2004; Saunders, 1999.

clearly reached for a teddy bear and whined, the parent might say "Want teddy" and hand it to the child. Some of the principles of functional intervention are discussed in the following sections.

Train in the Natural Environment.   Individuals with MR have great difficulty generalizing training to novel contexts. Although highly structured training may increase the rate of learning, especially for individuals with severe MR, such training may be limited to the training context (Salzberg & Villani, 1983). In other words, it is difficult to teach the spontaneous use of skills in untrained situations. Highly structured settings offer a limited variety of communication situations. Difficulties in generalization can be minimized if training occurs using familiar materials within daily activities that occur in everyday locations of the client (Gullo & Gullo, 1984; McCormick, 1986; Stowitschek, McConaughy, Peatross, Salzberg, & Lignngaris/Kraft, 1988).

Language training is more functional if taught in situations where there is actually a need for language to be used. The general result is more spontaneous usage, which in turn motivates the individual to learn more language. The natural stimuli present in the training environment become signals associated with the behavior trained.

Everyday routines also provide an excellent vehicle for training and facilitating generalization. Routines provide a familiar script or scaffolding that enables the client to participate more fully by freeing cognitive energy that might otherwise be used to aid participation. Children with MR seem to produce more speech and more diverse vocabulary in routine situations than in other less familiar situations (Yoder & Davies, 1992).

Caregivers Can Be Trained as Language Facilitators.   Families can play a key role, especially in early intervention. SLPs in early intervention need to value the knowledge the family possesses about their child and their child's syndrome. Compared to parents of children with lesser known syndromes, parents of children with DS usually have more in-depth understandings of their children's strengths and weaknesses (Fidler, Hodapp, & Dykens, 2002). A further resource is nationally based parent–professional organizations, many of which have chapters in different regions and states, publish literature, hold conferences, and have websites, such as the following:

National Down Syndrome Society   www1.ndss.org

Williams Syndrome Association   www.williams-syndrome.org

National Fragile X Foundation   www.fragilex.org/html/what.htm

People within the natural environment, such as parents, teachers, and aides, should be included in the training as language trainers/facilitators and as clients themselves (Owens, 2004). In short, greater involvement by caregivers yields greater results for generalization to the home and other settings.

The effective use of parents as agents of behavioral change is well established (Heifetz, 1980). Infant stimulation programs conducted in the home by trained parents can significantly improve the functioning of children with MR (Sharav & Shlomo, 1986). Several parent variables can affect the outcome, however. Parent socioeconomic status, pretraining skills, and experience positively correlate with the short-term learning outcomes (Clark, Baker, & Heifetz, 1982). Mothers with low socioeconomic status also can make positive strides with their children, because prior to training, these mothers often overlook natural teaching situations used by mothers from middle and upper socioeconomic levels. The key to success with language trainers is to consider individual trainer differences and learning styles and to individualize the techniques these trainers use (Reese & Serna, 1986).

Although maternal responses to their infants' intentional communications vary with maternal education level, mothers can be taught to respond in ways that foster their children's communication development (Yoder & Warren, 2001b). Direct care staff in community residences can also be trained to provide opportunities for communication to nonspeaking children through a combination of a workshop and nondirective consultation (Schlosser, Walker, & Sigafoos, 2006). Training can result in providing more opportunities to children and concurrent increases in children's initiation of communication.

The variables that control transfer of parental skills to natural settings are not fully understood, although transfer increases with the similarity of the tasks and training structure to the natural environment. Feedback from the SLP regarding application of newly acquired training skills is also important.

Successful use of parents as language facilitators seems to depend on three components (Salzberg & Villani, 1983).

1. Parents must use their training skills at home.
2. Parents must be specifically taught to adapt training techniques to these more informal situations.
3. Parents need to receive professional feedback.

Interactive models that train parents in general interactive strategies may result in parents becoming more responsive, less directive, and better able to model language but may have little effect on the children's development (Tannock, Girolametto, & Siegel, 1992). Specific skills training is needed by parents if more specific learning is to be expected.

Preintervention child–parent and client–caregiver interactional patterns may be nurturing but insufficient to effect real change. These interactions can be systematically modified. There is still no guarantee that the new interactional patterns will be used in the home, however. Several suggestions are offered in Table 6.6 for facilitating language development in both clinical and more natural settings. Effective parent training requires the use of parental skills in the home. Generalization does not just happen. The environment must be modified systematically to increase the likelihood of generalization.

INITIAL COMMUNICATION AND LANGUAGE TRAINING

For many individuals with MR, training begins at a presymbolic or early symbolic level, often in early intervention programs. Many young children participate in infant stimulation or preschool programs. Nonspeaking adults with profound MR may also be trained at this level. Training should begin as soon as it is recognized that a child may be at risk for communication or language impairment (Mahoney & Snow,

Table 6.6   **Suggestions for Facilitating Language Generalization**

In the natural environment:

1. Arrange the environment to accomplish with language what cannot be accomplished easily in other ways.
2. Delay reinforcement and provide cues when the appropriate verbal response is obvious.
3. Be responsive to communication attempts.
4. Restructure the environment to create opportunities for a particular response to occur.

In the language training environment:

1. Teach language skills generalizable outside the clinic.
2. Vary the contexts, trainers, and training materials.
3. Use the consequences that are varied and related to the language use being taught.
4. Reduce the density of reinforcement as performance improves.

Adapted from Spradlin & Siegel, 1982.

1983). SLPs can work with caregivers to help them fine-tune the infant–caregiver interaction to better facilitate language learning.

Behaviors observed in typical development can serve as a basis for training with children with MR. Development or change follows a developmental hierarchy. Children use single-word verbalizations and then short, multiword utterances. In addition, behavioral change goes from simple to complex. Short word-order rules appear before complex syntactic systems. Complex behavior results from coordination or modification of simpler responses.

Professional caregivers and parents cannot teach all of the complex behaviors found among humans; rather, they must determine which behaviors to target. Selection of appropriate training targets is critical. Because development is rarely linear, educators must also determine the sequence of trained skills. In addition, intervention must consider the individual needs of the child and family.

Overall Model

In communication intervention with nonspeaking children, SLPs often use a dual approach, with major emphasis on establishing an initial communication system and secondary emphasis on training presymbolic skills (see Figure 6.3). These two paths merge when a child begins to use symbols. The child who does not reach this point still has a communication system, even if it is limited to gestures or a generalized request signal.

Assessment

The goal of assessment is to identify a child's communication behaviors and to identify the contexts, times, and individuals that affect that child's communication (Mahoney & Weller, 1980). This goal is based on the assumption that all individuals communicate, that each communication occurrence offers an opportunity for reciprocity, and that the

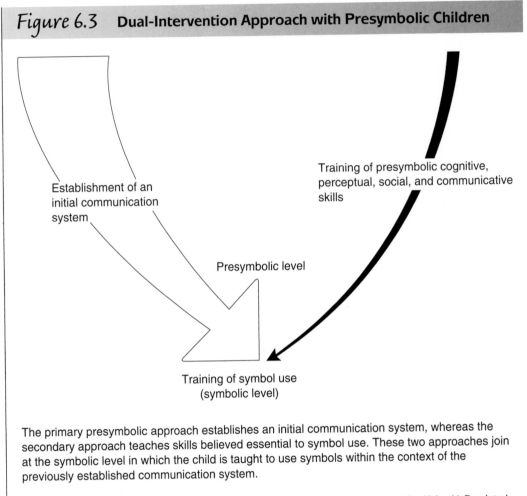

Figure 6.3   **Dual-Intervention Approach with Presymbolic Children**

Establishment of an initial communication system

Training of presymbolic cognitive, perceptual, social, and communicative skills

Presymbolic level

Training of symbol use (symbolic level)

The primary presymbolic approach establishes an initial communication system, whereas the secondary approach teaches skills believed essential to symbol use. These two approaches join at the symbolic level in which the child is taught to use symbols within the context of the previously established communication system.

From R. Owens, *Language Disorders, a Functional Approach to Assessment and Intervention* (4th ed.). Reprinted with permission of Allyn & Bacon, an imprint of Pearson Education. Copyright © 2004 by Allyn & Bacon.

behaviors of each communication partner affect the other (MacDonald, 1985). In addition, the SLP is interested in the level of presymbolic functioning and the content of communication.

For presymbolic children, it is essential that background data be integrated with observational and testing data to form an overall image of communication characteristics. Initial information can be gathered by observation and then supplemented through interviews with the child's caregivers. The SLP should attempt to obtain the following information (Calculator, 1988; Owens & Rogerson, 1988):

1. How does the child communicate primarily?
2. Does the child demonstrate any turn-taking behaviors?

3. What situations seem to be high-communication contexts?
4. What high-interest items does the child have?
5. Do caregivers provide enough time for the child to respond? How do caregivers cue the child to respond? How do they evaluate his or her responses?
6. Which caregivers seem to elicit the most client responses? Why?
7. Does the child seem to enjoy making sounds? Give examples. How often does the child vocalize? Which situations elicit maximum vocalization? Imitated vocalizations?
8. Which daily situations result in the most client–caregiver interactions? Describe these interactions. When do these occur daily? Are the child's responses consistent?
9. Does the child ever initiate communication? How? In what situations?
10. Does the child

> make wants known? How?
>
> request help? How?
>
> point to things, name them, or both? Does the child look at the object and/or partner while pointing or naming?
>
> ask questions or seek information? How?
>
> indicate emotions (pain, happiness, like/dislike)? How?
>
> seek attention? How? What happens if attention doesn't follow?

This general information can be supplemented by specific questions related to the functioning level of the child. Several language assessment tools are available for this purpose, as listed in 6.7. Many of these tools contain parental reports and questionnaires.

Data from such parental reports compare favorably to clinical data and increase the validity of assessment results (Miller, Sedey, & Miolo, 1995). The SLP's goal is to obtain an estimate of client functioning in order to provide a more thorough assessment. In addition, such probing familiarizes the caregiver with the behaviors to be tested and taught. This familiarization is vital if caregivers are to become fully participating members in the intervention process. These tools are best used as guides for describing a child's behavior; the goal should not be to fix a developmental age.

Children should also be observed by and with the caregiver and the SLP to verify information from questionnaires and interviews and to enhance the validity of the overall assessment. Of interest are the methods used by the child to communicate and the contexts in which these behaviors occur. Many of the tools listed in Table 6.7 offer formats for structured collection of observational data.

Children who communicate in a nonstandard manner should be observed carefully to determine the intent of such communication (Houghton, Bronicki, & Guess, 1987). For example, a child who bashes her head with her fist might be attempting to communicate. By observing the times and circumstances of this behavior, the SLP can form hypotheses about the child's intended meaning (Robinson & Owens, 1995).

Not all such behaviors contain communicative content, although consistent, predictable behaviors are likely to be meaningful. Hypotheses on the intent of such behaviors can be tested by carefully manipulating the events that precede and follow the behavior and carefully recording the effect on the behavior. For example, it might be hypothesized that head bashing before meals indicates a request for help. If aid given before or after the behavior results in nonperformance or cessation of the behavior,

Table 6.7 Assessment Protocols for Clients Functioning below Three Years

Assessment Tool	Infant–Preschool	School Age–Adult
Ages and Stages Questionnaires (ASQ): A Parent-Completed Child-Monitoring System. Bricker, D., Squires, J., & Mounts, L. (1995).	X	
Assessing Linguistic Behavior (ALB). Olswang, L., Stoel-Gammon, C., Coggins, T., & Carpenter, R. (1987a).	X	
Assessment, Evaluation, and Programming Systems: AEPS Measurement for Birth to Three Years (Volume 1). Bricker, D. (1993).	X	
Birth to Three Developmental Scales. Bangs, T., & Dodson, S. (1979).	X	
Carolina Curriculum for Infants and Toddlers with Special Needs. Johnson-Martin, N., Jens, K., Attermeier, S., & Hacker, B. (1991).	X	
Communication and Symbolic Behavior Scales. Wetherby, A., & Prizant, B. (1993).	X	X
Comprehension of Social-Action Games in Prelinguistic Children: Levels of Participation and Effect of Adult Structure. Platt, J., & Coggins, T. (1990).	X	
Developmental Activities Screening Inventory. Fewell, R., & Langley, M. (1984).	X	
Early Language Milestone Scale. Coplan, J. (1987).	X	
Family Administered Neonatal Activities. Cardone, I., & Gilkerson, L. (1989).	X	
Infant-Toddler Language Scale. Rossetti, L. (1990).	X	
Language Development Survey. Rescorla, L. (1989).	X	X
MacArthur Communicative Development Inventories. Fenson, L., Dale, P., Reznick, S., Thal, D., Bates, E., Hartung, J., Pethnick, S., & Reilly, J. (1993).	X	X
Observation of Communicative Interactions. Klein, M., & Briggs, M. (1987).	X	
Parent/Professional Preschool Performance Profile (5Ps). Variety Pre-Schooler's Workshop. (1987).	X	
Receptive Expressive Emergent Language Test. Bzock, K., & League, R. (1978).	X	

respectively, this may confirm the hypothesis. The SLP is interested in the range of communication needs expressed and in the modes of communication (visual, manual, vocal, tactile) used receptively and expressively (Caro & Snell, 1989; Owens, 2004).

More formal assessment of presymbolic skills might include the content listed in Table 6.8. This type of assessment requires real skill by the SLP, because standardized testing with children below age 3 is unreliable, forcing professionals to use less formal data collection methods. Skills essential to language acquisition can be grouped as cognitive, perceptual, social, and communicative (McLean & Snyder-McLean, 1978; Owens, 2008). For example, symbolic play and symbolic comprehension are significantly correlated with each other and with early expressive and receptive language in

Table 6.8 Possible Presymbolic Targets

Behavior	Cognitive	Perceptual	Social	Communicative
Physical imitation—imitating behaviors of others	X		X	
Imitation with objects—using extension of self for imitation	X			
Deferred imitation—retrieving a behavior for imitation	X			
Repetitive and sequential imitation—retrieving patterns	X	X		
Object permanence—retrieving object form from memory	X			
Turn taking—using motor imitation or eye contact in turn				X
Functional use—using objects for intended purpose in order to gain functional knowledge of meaning	X			
Means–ends—using one object or person to attain another	X		X	
Communicative gestures—displaying early intentions				X
Auditory memory—remembering sound patterns	X	X		
Word recognition—pairing names with entities				X
Vocal response—vocalizing in response to another person			X	X
Vocal turn taking—vocalizing turns			X	X
Vocal imitation—shaping vocalizations to resemble a model		X		X
Sequencing vocal imitation—imitating vocal sequences		X		X

Program for the Acquisition of Language with the Severely Impaired (PALS), by R. Owens, 1982, San Antonio: Psychological Corporation. Copyright 1982 by The Psychological Corporation. Adapted by permission.

children with DS (O'Toole & Chiat, 2006). A child's level of play, however, will differ with different play partners (DeKroon, Kyte, & Johnson, 2002). Children using symbols, such as words, signs, pictures, or pictographs, should be evaluated for the range of semantic and illocutionary functions expressed by these symbols (see Table 6.8). This can be done using both formal testing and sampling, although the latter is more valuable as a source of information about typical performance. Several of the assessment tools listed in Table 6.8 use data collected by a variety of methods, including direct testing, observation, and parental report.

Communication and language sampling may occur in a free-play situation with caregivers or in a combination of free play and structured sampling. Fifty utterances—whether spoken, signed, or picture indicated—should provide an adequate sample, unless a child repeats frequently. The SLP should be interested in both the breadth and depth of semantic and illocutionary functions. Of particular interest are the nonexistence of certain functions, the low incidence of others, and the length of each function. This can be assessed using a short rated sample (Owens, 1982d) or a more descriptive analysis (Wilcox & Campbell, 1983).

Early single-word and early multiword utterances are organized following simple word order rules based on semantics and early prelinguistic and single-word semantic functions (see Table 6.9). These semantic functions are expanded or combined into two-, three-, and four-word utterances by typically developing children, and these expansions can provide targets for training with minimally symbolic children with MR.

Likewise, specific illocutionary acts and communicative intentions can be found in early vocalizations, gestures, and single-word utterances. A language sample can be analyzed to determine the range of such intentions. The most valid results may be attained if caregivers participate with the child and if the child uses familiar objects, possibly in a play format (Westby, 1980). The SLP should be cautioned that although these semantic and illocutionary categories represent what linguists believe children mean or intend by their early vocalizations, gestures, and verbalizations, there is no way of knowing the actual meaning or intention. In addition, these categories are predetermined and may not accurately reflect the behavior of communicators with MR (Leonard, Steckol, & Panther, 1983).

Because caregivers act as language facilitators, the child–caregiver interaction is important in assessment. A sample might range from a ten-minute rated play sample (Owens, 1982d) to a more descriptive, lengthier analysis (Wilcox & Campbell, 1983). Analysis might involve the physical distance of the communicators; the use of reinforcement, responses, and cues by the caregiver; appropriate language by the caregiver for the perceived language skills of a child; turn taking, body posture, and movement; and the termination and reengagement of the interaction (MacDonald & Gillette, 1982; Owens, 1982d; Wilcox & Campbell, 1983). Also of interest are reciprocal behaviors of both the child and caregiver and the consistency and timeliness of the caregiver's responses to the child's attempts to communicate. These behaviors should be observed in several contexts, such as play and feeding, given the effect of context on interactive behaviors (Girolametto & Weitzman, 2002).

Once the initial evaluation has been completed, the SLP should understand the child's interactional strategies, most frequent topics, communication partners, and functioning level and the quality of the child–caregiver interaction. For nonverbal or

Table 6.9   **Semantic and Illocutionary Targets of Early Childhood**

Functions	Examples
Semantic	
Nomination—naming a person or object using a single- or multiword name or a demonstrative-plus as a name.	Doggie, Choo-choo This horsie
Location—marking spatial relationships. Utterances may contain single location words or two-word utterances containing an agent, action, or object plus a location word. The function can be demonstrated in response to *where* questions.	PARTNER: Where's doggie? CLIENT: Chair. Ball table, Doggie chair, Throw me, Throw here (X + locative)
Negation—marking of nonexistence, rejection, and denial using single negative words or a negative followed by another word (negative + X).	All gone (count as a single word), Away, No milk (client drank it), All gone car (the ride is over), No
Nonexistence generally develops first and marks the absence of a once-present object.	PARTNER: Time for bed. CLIENT: No (or No bed).
Rejection marks an attempt to prevent or to stop an event.	Stop it. No milk (pushes glass away).
Denial marks rejection of a proposition.	PARTNER: See the bear? CLIENT: No bear.
Modification	
Possession—appreciating that an object belongs to or is frequently associated with someone. Single-word utterances signal the owner's name. In two-word utterances, stress is usually on the initial word, the possessor.	Mine, My dollie, Johnnie bike (modifier + head) Dollie (client clutches doll)
Attribution—using descriptors for properties not inherently part of the object.	Yukky, Big doggie, Little baby (modifier + head)
Recurrence—understanding that an object can reappear or an event can be reenacted.	More, More milk, 'Nuther cookie (modifier + head)
Notice—signaling that an object has appeared, an event has happened, or an attempt to gain attention.	Hi Mommy, Bye-bye, Look Jim
Action—marking an activity.	
Action—single action words.	Jump, Eat
Agent + action—two-word signal that an animate initiated an activity.	Mommy throw, Doggie eat, Baby sleep
Action + object—two-word signal that an animate or inanimate object was the recipient of action.	Eat cookie, Throw ball

(continued)

Table 6.9 **Continued**

Functions	Examples
Illocutionary	
Answer—client responds to questions. The questioner's behaviors are a cue for the client's response; the response probably would not be produced without this cue. The client's responses are cognitively related to the question, although they may be incorrect.	PARTNER: (*holding doll*) What's this? CLIENT: Baby. PARTNER: Is this a mirror? CLIENT: No.
Question—client asks for information or verification by addressing the other person verbally. The client's behavior is a stimulus or cue and indicates that she expects an answer. The client can ask herself questions when engaged in egocentric play.	CLIENT: (*picks up toy telephone*) Phone? CLIENT: What this?
Reply—client makes meaningful response to the content of the other speaker's previous utterance, a verbal cue external to the client. The client may continue to build on the content and ignore the form of the utterance, such as responding to a word or thought in a question without answering the question. In many cases, the client will build on the content *and* respond with an appropriate form. This category does not include mere repetition.	PARTNER: Johnny, bring me the scissors. (command) CLIENT: No. PARTNER: May I have the keys? (request) CLIENT: In a minute. PARTNER: This is a cute dog. (declaration) CLIENT: My doggie.
Elicitation—client self-repeats in response to a request for repetition or clarification or in response to "Say X."	CLIENT: Kitty go. (declaration) PARTNER: What? CLIENT: Kitty go. PARTNER: Mary, say "ball." CLIENT: Ball.
Continuant—client signals that she is listening and wants to continue the interchange, or that she missed what was said.	Uh-huh, Okay, I see, Yes, What? Huh?
Declaration—client makes a statement that is situationally related and for communication but is not in response to another speaker. The utterance is more like a commentary. Cues are internal or situational but not verbal. This category also includes situationally related phonemic exclamations.	CLIENT: (*playing game with mother and glances out*) It raining out. CLIENT: (*playing with car*) Car go up. PARTNER: This is a cute doggie. CLIENT: My doggie. (reply) He lives in a house. (declaration) PARTNER: This is a cute doggie. CLIENT: My doggie. (reply) I have kitty, too. (declaration)

Functions	Examples
Practice—client repeats or imitates in whole or part what she or another person says with no change in intonation that would indicate a change of intent. In addition, internal replay without added new information is considered practice. This category also includes counting, singing, babbling, or rhyming behaviors in which the client seems to be experimenting or rehearsing.	PARTNER: Ball. CLIENT: Ball. PARTNER: See the red ball. CLIENT: Red ball. PARTNER: See the red ball. CLIENT: See ball. (practice) Ball, ball, ball. (practice)
Perseverative responses, even if the other person interjects an utterance between them, are considered practice as long as they do not mark discrete events or objects.	
Name—client labels an object or event that is present, but the label is not in response to a question. This verbal behavior is usually accomplished by pointing or nodding.	CLIENT: (*picks up ball*) Ball. CLIENT: (*points to ball*) That ball.
Suggestion, command, demand, request—The primary function of the client's utterance is to influence another person's behavior by getting that person to do something or to give the client permission. The form may be imperative, declarative, or interrogative.	CLIENT: Gimmie cookie. CLIENT: Stop that. CLIENT: Mommy. CLIENT: Throw ball. (*parent throws ball*) Throw ball. (*parent throws ball*) Throw ball.

Program for the Acquisition of Language with the Severely Impaired (PALS), by R. Owens, 1982, San Antonio: Psychological Corporation. Copyright 1982 by The Psychological Corporation. Adapted by permission.

minimally verbal children with severe communication delays, the levels of receptive and expressive language ability seem to be the best predictors of success in communication intervention (Brady, Steeples, & Fleming, 2005). Throughout the clinical intervention phase, the SLP should test and probe in order to fine-tune training techniques.

Intervention

The first step in training is to decide what to teach, who will teach it, and under what circumstances. In the previous section, a number of training targets were suggested for early intervention. The participants and the circumstances are related and will significantly shape the intervention program.

It is essential in initial language programming to include the natural environment of the child. In establishing early communication, the SLP must enlist the aid of the child's caregivers in the intervention process. Typically, the professional trains client responses, and the parents train and elicit these responses within the home (Wulz, Hall, & Klein, 1983). The components are environmental manipulation and teaching interaction. In *environmental manipulation,* the caregivers restructure needs-meeting situations so their child's needs are not anticipated but are dependent on his or her communication behavior. Within the teaching phase, the child is taught to respond to need-to-communicate situations. The purposes of the training are to expand the child's communication repertoire and stimulate responding.

Home-based training should not be disruptive. The goal is not to give parents added responsibilities but rather to help them make use of teaching opportunities in daily routines by restructuring these ongoing activities (Wulz et al., 1983). Called **incidental teaching,** this type of training should be given primacy as an early communication training strategy (Owens, 1982d). If, for example, the parent is training object permanence (the knowledge that unseen entities still exist), nonfloating soap and toys can be incorporated into the bathing routine. Because almost any routine can be adapted for language training, there is no need to rely solely on formal, out-of-context training modes. With children, the modality for training may be play. Play is child centered, and the child's activity can provide the focus of training. Training should occur in short, repetitive, daily activities in which the reinforcer is part of the activity, such as requesting another cookie at snack time (Halle, Alpert, & Anderson, 1984). The content should be meaningful in the situation and result in real consequences.

Environmental rules can also be used to restructure client–caregiver interactions (MacDonald, 1978b). Once children have learned a skill, they can be required to perform that skill in order to obtain desired entities or privileges. For example, if a child can sign *cookie,* the sign will be required to get a cookie. Previously accepted pointing or whining will not be acceptable. Environmental rules affect both client and caregiver behaviors.

Although insufficient when used alone, language stimulation techniques can also be used in the natural environment (Owens, 1982d). Ideally, such stimulation slightly precedes a child's actual level of functioning. Stimulation can take the form of "Motherese." It is important that language trainers maintain an interactive style to avoid occurrence of the solitary nonlanguage activities common among children with MR (Smith & Hagen, 1984).

The importance of formal or structured training cannot be overlooked but should be minimized when possible (MacDonald, 1985; Owens, 1982d). Often, this training can be adapted to a play modality (Manolson, 1983). Two trainers can facilitate client responding (Richmond & Lewallen, 1983). One trainer cues a child while the second trainer models or prompts the appropriate response. For maximum generalization, formal training should occur in as natural a manner as possible, employing a child's caregivers and the natural environment of the home or classroom.

It is not always possible to train within the home. An alternative is the classroom (Brightman, Ambrose, & Baker, 1980). Within residential settings, aides, direct care staff, or foster grandparents may serve as language facilitators (Owens, McNerney, Bigler-Burke, & Lepre-Clark, 1987). The behaviors of direct care staff can be modified by having them provide simple praise or feedback plus praise (Realon, Lewallen, & Wheeler, 1983).

Early communication in the form of basic signal systems can be established using **behavior chain interruption** techniques (Goetz, Gee, & Sailor, 1985; Hunt, Goetz, Alwell, & Sailor, 1986; Romer & Schoenberg, 1991; Sternberg, Pegnatore, & Hill, 1983). There are two basic elements to behavior chain interruption: (1) the child engages in a pleasurable activity that the trainer interrupts, and (2) the child is prompted to give a communicative response, such as a touch, to have the activity begin again. The communicative response or signal can be modified or expanded into a more conventional gesture or sign.

Communication systems can also be initiated through the use of pictures or signs to signal a generalized or nonspecific request, such as a cup to indicate *drink* (Reichle, 1990). (This procedure will be discussed in more detail in the next section on augmentative communication.)

Natural behaviors, such as reaching, can be modified into a requesting gesture or a point to a printed symbol (Reichle & Sigafoos, 1991). All spontaneous vocalizations and other attempts to communicate should be encouraged and reinforced. The amount of vocalizing can be increased through reinforcement and modified into meaningful communication (Drash, Raver, Murrin, & Tudor, 1989; Poulson, 1988).

Once trained in imitation, a single word or sign can be trained within a variety of semantic functions and communication intentions. Thus, a single word or sign can be trained to be used to express several meanings and intentions. Single words trained solely in response to "What's this?" have only limited use for a child. Possible semantic and illocutionary training targets appear in Table 6.9. Using this table, the SLP may pair each semantic category with each of the illocutionary acts. For example, a "location" response might follow the cue "Where is baby?" A "nomination" question might consist of "Cup?" or "What?" A "location" question might also consist of "Cup?" if a child is trying to guess the location of some small object. Within these category combinations, longer utterances may also be learned. It has been demonstrated that children continue to use combinations of the semantic rules in utterances of up to four words. Programming possibilities are presented in Figure 6.4. After this point, learning focuses on internal sentence reorganization and new structures are learned.

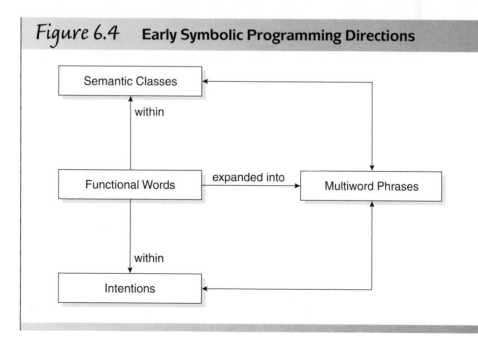

Figure 6.4 **Early Symbolic Programming Directions**

Some developmental guidelines exist for the semantic functions. In general, the order of appearance is nomination, negation, action, objects, state or attribution, change in state or attribution, possession and location, experiencer of action, and agent (Menyuk, 1974). Initial two-word functions include nomination ("that _____"), recurrence ("more _____"), and nonexistence ("no _____"). Next, separate semantic classes are combined to produce utterances to indicate agent plus action ("Mommy eat"), possession ("Baby cookie"), and location ("Doggie bed").

Again, SLPs must be cautious not to slavishly follow developmental data. Such information provides a useful guideline, but decisions must be based on careful assessment of a child and data collected during intervention.

Augmentative and Alternative Communication (AAC)

Some individuals with MR, particularly those with more severe impairment, experience great difficulty with speech and the use of symbols. For these nonspeaking children, augmentative and alternative communication (AAC) may be necessary. Augmentative and alternative forms can increase or expand the symbolic communication capabilities of these nonspeaking individuals. Common forms of AAC include manual communication, communication boards, and electronic- or computer-based communication. These forms will be discussed briefly along with assessment and programming considerations.

Contrary to a common misconception, the use of AAC systems does not deter further development of speech. AAC facilitates symbol learning; increases verbalization of trained symbols; increases attention, intentional communication, and sociability; facilitates spontaneous verbal communication; increases communication initiations; and increases the range of meanings and communication partners. In a comprehensive study of published research on speech production before, during, and after AAC intervention that involved instruction in manual signs or nonelectronic aided systems, no subjects demonstrated decreases in speech production as a result of AAC intervention, 11 percent showed no change, and the majority (89 percent) demonstrated modest gains in speech (Millar, Light, & Schlosser, 2006). Even challenging behaviors, such as those that are self-injurious, can reportedly be reduced by a positive AAC support plan (Hetzroni & Roth, 2003).

These outcomes are not guaranteed, however, and only occur in the presence of thorough assessment and well-planned and executed intervention that includes natural communication settings and partners. Nothing destroys the effectiveness of AAC use more quickly than nonuse by others in the home or school.

Types of AAC. There are two types of augmentative and alternative communication systems: aided and unaided. *Aided* AAC uses a device such as a communication board or an electronic means of communication. *Unaided* systems consist of manual communication, such as gestures, signs, and finger spelling.

Communication boards come in many different shapes and varieties. In general, boards are easy to make and are portable and very adaptable. The visual symbols used may include, from least to most symbolic, models or miniatures, pictures, drawings, Rebus symbols, Blissymbols, and letters and words. Examples are presented in Figure 6.5. Preschool children with DS find gestures significantly easier to

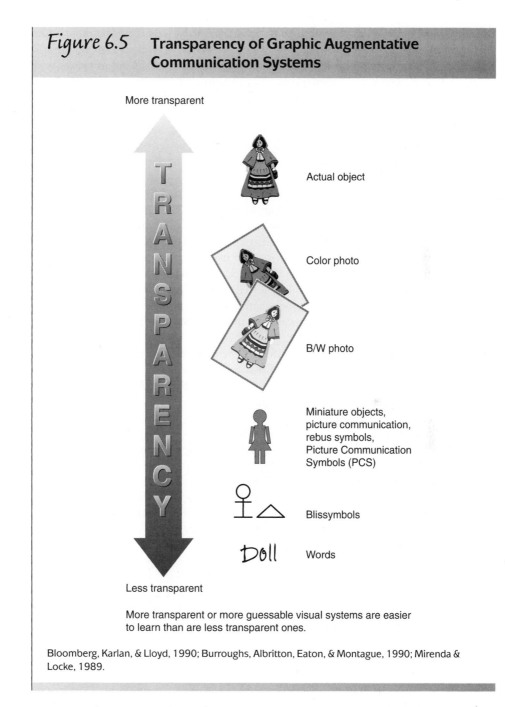

Figure 6.5 **Transparency of Graphic Augmentative Communication Systems**

More transparent

TRANSPARENCY

Actual object

Color photo

B/W photo

Miniature objects, picture communication, rebus symbols, Picture Communication Symbols (PCS)

Blissymbols

Words

Less transparent

More transparent or more guessable visual systems are easier to learn than are less transparent ones.

Bloomberg, Karlan, & Lloyd, 1990; Burroughs, Albritton, Eaton, & Montague, 1990; Mirenda & Locke, 1989.

understand than miniatures or substitute objects used as abstract symbols to represent other objects (O'Toole & Chiat, 2006). Rebus symbols are pictographic represent
of concepts. Blissymbols are generally less iconic than Rebus symbols but allow for
more generative language use. For example, the Rebus symbol for the word *book* is
a pictograph showing simplistic details of an open book; the Blissymbol is a square
with a vertical line through its center that represents an open book schematically.
These encoding forms are not exclusive and may be used in combination. In general,
the more iconic or "guessable" the encoding system, the easier it is to learn. In turn,
the less iconic systems are more flexible and generative, allowing more adultlike
representation.

The tremendous growth of computer technology is opening many new possibilities for the nonspeaking. Input systems may be as varied as a simple one-direction
switch or as complex as a computer keyboard, and output may include print, graph-
ics, and/or prerecorded or synthesized speech. In general, three types of indicating
methods are used by children: scanning, encoding, and direct selection. In the scanning method, the device continually scans the display of symbols, and the child stops
the scan on the desired symbol. With encoding, a code such as numbers or digits is
used to access the computer's memory. Finally, in direct selection, the child moves a
cursor or pointer to the desired symbol or may, if possible, type the message.

Accessing computers may be the most difficult problem, particularly for individuals with severe motor limitations. The interface switch between the child and microcomputer must often be modified or custom designed to the motor abilities of an
individual client. The slowness of use of an interface device may actually negate some
of the speed advantages associated with microcomputers.

There are several types of unaided sign systems, including American Sign Language (ASL), which is a language of its own, and Seeing Essential English (SEE$_1$) or
Signing Exact English (SEE$_2$), which closely approximate English syntax. Signed English, the most widely taught system, uses signs from other systems but does not adhere as closely to English morphological rules as SEE$_1$. American Indian sign
language (Amer-Ind) has also been used successfully with persons with MR, perhaps
because of its transparency. *Transparency* is the ease of understanding a sign once its
origin is explained. It may be advantageous for some children to have more than one
type of augmentative system. Different systems may have application in different
environments.

Evaluation.   Evaluative decisions on client use of AAC are made by a team of professionals, usually consisting of an SLP, psychologist, physical therapist, occupational
therapist, special education teacher, a client advocate such as a parent, and, when appropriate, the client. Assessment is a continuing process, which, in this case, is essential to adapt the AAC system to the child's changing needs and abilities.

The American Speech–Language–Hearing Association (ASHA) Ad Hoc Committee on Communication Processes and Non-Speaking Persons (1980) identified three
components of the assessment for augmentative communication. First, the team must
assess the appropriateness of an augmentative system. Not all nonspeaking individuals are candidates for augmentative communication. For example, the cognitive
abilities needed for spontaneous symbol use apply to augmentative communication

as well as to verbal language (Bryen, Goldman, & Quinlisk-Gill, 1988; Goossens, 1984; Owens & House, 1984; Shane & Bashir, 1980; Silverman, 1980). The environment also must be supportive of the use of augmentative systems (Owens & House, 1984; Shane, Lipshultz, & Shane, 1982).

The second component of an evaluation is selection of the appropriate communication mode. The team must decide which type or types of AAC will be appropriate for the nonspeaking individual. Of particular importance are the motor abilities of a child in the context of the body's total movement patterns (Bottorf & DePape, 1982). The evaluative team is interested in the range, speed, strength, and consistency of movement. Children with good motor skills may be candidates for manual systems, whereas those with less ability may use communication boards or electronic systems. For electronic devices, decisions should be based on a task analysis that includes the child's present skills and those behaviors needed to operate the communication aid.

Finally, the team must select the appropriate symbol system or systems. Questions of appropriateness relate to cognitive ability, visual acuity, and environmental receptivity. For example, greater cognitive skills and visual discrimination abilities are needed for word use than for picture use. Pictures are generally easier to discriminate than lexigrams (picture–letter combinations), which are in turn easier than printed words (Romski, Sevcik, Pate, & Rumbaugh, 1985). In addition, the use of a symbol system such as Blissymbols might hinder communication in a nonreceptive environment.

Intervention.   The focus of intervention should be increasing successful interactions (Bottorf & DePape, 1982). In general, communication interactions can be fostered by adapting the augmentative system to the individual client and the communication environment.

The SLP should establish an augmentative environment around the child. The AAC system is available at all times, and others are encouraged to use it. Signs are always available, but others may not use them when talking to the child. Their use by others may facilitate comprehension and help establish an atmosphere of sign. In addition, the unique daily routine of each client can foster AAC use. Lack of generalization of augmentative systems may be related to lack of knowledge and infrequent use by caregivers (Bryen & McGinley, 1991).

Selection of individualized content should reflect client routines, interests, and needs. The vocabulary selected will affect the types of interactions in which it is used (Bottorf & DePape, 1982). The initial vocabulary should be based on the client's individual interests, routines, and basic needs and on the recommendations of others within the environment. In addition, signs may be chosen on the basis of symmetry, taction, and iconicity. Individuals with severe MR can learn signs more rapidly if the signs are symmetrical or contain identical hand movements, have some contact with the body (taction), and are iconic or highly representational (Kohl, 1981).

AAC is not a panacea, and the results are not always favorable. The average client with severe or profound MR may learn to produce only a few signs spontaneously after years of training (Bryen et al., 1988). Lack of progress seems to be related to overuse of imitative training with little thought toward spontaneous use, unmeaningful training situations, inappropriate vocabulary or augmentative systems, and little environmental support by caregivers. Professional sensitivity toward child-specific issues of ethnicity and disability and parental involvement in parent–professional partnerships can help families learn how to use AAC devices (Parette, Brotherson, & Blake Huer, 2000).

Successful intervention builds on a child's current communication base and employs a multimodality strategy that uses all of a child's means of communication (Paul, 2000). Thus, some children may rely on a communication board supplemented by a few signs and vocalizations. The SLP attempts to open new avenues of communication while strengthening and building existing ones.

The environment should be modified systematically to encourage the use of AAC. Nonspeaking children must be given opportunities to use their augmentative systems. Teachers and caregivers need to be cautioned not to dominate communication. Communication partners must be patient and await client responses. Children should also be given choices in their daily routines and among alternative activities to foster active system use. Even individuals with severe MR can retain symbol vocabularies well over long periods of time if they use these symbols to control their daily environment (Romski, Sevcik, & Rumbaugh, 1985).

Initial AAC use can be challenging for both the child and the caregivers who communicate with the child. Common challenges include the following (Johnston, Reichle, & Evans, 2004):

- The child doesn't use the AAC system.
- Communication partners don't use the AAC system.
- The child uses socially or contextually unacceptable communicative behaviors.

In the first two instances, an SLP can address issues relative to the response effort, rate, immediacy, and quality of reinforcement and the interaction efficacy of these variables. In the third situation, social and contextual variables must be addressed. Table 6.10 presents issues to consider for each challenge.

Augmentative communication systems can be part of a nonspeaking individual's effective interaction system if continually evaluated and adapted to his or her communication needs. As noted in the discussion of early intervention, an SLP must be concerned with semantic categories and communicative intentions and with the use of the AAC system within the child's natural communication environment.

LANGUAGE RULE TRAINING

Once a child begins to use symbols meaningfully, training targets become the rule systems used with these symbols. The SLP should be knowledgeable about the rules used in the five generally recognized areas of language: syntax, morphology, phonology, semantics, and pragmatics.

Children with language impairment differ in their comprehension of sentences according to linguistic stage (Page & Horn, 1987). For example, the child who utters four-word sentences or less is using semantic comprehension strategies, not syntactic ones. Therefore, the SLP must be concerned with selecting the appropriate level of linguistic input to facilitate both comprehension and production. It is best to present examples of the language code that slightly exceed the child's expressive language skills.

Table 6.10   Challenges and Issues in Supporting Beginning AAC Users

Challenge	Issue	Consideration
Child doesn't use the AAC system	System requires too much physical or cognitive effort by the child	Reassess effort needed and change or modify system (i.e., selection mode or symbol system)
	Issues of motor ability, visual acuity, speed, and memory	Use most efficient mode of communication, even if result is multimodality responding
	Child's reinforcement is too infrequent	Structure environment to encourage or require use
		Train partners to respond, especially to spontaneous AAC use
		Emphasize content highly likely to occur to increase chances for reinforcement
	Child's reinforcement is delayed	Structure environment to encourage or require use
		Teach partners to respond
	Child's reinforcement is not motivating	Teach child to request
		Teach signs/symbols for desirable items and actions
		Train functional communication emphasizing the child's content
Communication partners don't use the AAC system	System requires too much physical or cognitive effort by the partner to interpret the message	Include partners in all decisions regarding their child's AAC assessment and training
		Teach partners to be partners
		Select more easily comprehended AAC method
	Partner's reinforcement is too infrequent	Structure environment to encourage or require use
	Partner's reinforcement is delayed	Teach partners to be patient with child and to expect delay
		Schedule times when partner can devote self to child's communication
	Partner's reinforcement is not motivating	Ensure partners collect data so they can see change
Child uses socially or contextually unacceptable communicative behaviors	Unacceptable behavior is easier for child to do	Simplify AAC method
		Strongly reinforce simplified AAC method
		Don't respond to unacceptable behavior
		Maximize the efficacy of the AAC method
		Provide contexts to elicit acceptable AAC behaviors and respond to these behaviors

Adapted from Johnston, Reichle, & Evans, 2004.

Professionals sometimes assume that only the adult forms of these rules are acceptable training targets. A typical 2-year-old who asks "What Mommy eating?" is not considered to be language disordered but to be following an age-appropriate rule. Likewise, individuals with MR follow rules that generally reflect their level of cognitive functioning.

Evaluation

The initial evaluation should attempt to determine which rule systems a child uses expressively and which ones he or she comprehends. Assessment ideally should include both formal testing and informal evaluation.

Very few formal tests were designed for and normed on the retarded population. Most commercially available tests were developed and normed on typically developing children. Before an SLP uses a standardized speech-language test with a student with intellectual disability (ID), he or she should carefully consider the design and purpose of the test and whether it includes students with ID in the normative group. In a study of 49 tests published between 1994 and 2004, only 23 included children with mild ID in the norm group (Cascella, 2006). No tests included students with more significant ID. Although separate norms for students with mild ID were included in 15 tests, none included a large group of children, making comparisons difficult. It is imperative, therefore, that the SLP supplements standardized tests with nonstandardized procedures.

An SLP must consider multiple conditions and a child's motor and cognitive abilities before choosing a language test or tests. The means of responding may need to be modified for children with oral motor difficulties or those who use AAC. These individuals may also need more time to complete timed tests.

In addition, test norms may be inappropriate for children with MR. It is of little value for intervention planning to demonstrate that a child with MR is in fact delayed in language. Testing will be of more value when it is used to help describe a child's language features and behavior. This will necessitate going behind scores and trying to analyze behavior.

Existing materials can be modified and new assessment tools developed (Owings & Guvette, 1982). Many SLPs supplement formal tests with their own locally prepared instruments (Pickett & Flynn, 1983). Formal testing situations are artificial and generally lack the natural cues available in a conversational setting. Additional sources of information are needed. Informally collected language samples can provide valuable information. Language varies with context and partners, requiring more than one sample for an adequate analysis. For example, the use of pictures in storytelling tasks increased the MLU of adolescents with Down syndrome (Miles, Chapman, & Sindberg, 2006).

Samples can be analyzed in a number of ways. Initially, an SLP should determine the mean length of utterance (MLU). An increasing MLU correlates with increasing complexity up to an MLU of 4.0 morphemes. Table 6.11 contains MLU values and equivalent ages for typically developing children.

Of the commercially available analysis methods, the Systematic Analysis of Language Transcripts (SALT) (www.saltsoftware.com), seems to be the most functional and easily accessible. Others, such as Developmental Sentence Scoring (Lee, 1974),

Table 6.11   **MLU and Approximate Age**

MLU	Predicted Chronological Age in Months	Predicted Age in Months ± 1 SD
1.5	23.0	18.5–27.5
2.0	26.9	21.5–32.3
2.5	30.8	23.9–37.7
3.0	34.8	28.0–41.6
3.5	38.7	30.8–46.6
4.0	42.6	36.7–48.5
4.5	46.6	40.3–52.9
5.0	50.5	42.1–58.9
5.5	54.4	46.0–62.8
6.0	58.3	49.9–66.7

Adapted from Miller, 1980.

result in a normative score but provide little direction for intervention. Language samples may also be analyzed using less formal, more descriptive methods (Owens, 2004). An SLP should attempt to describe all aspects of language. Pragmatic concerns, such as inappropriate communication, are difficult to measure directly but very important for overall communication effectiveness.

Intervention

Again, generalization is best ensured by use of the natural environment for language training. Caregivers can be instructed in the use of evaluative feedback and expansion techniques. For example, caregivers can provide corrective feedback in the form of modeling the correct production. Incomplete or primitive responses can be expanded into a more adultlike forms. The conversational context should not be overlooked for the training opportunity that it provides. As noted previously, generalization to spontaneous conversational use does not happen automatically for many children with MR. Training within structured conversations familiarizes the child with the situations and contexts that govern language feature use.

The primary criterion for selecting training targets should be usefulness to the child of the language features targeted. Targets should include those language features or behaviors that facilitate communication, such as asking questions, or that offer more communication options to the child, such as using the telephone.

It is best if the trainer does not introduce too many new items into the training task. Training cues, prompts, and materials should change gradually. Previously trained information should be used to aid new learning. For example, knowledge of the semantic categories and rules previously discussed can be used to train syntax. Agent words (*mommy, doggie*), because of their position in the utterance and their use, can become subjects. Possession, previously expressed by word order, can be expanded through the training of the possessive marker (*'s*).

Miniature linguistic systems may be helpful in training word order (Bunce, Ruder, & Ruder, 1985). Table 6.12 demonstrates a miniature system matrix in which one language feature occupies each axis. The child can learn a word order rule by combining words from each grouping. Good generalization has been reported with miniature systems from training of some but not all possible combinations. The Xs in Table 6.12 identify the combinations most effective in training.

New language features can be introduced using focused stimulation in which examples of the feature are given frequently in context. For example, when introducing the present progressive verb form (verb + -*ing*), the trainer might use self-talk to describe what he or she is doing or parallel talk to describe what the child is doing. Repeated use in context will highlight the feature for the child and help focus attention.

When attempting to elicit full sentences, the SLP should be very careful to use cues that make sense pragmatically and reflect general language use. For example, the cue "What do you want?" is most likely to elicit a single-word or short-phrase response, such as "Cookie." Demanding "I want cookie" as a response is inappropriate pragmatically.

Vocabulary, often a deficit area, can also be trained within the context of daily events in which the symbols have some relevance. The use of key words or pictures can facilitate learning and ensure memory better than direct instruction (Scruggs, Mastropieri, & Levin, 1985). For example, the word *popover* contains the key word *pop*; pictures that show the word *popover* or a toaster pastry "popping" out of a toaster may aid word recall. Stories can also be used to facilitate recall of single words or series of words (Glidden & Warner, 1985).

Table 6.12 **Miniature Linguistic Systems**

	Cookie	Cake	Pudding	Pie	Bread
Eat	X	X	X	X	X
Bake	X				
Mix	X				
Want	X				
Give	X				

	Pet	Dog	Cat	Horse	Ferret
Feed	X	X			
Bathe		X	X		
Groom			X	X	
Walk				X	X
Brush	X				X

Verbs on one axis are combined with nouns on the other to form short phrases. Each combination taught is marked with an X. Rule learning will generalize to the untrained combinations.

Many children with mild MR will learn to read. Although the reading of children with MR who are ages 7 to 12 can benefit from phonological reading instruction, those with better language skills will make the most progress (Conners, Rosenquist, Sligh, Atwell, & Kiser, 2006). Children with moderate to severe MR benefit from a combination of traditional and modified orthography in sight-word reading instruction in which they are taught to recognize words visually (Van der Bijl, Alant, & Lloyd, 2006). Traditional instruction teaches letter–sound relationships. In this modified orthographic instruction, the word to be learned is embedded in a picture that represents it or a figure is embedded into the word. It is assumed that if written words are accentuated visually to closely resemble the objects they represent, their meanings or symbolic functions will be easier for the child to understand.

SLPs should be aware of the special learning needs of those with MR. Cognitive operations should be trained before the linguistic skills that express those operations. For example, a child should understand reversibility of processes and time relationships before learning linguistic concepts such as *before, after,* and *because.* Children such as those with DS may need help with successive processing skills. Simultaneous skills related to overall meaning may be employed to facilitate sequential operations.

Finally, some individuals, such as those with DS, will require additional input beyond auditory symbols. Visual and tactile input can enhance their learning. The use of pictures or experiential activities might facilitate concept learning and elicit more client responses. The child's involvement in activity will result in more verbal responsiveness than involvement by the SLP or the use of pictures (Cook & Seymour, 1980). Likewise, active participation by the severely retarded client will become a cue for verbal behavior that was situationally appropriate (Spiegel, 1983).

LANGUAGE USE

With higher-functioning teenagers with MR in prevocational or vocational training programs, the focus of training should be language use. Although a minimum of language structure is required, language forms are not as critical to life success. The main difference between occupationally and socially successful and nonsuccessful adults with MR seems to be integration at work and in society. Further, there is a great need among individuals in the retarded population to attain regular employment and have nonretarded friends. One difference between the successful and unsuccessful person is found in the area of social skills, including language. Therefore, more appropriate language use is a desirable training target.

Some language factors, such as following directions and asking questions, may be more important than others, particularly in the work setting. Adults with MR are less likely to be employed if their language use is inappropriate, such as being abusive, argumentative, vulgar, bossy, loud, interruptive, or irrelevant. Additional skills for training might also include conversational abilities and direction following.

These vocational–interpersonal skills can be modified through a combination of modeling, coaching, and behavior rehearsal Appropriate verbal behavior can be modeled while children are trained in appropriate use. Rehearsal and role-playing in situations close to those of actual use can be beneficial. Social feedback in the forms of praise, instruction, and reprimands has been more effective than reprimands and instruction in reducing inappropriate verbalizations.

Other conversational skills may also be taught. Teenagers who are mentally retarded may have particular difficulties communicating with their parents and expressing their feelings. As conversational partners, adults, including those with MR, are expected to observe the rules of turn taking and to be able to introduce, sustain, and contribute to the topic of conversation. In addition, they should be able to take their communication partner's perspective and to vary their own role and informational contribution accordingly. Pragmatic abilities of those functioning at school-age or adult levels may also be assessed and trained for a range of intentions and forms of expression (Prutting & Kirchner, 1983). Normally developing peers can serve effectively as models and elicit appropriate conversational responses (Wilkinson & Romski, 1995).

Critical social and communication skills can be taught within the classroom, home, or workplace (Stowitschek et al., 1988). Adolescents and adults with severe MR can be taught to successfully answer the telephone and respond to a variety of messages and callers (Karen, Astin-Smith, & Creasy, 1985). Even individuals with MR recognize the need for these conversational skills. In a social room in a day training program, the clients established the following rules:

- Stay on topic.
- Be quiet when others are talking.
- Listen to what you hear.
- Don't interrupt others.
- Take turns—give everyone a chance.
- Speak so others can hear you.
- Don't talk to yourself.

Summary

The definition of mental retardation explored in this chapter considers cognitive functioning and adaptive behavior. Overall, this definition reflects empirical findings that individuals with MR are developmental beings whose behavior is characterized by both delay and difference. This finding is also true for the language development of the retarded population, with special modification.

These characteristics suggest a developmental language intervention approach. The wise SLP will use typical development as a guide for creative programming. The language intervention targets will differ with the language skills of the client. Initial training should focus on cognitive, perceptual, social, and communicative skills and on establishing early communication. Early building blocks will be semantic and pragmatic. Once short multiword utterances have been trained, the SLP should target language rule systems. As the client becomes more capable in using language rules, language use should become a tool for normalization training. Such training is particularly true of clients in vocational training programs.

We began this chapter with a quote from Nigel Hunt (1967) and will end with one as well:

Thank you ever so much for letting me write this book. I am most delightful. (p. 124)

Case Study **Catherine**

Catherine is a 33-year-old with severe MR who resides in a developmental center but attends a day training program in the community. She has been institutionalized since early childhood. The cause of her MR is unknown. Her mental age, as measured on the Wechsler Intelligence Scale for Children—Revised, is slightly above age 6, although her language performance is lower. She experiences seizures, primarily of the petitmal type. During seizure activity, Catherine usually stares and has a blank expression. Such episodes are usually a few seconds in duration, although on a few occasions, Catherine has lost consciousness. Currently, her seizures are controlled through medication. At times, Catherine becomes violent and strikes other clients for no apparent reason. Her placement in a community residence depends on controlling this behavior. She has good self-help skills, such as dressing and feeding, but poor language, money, and time skills.

Catherine's receptive vocabulary age is approximately 5 years, as measured on the Peabody Picture Vocabulary Test. Although she can point to pictures named, she has difficulty explaining word meanings. Her equivalent receptive language age, as measured by the Test for Auditory Comprehension of Language—Revised (TACL—R), is 4 years, 2 months. This score was corroborated for her expressive language by the Carrow Elicited Language Inventory. In this sentence imitation test, Catherine received an age equivalent of 46 months. Her performance was characterized by sentence simplification, omission of articles, and difficulties with verb tensing and pronouns. On the TACL—R, she also made several errors in verb tensing and pronouns. A free sample analyzed using Miller's Assigning Structural Stage indicated that Catherine's language skills are primarily those found in Brown's stage IV. Her MLU is approximately 3.67. Her language is primarily responsive and characterized by short sentences; a scarcity of complex or compound sentences; little use of pronouns beyond *you, me, he, she,* and *him;* and absence of tensing markers. Some auxiliary verbs and modals are present, but there is some confusion with the verb *to be.* Most sentences are simple declaratives or negatives.

In the vocational training program, Catherine's communication behavior is mostly responsive, although staff report that she also exhibits perseverative verbal behavior. While in vocational training, she will continually repeat the instructions she has been given or the statements made to her. This behavior is whispered but still annoys others around her. Staff report that it is difficult to stop this behavior.

Catherine is seen by the SLP twice weekly for individual programming and once a week for group training. Within the individual sessions, the SLP works primarily on verb tensing, focusing on the regular and irregular past and the future tense. Once Catherine gives a correct response, the SLP attempts to gain a longer verbalization from her. Group work attempts to encourage the initiation of conversation and use of longer utterances. In her vocational training program, Catherine is expected by the staff to provide longer responses in conversation. A questioning technique is used to elicit expansion of previous utterances. In addition, Catherine is reinforced for short periods without perseverative whispering.

Study Questions

1. What is the AAMR (1992) definition of mental retardation? Explain each portion of this definition.
2. How does the cognitive functioning of someone with MR differ from that of a nonretarded person? How might these differences relate to general intervention considerations?
3. Compare five aspects of the language abilities of the retarded and nonretarded populations.
4. Explain the developmental model of intervention and its relation to language training with persons with MR.
5. What are some of the targets for language intervention with persons with MR?

References

Abbeduto, L., Davies, B., Solesby, S., & Furman, L. (1991). Identifying the referents of spoken messages: Use of context and clarification requests by children with and without mental retardation. *American Journal on Mental Retardation, 95,* 551–562.

Abbeduto, L., Furman, L., & Davies, B. (1989). Relation between the receptive language and mental age of persons with mental retardation. *American Journal on Mental Retardation, 93,* 535–543.

Abbeduto, L., & Rosenberg, S. (1980). The communicative competence of mildly retarded adults. *Applied Psycholinguistics, 1,* 405–426.

Abbeduto, L., Short-Meyerson, K., Benson, G., & Dolish, J. (1997). Signaling of noncomprehension by children and adolescents with mental retardation: Effects of problem type and speaker identity. *Journal of Speech, Language, and Hearing Research, 40,* 20–32.

Abbeduto, L., Short-Meyerson, K., Benson, G., Dolish, J., & Weissman, M. (1998). Understanding referential expressions in context: Use of common ground by children and adolescents with mental retardation. *Journal of Speech, Language, and Hearing Research, 41,* 1348–1362.

Abrahamsen, A., Romski, M., & Sevcik, R. (1989). Concomitants of success in acquiring an augmentative communication system: Changes in attention, communication, and sociability. *American Journal on Mental Retardation, 93,* 475–496.

Affleck, G., Allen, D., McGrade, B., & McQueeney, M. (1982). Home environments of developmentally disabled infants as a function of parent and infant characteristics. *American Journal of Mental Deficiency, 86,* 445–452.

Alanay, Y., Unal, F., Turanli, G., Alikasifoglu, M., Alehan, D., Akyol, U., Belgin, E., Sener, C., Aktas, D., Boduroglu, I., Utine, E., Volkan-Salanci, B., Ozusta, S., Genc, A., Basar, F., Sevinc, S., & Tuncbilek, E. (2007). A multidisciplinary approach to the management of individuals with fragile X. *Journal of Intellectual Disability Research, 51,* 151–161.

Alvares, R. L., & Downing, S. F. (1998). A survey of expressive communication skills in children with Angelman syndrome. *American Journal of Speech-Language Pathology, 7*(2), 14–24.

American Association on Mental Retardation. (1992). *Mental retardation: Definition, classification, and systems of support* (9th ed.). Washington, DC: Author.

ASHA Ad Hoc Committee on Communication Processes and Nonspeaking Persons. (1980). Nonspeech communication: A position paper. *ASHA, 22,* 267–272.

Bangs, T., & Dodson, S. (1979). *Birth to Three Developmental Scales.* Seattle: University of Washington Press.

Bender, N., & Carlson, J. (1982). Prosocial behavior and perspective-taking of mentally retarded and nonretarded children. *American Journal of Mental Deficiency, 86,* 361–366.

Berger, J., & Cunningham, C. (1983). The development of early vocal behaviors and interactions in Down syndrome and non-handicapped infant-mother pairs. *Developmental Psychology, 19,* 322–331.

Berry, P., Groeneweg, G., Gibson, D., & Brown, R. (1984). Mental development of adults with Down's syndrome. *American Journal of Mental Deficiency, 89,* 252–256.

Bilsky, L., Walker, N., & Sakales, S. (1983). Comprehension and recall of sentences by mentally retarded and nonretarded individuals. *American Journal of Mental Deficiency, 87,* 558–565.

Bishop, D. V. M. (1999). An innate basis for language? *Science, 286,* 2283–2284.

Blacher, J. (1982). Assessing social cognition of young mentally retarded and nonretarded children. *American Journal of Mental Deficiency, 86,* 473–484.

Bleile, K., & Schwartz, I. (1984). Three perspectives on the speech of children with Down's syndrome. *Journal of Communication Disorders, 17,* 87–94.

Bloomberg, K., Karlan, G., & Lloyd, L. (1990). The comparative translucency of initial lexical items represented in five graphic symbol systems and sets. *Journal of Speech and Hearing Research, 33,* 717–725.

Bottorf, L., & DePape, D. (1982). Initiating communication systems for severely speech-impaired persons. *Topics in Language Disorders, 2,* 55–72.

Bowler, D. (1991). Rehearsal training and short-term free-recall of sign and word labels by severely handicapped children. *Journal of Mental Deficiency Research, 35,* 113–124.

Brady, N. C., Steeples, T., & Fleming, K. (2005). Effects of prelinguistic communication levels on initiation and repair of communication in children with disabilities. *Journal of Speech, Language, and Hearing Research, 48,* 1098–1113.

Bricker, D. (1993). *Assessment, Evaluation, and Programming Systems: AEPS Measurement for Birth to Three Years* (Vol. 1). Baltimore: Paul H. Brookes.

Bricker, D., Squires, J., & Mounts, L. (1995). *Ages and Stages Questionnaire (ASQ): A parent-completed child-monitoring system.* Baltimore: Paul H. Brookes.

Brownell, M. D., & Whiteley, J. H. (1992). Development and training of referential communication in children with mental retardation. *American Journal on Mental Retardation, 97,* 161–172.

Bryen, D., & McGinley, V. (1991). Sign language input to community residents with mental retardation. *Education and Training in Mental Retardation, 26,* 207–214.

Bryen, D., Goldman, A., & Quinlisk-Gill, S. (1988). Sign language with students with severe/profound mental retardation: How effective is it? *Education and Training in Mental Retardation, 23*, 129–137.

Bunce, B., Ruder, K., & Ruder, C. (1985). Using the miniature linguistic system in teaching syntax: Two case studies. *Journal of Speech and Hearing Disorders, 50*, 247–253.

Burger, A., Blackman, L., & Clark, H. (1981). Generalization of verbal abstraction strategies by EMR children and adolescents. *American Journal of Mental Deficiency, 85*, 611–618.

Burger, A., Blackman, L., Clark, H., & Reis, E. (1982). Effects of hypothesis testing and variable format training on generalization of a verbal abstraction strategy by EMR learners. *American Journal of Mental Deficiency, 86*, 405–413.

Burroughs, J., Albritton, E., Eaton, B., & Montagne, J. (1990). A comparative study of language delayed preschool children's ability to recall symbols from two symbol systems. *Augmentative and Alternative Communication, 6*, 202–206.

Bzock, K., & League, R. (1978). *Receptive Expressive Emergent Language Scale.* Austin, TX: Pro-Ed.

Calculator, S. (1988). Exploring the language of adults with mental retardation. In S. Calculator & J. Bedrosian (Eds.), *Communication assessment and intervention for adults with mental retardation* (pp. 95–106). San Diego, CA: College-Hill.

Cardone, I., & Gilkerson, L. (1989). *Family administered neonatal activities.* Washington, DC: Bulletin of the National Center for Clinical Infant Programs.

Cardosa-Martins, C., & Mervis, C. (1990). Mothers' use of substantive deixis and nouns with their children with Down syndrome: Some discrepant findings. *American Journal on Mental Retardation, 94*, 633–637.

Cardosa-Martins, C., Mervis, C., & Mervis, C. (1985). Early vocabulary acquisition by children with Down's syndrome. *American Journal of Mental Deficiency, 90*, 177–184.

Caro, P., & Snell, M. (1989). Characteristics of teaching communication to people with moderate and severe disabilities. *Education and Training in Mental Retardation, 24*, 63–77.

Caron, J. (1994). Male-female characteristics of Fragile X syndrome. Typescript.

Cascella, P. W. (2006). Standardised speech-language tests and students with intellectual disability: A review of normative data. *Journal of Intellectual and Developmental Disability, 31*, 120–124.

Caselli, M. C., Vicari, S., Longobardi, E., Lami, L., Pizzoli, C., & Stella, G. (1998). Gestures and words in early development of children with Down syndrome. *Journal of Speech, Language, and Hearing Research, 41*, 1125–1135.

Cegelka, P., & Prehm, H. (1982). *Mental retardation: From categories to people.* Columbus, OH: Merrill/Macmillan.

Centers for Disease Control (CDC) (2006). Improved national prevalence estimates for eighteen selected major birth defects, United States, 1999–2001. *Morbidity and Mortality Weekly Report, 54*, 1301–1305.

Chapman, R. S., Kay-Raining Bird, E., & Schwartz, S. E. (1990). Fast mapping of words in event contexts by children with Down syndrome. *Journal of Speech and Hearing Disorders, 55*, 761–770.

Chapman, R. S., Schwartz, S. E., & Kay-Raining Bird, E. (1988, November). *Predicting comprehension of children with Down syndrome.* Paper presented at the Annual Convention of the American Speech-Language-Hearing Association, Boston.

Chapman, R. S., Seung, H.-K., Schwartz, S. E., & Kay-Raining Bird, E. (1998). Language skills of children and adolescents with Down syndrome: II. Production deficits. *Journal of Speech, Language, and Hearing Research, 41,* 861–873.

Clark, D., Baker, B., & Heifetz, L. (1982). Behavioral training for parents of mentally retarded children: Prediction of outcome. *American Journal of Mental Deficiency, 87,* 14–19.

Conners, F. A., Rosenquist, C. J., Sligh, A. C., Atwell, J. A., & Kiser, T. (2006). Phonological reading skills acquisition by children with mental retardation. *Research in Developmental Disabilities: A Multidisciplinary Journal, 27,* 121–137.

Coplan, J. (1987). *Early Language Milestone Scale.* Tulsa, OK: Modern Education.

Cupples, L., & Iacono, T. (2000). Phonological awareness and oral reading skills in children with Down syndrome. *Journal of Speech, Language, and Hearing Research, 43,* 595–608.

Danforth, S., & Navarro, V. (1998). Speech acts: Sampling the social construction of mental retardation in everyday life. *Mental Retardation, 36,* 31–43.

Davis, H., Stroud, A., & Green, L. (1988). Maternal language environment of children with mental retardation. *American Journal on Mental Retardation, 93,* 144–153.

Day, J., & Hall, L. (1988). Intelligence-related differences in learning and transfer and enhancement of transfer among mentally retarded persons. *American Journal on Mental Retardation, 93,* 125–137.

DeKroon, D. M. A., Kyte, C. S., & Johnson, C. J. (2002). Partner influences on the social pretend play of children with language impairments. *Language, Speech, and Hearing Services in Schools, 33,* 253–267.

Domingo, R. A., Barrow, M. B., & Amato, J. (1998). Exercise of linguistic control by speakers in an adult day treatment program. *Mental Retardation, 36,* 293–302.

Drash, P., Raver, S., Murrin, M., & Tudor, R. (1989). Three procedures for increasing vocal response to therapist prompt in infants and children with Down syndrome. *American Journal on Mental Retardation, 94,* 64–73.

Dykens, E. M., Rosner, B. A., & Ly, T. M. (2001). Drawings by individuals with Williams syndrome: Are people different from shapes? *American Journal on Mental Retardation, 106,* 94–107.

Eheart, B. (1982). Mother–child interactions with nonretarded and mentally retarded preschoolers. *American Journal of Mental Deficiency, 87,* 20–25.

Ellis, N., Deacon, J., & Wooldridge, P. (1985). On the nature of short-term memory deficit in mentally retarded persons. *American Journal of Mental Deficiency, 89,* 393–402.

Ellis, N., Deacon, J., Harris, L., Poor, A., Angers, D., Diorio, M., Watkins, R., Boyd, B., & Cavalier, A. (1982). Learning, memory, and transfer in profoundly, severely, and moderately mentally retarded persons. *American Journal of Mental Deficiency, 87,* 186–196.

Ellis, N., Woodley-Zanthos, P., & Dulaney, C. (1989). Memory for spatial location in children, adults, and mentally retarded persons. *American Journal on Mental Retardation, 93,* 521–527.

Ezell, H., & Goldstein, H. (1991). Comparison of idiom comprehension of normal children and children with mental retardation. *Journal of Speech and Hearing Research, 34,* 812–819.

Fenson, L., Dale, P., Reznick, S., Thal, D., Bates, E., Hartung, J., Pethnick, S., & Reilly, J. (1993). *MacArthur Communicative Development Inventories.* San Diego, CA: Singular.

Fewell, R., & Langley, M. (1984). *Developmental Activities Screening Inventory.* Austin, TX: Pro-Ed.

Fey, M. E., Warren, S. F., Brady, N., Finestock, L. H., Bredin-Oja, S. L., Fairchild, M., Sokol, S., & Yoder, P. J. (2007). Early effects of reactivity education/prelinguistic mileau teaching for children with developmental delays and their parents. *Journal of Speech, Language, and Hearing Research, 49,* 526–547.

Fidler, D. J. (2003). Parental vocalizations and perceived immaturity in Down syndrome. *American Journal on Mental Retardation, 108,* 425–34.

Fidler, D. J., Hodapp, R. M., & Dykens, E. M. (2002). Behavioral phenotypes and special education: Parent report of educational issues for children with Down syndrome, Prader-Willi syndrome, and Williams syndrome. *Journal of Special Education, 36,* 80–88.

Geschwind, D. H., & Dykens, E. (2004). Neurobehavioral and psychosocial issues in Klinefelter syndrome. *Learning Disabilities Research and Practice, 19,* 166–173.

Girolametto, L., & Weitzman, E. (2002). Responsiveness of child care providers in interactions with toddlers and preschoolers. *Language, Speech, and Hearing Services in Schools, 33,* 268–281.

Glidden, L., & Warner, D. (1985). Semantic processing and serial learning by EMR adolescents. *American Journal of Mental Deficiency, 89,* 635–641.

Goetz, L., Gee, K., & Sailor, W. (1985). Using a behavior chain interruption strategy to teach communication skills to students with severe disabilities. *Journal of the Association for Persons with Severe Handicaps, 10,* 21–30.

Goossens, C. (1984). *Assessment for nonspeech.* Paper presented at the annual conference of American Association on Mental Deficiency, Minneapolis, MN.

Greenwald, C., & Leonard, L. (1979). Communicative and sensorimotor development of Down's syndrome children. *American Journal of Mental Deficiency, 84,* 296–303.

Gullo, F., & Gullo, J. (1984). An ecological language intervention approach with mentally retarded adolescents. *Language, Speech and Hearing Services in Schools, 15,* 182–191.

Gutowski, W., & Chechile, R. (1987). Encoding, storage, and retrieval components of associative memory deficits of mildly mentally retarded adults. *American Journal of Mental Deficiency, 92,* 85–93.

Hagerman, R., Kemper, M., & Hudson, M. (1985). Learning disabilities and attentional problems in boys with the Fragile X syndrome. *American Journal of Diseases of Children, 139,* 674–678.

Halle, J., Alpert, C., & Anderson, S. (1984). Natural environment language assessment and intervention with severely impaired preschoolers. *Topics in Early Childhood Special Education, 4,* 36–56.

Harding, C. (1984). Acting with intention: A framework for examining the development of the intention to communicate. In L. Feagans, C. Garvey, & R. Golinkoff (Eds.), *The origins and growth of communication.* Norwood, NJ: Ablex.

Harris, D. (1982). Communicative interaction processes involving nonvocal physically handicapped children. *Topics in Language Disorders, 2,* 21–38.

Heifetz, L. (1980). From consumer to middleman: Emerging roles for parents in the network of services for retarded children. In R. Abidin (Ed.), *Parent education and intervention handbook*. Springfield, IL: Charles Thomas.

Hetzroni, O. E., & Roth, T. (2003). Effects of a positive support approach to enhance communicative behaviors of children with mental retardation who have challenging behaviors. *Education and Training in Mental Retardation and Developmental Disabilities, 38,* 95–105.

Hodapp, R. M. (1997). Direct and indirect behavioral effects of different genetic disorders of mental retardation. *American Journal on Mental Retardation, 102,* 67–79.

Hodapp, R. M., DesJardin, J. L., & Ricci, L. A. (2003). Genetic syndromes of mental retardation: Should they matter for the early interventionist? *Infants and Young Children, 16,* 152–161.

Hodapp, R. M., & Dykens, E. M. (1994). Mental retardation's two cultures of behavioral research. *American Journal on Mental Retardation, 98,* 675–687.

Hodapp, R. M., Dykens, E. M., Ort, S. I., Zelinsky, D. G., & Leckman, J. F. (1991). Changing patterns of intellectual strengths and weaknesses in males with fragile X syndrome. *Journal of Autism and Developmental Disorders, 21,* 503–516.

Houghton, J., Bronicki, G., & Guess, D. (1987). Opportunities to express preferences and make choices among students with severe disabilities in classroom settings. *Journal of the Association for Persons with Severe Handicaps, 12,* 18–27.

Hunt, N. (1967). *The world of Nigel Hunt: The diary of a mongoloid youth.* New York: Garret.

Hunt, P., Goetz, L., Alwell, M., & Sailor, W. (1986). Using an interrupted behavior chain strategy to teach generalized communication responses. *Journal of the Association for Persons with Severe Handicaps, 11,* 196–204.

Johnson-Martin, N., Jens, K., Attermeier, S., & Hacker, B. (1991). *Carolina Curriculum for Infants and Toddlers with Special Needs.* Baltimore, MD: Paul H. Brookes.

Johnston, S. S., Reichle, J., & Evans, J. (2004). Supporting augmentative and alternative communication use by beginning communicators with severe disabilities. *American Journal of Speech-Language Pathology, 13,* 20–30.

Kamhi, A. (1981). Developmental vs. different theories of mental retardation: A new look. *American Journal of Mental Deficiency, 86,* 1–7.

Kamhi, A., & Masterson, J. (1989). Language and cognition in mentally handicapped people: Last rites for the difference-delay controversy. In M. Beveridge, G. Conti-Ramsden, & I. Leudar (Eds.), *Language and communication in mentally handicapped people*. London, England: Chapman & Hall.

Karen, R., Astin-Smith, S., & Creasy, D. (1985). Teaching telephone-answering skills to mentally retarded adults. *American Journal of Mental Deficiency, 89,* 595–609.

Kernan, K. (1990). Comprehension of syntactically indicated sequence by Down's syndrome and other mentally retarded adults. *Journal of Mental Deficiency Research, 34,* 169–178.

Klein, M., & Briggs, M. (1987). *Observation of Communicative Interactions.* Los Angeles: Mother–Infant Communication Project, California State University.

Klink, M., Gerstman, L., Raphael, L., Schlanger, B., & Newsome, L. (1986). Phonological process usage by young EMR children and nonretarded preschool children. *American Journal of Mental Deficiency, 91,* 190–195.

Kohl, F. (1981). Effects of motoric requirements on the acquisition of manual sign responses by severely handicapped students. *American Journal of Mental Deficiency, 85,* 396–403.

Lamberts, F. (1981). Sign and symbol in children's processing of familiar auditory stimuli. *American Journal of Mental Deficiency, 86,* 300–308.

Lee, L. (1974). *Developmental sentence analysis.* Evanston, IL: Northwestern University Press.

Leonard, L. B. (1987). Is specific language impairment a useful construct? In S. Rosenburg (Ed.), *Advances in applied psycholinguistics* (Vol. 1, pp. 1–39). Cambridge, England: Cambridge University Press.

Leonard, L., Steckol, K., & Panther, K. (1983). Returning meaning to semantic relations: Some clinical applications. *Journal of Speech and Hearing Disorders, 48,* 25–35.

Levine, H., & Langness, L. (1985). Everyday cognition among mildly mentally retarded adults: An ethnographic approach. *American Journal of Mental Deficiency, 90,* 18–26.

Lewis, P., Abbeduto, L., Murphy, M., Richmond, E., Giles, N., Bruno, L., & Schroeder, S. (2006). Cognitive, language and social-cognitive skills of individuals with fragile X syndrome with and without autism. *Journal of Intellectual Disability Research, 50,* 532–545.

Lincoln, A., Courchesne, E., Kilman, B., & Galambos, R. (1985). Neuropsychological correlates of information-processing by children with Down syndrome. *American Journal of Mental Deficiency, 89,* 403–414.

Lobato, D., Barrera, R., & Feldman, R. (1981). Sensorimotor functioning and prelinguistic communication of severely and profoundly mentally retarded individuals. *American Journal of Mental Deficiency, 85,* 489–496.

Love, R. J., & Webb, W. G. (1986). *Neurology for the speech-language pathologist.* Stoneham, MA: Butterworth.

Luftig, R., & Johnson, R. (1982). Identification and recall of structurally important units in prose of mentally retarded learners. *American Journal of Mental Deficiency, 86,* 495–502.

MacDonald, J. (1978). *Environmental Language Intervention Program.* Columbus, OH: Merrill/Macmillan.

MacDonald, J. (1985). Language through conversation: A model for intervention with language-delayed persons. In S. Warren & A. Rogers-Warren (Eds.), *Teaching functional language* (pp. 89–122). Baltimore, MD: University Park Press.

MacDonald, J., & Gillette, Y. (1978). *Environmental Communication System (ECO).* San Antonio, TX: Psychological Corporation.

Mahoney, G., Glover, A., & Finger, I. (1981). Relationship between language and sensorimotor development of Down syndrome and nonretarded children. *American Journal of Mental Deficiency, 86,* 21–27.

Mahoney, G., & Snow, K. (1983). The relationship of sensorimotor functioning to children's response to early language training. *Mental Retardation, 21,* 248–254.

Mahoney, G., & Weller, E. (1980). An ecological approach to language intervention. *New Directions for Exceptional Children, 2,* 17–33.

Manolson, A. (1983). *It takes two to talk.* Toronto: Hanen Early Language Resource Centre.

Marcell, M., & Jett, D. (1985). Identification of vocally expressed emotions by mentally retarded and nonretarded individuals. *American Journal of Mental Deficiency, 89,* 537–545.

Marcell, M., & Weeks, S. (1988). Short-term memory difficulties and Down's syndrome. *Journal of Mental Deficiency Research, 32,* 153–162.

Maurer, H., & Sherrod, K. (1987). Context of directives given to young children with Down syndrome and nonretarded children: Development over two years. *American Journal of Mental Deficiency, 91,* 579–590.

McCormick, L. (1986). Keeping up with language trends. *Teaching Exceptional Children, 18,* 123–129.

McLean, J., & Snyder-McLean, L. (1978). *A transactional approach to early language training.* Columbus, OH: Merrill/Macmillan.

McLean, L. K., Brady, N. C., McLean, J. E., & Behrens, G. A. (1999). Communication forms and functions of children and adults with severe mental retardation in community and institutional settings. *Journal of Speech, Language, and Hearing Research, 42,* 231–240.

McLeavey, B., Toomey, J., & Dempsey, P. (1982). Nonretarded and mentally retarded children's control over syntactic structures. *American Journal of Mental Deficiency, 86,* 485–494.

Meador, D. (1984). Effects of color on visual discrimination of geometric symbols by severely and profoundly mentally retarded individuals. *American Journal of Mental Deficiency, 89,* 275–286.

Merrill, E. (1985). Differences in semantic processing speed of mentally retarded and nonretarded persons. *American Journal of Mental Deficiency, 90,* 71–80.

Merrill, E., & Bilsky, L. (1990). Individual differences in the representation of sentences in memory. *American Journal on Mental Retardation, 95,* 68–76.

Merrill, E. C., & Jackson, T. S. (1992). Degree of associative relatedness and sentence processing by adolescents with and without mental retardation. *American Journal on Mental Retardation, 97,* 173–185.

Merrill, E., & Mar, H. (1987). Differences between mentally retarded and nonretarded persons' efficiency of auditory sentence processing. *American Journal of Mental Deficiency, 91,* 406–414.

Mervis, C. B. (1988). Early lexical development: Theory and application. In L. Nadel (Ed.), *The psychology of Down's syndrome* (pp. 104–144). Cambridge, MA: MIT Press.

Mervis, C. B., Morris, C. A., Bertrand, J. M., & Robinson, B. F. (1999). Williams syndrome: Findings from an integrated program of research. In H. Tager-Flusberg (Ed.), *Neurodevelopmental disorders* (pp. 65–110). Cambridge, MA: MIT Press.

Miles, S., Chapman, R., & Sindberg, H. (2006). Sampling context affects MLU in the language of adolescents with Down syndrome. *Journal of Speech, Language, and Hearing Research, 49,* 325–337.

Millar, D. C., Light, J. C., & Schlosser, R. W. (2006). The impact of augmentative and alternative communication intervention on the speech production of individuals with developmental disabilities: A Research Review. *Journal of Speech, Language and Hearing Research, 49,* 248–264.

Miller, A., & Newhoff, M. (1978). *Language disordered children: Language disordered mothers?* Paper presented at the American Speech and Hearing Association Annual Conference, San Francisco.

Miller, J. (1980). *Assessing language production in children.* Baltimore, MD: University Park Press.

Miller, J., Chapman, R., & MacKenzie, H. (1981). Individual differences in the language acquisition of mentally retarded children. *Proceedings from the Second Wisconsin Symposium on Research in Child Language Disorders.* Madison: University of Wisconsin.

Miller, J., Sedey, A. L., & Miolo, G. (1995). Validity of parent report measures of vocabulary development for children with Down syndrome. *Journal of Speech and Hearing Research, 38,* 1037–1044.

Mirenda, P., & Locke, P. (1989). A comparison of symbol transparency in nonspeaking persons with intellectual disabilities. *Journal of Speech and Hearing Disorders, 54,* 131–140.

Mirrett, P. L., Roberts, J. E., & Price, J. (2003). Early intervention practices and communication intervention strategies for young males with fragil X syndrome. *Language, Speech, and Hearing Services in Schools, 34,* 320–331.

Moran, M., Money, S., & Leonard, D. (1984). Phonological process analysis of the speech of mentally retarded adults. *American Journal of Mental Deficiency, 89,* 304–306.

Mundy, P., Kasari, C., Sigman, M., & Ruskin, E. (1995). Nonverbal communication and early language acquisition in children with Down syndrome and in normally developing children. *Journal of Speech and Learning Research, 38,* 157–167.

Murphy, M. M., & Abbeduto, L. (2007). Gender differences in repetitive language in fragile X syndrome. *Journal of Intellectual Disability Research, 51,* 387–400.

Nigro, G., & Roak, R. (1987). Mentally retarded and nonretarded adults' memory for spatial location. *American Journal of Mental Deficiency, 91,* 392–397.

Nugent, P., & Mosley, J. (1987). Mentally retarded and nonretarded individuals' attention allocation and capacity. *American Journal of Mental Deficiency, 91,* 598–605.

Ogletree, B. T., Wetherby, A. M., & Westling, D. L. (1992). Profile of the prelinguistic intentional communicative behavior of children with profound mental retardation. *American Journal on Mental Retardation, 97,* 188–196.

Oller, D., & Seibert, J. (1988). Babbling of prelinguistic mentally retarded children. *American Journal on Mental Retardation, 92,* 369–375.

Olswang, L., Stoel-Gammon, C., Coggins, T., & Carpenter, R. (1987a). *Assessing Linguistic Behavior (ALB).* Seattle: University of Washington Press.

Opitz, J. M. (1996, March). *Historiography of the causal analysis of mental retardation.* Paper presented at the Annual Gatlinburg Conference on Research and Theory in Mental Retardation, Gatlinburg, TN.

O'Toole, C., & Chiat, S. (2006). Symbolic functioning and language development in children with Down syndrome. *International Journal of Language and Communication Disorders, 41,* 155–171.

Owens, R. (1982). *Program for the Acquisition of Language with the Severely Impaired (PALS).* San Antonio, TX: Psychological Corporation.

Owens, R. (2004). *Language disorders, A functional approach to assessment and intervention* (4th ed.). Boston: Allyn & Bacon.

Owens, R. (2008). *Language development: An introduction* (7th ed.). Boston: Allyn & Bacon.

Owens, R., & House, L. (1984). Decision-making processes in augmentative communication. *Journal of Speech and Hearing Disorders, 49,* 18–25.

Owens, R., & MacDonald, J. (1982). Communicative uses of the early speech of nondelayed and Down syndrome children. *American Journal of Mental Deficiency, 86,* 503–510.

Owens, R., McNerney, C., Bigler-Burke, L., & Lepre-Clark, C. (1987). The use of language facilitators with residential retarded populations. *Topics in Language Disorders, 7*(3), 47–63.

Owens, R. E., & Rogerson, B. S. (1988). Adults at the presymbolic level. In S. Calculator & J. Bedrosian (Eds.), *Communicative assessment and intervention for adults with mental retardation* (pp. 189–230). San Diego, CA: College-Hill.

Owings, N., & Guvette, T. (1982). Communication behavior assessment and treatment with the adult retarded: An approach. In N. Lass (Ed.), *Speech and language: Advances in basic research and practice* (Vol. 7). New York: Academic Press.

Page, J., & Horn, D. (1987). Comprehension in developmentally delayed children. *Language, Speech and Hearing Services in Schools, 18,* 63–71.

Parette, H. P., Brotherson, M. J., & Blake Huer, M. (2000). Giving families a voice in augmentative and alternative communication decision making. *Education and Training in Mental Retardation and Developmental Disabilities, 35,* 177–190.

Papania, N. (1954). A qualitative analysis of vocabulary responses of institutionalized mentally retarded children. *Journal of Clinical Psychology, 10,* 361–365.

Paul, R. (2000). Facilitating transitions in language development for children using AAC. *Augmentative and Alternative Communication, 13,* 139–148.

Peter, D. (2000). Dynamics of discourse: A case study illuminating power relations in mental retardation. *Mental Retardation, 38,* 354–362.

Petersen, G., & Sherrod, K. (1982). Relationship of maternal language to language development and language delay of children. *American Journal of Mental Deficiency, 86,* 391–398.

Philofsky, A., Hepburn, S. L., Hayes, A., Hagerman, R., & Rogers, S. J. (2004). Language and cognitive functioning and autism symptoms in young children with fragile X syndrome. *American Journal on Mental Retardation, 109,* 208–218.

Pickett, J., & Flynn, P. (1983). Language assessment tools for mentally retarded adults: Survey and recommendations. *American Journal of Mental Deficiency, 21,* 244–247.

Platt, J., & Coggins, T. (1990). Comprehension of social-action games in prelinguistic children. *Journal of Speech and Hearing Disorders, 55,* 315–326.

Poulson, C. (1988). Operant conditioning of vocalization rate of infants with Down syndrome. *American Journal on Mental Retardation, 93,* 57–63.

Prater, R. (1982). Functions of consonant assimilation and reduplication in early word productions of mentally retarded children. *American Journal of Mental Deficiency, 86,* 399–404.

Price, J., Roberts, J., Vandergrift, N., & Martin, G. (2007). Language comprehension in boys with fragile X syndrome and boys with Down syndrome. *Journal of Intellectual Disability, 51,* 318–326.

Pruess, J., Vadasy, P., & Fewell, R. (1987). Language development in children with Down syndrome: An overview of recent research. *Education and Training in Mental Retardation, 22,* 44–55.

Prutting, C., & Kirchner, D. (1983). Applied pragmatics. In T. Gallagher & C. Prutting (Eds.), *Pragmatic assessment and intervention issues in language*. San Diego, CA: College-Hill.

Realon, R., Lewallen, J., & Wheeler, A. (1983). Verbal vs. verbal feedback plus praise: The effects on direct care staff's training behaviors. *Mental Retardation, 21,* 209–213.

Reese, R., & Serna, L. (1986). Planning for generalization and maintenance in parent training: Parents need IEPs too. *Mental Retardation, 24,* 87–92.

Reichle, J. (1990). *Intervention with presymbolic clients: Setting up an initial communication system.* Paper presented at the New York State Speech-Language-Hearing Association Annual Convention, Kiamesha Lake, NY.

Reichle, J., & Sigafoos, J. (1991). Establishing an initial repertoire of requesting. In J. Reichle, J. York, & J. Sigafoos (Eds.), *Implementing augmentative and alternative communication*. Baltimore, MD: Paul H. Brookes.

Reid, G. (1980). Overt and covert rehearsal in short-term motor memory of mentally retarded and non-retarded persons. *American Journal of Mental Deficiency, 85,* 69–77.

Rein, R., & Kernan, K. (1989). The functional use of verbal perseverations by adults who are mentally retarded. *Education and Training in Mental Retardation, 24,* 381–389.

Rescorla, L. (1989). The Language Development Survey: A screening tool for delayed toddlers. *Journal of Speech and Hearing Disorders, 54,* 587–599.

Richmond, G., & Lewallen, J. (1983). Facilitating transfer of stimulus control when teaching verbal labels. *Education and Training of Mentally Retarded, 18,* 111–115.

Roberts, J. E., Hatton, D. D., & Bailey, D. B. (2001). Development and behavior of male toddlers with fragile X syndrome. *Journal of Early Intervention, 24,* 207–23.

Roberts, J. E., Hennon, E. A., Price, J. R., Dear, E., Anderson, K., & Vandergrift, N. (2007). Expressive language during conversational speech in boys with fragile X syndrome. *American Journal on Mental Retardation, 112,* 1–17.

Roberts, J. E., Long, S. H., Malkin, C., Barnes, E., Skinner, M., Hennon, E. A., & Anderson, K. (2005). A comparison of phonological skills with fragile X syndrome and Down syndrome. *Journal of Speech, Language, and Hearing Research, 48,* 980–995.

Roberts, J. E., Martin, G. E., Maskowitz, L., Harris, A. A., Foreman, J., & Nelson, L. (2007). Discourse skills of boys with fragile X syndrome in comparison to boys with Down syndrome. *Journal of Speech, Language, and Hearing Research, 50,* 475–492.

Roberts, J. E., Mirrett, P., & Burchinal, M. (2001). Receptive and expressive communication development in young meales with fragile X syndrome. *American Journal of Mental Retardation, 106,* 216–231.

Robinson, L. A., & Owens, R. E. (1995). Functional augmentative communication and positive behavior change. *Augmentative and Alternative Communication, 11,* 207–211.

Romer, L., & Schoenberg, B. (1991). Increasing requests made by people with developmental disabilities and deaf-blindness through the use of behavior chain interruption strategies. *Education and Training in Mental Retardation, 26,* 70–78.

Romski, M., Sevcik, R., & Rumbaugh, D. (1985). Retention of symbolic communication skills by severely mentally retarded persons. *American Journal of Mental Deficiency, 89,* 441–443.

Romski, M., Sevcik, R., Pate, J., & Rumbaugh, D. (1985). Discrimination of lexigrams and traditional orthography by nonspeaking severely mentally retarded persons. *American Journal of Mental Deficiency, 90,* 185–190.

Rondal, J., Ghiotto, M., Bredart, S., & Bachelet, J. (1988). Mean length of utterance of children with Down syndrome. *American Journal on Mental Retardation, 93,* 64–66.

Rosin, M., Swift, E., Bless, D., & Vetter, D. (1988). Communication profiles of adolescents with Down syndrome. *Journal of Childhood Communication Disorders, 12,* 49–64.

Rossetti, L. (1990). *Infant–Toddler Language Scale.* East Moline, IL: LinguiSystems.

Salzberg, C., & Villani, T. (1983). Speech training by parents of Down syndrome toddlers: Generalization across settings and instructional contexts. *American Journal of Mental Deficiency, 87,* 403–413.

Saunders, S. (1999). Teaching children with fragile X syndrome. *British Journal of Special Education, 26*(2), 76–79.

Schlosser, R.W., Walker, E., & Sigafoos, J. (2006). Increasing opportunities for requesting in children with developmental disabilities residing in group homes through pyramidal training. *Education and Training in Developmental Disabilities, 41,* 244–252.

Scruggs, T., Mastropieri, M., & Levin, J. (1985). Vocabulary acquisition of mentally retarded students under direct and mnemonic instruction. *American Journal of Mental Deficiency, 89,* 546–551.

Shane, H., & Bashir, A. (1980). Election criteria for the adoption of an augmentative communication system: Preliminary considerations. *Journal of Speech and Hearing Disorders, 45,* 408–414.

Shane, H., Lipshultz, R., & Shane, C. (1982). Facilitating the communicative interaction of nonspeaking persons in large residential settings. *Topics in Language Disorders, 2,* 73–84.

Sharav, T., & Shlomo, L. (1986). Stimulation of infants with Down syndrome: Long-term effects. *Mental Retardation, 24,* 81–86.

Shriberg, L., & Widder, C. (1990). Speech and prosody characteristics of adults with mental retardation. *Journal of Speech and Hearing Research, 33,* 627–653.

Slonims, V., & McConachie, H. (2006). Analysis of mother–infant interaction in infants with Down syndrome and typically developing infants. *American Journal on Mental Retardation, 111,* 273–289.

Smith, L., & Hagen, V. (1984). Relationship between the home environment and sensorimotor development of Down syndrome and nonretarded infants. *American Journal of Mental Deficiency, 89,* 124–132.

Sokolov, J. L. (1992). Linguistic imitation in children with Down syndrome. *American Journal on Mental Retardation, 97,* 209–221.

Sommers, R., Patterson, J., & Wildgren, P. (1988). Phonology of Down syndrome speakers, ages 13–22. *Journal of Childhood Communication Disorders, 12,* 65–91.

Spiegel, B. (1983). The effect of context on language learning by severely retarded young adults. *Language, Speech and Hearing Services in Schools, 14,* 252–259.

Spradlin, J., & Siegel, G. (1982). Language training in natural and clinical environments. *Journal of Speech and Hearing Disorders, 47,* 2–6.

Steffens, M. L., Oller, D., Lynch, M., & Urbano, R. C. (1992). Vocal development in infants with Down syndrome who are developing normally. *American Journal on Mental Retardation, 97,* 235–246.

Stephenson, J., & Dowrick, M. (2005). Parents' perspectives on the communication skills of their children with severe disabilities. *Journal of Intellectual and Developmental Disability, 30,* 75–85.

Sternberg, L., Pegnatore, L., & Hill, C. (1983). Establishing interactive communication behaviors with profoundly mentally handicapped students. *TASH Journal, 8,* 39–46.

Stowitschek, J., McConaughy, E., Peatross, D., Salzberg, C., & Lignngaris/Kraft, B. (1988). Effects of group incidental training on the use of social amenities by adults with mental retardation in work settings. *Education and Training in Mental Retardation, 23,* 202–212.

Stromme, P., & Hagberg, G. (2000). Etiology in severe and mild mental retardation: A population-based study of Norwegian children. *Developmental Medicine and Child Neurology, 42,* 76–86.

Sudhalter, V., & Belser, R. C. (2001). Conversational characteristics of children with fragile X syndrome: Tangential language. *American Journal on Mental Retardation, 106,* 389–400.

Sudhalter, V., Cohen, I., Silverman, W., & Wolf-Schein, E. (1990). Conversational analysis of males with Fragile X, Down syndrome, and autism: Comparison of the emergence of deviant language. *American Journal on Mental Retardation, 99,* 431–441.

Tannock, R. (1988). Mothers' directiveness in their interactions with their children with and without Down syndrome. *American Journal on Mental Retardation, 93,* 154–165.

Tannock, R., Girolametto, L., & Siegel, L. S. (1992). Language intervention with children who have developmental delays: Effects of an interactive approach. *American Journal on Mental Retardation, 97,* 145–160.

Turner, L., & Bray, N. (1985). Spontaneous rehearsal by mildly mentally retarded children and adolescents. *American Journal of Mental Deficiency, 90,* 57–63.

Van Borsel, J. (1988). An analysis of the speech of five Down's syndrome adolescents. *Journal of Communication Disorders, 21,* 409–421.

Van der Bijl, C., Alant, E., & Lloyd, L. (2006). A comparison of two strategies of sight word instruction in children with mental disability. *Research in Developmental Disabilities: A Multidisciplinary Journal, 27,* 43–55.

Van Der Gagg, A. (1989). The view from Walter's window: Social environment and the communicative competence of adults with a mental handicap. *Journal of Mental Deficiency Research, 33,* 221–227.

Variety Pre-Schooler's Workshop. (1987). *Parent/Professional Preschool Performance Profile (5Ps).* Syosset, NY: Variety Pre-Schooler's Workshop.

Westby, C. (1980). Assessment of cognitive and language abilities through play. *Language, Speech and Hearing Services in Schools, 11,* 154–168.

Wetherby, A., & Prizant, B. (1993). *Communication and Symbolic Behavior Scales.* Chicago: Riverside.

Wilcox, M., & Campbell, P. (1983). *Assessing communication in low-functioning multihandicapped children.* Paper presented at the American Speech-Language-Hearing Association Annual Convention, Cincinnati, OH.

Wilkinson, K. M., & Romski, M. A. (1995). Responsiveness of male adolescents with mental retardation to input from nondisabled peers: The summoning power of comments, questions, and direct prompts. *Journal of Speech and Hearing, 38,* 1045–1053.

Wolf-Schein, E., Sudhalter, V., Cohen, I., Fisch, G., Hansen, D., Pfadt, A., Hagerman, R., Jenkins, E., & Brown, W. (1987). Speech-language and Fragile X syndrome. *ASHA, 29,* 35–38.

Wulz, S., Hall, M., & Klein, M. (1983). A home-centered instructional communication strategy for severely handicapped children. *Journal of Speech and Hearing Disorders, 48,* 2–10.

Yoder, P. J., & Davies, B. (1992). Do children with developmental delays use more frequent and diverse language in verbal routines? *American Journal on Mental Retardation, 97,* 197–208.

Yoder, P. J. & Feagans, L. (1988). Mothers' attributions of communication to prelinguistic behavior of developmentally delayed and mentally retarded children. *American Journal on Mental Retardation, 93,* 36–43.

Yoder, P. J., & Warren, S. F. (1998). Maternal responsivity predicts the prelinguistic communication intervention that facilitates generalized intentional communication. *Journal of Speech, Language, and Hearing Research, 41,* 1207–1219.

Yoder, P. J., & Warren, S. F. (2001a). Intentional communication elicits language-facilitating maternal responses in dyads with children who have developmental disabilities. *American Journal on Mental Retardation, 106,* 327–35.

Yoder, P. J., & Warren, S. F. (2001b). Relative treatment effects of two prelinguistic communication interventions on language development in toddlers with developmental delays vary by maternal characteristics. *Journal of Speech, Language, and Hearing Research, 45,* 224–237.

Yoder, P. J., & Warren, S. F. (2002). Effects of prelinguistic milieu teaching and parent responsivity education on dyads involving children with intellectual disabilities. *Journal of Speech, Language, and Hearing Research, 45,* 1297–1310.

Yoder, P. J., & Warren, S. F. (2004). Early predictors of language in children with and without Down syndrome. *American Journal on Mental Retardation, 109,* 285–300.

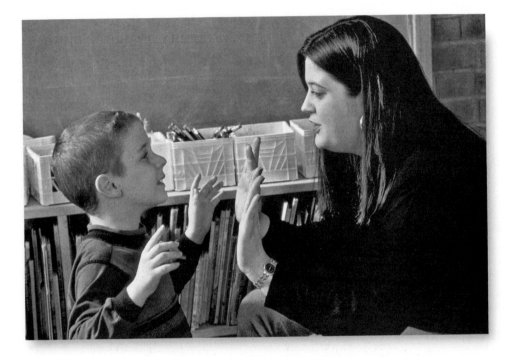

CHAPTER 7

Autism Spectrum Disorders
Learning to Communicate

Ellenmorris Tiegerman-Farber
Adelphi University

When you finish this chapter, you will be able to

- Identify theoretical and etiological perceptions of the underlying causes of autism spectrum disorders (ASD).
- Understand therapeutic programming provided for children with autism.
- Discuss the settings within which children with autism are educated and the reality of inclusion.
- Discuss the changing role of the speech-language pathologist in serving children with autism across multiple settings.

- Discuss the changing role of the parent as a primary teacher for the child with autism spectrum disorders.
- List expectations of how the individual with autism can function in society.
- Understand the relationship between autism and language acquisition theory.

Each child with autism has unique learning needs. Just as there are differences in normal language learners, so, too, are there individual differences in children with language disorders. It is unrealistic, therefore, to view children with autism spectrum disorders (ASD) as a homogeneous population. Children with autism spectrum disorders present language, cognitive, communicative, behavioral, and social learning problems.

Autism spectrum disorders include five disorders that share varying degrees of deficit across three domain areas: social, communication, and behavioral functioning. The disorders are autism, Rett's disorder, childhood disintegrative disorder (CDD), Asperger syndrome, and pervasive developmental disorder (PDD). Macintosh and Dissanayake (2006) have proposed that autism and Asperger syndrome belong on a single spectrum of disorder. Reported rates of autism for boys are significantly higher than for girls—approximately four times higher (Williams, Higgins, and Brayne, 2006).

Kanner (1943) was the first to describe children with autism as being a distinct category. Since that time, autism has been the subject of much clinical investigation and research, yet the nature of its causes, manifestations, and treatments remains in dispute. Kanner defined the cause as an innate inability to form biologically affective contact with people. He attributed this inability to an emotional deprivation resulting from rigidity of the parents, who were characterized by obsessive meticulousness and intellectualization. Controlled studies have failed to demonstrate significant differences in parental psychopathology and early mother–child interaction between groups of children with and without psychotic brain damage. For a long time, the psychoanalytic view that the mother–child relationship was the cause of autism was widely accepted; however, support for that view has gradually declined as newer research has uncovered evidence of an organic basis for the disorder.

Greenspan and Wieder (1997) proposed that the symptoms that characterize ASD may be due to an underlying neuropsychological dysfunction in the connection between affect (or intent) and the sequencing of motor patterns and verbal symbols. Autism spectrum disorders, which include a range of affective and communicative disorders from more (autism) to less (pervasive developmental disorder) severe, have been increasing. In the last ten years, the incidence has increased from 1 in 2,500 to 1 in 150 live births (Bradley, 2007). The criteria described by Kanner (1943) have been more broadly defined in the *Diagnostic and Statistical Manual of Mental Disorders (DSM-IV-TR)*, published by the American Psychiatric Association (APA, 2000), to include degrees of dysfunction in reciprocal interaction, relating, and symbolic communication.

One related issue involves how children are classified with developmental disabilities. Within the medical model, the underlying cause for a disorder is considered of primary importance. Historically, this point of view has carried over to the public school domain. As a result, many children with disabilities are assigned to educational placements based on etiological labels (mental retardation, autism, neurological impairment, etc.). Certainly, there are advantages and disadvantages to both the etiological and the nonetiological models. One advantage of the nonetiological approach to disorders in the schools might be the classification of children by characteristics such as communication and language behaviors—the approach described in this chapter. The identification of language/communication deficits provides critical information about the unique educational needs of children with autism spectrum disorders.

A discussion of autism research, more than research concerning any other population within the educational system, reveals the many theoretical and therapeutic changes that have occurred recently in the area of child language acquisition. In addition, it is my theoretical position that children with autism are severely language-disordered learners, rather than behaviorally impaired children. It should also be noted that the language learning characteristics of children with autism are evident in the language patterns of other language-disordered children. To the extent that their language needs are the same, children with autism should be educated in the same manner as other children with language and communication disorders. While studying the chapters in Part II, it is important to compare the language/communication characteristics across children with different educational labels.

Etiology: Central Language Disorder

Specific theories relating to the cause of ASD have been proposed but not proven (Wing, 1997). The range of etiological views of autism extends from a psychoanalytic perspective of the parent–child relationship to neurological, genetic, and biochemical causes. Bettelheim, in *The Empty Fortress* (1967), also proposed a psychological model. He suggested that the mother does not produce autism but rather that autism is the child's reaction to the mother's attitudes. The child with autism fears maternal destruction and rejects his or her mother. The child retreats within himself or herself even further, and reality becomes so fearful that inactivity is the only available response. Autism develops. The symptoms of autism have been attributed to problems with early interpersonal relationships, motivation, and emotionality resulting in a diagnosis of emotional disturbance.

About 75 percent of the children with autism have IQs in the severely retarded range; as a result, mental retardation is often associated with this disorder. Wetherby and Gaines (1982), however, did not observe the similarity in levels of cognitive and linguistic ability that is typical in children with mental retardation. In the children with autism, cognitive abilities exceeded linguistic abilities in several areas. The authors suggested that the relationship between cognition and language is dynamic, rather than static; the interdependence varies over time with development. Whereas cognitive development may be necessary for intentional communication, "cognitive development may not be sufficient for more advanced language development" (p. 69).

Loveland, Landry, Hughes, Hall, and McEvoy (1988) described autism as a pervasive developmental disorder characterized by severe deficits in language, cognition, and social development. The language of children with autism is severely delayed and is often described as disordered. In many cases, functional language does not develop at all. Verbal language, when it does develop, is usually rigid, ritualistic, and stereotypical. Children with autism develop verbal routines that rarely change in form and are used over and over in a variety of related and somewhat related contexts.

Even though the language and gestures of children with autism are pragmatically deficient, they can be communicative despite the use of unconventional forms. Loveland and colleagues (1988) showed that, when compared to children of similar mental age and language level, children with autism presented a different pattern of use of gesture and language. Children with autism produced fewer communicative acts than children with language delays. In addition, the children with autism showed some performance heterogeneity in their ability to produce communicative acts and to produce acts that served a range of interactive functions. The researchers suggested that although children with autism have difficulties initiating interaction, they seem to have less difficulty responding to the directions of another communicator. Their data support the idea that children with autism are relatively poor at engaging another person's attention, introducing a topic, or taking turns in an interaction.

In the child with autism who is learning language, the degree of communication initiation may reflect the degree of social-pragmatic impairment. In the Loveland et al. (1988) study, children with autism had a lower level of pragmatic abilities than normally developing 2-year-olds. Language level, mental age, and IQ could not account for the children's pragmatic interactional deficits. The researchers concluded that there is an asynchrony in development between content areas (pragmatic and semantic) and structural areas (syntax and phonology). The language development of children with ASD follows a sequence quite different from that of other children with disabilities.

Along with the discussions of underlying central language disorder and heterogeneity of language characteristics in children with autism is their relationship to children with specific language impairment (SLI). Miller (1996) noted that SLI is not a static but a dynamic condition that evolves with development. Although the patterns of strengths and weaknesses change as a function of intervention, there are only a limited number of profiles of language strengths and weaknesses in children with SLI. Conti-Ramsden and Botting (1999) noted in their investigation of children with specific language impairment that the profiles of difficulties in language impairment were stable, even though individual children may have moved across subgroups. As noted by the authors, "When changes occurred and children moved to a different subgroup, the profiles of such children became similar to the profiles of the children belonging to a different group . . . children's profiles of difficulties continued to fall into a limited number of patterns already observed" (p. 8).

RELATED FACTORS

Four factors have contributed to the changing ways in which children with ASD have been viewed in the past several years. First, the Autism Society of America has heightened general awareness of the needs of children with autism. This awareness has affected the direction of legislation in state and federal funding of educational programs. Second, passage of Public Laws 94-142 (1975) and 99-457 (1986) has had profound implications for the development of curricula due to the mandate that children with disabilities be educated in the least restrictive environment (LRE). As a result, increasing funds have been available for the development of educational programs for children with autism spectrum disorders in early intervention programs and public school settings.

Third, recent developments in research have suggested neurological differences in processing (visual, auditory, linguistic, and cognitive) between children with ASD and other populations of children (Bailey, Phillips, & Rutter, 1996). Neurological differences suggest an etiological explanation other than emotional disturbance; specifically, that the underlying cause of the disorder relates to perceptual, cognitive, and information-processing differences. These characteristic differences result in language patterns that develop differently.

Although it is still unclear whether specific aspects of language are inherited and specieswide, regardless of environmental variations, questions are being raised about a genetic etiology for ASD (Volkmar, Lord, Bailey, Schultz, & Klin, 2004). Folstein and Mankoski (2000) stated that the evidence from twin and family studies indicated that both autism and SLI are genetically mediated. More families than expected had children with both disorders, and in some cases, the features of autism and SLI overlapped. Other studies demonstrated the familiality of speech and language problems (Bishop, North, & Dolan, 1995; Lewis, Cox, & Byard, 1993). As stated by Gilger (1995),

> In studies where families were selected through an individual with language impairment (i.e., the proband), an overage of approximately 20% to 50% of the first degree relatives of the proband also exhibited or reported a history for speech and language difficulties clearly above expectations for the normal population (i.e., 2% to 7%). Brothers and sisters of language impaired probands were, respectively, 30 and 16 times more likely to have language problems than siblings of control probands. (p. 14)

The fourth and final factor involves recent research in child language development. The changing perspectives in language theory and therapy have affected the view that the communication and language deficits in children with autism are of critical importance, suggesting that pragmatic/semantic deficits may explain behavioral problems. The interplay among these factors has resulted in the progressive attempt to develop language and educational programs for children with ASD in more natural environments.

Since the goal of this chapter is to describe children with autism spectrum disorders in terms of characteristic behaviors, many aspects of developmental learning are presented: language, cognition, play, social interaction, and so forth. These characteristics provide a comprehensive picture of the child with autism spectrum disorders as one who has a language/communication disorder. The chapter also provides comparisons between children with ASD and children with typical language development.

Behavioral Characteristics

The population of individuals with ASD is heterogeneous (Folstein, 2006). Children vary in the number and severity of characteristics exhibited, so for the sake of description, all of the characteristics presented in this chapter are discussed in terms of Adam, who has been diagnosed as a preschool child with autism. As children exhibit fewer of the characteristics, they may be classified as having high-functioning autism (HFA) or Asperger syndrome (AS). Children with Asperger syndrome appear to have appropriate language skills but are highly rigid behaviorally and socially (Rubin, 2007). Some of these characteristics will be discussed more fully in later sections dealing with communication and language.

GAZE AVERSION

Bornstein and Brown (1996) described the development of attention in early infancy. Between 3 and 5 months after birth, infant attention patterns become stable. Whether the explanation is attributed to endogenous aspects within the child, such as perceptual acumen or persistent temperament style, or to exogenous influences, such as maternal responsiveness, attention behavior serves a critical communication function in child language development. Looking, or gaze behavior, serves as a signal to the adult that the child is ready to engage in interaction. In a similar fashion, when the child looks away or averts his or her gaze, the child communicates that the interaction has been terminated. Gaze interaction is one of the earliest dyadic means of communicative exchange between the mother and child. In addition, the mother functions as a continuously gazing listener who is "turned on and off" by the infant. Later on, linguistic forms are mapped onto this early conversational exchange with the eyes (Maestro et al., 2002). This earliest of communicative dialogues does not seem to occur or progress in children with autism. The clinical data needed at 3 to 6 months would require early identification of diagnostically significant atypical gaze patterns in infants.

Perhaps the most salient characteristic of autism is the lack of eye contact with other people during the communication exchange process. This characteristic, more than any other, has resulted in children with autism being described as aloof, distant, withdrawn, and nonrelating. Children with autism do not look at or facially orient their gaze toward another person; they avert their eyes when someone talks to them. In fact, attempts by a communication partner to get the child to look are met with physical resistance, particularly when that person is physically near the child. As the child with autism moves farther away from another person, he exhibits a greater number of gazes oriented to that person. Another difference concerns the physical orientation of the child. Unless one is sneaking a look, the bodies of both speaker and listener are normally lined up shoulder to shoulder. The child with autism turns his or her entire body (and head) away from the speaker and emits infrequent, fleeting gazes from the corners of his or her eyes.

Consider Adam's gaze pattern during an interactional exchange. Even after having been trained to look at the speaker, Adam would change the orientation of his body. The more he focused on the speaker facially, the more his body was turned away. When the speech-language pathologist (SLP) held Adam's head so face-to-face interaction could take place, his eyes shifted from corner to corner (side to side).

RITUALISTIC BEHAVIOR

Rituals are a normal part of the daily routines and patterns of life for most children and adults. There are, however, differences between the rituals exhibited by typical children (Jeremy) and children with autism. For the child with autism, the ritual is a sequence or pattern of behavior that must be exhibited in the same way and in the same order; there is little room for change. The chair must be placed just so in the living room. The child can only drink from the Snoopy cup. When there is a change in the environment, the child may spin records, twirl wires, bang objects, and turn lights on and off incessantly. Children with ASD do not manipulate objects appropriately in a functional way; they often repeat an object manipulation (twirling the telephone wire) for hours. There are also rituals in which the child rocks back and forth in a corner. These repetitive behaviors are frequently referred to as *self-stimulatory behaviors;* they are presumably the child's attempt to maintain sameness (Green et al., 2006). Consider several examples of rituals:

- *Jeremy's nightly ritual:* Take bottles and Binkies (pacifiers) upstairs. Put bottles and Binkies in bed. Put Superdog in bed. Cover Superdog. Give Superdog his bottle. Give Superdog his Binky. Jeremy drinks bottle. Jeremy takes his own Binky.
- *Ellenmorris's pretherapy session ritual:* "Hi, Adam. Come on, let's go play." Offers hand to Adam. Walk hand-in-hand to therapy room.

What are the differences between normal ritual patterns and those that characterize autism? First, with a child who is developing normally, the ritual pattern represents only a small part of his performance or interaction repertoire. Because children with autism have very restricted performance repertoires, their ritual patterns constitute a much larger proportion. Children with autism develop many ritualized patterns of behavior. "Everything becomes a ritual," noted Adam's mother.

The second difference is that it is very difficult to change the ritualized patterns in the child with autism. Any minute change in a ritual can result in a catastrophic reaction from the child. Many parents note that the resulting violent temper tantrums are so aversive that they hesitate to, and often do not, change environmental sequences or events. Jeremy might balk a bit if something is performed differently or left out of his nightly sequence (e.g., not giving Superdog his Binky), but his reaction would not be a catastrophic.

The third difference is that ritualized patterns, referred to as *adultomorphisms* by Piaget (1962), are indicative of a child's relational knowledge of experiences and events within his or her environment. The child's ritualized patterns show progressive and developmental changes; they incorporate the child's changing perceptions and conceptions of the world. Therefore, for the typically developing child, the ritual indicates an attempt to integrate and synthesize observed environmental sequences. For the child with autism, however, the ritualized pattern represents an attempt to maintain a systematic order within the environment.

TEMPER TANTRUMS

There are responses to the natural environment that develop and maintain ritualized patterns. Reconsider Ellenmorris's ritual, described previously, with regard to temper tantrums:

> *Ellenmorris's ritual:* One afternoon, therapy was running late. Because I was getting ready to see Adam, a graduate student volunteered to meet Adam in the waiting room of the Speech and Hearing Center. A few minutes later, Adam was wildly screaming in the hall. I walked into the hall to see Adam pounding the sides of his head with his fists. The therapy session was, to say the least, difficult. Before Adam's mother left, she was asked if anything had happened on the way to the center and if Adam were feeling all right. She said that he was perfectly all right until the graduate student had met him in the waiting room.

For the two years that Adam had been enrolled at the Speech and Hearing Center, I had gone to the waiting room to bring him to the therapy room. In essence, a ritualized pattern had developed. As a result of this experience, my clinical staff attempted to identify the existence of other ritual patterns in their interactions with Adam. The purpose of the investigation was to modify the staff's and the child's patterns of ritualized interaction. Adam's response (a temper tantrum) was typical of how children with autism react to attempts to introduce change into their world. The temper tantrum is the autistic child's catastrophic reaction to change (Shriver, Allen, & Mathews, 1999a).

Temper tantrums can be either self-abusive or aggressive in form. Self-abusive and aggressive behaviors exhibited by children can include any of the following: pulling hair, biting, scratching, head banging, pinching, head butting, and so on. The difference between self-abusive and aggressive behaviors is the direction of the behavior—toward the self or toward others. One of the difficulties related to temper tantrums is the intensity of the child's reaction to even a slight environmental change; a minute change in a ritual can result in a violent outburst. Children with autism can become physically uncontrollable; obviously, the older and bigger the child gets, the harder it is for a parent or a teacher to manage such behaviors (Kobayashi & Murata, 1998).

SELF-STIMULATORY BEHAVIOR

Self-stimulation includes high-frequency behaviors that have been traditionally described as noncommunicative and noninteractional (MacDonald et al., 2007; Richler, Bishop, Kleinke, & Lord, 2007; Wimpory, Hobson, Williams, & Nash, 2000). They are often emitted when the child seeks to withdraw from the environment. This withdrawal pattern occurs when the child with autism cannot cope with direct input from teaching or instruction. Self-stimulatory behaviors are nonprogressive. They interfere with the child's learning, especially in the classroom.

What should the SLP or teacher do about these behaviors? Behavioral approaches to training have proposed eliminating or decreasing the frequency of self-stimulatory behaviors by means of aversive consequences. However, the child's repertoire includes so many self-stimulatory behaviors that eliminating them would leave very few emitted behaviors.

HYPO- VERSUS HYPERSENSITIVITY TO STIMULI

Children with autism do not have the same response threshold to environmental stimuli as other children with and without disabilities. A reduced sensitivity to stimuli is called *hyposensitivity.* Adam's mother has said, "I could clap a pair of cymbals next to my child's ears and he would not blink." Children with autism do not react to or seem in any way to recognize sounds and environmental stimuli consistently. It is not surprising that many of these children, at some point in their history, have been identified as having hearing loss or deafness. Many parents describe the child with autism as being "here and there." Whenever Adam was responsive during a therapy session, his mother would say, "He's come in for a landing."

The child's inconsistent responding is complicated by his inconsistent and often extreme reaction to even the slightest change in input. Heightened or excessive sensitivity to stimuli is called *hypersensitivity.* Adam would place his hands over his ears and eyes to block out input. The inconsistency in responding, with the ever-present possibility of a catastrophic temper tantrum, reduces the child's behavior (i.e., determining how he or she is going to react) to a guessing game for parents, speech-language pathologists, and teachers.

MUTISM

Mutism includes a range of behavior, from periods of total silence to the production of meaningless sounds (i.e., used for self-stimulatory rather than communicative purposes). Most, if not all, children with autism progress through a period of mutism. Some autistic children remain mute all their lives.

Hurford (1991) posited that there is a critical period for language acquisition. The clinical and developmental concern is that if a functional language system is not acquired by 5 years of age, there is little probability of it developing thereafter. Often, when the child becomes verbal, his or her initial words and phrases are quite intelligible. There seems to be a quantum leap or change in the child's performance that cannot as yet be explained. The child with autism does not demonstrate the progressive developmental changes in pragmatics, phonology, semantics, and syntax during the first 36 months that are seen in the typically developing child.

Most of the information accumulated about this time comes from parent interviews. Parents provide critical information about their children's behavior and skills in natural settings with adults and peers that may not be directly observable by the SLP, teacher, or psychologist. Parents can also provide information on developmental history, because the age of onset is an important diagnostic factor. The child's medical history may assist in ruling out other developmental disabilities, such as traumatic brain injury, deafness, and cerebral palsy (Shriver, Allen, & Mathews, 1999b).

Researchers are not sure why some children progress to the next stage—echolalic behavior—and some do not, nor do they agree about the prerequisite changes within the child that result in transition to the next stage. For example, Adam's developmental history represents a dramatic and unexplainable change from one stage to another. Mute until the age of 4 years, 3 months, Adam produced only meaningless grunts. When he started to speak, his productions were long, imitated utterances, such as "Open door please" and "Time go home now." His productions were, as his mother described, "as clear as a bell."

It is important to note that during this phase, many SLPs and parents discuss the use of alternative systems of communication (see the section on alternative therapies). In Adam's case, a sign language system was introduced and used for many months quite successfully. Adam did acquire a core lexicon of signs, which he used appropriately to communicate his basic needs.

In Adam's case, the transition from the use of sign language to verbal language was difficult to explain. The result of this mute period was echolalic behavior. Adam's "eureka" experience, as his mother called it, occurred one day when he came to language therapy producing (very clearly) a verbal label in place of a learned sign. In the next four weeks, he replaced his sign productions with verbal productions. Sign training seemed to have facilitated Adam's development of verbal production. Once a sign was replaced with a verbal production, the sign was never used again. His communication system, therefore, consisted of several forms: words, sign forms, and interchangeable sign/verbal forms. These interchangeable forms indicated a transition—a replacement of a sign by a word. Use of each new word form increased as use of the sign decreased. This replacement process emphasizes that Adam utilized a systematic learning pattern, albeit different from typical learners. Adam's pattern of learning provided some insight into how he learned.

Some children with autism never develop speech or language. The incidence of muteness ranges from 28 percent (Lotter, 1967) to 61 percent (Fish, Shapiro, & Campbell, 1966); the variability is a function of the difficulties with terminology and the issues discussed at the beginning of this chapter. Bartak and Rutter (1976) found that approximately 80 percent of all children with ASD were misdiagnosed as deaf at one time in their developmental history. DeMyer and colleagues (1973) noted that about 65 percent of the children who were mute at age 5 were still mute several years later. A large proportion of children with autism never develop conventional communicative and/or linguistic interactions within the environment.

ECHOLALIA

Echolalia has been defined traditionally as the meaningless repetition of someone else's words. As a result, some researchers have advocated that the behavior should be eliminated or decreased through therapy. Echolalia also has been described traditionally as a transition period between muteness and evidence of linguistic knowledge, but research on children's progress through the various learning stages is limited.

Prizant and Duchan (1981) noted that to determine what echolalic utterances mean, they must be analyzed within a natural communicative environment. It is important to understand how the child functions within the communicative context—specifically, how the child with autism uses whatever behavior he has developed for the purpose of communication. To determine the communicative intent of the child's message, the SLP and parent must analyze the communicative context within which the utterance occurs. In such cases, eliminating echolalia would actually decrease the occurrence of communicative behavior. It thus becomes important to determine if the echolalic form represents the child's communicative intention.

The following interactions illustrate that Adam's dramatic jump to an echolalic period revealed the need to assess his meaning within context. The examples indicate how this child manipulated various linguistic and nonlinguistic behaviors to convey communicative intentions. Adam's mother was, to say the least, thrilled when her son started to "talk"; however, her exuberance quickly wore away. She described Adam as her "talking shadow." A typical exchange between mother and child is presented to highlight the difficulty, confusion, and frustration in an exchange with a child who is echolalic:

Mother: Adam, are you ready?

Adam: Adam, are you ready?

Mother: Go open the door.

Adam: Go open the door.

Mother: Where is your coat?

Adam: Your coat.

To determine if Adam's imitations were meaningful, several aspects of his behavior could be analyzed within the context. For example, consider the following exchange:

Mother: Go open the door.

Adam: Go open the door.

Nonverbal behavior: Adam looks at the door and then gets up and opens it.

Adam indicated by means of his behavior that, although he echoed his mother's production, he understood the meaning of her message and its related action. The nonverbal behavior (i.e., gaze behavior, gestures, and actions) of children with ASD indicates their understanding of the linguistic message and whether their echoic utterance was meaningful (Tiegerman-Farber & Radziewicz, 1998).

Consider another exchange:

Mother: Where is your coat?

Adam: Your coat.

Nonverbal behavior: Adam looks at the coat and then goes to pull on the coat, which is lying across a chair.

In this exchange, Adam's nonverbal behavior indicated his interpretation of the context. The interchange provides additional information as well. First, the linguistic form of Adam's production was slightly different from that of his mother's utterance. Second, his intonation pattern, which was different from his mother's (upward inflection), indicated his ability to make changes in suprasegmental features. Third, he exhibited nonverbal behaviors that signaled he understood his mother's message. This exchange indicates several ways in which the child with autism can manipulate some of the components of the language process. These exchanges indicate how the form and function of the child's communicative behavior can be analyzed within the ongoing natural context (Tiegerman-Farber & Radziewicz, 2007d).

Prizant and Wetherby (1987) proposed that ordinarily, intentionality must combine with conventionality to develop communication. A close analysis of communicative intent might highlight the social and communicative functions in children with autism. Although they may not use conventional forms, such as pointing or showing, children with autism may use idiosyncratic behaviors, such as echolalia and self-stimulation, to signal various communicative functions. One cannot assume that because the child with ASD does not use conventional forms of communication, he or she cannot communicate. This position is as inappropriate as the one that assumes that the child's use of conventional forms automatically indicates his or her intention to communicate. The meaning of the child's interaction can be determined only by analyzing his or her behavior within a social context. Such analysis of a child's unconventional communicative forms and functions requires multiple observations across different contexts; the ultimate challenge is to determine if the unconventional forms actually express communicative intentions.

Prizant and Rydell (1984) investigated the functions of delayed echolalia in children with autism. In delayed echolalia, children repeat utterances long after they originally hear them. The authors noted that "echolalic behaviors, both immediate and delayed, are best described as a continuum of behaviors in regard to exactness of repetition, degree of comprehension, and underlying communicative intent" (p. 183). Delayed echolalia has also been referred to as "old forms applied to new situations." The use of echolalia as a form of communication is an unusual strategy in the typically developing child, but it serves several important functions in the child with autism. The fact that the child with autism uses old forms in new contexts indicates that on some associative level, he establishes a relationship between a linguistic form (as rigid as it is) and an event. That is, the production of a delayed echolalic response indicates that the child perceived a relationship between a verbal utterance and a context. As the child's linguistic abilities increase, he or she is able to substitute, delete, and/or conjoin elements in the echoed response (delayed mitigated echolalia).

In addition, the child's unique ability to imitate sophisticated linguistic sentences and paragraphs verbally is often quite deceptive in terms of his actual spontaneous ability. In the Prizant and Rydell (1984) study, a production was considered a delayed echolalic utterance if it satisfied one or both of the following criteria: (1) the repetition was beyond the child's syntactic abilities, and (2) the utterance consisted of a rigid and routinized string. The children in the study showed a marked discrepancy between the mean length of utterance (MLU) for echolalic and spontaneous productions. Whereas the children's spontaneous productions were primarily at a phase 1 level of linguistic complexity, the echolalic utterances represented a much more sophisticated linguistic ability.

Whether the child uses immediate or delayed echolalia, his or her productions are generated for interactive purposes. Echolalia is not a simplistic or unitary form; it represents a continuum of interaction and comprehension. The adult's interpretation of the echolalic utterance will be based on knowledge of the child and characteristics of their shared context. For the child with autism, the use of unconventional language forms interferes with the development of conventional forms and higher-order metalinguistic abilities. One of the most interesting findings of the Prizant and Rydell (1984) study was that some of the noninteractive echolalic utterances—those produced without communicative intent by the child—did serve meaningful purposes. Although some of the utterances served no specific functions, others served cognitive and/or conversational or turn-taking functions.

Echolalia has been described as a transitional phase of development that signals movement from (1) echolalia without communicative intent, to (2) echolalia with the intent but limited linguistic competence, to (3) echolalia with intent and linguistic ability. This developmental pattern of linguistic and comprehension changes is similar to the communicative sequence exhibited by the typical child as he or she learns language.

EARLY ONSET/ASSESSMENT

The onset of autism relates to a parent's awareness of a problem. The diagnosis of autism becomes difficult if parents and professionals do not have access to standardized assessment tools (Lord & Luyster, 2006; Zwaigenbaum et al., 2007). Assessing a child that may have autism requires evaluation of several areas: language/communication, cognition, motor, and social skills. Public Law 99-457 (1986), which established the early intervention system, emphasizes a family-oriented approach to assessment and treatment. Part of the process is a family assessment that identifies the needs of the entire family as an ecological unit to support the child (Tiegerman-Farber & Radziewicz, 2007b). The following tests can be used by the inter/transdisciplinary team as part of an assessment protocol:

1. *Childhood Autism Rating Scale (CARS)* (Schopler, Reichler, & Rennet, 1998). The CARS is composed of fifteen four-point scales on which a child's behavior is rated on a continuum from within normal limits (1) to severely abnormal (4). The CARS is best used as a screening measure.

2. *Autism Diagnostic Interview–Revised (ADI–R)* (Lord, Rutter, & LeCouteur, 1994). The ADI–R is described as a semistructured, investigative-based interview for caregivers of children and adults for whom autism or pervasive development disorders is a possible diagnosis.

3. *Autism Behavior Checklist (ABC)* (Krug, Arick, & Almond, 1993). The ABC is a behavior-rating checklist that is used when interviewing parents and teachers. It is considered most effective to use in contexts with direct observations across multiple domains.

4. *Psychoeducational Profile–Revised (PEP–R)* (Schopler, Reichler, Bashford, Lansing, & Marcus, 1990). The PEP–R provides information on developmental functions as well as degrees of abnormality in relating and affect, play and interest in materials, sensory responses, and language. The PEP–R is designed for children 6

months to 7 years of age or children under 12 years of age with developmental delays.

5. *Pre-Linguistic Autism Diagnostic Observation Schedule (PL-ADOS)* (DiLavore, Lord, & Rutter, 1995). The PL-ADOS is designed for children under 6 years of age and as a standardized observational measure in which the examiner interacts with the child in structured situations.

Some parents have described their early awareness of a problem during the infant's first months of life. They noted that the infant "could not be comforted." Other parents have described a normal developmental sequence during the first 24 months of life followed by a period of regression or a failure to progress (Bernabei, Cerquiglini, Cortesi, & D'Ardia, 2007; Osterling, Dawson, & Munson, 2002; Siperstein & Volkmar, 2004). The information concerning behavioral and communication development before the time of diagnosis is subjective and a function of the parents' interpretation and memory of early experiences with the child, although parents are reliable reporters. The fact that communication behaviors are not present at 30 months of age does not mean that the behaviors were not present earlier. It is possible that early communication behaviors did develop during the first 9 to 12 months but deteriorated due to neurological deficits.

Current diagnostic tools are not adequate to identify the communication behaviors—gaze, vocalization, and gesture—that are critical to the early identification of ASD. Research analyses and investigations of infants who are not acquiring early communication behaviors between birth and 12 months will eventually result in the identification and diagnosis of ASD in younger and younger children.

The younger the infant, the more difficult the determination of disorder, unless there are neurological signs of impairment. Generally, parents proceed through the frustrations of a diagnostic evaluation as their child approaches his second birthday. One of the most important diagnostic variables—language—is often difficult to assess by standardized means before 24 months (Volkmar, Chawarska, & Klin, 2005). Only within the past few years has early identification, focusing on the child between 2 and 3 years of age, resulted in intervention (Wing & Potter, 2002). Educational options are still rather limited for the preschool child with autism (Tiegerman-Farber & Radziewicz, 2007a).

Onset before age 30 months has been a central criterion in the differential diagnosis of autism. A study indicated that in 76 percent of autism cases, parents identified a problem before their child was 24 months of age. In 94 percent of the cases, parents identified a problem before their child was 36 months old. Parents who recognized a problem earlier tended to seek help sooner. In addition, early onset is also related to developmental severity, particularly in behavioral functioning. Children with later developmental onset scored significantly higher on IQ tests than early onset children, suggesting that these later cases were less severe in terms of symptomatology characteristic of ASD (Volkmar, Chawarska, & Klin, 2005). The authors recommended the need for further research into the differential diagnosis of two distinct groups within the late-onset category: (1) children with autism who experience a developmental regression after 30 months of age and (2) children with autism who are identified at a much later developmental period because their symptomatology is relatively mild.

PLAY

It is generally acknowledged that play is important to the development of adaptability, learning, cognition, and social behavior (Lifter, Sulzer-Azaroff, Anderson, & Cowdery, 1993). The function of play is to exercise and develop manipulative and interactional strategies that children will later integrate into more sophisticated task-oriented sequences. A more general theory suggests that in play, children learn to affect and control activities they are unable to execute or dominate in other contexts. In play, children develop control over animate and inanimate objects and contexts. Recent analyses of early social interactions suggest that play behavior influences the physical and interactional behaviors of all children involved in the experience (Maestro et al., 2005). Thus, play has cognitive, social, and integrative functions in early development.

The underlying theory proposes that play begins with action manipulations directed by the child. As manipulative and physical abilities expand, children develop an increasing capacity to deal with objects and peers more actively (Maestro et al., 2002; Osterling et al., 2002). Children with autism, however, are limited in their social interaction with the environment, and because of their restricted experiences, they share many behavioral/learning problems with other children, whether the specific diagnosis is mental retardation, cerebral palsy, or brain damage. Children with ASD withdraw from interactional experiences and learn to manipulate by means of temper tantrums and disruptive behaviors. Withdrawal from the environment makes it difficult to determine if these children do not know how to play, if they lack the opportunity to do so, or both. Many researchers have suggested that there is a cyclical relationship between the child's bizarre manipulative performances and inability to integrate experiences within the environment, causing even further withdrawal. The child's creation of an inner world is an attempt to establish and maintain an internal order that he or she cannot establish in the outside world; self-stimulatory and ritualistic behaviors may be a result of socio-affective deficits (Kasari, Freeman, & Paparella, 2007).

Play is a natural means of teaching children with autism social interactional skills. Play is a child-directed, rather than a teacher-directed, activity. Play facilitates children's choices of materials, activities, and peer partners. Within a play setting, the child with autism learns that specific behaviors lead to responses from peers. Communicative behaviors and interactional exchanges are more likely to be learned and used in social settings if they lead to naturally reinforcing consequences for children with autism (Olley, 1999). Functional and symbolic play skills are associated with language abilities. In addition, specific nonverbal communication skills, such as gestures, are also correlated with language acquisition.

Social interactional skills can be facilitated by typical peers-integrated preschool programs. The integrated classroom relies on play activities that involve child-based preferences for objects, creative interactions, and peer partners. The early childhood curriculum emphasizes independent play and social interaction in naturally occurring routines. Social skills can be facilitated in play and in groups rather than the one-to-one instruction methodology described by behavioral specialists such as Lovaas and Buch (1997). The early childhood curriculum becomes part of an inclusion training model that uses circle time, story time, and activity centers to facilitate the development of communication (Strain & Cordisco, 1994). (The controversy related to inclusive programming will be discussed later in the chapter.)

COGNITION

The relationships among perception, language, and cognition remain rather controversial. Current trends have been influenced by cognitive theories that stress the importance of early social and interactional experiences within the environment. In discussing cognitive development in children with ASD, it is important to consider perceptual and cognitive processes as well as social interactional experiences.

Harris, Handleman, Gordon, Kristoff, and Fuentes (1991) studied changes in intellectual and language functioning in children with autism and normally developing peers over the course of a year. The results indicated that, relative to their typical preschool peers, the preschool children with autism showed a greater increase in intellectual progress in the program. The typical preschool children maintained their cognitive functioning across the schoolyear, but the preschool children with autism showed a significant increase in functioning. The nineteen-point increase in IQ provides support for the effectiveness of early intervention programming and the ability of children with autism to benefit from comprehensive programming.

Approximately 75 percent of children with autism are reported to function within the mentally retarded range (APA, 1994). Differential diagnosis is further complicated by the fact that children with severe or profound mental retardation may exhibit behaviors similar to children with ASD. Children with mental retardation exhibit quantitative delays in social interaction, communication, and behavior that are commensurate with their developmental level. In contrast, children with ASD present qualitative differences in functioning that are not typically exhibited by other children with language delays.

In addition, children with autism demonstrate a wide variability of skills. Sometimes, the skill differences (i.e., splinter skills or savant abilities) result in exceptional abilities in one area but significant deficits in other areas. Adam, for example, had excellent memory and rote recall. His ability, however, should be viewed in terms of his use of the skill within the social context. His remarkable recall was often used for noncommunicative and self-stimulatory purposes. Information was frequently extracted as a whole and not used for interactional purposes. Adam would sit in a corner of his room and recite verbatim the news report presented the previous night.

Identifying strengths, skills, and abilities is only an initial step. It is also important to determine how children with ASD use and apply their skills within the learning context. (See the later sections on hyperlexia and phonology.) Children with autism display significantly higher abilities on tasks that require the discrimination of concrete visual spatial relations and significantly lower abilities on tasks that require abstraction or the ability to organize concrete information on the basis of subtle conceptual relationships between stimuli. Children with ASD also present integration deficits when stimuli increase in complexity and/or require cross-modal processing. Their difficulties identifying what is meaningful and relevant in a situation results in the rigid use of rules when interacting with the environment. Conceptual development is further compromised by their tendency to attend to or fixate on one aspect of a picture or story, often some irrelevant minutiae (Shriver et al., 1999a). All of these examples describe an idiosyncratic pattern of interaction within the environment.

Sigman and Ungerer (1984) discussed the early cognitive deficits specific to ASD. Although sensorimotor skills and language were positively correlated in children without disabilities, they were unrelated in the children with autism. The authors suggested that sensorimotor knowledge may be necessary but not sufficient for language development. The marked discrepancy between sensorimotor abilities and language disabilities in children with autism provides support for the argument that sensorimotor and symbolic knowledge may involve divergent development.

Several hypotheses may explain the variation in deficits. The first theory is that representational thought may require the interface of two subsystems. One such subsystem involves the development of sensorimotor skills with the ability to recall information for problem solving. The second subsystem involves the ability to translate experiences into symbols; this is difficult for children with autism. Cognitive deficits in children with autism are secondary to social deficits.

Sigman and Ungerer (1984) also noted that "all the areas of specific cognitive deficit identified to date depend on social interaction for their development" (p. 301). This finding highlights the significance of the social learning process to other areas of development. The social experience becomes the "field with developmental areas such as play, cognition, imitation, and language facilitated on this field" (p. 301).

PERCEPTION

Little is known about how children with ASD perceive their environments. Assumptions are made on the basis of their patterns of interaction in the environment—that is, the way in which they relate to agents, actions, and objects. The behavioral characteristics described previously provide some indication of the child's internal operations and resulting reactions to the impinging world.

What is it that the child with autism sees and hears? One can only infer, based on observed responses and reactions, the child's difficulties and confusions. The child's behavior suggests that very little of what he or she sees and hears makes sense. Words, voices, faces, and gestures are no more than rapidly changing stimuli, like changes in color that are transient and difficult to grasp. People handle the child and do things to him or her. What does it mean? All those faces and changing expressions. What do they mean? Few things are recognizable to the child, since everything is always changing.

That the world appears confusing to the child with autism is not surprising. Nor is it surprising that the child maintains a ritualized, ordered environment and indeed struggles to continue that order and sameness. Finally, when the environment impinges beyond the management point, the child fights back and throws tantrums, which are the result of frustration and confusion. The child tries to create an inner world that is more understandable and consistent (Tiegerman-Farber & Radziewicz, 2007a). Self-stimulation can be seen as an attempt to reestablish sameness. Many parents indicate that their child exhibits self-stimulatory behaviors when exposed to a new situation or experience. The child's perceptual deficits create further problems because they severely limit his or her interactional experiences with peers and adults. The child who sees the world in a distorted manner interacts with the world in a distorted manner. This cycle does not permit the child to experience the multiplicity of interactions that are the building blocks of conceptual development (Tager-Flusberg, 1999).

GENERALIZATION

Children with ASD also have difficulty generalizing learned behaviors from one context to another. Because these children cannot identify the relevant information within the complexities of a situation, they cannot identify what is important and what is not, creating a further problem in establishing conceptual or perceptual relationships. The ability to establish categories of any kind depends on the ability to discriminate differences as well as to determine how stimuli are related to one another. Perceptual deficits contribute to the failure to generalize learning and develop strategies for adapting to continually changing social contingencies. Social rigidity limits the ability of children with ASD to adjust to changing social contingencies, and perseverative responses interfere with the development of problem-solving skills (Prior & Hoffmann, 1990; Russell, Mauthner, Sharpe, & Tidswell, 1991).

Deficits in generalization indicate a cognitive impairment in children, a problem that seriously limits their ability to learn spontaneously. The inability to develop conceptual relationships—to extract and use similarities across situations and to learn from past experiences—condemns children with autism to repeated learning experiences. Typical children search for rules; in order to establish rules, they identify relevant and related stimuli within conceptual categories. Generalization involves the ability to identify the relationship between situation A and situation B and then to apply the rule to situations A′ and B′. Without rule-governed behavior, children have difficulty processing, categorizing, and interpreting social events (Tager-Flusberg, 1999).

The efficacy of any treatment program depends on incorporated strategies that will facilitate learning to and within the child's natural environment. Generalization from the therapy room to the classroom to the home requires specific training of family members, teachers, and peers (Goldstein, 2002; Green, Everhart, Gordon, & Gettman, 2006; Steege, Mace, Perry, & Longenecker, 2007; Yoder & Stone, 2006).

THEORY OF MIND AND META SKILLS

The development of a theory of mind involves the ability to represent mental states. Research indicates that typical children realize that the actions of other people are related to what they think and believe and not necessarily to factual occurrences. A child's ability to take the perspective of another person—to understand another's point of view—begins in early childhood. Theory-of-mind research in autism refers to the ability to attribute mental states such as desire, knowledge, and belief to oneself and other people as a means of explaining behavior.

Pennington and colleagues (1998) described a shift in theoretical perspective concerning the underlying origin of autism as a deficit in metarepresentation. *Meta skills*—metacognitive and metalinguistic—require intact language production and comprehension abilities in children. The metas involve the abilities to revise, reflect, and repair language rules. Metalinguistic skills represent a higher conceptual understanding of production and comprehension skills. When the child can "talk about talking," he or she is aware of language structures and can make judgments about their appropriateness. Metacognitive skills involve the ability to deal abstractly with one's thought processes in comprehension, memory, information processing, reasoning, and problem solving.

For the child with ASD, pervasive deficits in social interaction, language production, and comprehension limit the development of the more abstract meta skills (Mundy, Sigman, & Kasari, 1994). The majority of children with autism (60 to 70 percent) present limited development in the metarepresentational area. A minority (20 to 30 percent) appear to develop to a level equivalent to 3- to 4-year-old typical children by the time they reach their teenage years.

Investigations related to research in the area of theory of mind may provide another explanation: They propose that the communication, socialization, and mental imagery deficits characteristic of autism may be attributable to the inability to symbolize and conceptualize mental states—what Baron-Cohen (1995, 1998) refers to as "mindblindness." For example, children with ASD present conceptual difficulties in connected situations requiring judgments about joking, lying, persuasion, and pretense (Happe, 1994).

Children with ASD may also have difficulty developing the behavioral strategies that involve disengaging attention from focal objects. Research by Hughes and Russell (1993) indicated that subjects with autism failed a test of strategic deception because they had difficulty mentally disengaging from a focal object, not because they were unable to perform a theory-of-mind task. The ability to disengage attention from a focal object is one of many mental operations referred to as *executive functions*. According to Hughes and Russell (1993), these functions "are separately necessary and jointly sufficient for volitional goal directed behavior; inhibition of perceptually triggered or inappropriate responses; and monitoring the success and failure of current strategies." The researchers further suggested that the results achieved from the tests traditionally used to assess theory of mind may have been confounded by the executive difficulties exhibited in children with autism. The theory-of-mind deficit in autism is part of the broader deficit in higher-order cognitive processes (Russell, 1997).

Language Components

In describing autism as a language/communication disorder (LCD), several components of language will be discussed: pragmatics, semantics, syntax, and phonology. Studying the interrelationship among these components can provide insight into the unique learning needs of children with ASD. An asynchronous pattern of development has been described, with semantic and syntactic components progressing independently from one another. A child may evidence (1) more advanced or complex semantic skills while his or her syntactic abilities remain severely limited, or (2) more advanced syntactic skills while his or her semantic abilities remain severely limited. This uneven developmental pattern across language components is linked to the structures and functions of neuropsychology and to the development of different language processes (Rapin & Dunn, 2003; Tager-Flusberg, 1999). Uneven development indicates that different areas within the central nervous system are more or less impaired, which determines the level of functioning and the language abilities developed within the child.

Language represents an integrated system; every component contributes to the development of the whole system. To understand the learning needs of children with language disorders, particularly children with ASD, it is important to compare and contrast development within and across components. Table 7.1 describes the strengths and deficits of children with high-functioning autism (HFA) and Asperger syndrome (AS) for comparison purposes. The language and communication deficits evidenced in children with autism spectrum disorders might be caused by (1) uneven developments within and/or across the components of the learning system and (2) an inability to interface and/or exchange developmental information across the components of the system.

PRAGMATICS

For children with ASD, the use of language for communicative purposes remains severely impaired in spite of developments in other language areas. Part of the problem relates to the interrelationship between social interaction and communication. Most children with autism do not develop a range of communicative functions, and as a result, their communicative and social interactions are limited. Whereas the social context facilitates learning in the typically developing child, this is the environment that presents the most difficulty for the child with autism, who removes himself or herself from the very context that teaches about communication. Given the child's severe communication deficits, the social situation becomes of primary importance for further learning (Peppé, McCann, Gibbon, O'Hare, & Rutherford, 2006).

In addition, the few interactive behaviors exhibited by children with autism are often part of specific and unusual routines. As noted previously, having an established routine allows the child with autism to maintain some control within his or her rapidly changing environment. The routine establishes predictability by maintaining a contextual sameness. Although children with autism indicate a preference for building such routines, these ritualized patterns further restrict social interaction. This added social limitation serves to maintain the communication deficit.

By responding to a limited range of behaviors, children with ASD selectively reinforce certain aspects of adults' input. The adult's problem is the child's limited interactional responsiveness and tolerance for change. Frequently, for the sake of interaction, the adult continues to provide a highly restricted form of communication (Tiegerman-Farber & Radziewicz, 2007a). As a result, social interaction tends to be inflexible, ritualistic, and rigidly routinized. In turn, these limited social and interactional patterns further affect the following aspects of communication: (1) initiating and terminating interaction, (2) maintaining conversational topics, (3) functioning in speaker and listener roles, and (4) using behavior for the purpose of communication (Osterling et al., 2002).

In general, children with ASD present the following pragmatic problems:

1. They do not develop a range of communicative functions.
2. They do not develop gaze interaction skills.
3. They do not develop prototypical behaviors such as protodeclaratives and protoimperatives.
4. They do not develop attention and joint action schemes.
5. They do not develop an awareness of agent, action, or object contingencies.

Table 7.1   Characteristics of Children with High-Functioning Autism and Asperger Syndrome

	Strengths	Deficits
High-Functioning Autism (HFA)		
Language	Verbal imitation or echolalia indicates the use of a gestalt style of language processing. Can recall large chunks of information, which can often be associated with daily routines and activities. Hyperlectic skills result in an advanced ability to read and an interest in print-based materials such as books.	Language skills are limited. Emerging pragmatic functions relate to physical needs. Semantic word meanings are limited to concrete attributes. Syntactic and morphological structures are emerging but highly restricted due to the severe conceptual deficits. Range of sentences is limited since analytic language processing skills are limited. Emerging conversational skills including topic maintenance, turn taking, and eye contact. Responses are still nonrelated and/or tangentially related. Limited, if any, understanding of nonliteral and multiple meanings of words and sentences.
Social	Will remain near peers and tolerate their initiations to interact. Emerging use of language allows child to communicate needs and wants and to inform others of anxieties and frustrations. Use of verbal language may also decrease behavioral outbursts by regulating the behaviors of others and allowing the child to control aspects of the environment.	Insistence on sameness within the environment. Use of ritual patterns that are nonprogressive and inflexible to maintain contextual sameness. Exhibits aggressive and/or self-injurious behaviors. Stereotypical behaviors still interfere with learning.
Cognition	Excellent memory and visual spatial skills. Recalls details, dates, and numbers. May also have advanced mathematical abilities.	High level of stereotypical behaviors. Symbol and abstract conceptual abilities are limited. Standardized testing may indicate abilities within the mental retardation range of functioning.
Play	May present advanced motor and manipulative skills with objects.	Limited manipulation of objects for exploration or social purposes. Engages in parallel but not social or imaginative play.
Special Abilities	Some present unusual abilities in artistic representation and music instrumentation.	

	Strength	Deficit
Asperger Syndrome (AS)		
Language	Semantic, syntactic, and phonological skills are within average range. Usually Language, although advanced, is pragmatically deficient. Language is concrete included in regular academic subjects and may perform at the top of the class in specific subject areas. Verbal skills may be advanced, with strengths in narrating detailed information that is book based, rather than socially or experientially based.	and interpreted literally. Advanced acquisition of and interest in text/written materials. Socially, child limits conversational exchanges. Language is not used to advance or develop interpersonal relationships. Limited understanding of humor.
Social	Can manage limited social interactions and settings with specific training. Emerging self-regulatory skills are developing so child can manage and monitor own behaviors and actions in contexts in which the interactional requirements are minimal.	Requires specific training to develop and maintain prosocial behaviors. Requires clear contingencies and social predictability, since unanticipated or unexpected changes result in catastrophic behavioral responses. Limited understanding of social cues and nonverbal behaviors may result in poor social choices and decision making. Child may become the focus of teasing and bullying in school. Has few friends and may be socially isolated and alone. Social anxieties limit activities and choices.
Cognition	Average or above-average cognitive abilities. Accumulates a wealth of detailed information. Strengths in visual spatial areas, resulting in advanced abilities in science, mathematics, mechanical engineering, and technology. Verbal skills are higher than nonverbal skills on standardized cognitive assessments.	Major deficits in perspective taking to understand the behavioral actions and interactions of others. Requires specific training on recognition, interpretation, and use of gestures and facial expressions. Deficits in planning abstract problem solving, organizational skills, and multitasking. Executive dysfunctions result in an inability to engage and disengage actions given social/contextual requirements.
Play	Can engage and tolerate activities and games that do not require metacognitive or metalinguistic decision making, such as board games and computer games.	Limited ability to interact cooperatively to complete a task. The choice is to work alone and independently from others. Becomes anxious and socially inappropriate in a peer group setting.
Special Abilities	Highly focused in areas of interest acquiring information/knowledge. Performance skills may be in gifted range.	

Based on Bennett, Szatmani, Bryson, Volden, Zwaigenbaum, Vaccarella, Duku, & Boyle, 2008; Crooke, Hendrix, & Rachman, 2008; Macintosh & Dissanayake, 2004; and Rubin, 2007.

6. They do not develop turn-taking or reciprocal action skills.
7. They do not develop gestures or imitation behaviors.

Prelinguistic behaviors, such as pointing, showing, and turn taking, typically are not present, and as a result, the communicative behavior of children with ASD is different from that of typical children. In addition, the differential aspects of each child tend to promote different patterns of responding and contingencies for interaction in peers and adults within the child's environment (Folstein, 1999).

Bernard-Opitz (1982) demonstrated that communicative performance is related to specific variables within the communicative context. The author analyzed how a child with autism used language with his mother, his clinician, and a stranger. The child's communicative style was different with each communication partner. With his mother, the child initiated communication by using requests as the primary speech act, whereas with the clinician, the child used statements to interact. The communicative interaction with the stranger resulted in unintelligible and noncommunicative utterances. In addition, the adults had a tendency to use requests as the predominant speech act during interaction with the child. The author suggested that the differences in the child's communicative behavior might have been related to his familiarity with the listener. Also, the child did not typically respond to the requests of the adults but rather generated another request by imitating the adult's syntactic structure.

Another interesting aspect of Bernard-Opitz's (1982) study was the difference between the mother's and the clinician's responses to the child's echolalic behavior. The mother reinforced the echolalic pattern by answering or clarifying the child's behavior. The clinician's response to unrelated utterances was to introduce another topic, redirecting the discourse rather than responding directly to the child's utterance.

The description of children with autism as noncommunicative and noninteractive has not been supported by research. Even with a limited range of communicative behaviors within his or her repertoire, the child responded differently to different interactional partners. So it is not that a child with autism cannot interact but rather that his or her range of communicative options is limited (Kashinath, Woods, & Goldstein, 2006).

Children with ASD are quite diverse in their range of communication and language deficits. As already noted, children with autism appear to use various strategies in an attempt to interact, even with a limited repertoire of conventional forms. In addition, they develop a more limited range of communicative functions than typical children. In the typically developing child, communication does not occur consecutively from one function to another; some functions emerge concurrently. Linguistic structures develop from communicative functions; typical children talk about the interactional context and their manipulative experiences. It is the social process that provides the basis for the development of conventional forms.

The synchronous development of communicative functions evident in typical children appears as a nonsequential pattern in children with autism. This suggests that the communicative pattern developed by children with autism is qualitatively, as well as quantitatively, different from the normal prelinguistic sequence. Children with ASD acquire communicative functions in a different developmental sequence, and as a result, their linguistic abilities develop differently (Calloway, Myles, & Earles, 1999). The following communicative characteristics describe the child with autism:

1. Communicative intent in gestural and vocal areas develops asynchronously.
2. The communicative profile is different from the profiles of other children with language disorders.
3. The sequence of communicative development is different from that in typical children.
4. Communicative functions are limited.
5. Certain aberrant behaviors can be intentional, interactive, and communicative.
6. They develop many behaviors that result in an environmental consequence but few behaviors that result in a social consequence.

Children with autism do not readily develop the range of communicative intentions produced by typical children because of an inability to develop and coordinate the interactional behaviors, as described previously. If and when linguistic skills do develop, communicative deficits remain.

The typical language learner develops conventional behaviors to communicate his or her needs. The child with ASD uses unconventional behaviors and/or linguistic forms. The result is that the social communicators in the child's environment may misinterpret and misunderstand his or her intentions and meaning. Communicative functions and exchanges, rather than specific linguistic forms or structures, should be facilitated in children with autism. Given the learning style of these children, linguistic forms are often acquired as routinized chunks. Historically, clinical and educational programs have focused on teaching specific linguistic structures or forms, the result being that children with ASD learned to reproduce rigid or "frozen" strings without a semantic-syntactic understanding of these utterances. Schwartz and Carta (1996) suggested that programmatic and instructional goals should focus on teaching children with autism the process of interactional communication rather than teaching them responses to specific questions or forms.

Calloway, Myles, and Earles (1999) found that children with ASD used communication as a means of requesting objects or controlling the behaviors of peers and adults, rather than as a means of social initiation to show, share, comment, provide information, and/or request information. Their findings indicated that as children with autism continue to develop communicative functions and means, more primitive communicative forms were replaced with more advanced forms. Although the progression of specific communicative functions varied, children showed consistent progress and development, often following a pattern from behavior regulation to social interaction to joint attention.

The only way to determine intentional behaviors is to observe and analyze how children with ASD behave within the social situation. What should the SLP look for in a child's behavior? Even the child with the most severe deficits has behaviors that can be identified as communicative if they are analyzed within the context (Prizant et al., 1990). Several incidents with Adam highlight this point:

Situation 1

- *Clinician:* The clinician places a tightly sealed container of vanilla ice cream on the table.
- *Adam:* Adam walks over to the table, turns over the container, tries to pull open the top, bites on the container, and drops it on the table. He walks away for several moments. He walks back to the table and picks up the container. He brings the container to the clinician and puts it in her lap. He walks away from the clinician and looks at her from across the room. (The clinician, of course, does nothing.) Adam approaches the clinician from the side, takes her hand, and places it on the ice cream.
- *Interpretation:* Adam is requesting that the clinician perform an action (open the ice cream) that he cannot do himself.

Situation 2

- *Clinician:* The clinician approaches Adam and sits down next to him.
- *Adam:* Adam gets up and moves away from the clinician.
- *Interpretation:* Adam is rejecting interaction.

Situation 3

- *Clinician:* The clinician talks to Adam.
- *Adam:* Adam puts his hands over his ears and turns away from the clinician but does not move away. Periodically, he takes his hands off his ears. When the clinician stops talking, Adam turns back to her.
- *Interpretation:* Adam does not want to engage in verbal interaction. The clinician learned that during these periods, Adam participated in activities that could be maintained without discourse (e.g., puzzles, blocks, coloring).

Adam could communicate several different intentions and presented different combinations of behavior to indicate his responses to input from the environment. It becomes critical for adults and typical peers to read the child's behaviors within a contextual framework before attempting to interpret his or her reactions to the environment. In fact, the maternal variable of rich interpretation—in which the mother assumes that her infant reacts to the environment and treats the infant as an active listener and communicator—could facilitate the communication exchange process with the child with ASD. The assumption that children with autism do not have the ability to communicate results in a self-fulfilling prophesy. If it is believed that they cannot communicate, then they will not be treated as communicators and their behaviors will not be analyzed to identify communicative interactions (Tiegerman-Farber, 1995).

SEMANTICS

The linguistic term *semantics* refers to meaning as it is encoded in language. *Semantic knowledge,* therefore, refers to the meaning within a language that is linguistically coded. *Conceptual knowledge* affects the acquisition of the semantic component of language.

Tager-Flusberg (1999) suggested that conceptual knowledge in typical children is transformed into semantic knowledge. The difficult task for children is to determine which aspects of these concepts are encoded within their particular linguistic system. Children's interactional experiences with agents, actions, and objects develop semantic relationships that code the content of language. Children with ASD have difficulty developing complex relationships and, as a consequence, establishing the underpinnings for symbolic forms of behavior, which provide the foundations for language.

The ability to develop meaningful and relevant perceptual-conceptual relationships allows typical children to establish general categories—that is, to relate agents, actions, and objects to one another. Doing so enables children to make cohesive and consistent sense of an environment, stimuli in the environment, and experiences within the environment that would otherwise be continually novel and changing. Categorical and organizational abilities provide children with the means of developing a schematic framework for their experiences. Language, as a representation of reality, begins within the microcosm of the child's social world. At a very basic semantic level, children with ASD cannot understand how objects are functionally related or associated, and as a result, they cannot translate their real-world experiences into linguistic structures by using a semantically based processing strategy.

Ogletree and Fischer (1995) noted that the focus of research has shifted from the structural aspects of language (i.e., phonology, morphology, and syntax) to the development of meaning within social contexts. Brook and Bowler (1992) listed some of the semantic/pragmatic deficits presented by children with autism:

1. confusion specific to the intent of communicative acts
2. problems encoding meaning relevant to conversation
3. difficulty with verbal/nonverbal cues of partners
4. problems initiating or responding to questions
5. impaired language comprehension
6. too literal interpretations of verbal messages
7. poor turn taking and topic maintenance
8. inappropriate speech volume and intonational patterns
9. semantic confusion specific to temporal sequencing
10. poor sense of semantic relationships
11. low rates of conversational repairs
12. providing too little or too much information to conversational partners

Table 7.2 describes Adam's development of lexical items to express his semantic knowledge and ideas about the world. Adam's semantic development at this time (4 years, 9 months) indicates his limited or restricted developmental use of functions. Adam developed lexical items within four semantic categories. Most of the lexical items were food related—specifically, desserts. Fewer action performances than objects were coded, and two of the action performances related to food (e.g., *eat* and *drink*). Analyzing the child's corpus (language sample) in this way provides the SLP with insight into what is important to the child within his or her environment. The child's preferences can then be incorporated into therapeutic activities.

Old knowledge provides a framework for processing new information. With the analytic style, new information can be compared to old information to develop concepts—specifically, semantic concepts. Prizant (1983) noted that semantic memory involves the ability to conceptualize beyond any single or specific context. Here the child abstracts relevant information across situations to organize concepts for long-term memory. This semantic ability allows the child to represent and reconstruct

Table 7.2 **Adam's Early Lexicon**

Semantic Functions	Lexical Entries
Object	Car, cookie, pretzel, juice, ice cream, milk, chip, M&M, hot dog, lolly, soda, popcorn, puzzle, Slinky, block, shoe, raisin, grape
Action	Open, push, eat, drink, throw, give
Negation: rejection	No
cessation	No
Recurrence	(Repeat of item label)
Agent	—
Action + object	—

an event symbolically. So to learn language, a child must be able to reconstruct sentence elements, not merely imitate them. The analytic style allows for linguistic generation with an understanding of semantic meaning as well as the related structural forms to express it. Children with autism have a language pattern characterized by repetition of unanalyzed forms. This language pattern indicates an inability to use generative rules for production purposes and an inability to analyze the internal structure of another's production (Windsor & Doyle, 1994).

Prizant (1983) suggested that gestalt and analytic styles represent processing abilities on opposite ends of a continuum. Because children with autism have an extreme style of gestalt processing, generative language development becomes very difficult. In particular, "those who remain primarily echolalic demonstrate a failure to move along the continuum toward analytic processing due to cognitive imitations" (p. 303). As spontaneous utterances increase, echolalia decreases; spontaneous productions indicate more flexibility in the use of combinatorial rules. This movement toward the analytic end of the processing continuum is necessary for the development of semantic–syntactic relations. To understand further the impact of the child's processing pattern on language learning, splinter abilities may contrast with idiosyncratic deficits. Children with ASD have excellent memories, visual processing skills, visual–spatial abilities, numerical skills, and musical abilities. The gestalt learning style interferes with the analytic requirements for the development of semantic functions and semantic–syntactic relationships (Brook & Bowler, 1992).

Language development, production, and creativity depend on an analytic style of processing that offsets the gestalt processing style. Without a working knowledge of the meaningful units of language, the child with ASD can form only surface associations between long language chunks and contexts. Often, the semantic relationship between the memorized chunk and the context is tangential. The discrepancy between form and function presents a serious strain on the communication process. The listener must attempt to derive the child's communicative intent based on what the listener thinks the child means.

HYPERLEXIA

The term *hyperlexia* has been used to describe children with ASD who have highly developed word recognition skills but little or no comprehension of the words they recognize. There appears to be a disparity between this site-recognition ability and the underlying semantic comprehension that relates to the processing of meaning in language. Hyperlexia has been described as a strength in which the child has a preference for materials presented visually rather than orally (Craig & Telfer, 2005). Why certain children acquire this splinter skill and how it is related to other developmental areas of learning continue to be perplexing and interesting questions from an educational perspective.

Many of the characteristics of ASD involve highly idiosyncratic and fragmented abilities, including hyperlexia. These splinter skills present learning problems over time, because they are not well integrated or cross-referenced with other areas of the child's learning. These skills do not represent functional behaviors that serve a social or communicative process (Patti & Lupinetti, 1993). Hyperlectic readers appear to be highly attuned to orthographic and phonological features; this visual–verbal decoding ability needs to be integrated with semantics and reading materials to enhance comprehension. As a result, the hyperlectic process in children with autism should be contrasted with their pervasive semantic deficits. Savant abilities and splinter skills highlight uneven and nonintegrated aspects of developmental learning, which appear to develop independently from areas of social communicative learning. If the savant skill does not serve to facilitate communicative interaction, then it poses an interesting problem for parents and teachers. In trying to understand an advanced reading ability or any savant skill in a child with ASD, the question becomes, How can this splinter skill be utilized educationally to facilitate the child's interactional abilities within the social context (Tiegerman-Farber & Radziewicz, 2007g)?

SYNTAX

The development of a normal linguistic system, in which structure is related to meaning, requires an interfacing of linguistic and nonlinguistic cognitive development. In typical children, lexical and relational semantic abilities are linked to broader conceptual developments, but morphological and syntactic abilities are not. The aspects of language that are conceptually based and reflect pragmatic/semantic functioning are significantly impaired in children with ASD.

The language/communication deficits presented by children with ASD are a result of a disintegrated developmental system in which advances in one component of language do not seem to affect developments in other component of language (Conti-Ramsden & Botting, 1999). The language pattern in children with ASD indicates that pragmatic/semantic development occurs independently from the structural development of language. The separate development of components highlights the devastating impact of two language subsystems that do not communicate with each other. Linguistic aspects such as verb endings, past tense, and present progressive, which require syntactic structures, present significant difficulties to children with ASD because of their inability to understand the underlying meaning of past tense.

The more basic problem for children with autism is that they do not understand the concepts that underlie the formulation of language. They have difficulties using or manipulating certain linguistic forms of language because they do not understand their semantic counterparts. Bartak, Rutter, and Cox (1975) compared autistic with dysphasic children and found both groups comparable in MLU and grammatical complexity. On a test of comprehension, however, the children with autism performed more poorly than the children with dysphasia.

It seems that the syntactic delays in children with ASD are related to their general developmental delays. These children present syntactic-processing skills similar to those evidenced by children with other types of disorders. Linguistic analyses indicated the use of rule-governed behavior, however, despite their limited production and comprehension of language.

Adam's productions are presented within the framework of various contextual and interactional situations to highlight his limited linguistic-processing abilities. Consider Adam's use of the following morphemes: present progressive, past tense, personal pronouns, relative pronouns, copula, articles, and plurals.

Clinician: What is Mommy doing?

Adam: Mommy is opening juice.

Within the framework of an interaction with the adult, Adam was able to use the copula and present progressive morphemes within his own speech. He also responded to the adult's question by altering the inflectional form of the adult's utterance (i.e., he did not imitate the question's inflectional pattern).

Clinician: What did you do?

Adam: Adam ate three cookie.

Within the framework of this interaction with the adult, Adam responded to the question by referring to himself as Adam; he did not use any personal pronouns. He was not able to code (or use) the past-tense form. When Adam was not able to code the morphemic structures presented within the adult's production, he reduced his own utterance or reverted to a string of content words. Plural forms were coded by the use of number without the plural *-s*.

In the preceding examples, there was a structural relationship between the linguistic input provided by the adult and the child's linguistic response: Adam based his response on the structure of the adult's input. The following interaction shows what happened to Adam's linguistic structure when the adult input was not provided:

Clinician: (has just poured Adam some juice)

Adam: Drink juice. (describing his own action)

Adam: More. (requesting more juice)

Adam: Pour juice. (directing clinician to perform an action)

Adam: Give. (requesting cup from clinician)

In this interaction, the clinician responded nonverbally to all of Adam's requests and directions. Adam did not, therefore, have the adult's linguistic input to rely on to structure his own utterances. The result was a reduction to the minimum use of forms that would get the message across effectively. This reduction process was quite typical of Adam's spontaneous, or self-initiated, speech.

To understand the structural/syntactic abilities of children with autism, it is important to analyze if and how their linguistic structures change within various interactional situations. For Adam, the adult's input provided a syntactic framework for his responses. Finally, Adam's productions required a close analysis of the context to clarify the meanings of his utterances. He rarely provided gestural support for his verbal productions.

During the third year of life, the typical language learner begins to encode meaning syntactically in the forms of phrases, sentences, and finally narratives. In the process of combining words, the child learns that words must be organized into sentences given specific linguistic rules. The child learns that ideas can be expressed by using specific sentence structures, such as a question, negation, coordination, sequence, causality, and temporality. Conventional forms are important to the expression of ideas. By 3 years of age, the typical language learner has already integrated aspects of formal structure, semantic meaning, and communicative interaction. This can be contrasted with some striking statistics on children with autism. Newsom, Carr, and Lovaas (1979) estimated that 50 percent of all children with autism are mute and that 75 percent of those who become verbal are echolalic by 5 years of age.

PHONOLOGY

Few studies have been conducted investigating phonological abilities in children with ASD, possibly because speech-language production is so limited (Wolk & Edwards, 1993). Adams and Gathercole (1995) found that 3-year-old children with good phonological memory skills produced speech that was grammatically more sophisticated than children with poorer phonological memory skills. This appears to be consistent with the speech production of children with ASD, although their utterances are imitated rather than spontaneous. Many children with autism have savant memory skills, resulting in the reproduction of large chunks of syntactically sophisticated utterances.

Adams and Gathercole (1995) also demonstrated that typical children with better phonological memory abilities were able to produce a wider array of grammatical forms in spontaneous speech. In addition, the ability to imitate utterances and retain them in short-term memory before they are incorporated into the child's syntactic knowledge appears to influence the development of syntactic forms. This certainly is not the case in children with autism: Their spontaneous productions are severely limited and reflect significant semantic/syntactic deficits. Regardless, children with ASD have excellent memory skills:

1. Their sophisticated imitated utterances do not reflect their understanding of the structural aspects of language.
2. Their memory abilities appear to be separated from the required phonological/morphological processing that occurs in normal development. Phonological and morphological development require analytic processing to identify phonemic and morphemic building blocks. Phonological memory may be necessary, but it is not sufficient for the structural acquisition of language.
3. The imitation of new structural forms, no matter how many repetitions, is not conceptually understood by the child with autism. As a result, he or she does not readily incorporate new forms "into the store of knowledge about the syntactic forms of the native language" (Adams & Gathercole, 1995, p. 11).

The inability of the child with ASD to progressively develop more complex morphosyntactic structures relates to developments in subsystems—structure and meaning—that do not interface/overlap. Thus, the schism between structure and meaning or form and function creates developmental differences at the phonological level as well as the syntactic level. In this case, the child with autism acquires a sound system apart from its meaning and application. Large sound chunks are often tangentially related to contextual occurrences and social interactions. Long sound strings are produced like a foreign language student repeating an English phrase without understanding its meaning.

The inability to utilize an analytic processing style prevents the child with ASD from acquiring the basic elemental sound/symbol units, which are finite but can be combined to generate an infinite number of speech productions. Fragmented language development results in growth without integration. The highest percentage of errors involve phonemes that are generally acquired later in typical children. The order of phonemic acquisition in children with autism seems to follow the typical developmental pattern, in spite of the delay in the onset of speech. The phonological ability of children with autism contrasts markedly with their developmental delays in pragmatic/semantic areas.

Therapeutic Issues and Strategies

The clinical view of the child with ASD has changed in the past several years. Theoretical changes in the area of child language development have dramatically affected the content and context of therapeutic programs. With the focus on communication learning, several related issues have been investigated by speech-language pathologists: parent language training, home training, alternative language systems, and language socialization in inclusive classrooms. These components present a more holistic approach to the language learning experience of children with autism (Schwartz & Carta, 1996).

Therapeutic programming varies from child to child, family to family, and clinician to clinician. It is this variety in training approaches and styles that provides the profession with its clinical strength. The developmental differences and needs of children with ASD present a number of challenges for educators, parents, and public officials. Children with ASD require an integrated educational model that facilitates the development of a life cycle philosophical approach for home and school. ASD is, after all, a life-long developmental disability. For a child with ASD, each social context represents an ecology along life's continuum of learning (Kohler & Strain, 1997). Research in the area of therapeutic methodologies stresses the need for adaptive communication in multiple contexts, integration of services, and development of inclusive social learning models. This so-called systems view establishes programming and decision making across a long-term service continuum, from birth through adulthood. In addition, the professional collaborative network must enhance the child's transition from one learning context to another and from one developmental stage to another. Finally, programming itself should focus on the process of learning, rather than specific content (Pierce & Schreibman, 1997).

ALTERNATIVE THERAPIES

Controversies within clinical journals highlight a range of alternative therapies that have not been endorsed by medical or clinical practitioners (Romanczyk, Arnstein, Soorya, & Gillis, 2003). Consider the case of facilitated communication (Biklen, 1993), in which an adult facilitator provides physical support to help a child with autism overcome his or her neuromotor difficulties. This physical support may be provided by helping the child to isolate his or her index finger and/or stabilizing his or her hand, wrist, or arm during a typing process. What is interesting about the technique is its underlying therapeutic premise. The use of facilitated communication is based on the idea that the child with autism is not cognitively impaired but rather has a form of praxis. This motor-processing disorder interferes with the expression of language and communication, and the underlying etiology is clearly different from anything discussed earlier within this chapter (Bebko, Perry, & Bryson, 2003; Mostert, 2001).

Facilitated communication is a controversial form of therapeutic intervention for a number of reasons. As described by Calculator (1992), "This communication technique remains one that is characterized by its ambiguity (e.g., lack of specific teaching process), mystique, recording anecdotes and spiritual underpinning" (p. 18). Calculator noted that facilitated communication exploded on the therapeutic scene before its efficacy had been investigated experimentally. Thus, professionals and parents know little about how or why and/or with whom facilitated communication does and does not work. Calculator noted that experimental investigation is critical because this procedure suggests the need to reevaluate the perception of ASD as a social, cognitive disability. This clearly has important implications for children with autism and other nonverbal, developmentally disordered children.

In the process of analyzing results, advocates for facilitated communication must be responsible for their claims of success. This cannot be another panacea that over time leads parents, teachers, and professionals down a chaotic road. One important question involves how the child with ASD has learned to be literate despite severe communicative, behavioral, and social difficulties. Researchers describe ongoing theoretical and clinical issues related to methodological problems in facilitated communication that have implications for introducing other alternative treatments that have not undergone empirical scrutiny. Researchers must be held accountable for unsubstantiated claims. The chaos created by the successes claimed by "facilitators" has resulted in legal suits and damages.

The information-processing style of children with autism becomes an important issue when adaptive systems are being considered. There are no clear-cut conclusions on the efficacy of any of the intervention systems: sign language, blissymbols, pictorial and written words, communication boards, microcomputers, or facilitated communication. The highly individualized learning styles of children with ASD must also be taken into consideration. The introduction of an adaptive learning system does not mean that the communication learning problems will be resolved automatically. The gestalt processing style in children with autism suggests that the way information is processed must be incorporated into therapeutic decision making. The communication difficulties of children with autism are often offset by extraordinary abilities in memory, visual processing, hyperlectic reading abilities, and mathematical and musical talents. Given the marked discrepancy between the form and the function, the issue for SLPs is attempting to use and integrate the child's skills in teaching communication. The variability in the population is compounded by highly individualized splinter skills in each child; intervention procedures must be matched to the child's learning style and needs.

CREATING NATURAL LEARNING CONTEXTS

Adam's training reflected the pragmatic/semantic issues raised in the literature during the 1990s. In the program described in this section, an attempt was made to incorporate each environment (school, after-school therapy, home, and day care) within the educational process. A set of operating principles was developed to coordinate intervention goals and therapeutic programming with inclusive education in mind. The identified learning contexts and communication behaviors represented a means of recreating communication experiences for Adam. The communication behaviors learned in therapy could be generalized to his home, preschool special education classroom, and day care center.

Since Adam had been enrolled in the Speech and Hearing Center for early intervention services, I attended the Committee on Preschool Special Education (CPSE) meeting when he transitioned into the preschool system. The CPSE consisted of a special education teacher, a school psychologist, a speech/language pathologist from the local school district, Adam's mother, and me. The CPSE functioned as a collaborative team, reviewing all of Adam's evaluations and progress reports.

The language training program that I presented to other members of the team was discussed to determine implementation issues within the recommended special education classroom. The CPSE recommended that Adam's mother and I meet with Adam's preschool teacher to discuss instructional and organizational changes within the classroom that would be required to implement the language program. The team recommended that I function as a teacher consultant within the classroom to provide teacher training and support. The CPSE also asked that I work with Adam's SLP, because language therapy was recommended three times per week as a related service. Adam's mother informed the CPSE that in the afternoon, Adam would be attending an integrated/early childhood program. The coordination of programming and services was not only complicated but time consuming.

To ensure the implementation of the program, the generalization of skills from context to context, and the development of an inclusion program, I met with all of the professionals and the mother on a regular basis. It is important to know that because Adam was receiving programmatic services across diverse settings—preschool special education classroom, early childhood classroom, individual speech language therapy, and private speech language therapy—the collaborative team consisted of the special education teacher, the early childhood teacher, a parent, the SLP, and myself.

The following operating principles were used to develop Adam's learning contexts:

1. A *learning context* was defined as any activity that provided an interactional framework—that is, an opportunity for interchange between the adult and child. The

Table 7.3   **An Example of a Learning Context**

Place	Activity/Context	Materials	Routine	Communicative Behavior
Therapy room	Making bubbles	Bubbles	Get bubbles	Point to object
	Large bubble	Wand	Open bubbles	Gaze at object/adult
		Fan	Get wand	Sign for object
			Pour bubbles (or action)	Consistent vocalization for object (or action)
			Turn fan on	Word
			Make bubbles	Some combination of these behaviors

activity was then described in terms of the type of (a) interactions to be developed, (b) communicative behaviors to be learned, and (c) semantic functions to be closed (see Table 7.3).

2. Each learning context established a task structure to develop an anticipation and sequence of events in the routine.

3. The learning context facilitated action and interaction; it allowed for the development of reversible role relationships between the adult and child.

4. A core lexicon was developed within each learning context to consistently and systematically focus communication and language training across all the adults working with the child.

5. The core lexicon was based on the development of those communicative behaviors that appear earliest in child language. These communicative behaviors were used across a variety of learning contexts to generalize language and communication relations.

6. Communicative interaction was stressed above production of stereotypic/routinized utterances.

7. The learning contexts that were developed were relevant and functional to the child. To facilitate interaction and communication, the adult focused on activities the child preferred.

8. Input to the child was limited in complexity and mean length of utterance. Adult input was functional and relevant to the immediate context and semantically related to the child's vocal, verbal, and nonlinguistic behaviors.

9. The child was presented with a choice of learning contexts; at any time, he could maintain or terminate an activity. Verbal, vocal, and nonverbal behaviors were analyzed within the learning contexts to determine communicative intentions.

10. The child was trained first to participate and interact within the context and second to "talk" about his social experiences.

Table 7.4   **Example of a Communication/Language Description of a Learning Context (Context: Bubbles; Materials: Bottle of Bubbles, Bubble Maker, Fan)**

Semantic Functions	Forms Trained/Adult Input
1. Object	Bubbles, fan
2. Action	Open, blow, give, turn on
3. Agent	Ellen, Adam, Mommy, Daddy
4. Agent + action	Adam open, Ellen open Adam blow, Ellen blow
5. Action + object	Make bubbles, pour bubbles, open bubbles
6. Recurrence	Bubbles . . . bubbles . . . bubbles, more, more bubbles
7. Negation Rejection Cessation (action)	No, no bubbles Stop, no more, no more bubbles No pour, no blow
8. Agent + action + object	Adam open bubbles Ellen open bubbles Mommy open bubbles Adam pour bubbles Ellen pour bubbles Adam blow bubbles Ellen blow bubbles Mommy blow bubbles

11. Every adult working with the child was given a copy of the communication/language description of each learning context. Thus, each teacher provided consistent input within and across activities (see Table 7.4).

12. Echolalic behavior was used to develop language behaviors. With the knowledge that the child would imitate, the adult would code, for instance, a nonlinguistic event:

Event: *Adam opening the bubbles*

Adult: Adam open bubbles.

Adam: Adam open bubbles.

The clinical goals identified for Adam's training included the following:

1. development of imitative interaction skills
2. expansion of object manipulation skills (semantic knowledge)
3. development of sign/gesture forms
4. use of interactional behaviors that signal communicative intentions
5. generalization of communication behaviors

The goals and procedures described in this section were developed based on the need to individualize language and communication programming for Adam. The pragmatic/semantic content was applicable to other children with ASD as well as other children with language disorders. The skills developed in individual therapy needed to become part of the special education classroom curriculum. The primary goal within the classroom, which was highly structured, was to provide opportunities for Adam to engage in social interactions with peers. As a result, the preschool classroom was organized around group activities that facilitated communicative interactions, peer-related behaviors, and functional play.

Children with LCD who present disruptive behaviors tend to be less responsive to peers and do not initiate interactions; this was certainly the case with Adam. The development of social competence was critical if Adam was going to engage in positive interactions with typical peers in day care. Adam needed to develop a level of social performance comparable to children without disabilities if social interaction was going to occur. A social/pragmatic language intervention program is a starting point for children with ASD (Ingersoll, Dvortcsak, Whalen, & Sikora, 2005).

Communication interaction would be the result of predictable interaction routines between two or more people. Once Adam learned to operate within these familiar contexts, event sequences could be altered. Adam's awareness of the environment was noted by observing his reactions to unanticipated change and his attempts to repair the situation. This provided opportunities to facilitate the development of communicative behaviors and interactions between the adult and child or the child and child. It was important to provide Adam with opportunities to initiate and regulate actions, people, and events in his environment. Adam needed to develop a contingency relationship between his behavior and that of his peers; reciprocal interaction was based on such a consequence-based conceptualization.

In attempting to teach Adam to express his needs, the teacher manipulated contextual events to create the need and facilitate its expression. Consider this example:

Context: *Ice cream container cannot be opened by the child.*

Adult: Ellen open ice cream.

Adam: Ellen open ice cream.

Consequence: *Ellen performs action.*

It was important to identify a number of situational contexts that created communicative need. These situations provided Adam with the opportunity to intentionally direct the course of events within the environment. The ultimate goal was to teach Adam that language is a tool, a vehicle, a means to affect the behaviors of other interactants. To achieve this goal, Adam had to experience himself as an effective communicator with his peers.

Generalization of Communication Behaviors through Home Training

A home training program can be used to help children generalize the learning experience to various environments (Kashinath et al., 2006; Tiegerman-Farber & Radziewicz, 2007e). In Adam's case, the home provided a training experience within a more natural environment. Part of the home training program developed for Adam included training parents and siblings as communication facilitators. In addition, a dedicated group of volunteers was trained to work within the framework of the program and to provide extensive training seven days a week—after school and on weekends.

The home training program can be contrasted with the more traditional therapy experience provided for children with ASD in school. A home-based model with parents as facilitators supports a generalization process that cannot be achieved solely by a school-based learning model (Green et al., 2006). Adam's mother was present and integrated into the framework of each session. She was carefully trained by the speech-language pathologist to work with Adam at home.

The home-based program was developed to be a language training program for as long as Adam was awake. In school, the SLP provided language training outside the classroom for thirty minutes three times a week. Coordinating training goals with the classroom teacher was possible but difficult. Another difference concerned the nature of the training experience itself. The home training program focused on the development of language and communication behaviors within all of the training contexts (see Table 7.3). Activities were identified to facilitate interaction and communication. The activity provided a means to an end: adult–child interaction. Nothing had to be simulated. Activities were meaningful and relevant to the child's daily-living needs and the immediate context.

As a language learning experience, the home training program presented certain advantages for Adam:

1. Family members were trained to function as communication facilitators.
2. Various activities within the home provided the means to integrate language behavior with relevant nonlinguistic experiences.
3. The use of communicative behaviors was generalized across learning contexts.
4. The orientation of the program emphasized the child's language and communication needs.

These components were not available to Adam within the traditional special education classroom. Thus, the home training program proved to be an important supplement to traditional learning.

The educational setting has a responsibility to develop formal parent language training programs to provide parents with academic and procedural knowledge (Tiegerman-Farber, 1995). Training parents to function as communication facilitators for children with ASD extends the educational process beyond 3:00 PM to the home context. Parents need to understand language development, language disorders, and language intervention issues if they are going to assist in the educational development of their children. Teaching parents about language and the language needs of their children gives them the tools to do so. To teach parents to understand their children is both the greatest responsibility and the greatest gift of education (Brookman-Frazee, Stahmer, Baker-Ericzén, & Tsai, 2006; Ingersoll & Dvortcsak, 2006).

SOCIAL PROBLEMS AND BEHAVIORAL TECHNOLOGY

Because of the extensive behavioral difficulties characteristic of children with ASD, many clinicians and parents use behavioral procedures to train targeted behaviors, such as self-care and daily-living skills. Behavioral interventions are also used in educational programs to deal with inappropriate and injurious behaviors exhibited within the classroom (Risley, 1996). The classroom teacher may utilize a behavior modification model because of the need to operationalize classroom procedures and training goals. Underlying the behavioral approach is the identification of an observable and measurable targeted performance (e.g., sitting, looking, or vocalizing). For example, rather than target attention as a training performance, the clinician or teacher identifies all of the descriptive behaviors of attention: sitting, physical orientation, eye contact, and so on. These identified behaviors are then trained by means of a successive approximation procedure.

The management difficulties presented by children with ASD have a significant impact on the abilities of educators and parents to integrate them with peers and siblings (Yell & Drasgow, 2000). The behavior problems often exhibited by children with autism—aggression, self-injurious behavior, unanticipated explosive behaviors, self-stimulation, and extraneous verbal–vocal behaviors—often interfere with their acceptance by others within natural settings and complex community contexts (Carter, 2001). The management of severe behavior problems may initially require a combined treatment approach using highly individualized training schedules by means of behavior analysis. Children's behavior can be assessed and functionally analyzed to determine the most appropriate management schedule within the educational setting, the home, and the community. The management of intrusive behaviors requires identifying contingent stages that will be used by a multidisciplinary team of professionals across various learning settings. The combined behavioral approach emphasizes the identification of target behaviors and the need to develop appropriate social learning skills that will be maintained and reinforced by adults and peers (Lopata, Thomeer, Volker, & Nida, 2006). The disruptive behavior of children with ASD often results in social rejection by peers, which further interferes with the educational learning process in integrated settings.

The relationship between language and behavior has recently received a great deal of attention, given the increasing demand for behavioral programs and treatments (Lovaas & Buch, 1997). Some behavioral intervention programs emphasize the primacy of behavior by (1) defining language as just another form of behavior, (2) minimizing the complexity of the language learning process into discrete observable trials, (3) underestimating the significance of the language/communication deficits in children with autism by overemphasizing behavioral deficits, and (4) developing behavioral programs, rather than language learning programs (Tiegerman-Farber & Radziewicz, 2007f). As described by Gallagher (1997):

> Behavioral intervention programs for children who are perceived as habitually noncompliant that use reward systems to shape compliance have made the implicit assumption the children's noncompliance was due to oppositional behaviors, negativity or rebelliousness. The fact that at least some of the children's noncompliance could be due to their inability to understand instructions or directions or to use language to appropriately seek clarifications has been given insufficient attention. The relationship between language and noncompliance needs to be more fully understood given the prevalence of language disorders among children identified as having emotional/behavioral problems. (p. 7)

This position reflects the philosophical approach presented in this chapter.

The child with ASD has pervasive language deficits that limit his or her ability to express feelings, talk about thoughts, solve interpersonal problems, interpret the emotional behaviors of other communicators, and encode/decode interpersonal language (Bloomquist, August, Cohen, Doyle, & Everhart, 1997). Intrapersonal and interpersonal functioning are interrelated and language dependent. The limited emotional vocabulary negatively affects the child's abilities to control his or her emotions and regulate his or her behaviors. The child's emotional/behavioral problems should be viewed as a function of his or her pragmatic and semantic language deficits. This is not a minor issue considering the implications for treatment recommendations and programs.

Brinton and Fujiki (1993) noted that emotional/behavioral problems have been viewed as obstacles to language intervention that need to be addressed before the initiation of language training. The assumption that language problems will decrease if emotional/behavioral problems decrease has not been supported, however. Current studies emphasize the critical role that language serves in facilitating emotional/behavioral functioning (Gallagher, 1996; Prizant et al., 1990).

Given this perspective of the emotional/behavioral needs of children with autism spectrum disorders, the SLP should play a significant role on the inter-/transdisciplinary teams of professionals that are developing language programs for children. It may be time to rethink temper tantrums and self-stimulatory behaviors as indicative of the child's pragmatic/semantic problems. These behaviors are socially penalizing and serve specific communicative needs for the child. After identifying these needs, the SLP can then substitute communicative alternatives that are functionally equivalent but more socially appropriate (Gallagher, 1999).

PEER-MEDIATED COMMUNICATIVE INTERVENTION

The integration of children with ASD in least restrictive classrooms and early childhood programs requires a high degree of specialized programming and teacher training (Grey, Honan, McClean, & Daly, 2005; Scheuermann, Webber, Boutot, & Goodwin, 2003; Zhang & Griffin, 2007). Researchers who advocate for full inclusive programming propose peer-mediated social strategies as a mechanism for facilitating social skills and integration in children with autism. The process of teaching children to teach their peers provides the opportunity to integrate children with ASD in a socially meaningful way (Kalyva & Avramidis, 2005). The proviso, however, is the child's level of social performance comparable to other children without disabilities in the classroom. The greater the discrepancy, the greater the need for highly individualized instruction and the greater the possibility for peer rejection (Tiegerman-Farber & Radziewicz, 1998). If specialists seek to achieve social rather than physical integration of children with ASD, typical peers must be trained.

Guralnick (1999) noted that the point of "child benefit" is not clearly defined for either the child with a disability or his or her typical peer. Teachers are much more comfortable with the inclusion process when children with mild disabilities are involved. Adam was a challenge. Cooperative learning and peer tutoring, in which learners with and without disabilities are brought together to interact and socialize, provide an opportunity for students to develop a social awareness of peer roles, responsibilities, and skills as socialization becomes a primary focus for instruction (Tiegerman-Farber & Radziewicz, 2007f).

The typical language learner can provide peer instruction and modeling for the child with ASD. It becomes important, however, for teachers and adults to educate typical peers and ready them for this instructional opportunity (Odom, 2000). The early childhood classroom plays an important role in the social learning process for many children with developmental disabilities. The child with ASD presents a unique set of learning needs in social and communicative areas. In the effort to improve peer acceptance, it is important for early intervention programs to develop a peer training program; typical learners must be readied and trained to accept learners with different language and social skills (Odom & Diamond, 1998). Activities, interactional experiences, learning contingencies, and educational procedures must all be defined with peer partners in mind. The typical peer and a more socially challenging environment provide an opportunity for language learning and natural environmental contingencies.

The preschool classroom provides the opportunity for naturalistic learning. Milieu teaching approaches include naturalistic language intervention techniques (Hwang & Hughes, 2000). Communicative interactions are facilitated within the context of social activities and conversational interchanges. Clinical research has clearly demonstrated a change in intervention technologies to focus on child-specific, contextual, and interactional variables as the foundation for teaching communication between the child with ASD and typical peers (Frea, Craig, Odom, & Johnson, 1999).

For the child with severe language and communication deficits, early peer experiences by means of dyadic and triadic interchanges provide opportunities for social learning. Peer-mediated communicative interventions provide a means of facilitating social interactions in children with ASD (Odom, 2000). Children with autism usually remain on the outside of social play situations that would naturally provide the very learning stimulation needed. In addition, children with autism have few opportunities to interact with typical peers, given their pervasive behavioral deficits. Peers can be trained to use specific interactional strategies to engage children with autism in various activities and thereby facilitate the social learning process (Taylor & Levin, 1998).

Social scripts can provide the means for controlled interactions between children with and without ASD. Each child learns about the script and his or her own role in it. The script provides the format and the structure for the social interactions among the players (Adams, Gouvousis, VanLue, & Waldron, 2004). Rehearsing the script is very similar to playing the early social games that mothers engage in with their infants. The games provide a limited semantic domain and clearly defined roles for the interactants. With sociodramatic play scripts, typical children can model for the child with ASD and provide ongoing gestural and verbal cues. Research has demonstrated these results in integrated preschool classrooms:

1. Training peers to act as social agents resulted in higher rates of communicative interaction in preschoolers with disabilities.
2. Children with disabilities were equally responsive to teacher and peer input, suggesting that young children without disabilities can take on more directive responsibility for facilitating intervention with peers with ASD.

However, early childhood programs and schools that want to provide inclusive opportunities for children with autism will require organizational changes and funding supports for the following:

- the collaborative development of an inclusion mission for parents and teachers
- physical reconstruction of classrooms and buildings to remove structural barriers to inclusion (Tiegerman-Farber & Radziewicz, 1998)
- teacher training and staff development for regular education and special education teachers on instructional management of diverse learners (Bennett, DeLuca, & Bruns, 1997)
- development of an inclusion curriculum that provides modified instruction for children with autism in the general education classroom
- parent education programs that incorporate families within the educational decision-making process (Guralnick, 1999)

EDUCATIONAL TRENDS

The treatment of children with ASD has presented parents with significant emotional and financial problems, because many of the treatments are based on anecdotal reports, not experimental investigations. Treatments such as sensory integration therapy, auditory integration training, medications, diets, and megavitamins may improve some selected behaviors, but they do not consistently improve general areas of functioning for children with ASD (Heflin & Simpson, 1998).

The trend in educational programming involves the use of applied behavioral analysis (ABA) in early intervention and preschool special education programs, because there has been a great deal of scientific support for its limited effectiveness. Clearly, there are individual differences in children with autism that will affect how they respond to behavioral treatment. Many schools and parents feel that applied behavioral analysis is the treatment of choice because behavioral changes are observable and measurable and parents must be part of the training program to generalize results to natural settings. Also, aside from the management of disruptive behavior, another primary goal is independent functioning (Lovaas, 1999).

One issue, however, is the changing role of the speech-language pathologist. Since language/communication deficits are the central problem for children with ASD, any treatment must involve collaboration among the behavioral specialist, the SLP, and the parent. Applied behavioral analysis may provide a procedural methodology for how some children are taught, but a language learning curriculum determines what children are taught.

ABA is one methodological or instructional approach, and it is not effective for every child with ASD. Many other approaches should be considered, given the diversity of needs within the ASD population (Prizant & Rubin, 1999). Just as there is a continuum of severity within ASD, there should be a continuum of instructional approaches that incorporate the principles of evidence-based practice (Dollaghan, 2004). The SLP should work as a collaborator and consultant to ensure that language and communication behaviors are facilitated by other professionals. The underlying controversy with ABA can best be described by saying that language has structural form, but behavior is not language.

The California Departments of Education and Developmental Services Collaborative Work Group, described in Wolery and Winterling (1997), recommended organizing curriculum around normal developmental expectations by using predictable routines in areas such as social engagement, language, coping, and behavior management. The curriculum focused on skills that are typically deficient in children with ASD, such as socialization and communication. Often, a discussion of curriculum includes teaching methodology; in reality, educators need to develop curricula for early childhood through adolescence (Wolery & Winterling, 1997). In response to increasing demands from parents to provide inclusion and services within local public schools, some state departments of education have developed clinical guides for children with ASD to establish recommendations for best-practice procedures.

Given the fact that autism is now understood to be a severe language and communication disorder, the level of speech therapy services has been described as dramatically inadequate. Language learning must become the primary goal for classroom instruction and not just another related service. The educational curriculum and individualized education plan (IEP) should include language/communication goals and procedures.

Because special education teachers generally have limited academic training in language development and language disorders, many educational programs are now utilizing "push-in" services so that SLPs provide therapeutic services in classrooms. This creates the opportunity to implement collaborative and consultative teaching models. It also enhances a better understanding of instructional methods used by teachers and speech language pathologists. Currently, SLPs spend about 3 percent of their professional time working in classrooms (ASHA, 2002). Classroom-based interventions provide a more natural learning approach given language generalization problems. The push-in model also enhances opportunities for collaborative instruction with special and regular education teachers (Tiegerman-Farber & Radziewicz, 2007f).

Finally, the use of an etiological placement approach provides serious educational problems for children with ASD. Adam's mother noted that "a class of six autistic children is really six one-child classes." Six children who cannot interact and communicate also cannot serve as facilitators for one another. If the need is to develop communication skills, children with autism must be provided with child models who can facilitate such development. A nonetiological educational approach to placement would certainly address this issue. It would also provide children with a less restrictive educational placement and the opportunity to interact with higher-functioning social peers. Peer facilitation would allow for language modeling in the special education classroom.

The placement of children with ASD should be based on language level of functioning, rather than etiological label. To make this a reality, however, state education departments across the United States would have to change their disability categories and (etiologically based) educational placement processes. Enactment of Public Law 99-457 in 1986 mandated educational services for preschool children with disabilities, making the dream of early intervention a reality. Since then, research findings have proven that children with disabilities have a better prognosis the earlier intervention occurs.

THE INCLUSION MANDATE

Both legal support and educational controversy surround the inclusion of all students, including those with severe developmental disabilities, in regular classroom settings (Diehl, Ford, & Federico, 2005; Gena, 2006; Rock, Rosenberg, & Carran, 1995; Zhang & Griffin, 2007). Several research studies have supported the notion that students with severe developmental disabilities can be provided with appropriate educational services in general education classrooms. These studies have also documented the fact that students with severe disabilities can benefit from an inclusive setting, given the expanded opportunities for communication and social interactions between children with and without disabilities.

The Individuals with Disabilities Education Act (IDEA), which was passed in 1975 and amended in 1997 and 2004, emphasizes that inclusive programming during the preschool years, in which children with and without disabilities are integrated by means of socialization experiences, may provide the best opportunity to integrate and manage behavioral–social problems in children with ASD. The early childhood curriculum focuses on daily-living skills, language learning skills, play skills, peer interactions, self-awareness, and independence (Odom, 2000). Preschool programs also provide an important link in educational programming between the classroom and the home environment. Preschool programs often coordinate their goals across educational and therapeutic services by collaborating with parents. Educational and instructional needs identified at home and at school provide the basis for parent–teacher coordination of social and behavioral planning (Tiegerman-Farber & Radziewicz, 2007e).

Children with ASD have great difficulty generalizing learned behaviors to new contexts and situations, so educational programming must begin early. The focus on socialization, peer interactions, and communication behaviors will provide the child with a repertoire of social skills. The child's ability to function within the social context of the classroom, the restaurant, the playground, the mall, and other natural environments is based on the generalized use of social–communicative behaviors. Early intervention programs emphasize learning during a critical period for children with ASD (Ingersoll et al., 2005; NAICS, 2005; NRC, 2001).

Children with severe developmental disabilities can be provided with appropriate social and language models from age-appropriate peers. Children without disabilities will have the humanistic opportunity to acquire an understanding of social values that relate to learning differences between people. Children need to be provided with a curriculum that addresses positive attitudes about a variety of multicultural learners, including children with disabilities.

The failure to appropriately accommodate many students with severe disabilities underscores the difficulties within the public school system to implement and achieve full inclusion (Coffey & Obringer, 2004). Children with autism present severe language and communication deficits, social relational problems, and behavioral management problems (Tiegerman-Farber & Radziewicz, 2007g). The principle of *normalization* that is often raised about inclusive education suggests that the child with ASD will benefit from the regular education experience. Although there may be an attempt to include children with ASD in ongoing social and academic activities, such as reading, math, social studies, and science, their differences in learning require major modifications in teacher instruction, classroom procedures, and peer sensitivity awareness. Part of the decision concerning the appropriateness of a regular classroom for the child with autism should be the ability of educators to substantiate the educational benefit of inclusion for children with and without disabilities.

One criticism of educating children with ASD in the regular classroom is that their education may not be individualized to the same degree it would in a special education classroom. Parents and teachers must carefully consider the individual needs of the child by reviewing various learning options. Inclusion is one of many educational options. It is not the only option, and it certainly is not the option for every child. Parents should never be forced to place their child in a setting they believe will not benefit him or her educationally. The question for educators is whether the regular classroom can be redesigned and restructured as a learning environment that can handle the diverse needs of severely behaviorally impaired children.

Odom (2000) suggests that education must focus on identifying what is in the best interest of the child. Integrating the child with autism into the regular classroom requires a great deal of reorganization and commitment from parents, teachers, and administrators. One significant adaptation in the regular classroom would be to change the responsibilities of paraprofessionals from collecting data to facilitating the integration of children with autism into the least restrictive environment by teaching them functional skills. The paraprofessional's new role would involve implementing instructional programs in school and community environments where these skills will be used (Cook, Cameron, & Tankersley, 2007; Giangreco, Yuan, McKenzie, Cameron, & Fialka, 2005; Groom, 2006; Jameson, McDonnell, Johnson, Riesen, & Polychronis, 2007).

It will be interesting to see in the next several years whether speech assistants are utilized in the same way by SLPs. Given professional concerns about educational standards and requirements for licensure, SLPs may not agree with the idea that the speech assistant is a support to the speech/language program but not a replacement for the speech/language pathologist. In some communities, a licensed SLP supervises several speech assistants because it is cost effective. The instructional and financial demands of inclusive programming in schools may result in this kind of service delivery model. The more SLPs understand language development and learning, the greater the role they will play in educational decision making (Harn, Bradshaw, & Ogletree, 1999).

Summary

Children with ASD have unique language learning problems. Even though they have traditionally been described as a single population, research has stressed the heterogeneity exhibited within this group, suggesting that the etiological label is misleading. In addition, the use of this label detracts from the central problem related to the disorder: the inability to integrate communicative functions with other aspects of language.

The research describes a schism between form and function in children with basic language disturbances in pragmatic and semantic skills; phonological and syntactic skills develop relatively intact. In fact, the literature describing the language of higher-functioning children with ASD indicates severe communicative deficits in contrast to the almost normal acquisition of structural linguistic skills. Such communicative deficits include ongoing problems with initiating and terminating interaction, topic maintenance, and speaker/listener roles.

Finally, the changing role of the speech-language pathologist has changed dramatically over the past several years. SLPs are now working in schools, hospitals, homes, and many other settings to address the needs of children with ASD. SLPs must expand their knowledge to include skills related to collaboration, parent training, advocacy, and counseling.

Treatment of children with ASD must involve language-based educational programming during the infant and preschool years. The changes in child language theory have contributed greatly to the new therapeutic approaches used with children such as Adam. In a way, Adam is a product of the pragmatic era and the communication revolution. At this point, the impact of these theoretical and therapeutic changes on children with ASD can only be imagined.

Finally, the SLP has a central role to play in the educational programming developed for children with ASD. No other professional can better understand the language and communication deficits underlying this disorder.

Case Study   A. J.

The significance of language has broad implications not only for education but for other related areas, such as the law. I recently received a legal brief describing a young man (A. J.) diagnosed with Asperger syndrome who was being tried for murder and for whom the death penalty was being considered. A group of legal specialists contacted me concerning A. J.'s competency and sanity to stand trial, given his disorder.

Competency is a threshold requirement that involves an individual's ability to participate in his or her own defense and understand the implications of his or her actions. If the court deems that an individual is competent to stand trial, the next phase is the potential determination of mental illness: insanity by means of psychiatric evaluations. Competency is obviously a lower standard; an individual may be competent to stand trial but later found to be insane. The definition of *insanity* is as follows (New York Penal Law Section 40.15):

> A person is not criminally responsible for conduct if at the time of such conduct as a result of mental disease or defect, he lacks substantial capacity:
>
> a. to know or appreciate the wrongfulness of the conduct, or
> b. to conform his conduct to the requirements of the law.

Asperger syndrome is one of several disorders on the continuum of autism spectrum disorders (ASD). As discussed in this chapter, individuals with ASD have three primary areas of impairment: social behavior, language, and stereotypical patterns of behavior. The critical relationship between language and cognition is underscored by research findings related to theory of mind. The key question for consideration is, What do individuals with disabilities understand and think as a function of their language deficits?

Theory of mind refers to the ability to attribute mental states to oneself and other people as a means of understanding behavior. Research has indicated that children with ASD perform worse on theory-of-mind tests than language- or mental age–matched children. There is strong evidence that children with ASD have a specific impairment in interpreting human action within a mentalistic framework—what Baron-Cohen (1995) refers to as "mindblindness." In addition, the deficits in theory of mind are closely related to language deficits. Tager-Flusberg (1999) stated that "a deficit in theory of mind is central to how we interpret autism because human and social behavior depends on our understanding that people with whom we interact are intentional mental beings" (p. 4).

A. J., the young man with Asperger syndrome, had been diagnosed with a disability as a preschool child. Over the years, as his behavior became progressively more disruptive, he was reevaluated using various psychological measures.

It is my contention that the competency/insanity definitions cannot be applied to individuals with Asperger syndrome for the following reasons:

1. Competency to stand trial is based on an IQ test, and insanity is based on a psychiatric interview.
2. An IQ test does not adequately measure language deficits and certainly cannot determine specific impairments, such as mindblindness.
3. The determination of competency, based on an IQ test, does not identify a spectrum of language and social problems.
4. The assumption of competency is based on a performance level on an IQ test as well as the individual's understanding of his behavioral conformance.
5. An individual with a disability could have an average IQ but also a severe language/communication disorder (mindblindness) or other disability, which the IQ test would not measure or identify.

The present definition of competency should apply only to individuals who do not have a documented history of developmental disabilities, because it makes accommodations for (1) the individual with insanity (mental disease), who would be disqualified by means of a psychiatric evaluation, and (2) the individual with mental retardation (lacks capacity to understand), who would be disqualified by means of the IQ test. The problem for the individual with Asperger syndrome is that if a disorder such as mindblindness is not tested for, then it is not believed to exist. Thus, the individual would be considered competent to stand trial. This clearly discriminates against individuals with ASD and other disabilities. The issue is thus A. J.'s capacity to *understand.*

The legal history related to competency/insanity evolved prior to passage of IDEA in 1975. The competency/insanity standard was developed to rule out individuals who did not understand the implications of their actions. IDEA requires a multidisciplinary evaluation to determine disability. The tests utilized by the courts to determine competency—IQ tests and psychiatric evaluations, either individually or in combination—are not considered sufficient to determine a developmental disability by IDEA standards.

Given that A. J. was classified as developmentally disabled under IDEA, how can the court utilize (1) a less comprehensive standard of review to determine his competency (in fact, a lower standard) and (2) an assessment protocol that could not have been utilized to identify his disabilities to begin with? The IQ test and psychiatric evaluations cannot be used to determine that A. J. has a disability or his specific impairment of mindblindness. If A. J.'s disability cannot be identified by the present protocol, then is he competent to stand trial? The implication here is that the process of determination to stand trial and be considered for the death penalty is less comprehensive than the process of determination for a developmental disability.

Analyzing this scenario from another direction, consider that A. J. was classified as having a disability when he was a preschooler. Even with this information, the court used only an IQ test and psychiatric evaluation to determine his competency and sanity to stand trial. Should consideration also have been given to the fact that A. J. had a developmental disability and, more specifically, a condition referred to as *mindblindness* that could have affected his capacity to know the wrongfulness of his conduct and to conform to the requirements of the law? It is also important to remember that the theory-of-mind research, as well as the impairment mindblindness, represent relatively new areas of inquiry and investigation. There are only a few specialists who understand this impairment and even fewer assessment measures to identify the impairment.

Based on what little is known about mindblindness and the inadequacy of the competency/insanity protocol to identify such disabilities, should not the court reconsider its decision? The ability of the court to assess A. J.'s understanding was limited by tests that cannot evaluate his mindblindness impairment. I would have to argue that A. J.'s understanding and, as a result, his competency to stand trial should be reevaluated.

The terms *competency* and *insanity,* as they are presently defined, discriminate against individuals with disabilities, particularly those with language and social impairments that are not appropriately assessed by IQ tests and psychiatric evaluations and that result in deficits such as mindblindness. I recommend that the standard of competency, which is a lower standard of review, must be replaced by a more stringent IDEA standard of review for individuals with disabilities. Our expanding knowledge of language disorders presents a case for a legal reconsideration of what is meant by the phrase "competent to stand trial."

Study Questions

1. What is the definition of autism spectrum disorders and how has the definition changed over the past several years?
2. How do the behavioral characteristics of children with autism spectrum disorders affect their social relationships with peers in natural settings?
3. Compare the language characteristics of children with autism and children with mental retardation. Explain how these characteristics are the same and/or different in each population.
4. Describe the various intervention strategies that can be used to develop language in children with autism spectrum disorders.
5. Explain why parent training is important to the success of any therapeutic program developed for children with autism spectrum disorders served in clinical settings.

References

Adams, A., & Gathercole, S. (1995). Phonological working memory and speech. Production in preschool children. *Journal of Speech and Hearing Research, 38*(2), 403.

Adams, L., Gouvousis, A., VanLue, M., & Waldron, C. (2004). Social story intervention: Improving communication skills in a child with autism spectrum disorders. *Focus on Autism and Other Developmental Disabilities, 19*(2), 87–94.

American Psychiatric Association (APA). (2000). *Diagnostic and statistical manual of mental disorders* (text revision) (*DSM-IV-TR*). Washington, DC: Author.

American Speech-Language-Hearing Association (ASHA). (2002). *FAQ: Helping children with communication disorders in the schools—Speaking, listening, reading, and writing.* Retrieved May 14, 2007, from http://www.asha.org/public/speech/development/schools_faq.htm.

Bailey, A., Phillips, W., & Rutter, M. (1996). Autism: Towards an integration of clinical, genetic, neuropsychological, and neurobiological perspectives. *Journal of Child Psychology and Psychiatry, 37,* 89–126.

Baron-Cohen, S. (1995). *Mindblindness: An essay on autism and theory of mind.* Cambridge, MA: MIT Press.

Baron-Cohen, S. (1998). Does the study of autism justify minimal innate modularity? *Learning and Individual Differences, 10*(3), 179.

Bartak, L., & Rutter, M. (1976). Differences between mentally retarded and normally intelligent autistic children. *Journal of Autism and Childhood Schizophrenia, 6,* 109–120.

Bartak, L., Rutter, M., & Cox, A. (1975). A comparative study of infantile autism and specific developmental receptive language disorder. Vol. 1: The children. *British Journal of Psychiatry, 126,* 127–145.

Bebko, J. M., Perry, A., & Bryson, S. (2003). Commentary: Bebko, Perry, and Bryson on Mostert (2001), "Facilitated communication since 1995." *Journal of Autism and Developmental Disorders, 33*(2), 219.

Bennett, T., DeLuca, D., & Bruns, D. (1997). Putting inclusion into practice: Perspectives of teacher and parents. *Exceptional Children, 64,* 115–131.

Bennett, T., Szatmari, P., Bryson, S., Volden, J., Zwaigenbaum, L., Vaccarella, L., Duku, E., & Boyle, M. (2008). Differentiating autism and Asperger syndrome on the basis of language delay or impairment. *Journal of Autism and Developmental Disorders, 38*(4), 616–625.

Bernabei, P., Cerquiglini, A., Cortesi, F., & D'Ardia, C. (2007). Regression versus no regression in the autistic disorder: Developmental trajectories. *Journal of Autism and Developmental Disorders, 37*(3), 580–588.

Bernard-Opitz, V. (1982). Pragmatic analysis of the communicative behavior of an autistic child. *Journal of Speech and Hearing Disorders, 47,* 99–109.

Bettelheim, B. (1967). *The empty fortress: Infantile autism and the birth of the self.* New York: Free Press.

Biklen, D. (1993). *Communication unbound: How facilitated communication is challenging traditional views of autism and ability/disability* (Special Education Series no. 13). New York: Teachers College Press.

Bishop, D., North, T., & Dolan, C. (1995). Genetic basis of specific language impairment: Evidence from a twin study. *Developmental Medicine and Child Neurology, 37,* 56–71.

Bloomquist, M., August, G., Cohen, C., Doyle, A., & Everhart, K. (1997). Social problem solving in hyperactive-aggressive children: How and what they think in conditions of automatic and controlled processing. *Journal of Clinical Child Psychology, 26*(2), 127–180.

Bornstein, M., & Brown, E. (1996). Patterns of stability and continuity in attention across early infancy. *Journal of Reproductive and Infant Psychology, 14*(3), 195.

Bradley, A. (2007). Federal study documents rates of autism disorders in fourteen states. *Education Week, 26*(23), 6.

Brinton, B., & Fujiki, M. (1993). Language, social skills and socioemotional behavior. *Language, Speech, and Hearing Services in Schools, 24,* 194–198.

Brook, S., & Bowler, D. (1992). Autism by another name? Semantic and pragmatic impairments in children. *Journal of Autism and Development Disorders, 22,* 61–81.

Brookman-Frazee, L., Stahmer, A., Baker-Ericzén, M. J., & Tsai, K. (2006). Parenting interventions for children with autism spectrum and disruptive behavior disorders: Opportunities for cross-fertilization. *Clinical Child and Family Psychology Review, 9*(3/4), 181–200.

Calculator, S. (1992). Perhaps the emperor has clothes after all: A response to Biklen (1992). *American Journal of Speech Language Pathology,* 18–20.

Calloway, C., Myles, B., & Earles, T. (1999). The development of communicative functions and means in students with autism. *Focus on Autism and Other Developmental Disabilities, 14*(3), 140.

Carter, C. M. (2001). Using choice with game play to increase language skills and interactive behaviors in children with autism. *Journal of Positive Behavior Interventions, 3,* 131–151.

Coffey, K. M., & Obringer, S. J. (2004). A case study on autism: School accommodations and inclusive settings. *Education, 124*(4), 632–639.

Conti-Ramsden, G., & Botting, N. (1999). Classification of children with specific language impairment: Longitudinal considerations. *Journal of Speech, Language and Hearing Research, 42*(5), 1195. Retrieved from www.ehostvgw6.epnet.com.

Cook, B. G., Cameron, D. L., & Tankersley, M. (2007). Inclusive teachers' attitudinal ratings of their students with disabilities. *Journal of Special Education, 40*(4), 230–238.

Craig, H. K., & Telfer, A. S. (2005). Hyperlexia and autism spectrum disorder: A case study of scaffolding language growth over time. *Topics in Language Disorders. Language Disorders and Learning Disabilities: A Look across 25 Years, 25*(4), 364–374.

Crooke, P., Hendrix, R., & Rachman, J. (2008). Brief report: Measuring the effectiveness of teaching social thinking to children with Asperger syndrome (AS) and high functioning autism (HFA). *Journal of Autism and Developmental Disorders, 38*(3), 581–591.

DeMyer, M., Barton, S., DeMyer, E., Norton, J., Allen, J., & Steele, R. (1973). Prognosis in autism: A follow-up study. *Journal of Autism and Childhood Schizophrenia, 3,* 199–216.

Diehl, S., Ford, C., & Federico, J. (2005). The communication journey of a fully included child with autism spectrum disorder. *Topics of Language Disorders, 25*(4), 375–387.

DiLavore, P., Lord, C., & Rutter, M. (1995). The pre-linguistic autism diagnostic observation schedule. *Journal of Autism and Developmental Disorders, 25,* 355–379.

Dollaghan, C. (2004, April 13). Evidence-based practice: Myths and realities. *ASHA Leader,* 4–5, 12.

Fish, B., Shapiro, T., & Campbell, M. (1966). Long-term prognosis and the response of schizophrenic children to drug therapy: A controlled study of trifluoperazine. *American Journal of Psychiatry, 123,* 32–39.

Folstein, S. (1999). Autism: Autistic children. *International Review of Psychiatry, 11*(4), 269.

Folstein, S. (2006). The clinical spectrum of autism. *Clinical Neuroscience Research, 6*(3/4), 113–117.

Folstein, S., & Mankoski, R. (2000). Chromosome 7q: Where autism meets language disorder? *American Journal of Human Genetics, 67,* 278–281.

Frea, W., Craig, L., Odom, S., & Johnson, D. (1999). Differential effects of structured social integration and group friendship activities for promoting social interaction with peers. *Journal of Early Intervention, 22,* 230–242.

Gallagher, P. (1997). Promoting dignity: Taking the destructive D's out of behavior disorders. *Focus on Exceptional Children, 29*(9), 1–19.

Gallagher, T. (1996). Social-interactional approaches to child language intervention. In J. Beitchman & M. Konstatareas (Eds.), *Language, learning and behavior problems: Emerging perspectives* (pp. 418–435). Cambridge, England: Cambridge University Press.

Gallagher, T. (1999). Interrelationships among children's language, behavior, and emotional problems. *Topics in Language Disorders, 19*(2), 1–15.

Gena, A. (2006). The effects of prompting and social reinforcement on establishing social interactions with peers during the inclusion of four children with autism in preschool. *International Journal of Psychology, 41*(6), 541–554.

Giangreco, M. F., Yuan, S., McKenzie, B., Cameron, P., & Fialka, J. (2005). "Be careful what you wish for . . .": Five reasons to be concerned about the assignment of individual paraprofessionals. *Teaching Exceptional Children, 37*(5), 28–34.

Gilger, J. (1995). Behavioral genetics: Concepts for research and practice in language development and disorders. *Journal of Speech and Hearing Research, 38*(5), 1126–1142. Retrieved from http://www.ehostvgw6.epnet.com.

Goldstein, H. (2002). Communication intervention for children with autism: A review of treatment efficacy. *Journal of Autism and Developmental Disorders, 32*(5), 373–396.

Green, B. L., Everhart, M., Gordon, L., & Gettman, M. G. (2006). Including parent training in the early childhood special education curriculum for children with autism spectrum disorders. *Topics in Early Childhood Special Education, 26*(3), 179–187.

Green, V. A., Sigafoos, J., Pituch, K. A., Itchon, J., O'Reilly, M., & Lancioni, G. E. (2006). Assessing behavioral flexibility in individuals with developmental disabilities. *Focus on Autism and Other Developmental Disabilities, 21*(4), 2320–236.

Greenspan, S., & Wieder, S. (1997). Learning to interact. *Scholastic Early Childhood Today, 12*(3), 23–24.

Grey, I. M., Honan, R., McClean, B., & Daly, M. (2005). Evaluating the effectiveness of teacher training in applied behaviour analyses. *Journal of Intellectual Disabilities, 9*(3), 209–227.

Groom, B. (2006). Building relationships for learning: The developing role of the teaching assistant. *Support for Learning, 21*(4), 199–203.

Guralnick, M. (1999). The nature and meaning of social integration for young children with mild developmental delays in inclusive settings. *Journal of Early Intervention, 22,* 70–86.

Happe, F. (1994). *Autism: An introduction to psychological theory.* London: University College London Press.

Harn, W., Bradshaw, L., & Ogletree, B. (1999). The speech-language pathologist in the schools: Changing roles. *Intervention in School and Clinic, 34*(3), 163.

Harris, S., Handleman, J., Gordon, R., Kristoff, B., & Fuentes, F. (1991). Changes in cognitive and language functioning of preschool children with autism. *Journal of Autism and Developmental Disorders, 21,* 281–290.

Heflin, L., & Simpson, R. (1998). Interventions for children and youth with autism: Prudent choices in a world of exaggerated claims and empty promises. Part I: Intervention and treatment option review. *Focus on Autism and Other Developmental Disabilities, 13,* 194–211.

Hughes, C., & Russell, J. (1993). Autistic children's difficulty with mental disengagement from an object: Its implications for theories of autism. *Developmental Psychology, 29*(3), 498–510.

Hurford, J. (1991). The evolution of the critical period for language acquisition. *Cognition, 40,* 159–201.

Hwang, B., & Hughes, C. (2000). Increasing early social-communicative skills of preverbal preschool children with autism through social interactive training. *Journal of the Association for Persons with Severe Handicaps, 25,* 18–28.

Ingersoll, B., & Dvortcsak, A. (2006). Including parent training in the early childhood special education curriculum for children with autism spectrum disorders. *Journal of Positive Behavior Interventions, 8*(2), 79–87.

Ingersoll, B., Dvortcsak, A., Whalen, C., & Sikora, D. (2005). The effect of a developmental, social-pragmatic language intervention on expressive language skills in young children with autistic spectrum disorders. *Focus on Autism and Other Developmental Disabilities, 20,* 213–222.

Jameson, J. M., McDonnell, J., Johnson, J. W., Riesen, T., & Polychronis, S. (2007). A comparison of one-to-one embedded instruction in the general education classroom and one-to-one massed practice instruction in the special education classroom. *Education and Treatment of Children, 30*(1), 23–44.

Kalyva, E., & Avramidis, E. (2005). Improving communication between children with autism and their peers through the "circle of friends": A small-scale intervention study. *Journal of Applied Research in Intellectual Disabilities, 18*(3), 253–261.

Kanner, L. (1943). Autistic disturbances in affective contact. *Nervous Child, 2,* 217–250.

Kasari, C., Freeman, S., & Paparella, T. (2007). Interventions targeting joint attention and symbolic play can improve aspects of these skills in young children with autism. *Evidence-Based Mental Health, 10*(1), 21.

Kashinath, S., Woods, J., & Goldstein, H. (2006). Enhancing generalized teaching strategy use in daily routines by parents of children with autism. *Journal of Speech, Language and Hearing Research, 49*(3), 466–485.

Kobayashi, R., & Murata, T. (1998). Behavioral characteristics of 187 young adults with autism. *Psychiatry and Clinical Neuroscience, 52,* 383–390.

Kohler, F. W., & Strain, P. S. (1997). Combining incidental teaching and peer mediation with young children with autism. *Journal of Autism and Related Disorders, 12,* 196–206.

Krug, D., Arick, J., & Almond, P. (1993). *Examiner's manual. Autism Screening Instrument for Educational Planning* (2nd ed.). Austin, TX: Pro-Ed.

Lewis, B., Cox, N., & Byard, P. (1993). Segregation analysis of speech and language disorders. *Behavior Genetics, 23,* 291–299.

Lifter, K., Sulzer-Azaroff, B., Anderson, S., & Cowdery, G. (1993). Teaching play activities to preschool children with disabilities: The importance of developmental considerations. *Journal of Early Intervention, 17*(2), 139–159.

Lopata, C., Thomeer, M., Volker, M., & Nida, R. (2006). Effectiveness of cognitive-behavioral treatment on the social behaviors of children with Asperger disorder. *Focus on Autism and Other Developmental Disabilities, 21*(4), 237–244.

Lord, C., & Luyster, R. (2006). Early diagnosis of children with autism spectrum disorders. *Clinical Neuroscience Research, 6*(3/4), 189–194.

Lord, C., Rutter, M., & LeCouteur, A. (1994). Autism Diagnostic Interview—Revised (ADI—R): A revised version of a diagnostic interview for caregivers of individuals with possible pervasive developmental disorders. *Journal of Autism and Developmental Disorders, 24,* 659–685.

Lotter, V. (1967). Epidemiology of autistic conditions in young children: Some characteristics of parents and children. *Social Psychiatry, 1,* 163–181.

Lovaas, O. (1999). Experimental design and cumulative research in early behavioral intervention. In *Johns Hopkins Twentieth Annual Spectrum in Developmental Disabilities.* Timonium, MD: York.

Lovaas, O., & Buch, G. (1997). Intensive behavioral intervention with young children with autism. In N. N. Singh (Ed.), *Prevention and treatment of severe behavior problems: Models and methods in developmental disabilities* (pp. 61–86). Pacific Grove, CA: Brooks/Cole.

Loveland, K., Landry, S., Hughes, S., Hall, S., & McEvoy, R. (1988). Speech acts and the pragmatic deficits of autism. *Journal of Speech and Hearing Research, 31,* 593–604.

MacDonald, R., Green, G., Mansfield, R., Geckeler, A., Gardenier, N., Anderson, J., Holcomb, W., & Sanchez, J. (2007). Stereotypy in young children with autism and typically developing children. *Research in Developmental Disabilities, 28*(3), 266–277.

Macintosh, K. E., & Dissanayake, C. (2004). Annotation: The similarities and differences between autistic disorder and Asperger's disorder. A review of the empirical evidence. *Journal of Child Psychology and Psychiatry, 45,* 421–434.

Macintosh, K., & Dissanayake, C. (2006). Social skills and problem behaviours in school aged children with high-functioning autism and Asperger's disorder. *Journal of Autism and Developmental Disorders, 36*(8), 1065–1076.

Maestro, S., Muratori, F., Cavallaro, M. C., Pei, F., Stern, D., Golse, B., & Palacio-Espasa, F. (2002). Attentional skills during the first 6 months of age in autism spectrum disorder. *Journal of the American Academy of Child and Adolescent Psychiatry, 41*(10), 1239–1245.

Maestro, S., Muratori, F., Cavallaro, M. C., Pecini, C., Cesari, A., Paziente, A., Stern, D., Golse, B., & Palacio-Espasa, F. (2005). How young children treat objects and people: An empirical study of the first year of life in autism. *Child Psychiatry and Human Development, 35*(4), 383–396.

Miller, J. (1996). The search for the phenotype of disordered language performance. In M. Rice (Ed.), *Toward a genetics of language* (pp. 297–314). Mahwah, NJ: Lawrence Erlbaum.

Mostert, M. P. (2001). Facilitated communication since 1995: A review of published studies. *Journal of Autism and Developmental Disorders, 31*(3), 287–313.

Mundy, P., Sigman, M., & Kasari, C. (1994). Nonverbal communication, developmental level and symptom presentation in autism. *Development and Psychopathology, 6,* 389–401.

NAICS. (2005). The usage and perceived outcomes of early intervention and early childhood programs for young children with autism spectrum disorder. *Topics in Early Childhood Special Education, 25*(4), 195–207.

National Research Council (NRC). (2001). *Educating children with autism.* Washington, DC: National Academy Press.

Newsom, C., Carr, E., & Lovaas, O. (1979). The experimental analysis and modification of autistic behavior. In R. S. Davidson (Ed.), *Modification of pathological behavior.* New York: Gardner.

Odom, S. (2000). Preschool inclusion: What we know and where we go from here. *Topics in Early Childhood Special Education, 20*(1), 20.

Odom, S. L., & Diamond, K. E. (1998). Inclusion of young children with special needs in early childhood education: The research base. *Early Childhood Research Quarterly, 13*, 3–25.

Ogletree, B., & Fischer, M. (1995). An innovative language treatment for a child with high-functioning autism. *Focus on Autistic Behavior, 10*(3), 10.

Olley, J. (1999). Curriculum for students with autism. *School Psychology Review, 28*(1), 595.

Osterling, J. A., Dawson, G., & Munson, J. A. (2002). Early recognition of 1-year-old infants with autism spectrum disorder versus mental retardation. *Development and Psychopathology, 14*, 239–251.

Patti, P., & Lupinetti, L. (1993). Brief report: Implications of hyperlexia in an autistic savant. *Journal of Autism and Developmental Disorders, 23*(2), 397–404.

Pennington, B., Rogers, S., Bennetto, L., Griffith, E., Reed, D., & Shyu, V. (1998). Validity test of the executive dysfunction hypothesis of autism. In J. Russell (Ed.), *Executive functioning in autism.* Oxford, England: Oxford University Press.

Peppé, S., McCann, J., Gibbon, F., O'Hare, A., & Rutherford, M. (2006). Assessing prosodic and pragmatic ability in children with high-functioning autism. *Journal of Pragmatics, 38*(10), 1776–1791.

Piaget, J. (1962). *Play, dreams, and imitation in childhood.* New York: Norton.

Pierce, K., & Schreibman, L. (1997). Using peer training to promote social behavior in autism: Are they effective at enhancing multiple social modalities? *Focus on Autism and Other Developmental Disabilities, 12*(4), 207.

Prior, M., & Hoffmann, W. (1990). Brief report: Neuropsychological testing of autistic children through an exploration with frontal lobe tests. *Journal of Autism and Developmental Disorders, 20*, 581–590.

Prizant, B. (1983). Language acquisition and communicative behavior in autism: Toward an understanding of the "whole" of it. *Journal of Speech and Hearing Disorders, 46*, 241–249.

Prizant, B., Audet, L., Burke, G., Hummel, L., Maher, S., & Theadore, G. (1990). Communication disorders and emotional/behavioral disorders in children and adolescents. *Journal of Speech and Hearing Disorders, 55*, 179–192.

Prizant, B., & Duchan, J. (1981). The functions of immediate echolalia in autistic children. *Journal of Speech and Hearing Disorders, 46*, 241–249.

Prizant, B., & Rubin, E. (1999). Contemporary issues in interventions for autism spectrum disorders: A commentary. *Journal of the Association for Persons with Severe Handicaps, 24*(3), 199–208.

Prizant, B., & Rydell, P. (1984). Analysis of functions of delayed echolalia in autistic children. *Journal of Speech and Hearing Research, 27*, 183–192.

Prizant, B., & Wetherby, A. (1987). Communicative intent: A framework for understanding social-communicative behavior in autism. *Journal of the American Academy of Child and Adolescent Psychiatry, 26*, 472–479.

Rapin, I., & Dunn, M. (2003). Update on the language disorders of individuals on the autistic spectrum. *Brain and Development, 25*(3), 166–172.

Richler, J., Bishop, S., Kleinke, J., & Lord, C. (2007). Restricted and repetitive behaviors in young children with autism spectrum disorders. *Journal of Autism & Developmental Disorders, 37*(1), 73–85.

Risley, T. (1996). Get a life. In R. Koegel, L. Koegel, & G. Dunlap (Eds.), *Positive behavior support* (pp. 425–437). Baltimore, MD: Paul H. Brookes.

Rock, E., Rosenberg, M., & Carran, D. (1995). Variables affecting the reintegration rate of students with serious emotional disturbance. *Exceptional Children, 61*(3), 254–268.

Romanczyk, R. G., Arnstein, L., Soorya, L. V., & Gillis, J. (2003). The myriad of controversial treatments for autism: A critical evaluation of efficacy. In S. O. Lilienfeld, S. J. Lynn, & J. M. Lohr (Eds.), *Science and pseudoscience in clinical psychology* (pp. 363–395). New York: Guilford Press.

Rubin, E. (2007). A unique mind: Learning style differences in Asperger's syndrome and high-functioning autism. *ASHA Leader, 12*(1), 10–11.

Russell, J. (1997). How executive disorders can bring about an inadequate theory of mind. In J. Russell (Ed.), *Autism as an executive disorder.* Oxford, England: Oxford University Press.

Russell, J., Mauthner, N., Sharpe, S., & Tidswell, T. (1991). The "window task" as a measure of strategic deception in preschoolers and autistic subjects. *British Journal of Developmental Psychology, 9,* 331–349.

Scheuermann, B., Webber, J., Boutot, E. A., & Goodwin, M. (2003). Problems with personnel preparation in autism spectrum disorders. *Focus on Autism and Other Developmental Disabilities, 18*(3), 197–206.

Schopler, E., Reichler, R., Bashford, A., Lansing, M., & Marcus, L. (1990). *Psychoeducational Profile–Revised (PEP–R).* Austin, TX: Pro-Ed.

Schopler, E., Reichler, R., & Rennet, B. (1998). *The Childhood Autism Rating Scale (CARS).* Los Angeles: Western Psychological Services.

Schwartz, I., & Carta, J. (1996). Examining the use of recommended language intervention practices in early childhood special education classrooms. *Topics in Early Childhood Special Education, 16*(2), 251.

Shriver, M., Allen, K., & Mathews, J. (1999a). Effective assessment of the shared and unique characteristics of children with autism. *School Psychology Review, 28*(1), 538.

Shriver, M., Allen, K., & Mathews, J. (1999b). Introduction to the mini-series: Assessment and treatment of children with autism in the schools. *School Psychology Review, 28*(1), 535.

Sigman, M., & Ungerer, J. (1984). Cognitive and language skills in autistic, mentally retarded, and normal children. *Developmental Psychology, 20,* 293–302.

Siperstein, R., & Volkmar, F. (2004). Brief report: Parental reporting of regression in children with pervasive developmental disorders. *Journal of Autism and Developmental Disorders, 34*(6), 731–734.

Steege, M. W., Mace, F. C., Perry, L., & Longenecker, H. (2007). Applied behavior analysis: Beyond discrete trial teaching. *Psychology in the Schools, 44*(1), 91–99.

Strain, P., & Cordisco, L. (1994). LEAP preschool. In S. L. Harris & J. S. Handleman (Eds.), *Preschool education programs for children with autism* (pp. 225–244). Austin, TX: Pro-Ed.

Tager-Flusberg, H. (1999). A psychological approach to understanding the social and language impairments in autism. *International Review of Psychiatry, 11*(4), 235. Retrieved from http://www.ehostvgw6.epnet.com.

Taylor, B., & Levin, L. (1998). Teaching a student with autism to make verbal initiations: Effects of a tactile prompt. *Journal of Applied Behavior Analysis, 31*(4), 651–654.

Tiegerman-Farber, E. (1995). *Language and communication intervention in preschool children.* Boston: Allyn & Bacon.

Tiegerman-Farber, E., & Radziewicz, C. (1998). *Collaborative decision making: The pathway to inclusion.* Upper Saddle River, NJ: Prentice Hall.

Tiegerman-Farber, E., & Radziewicz, C. (2007a). Language disorders in infants and toddlers. In E. Tiegerman-Farber & C. Radziewicz (Eds.), *Language disorders in children: Real families, real issues, and real interventions* (pp. 37–74). Upper Saddle River, NJ: Prentice Hall.

Tiegerman-Farber, E., & Radziewicz, C. (2007b). Collaborative language assessment and decision making for infants and toddlers. In E. Tiegerman-Farber & C. Radziewicz (Eds.), *Language disorders in children: Real families, real issues, and real interventions* (pp. 75–110). Upper Saddle River, NJ: Prentice Hall.

Tiegerman-Farber, E., & Radziewicz, C. (2007c). Collaborative language assessment and decision making in preschool. In E. Tiegerman-Farber & C. Radziewicz (Eds.), *Language disorders in children: Real families, real issues, and real interventions* (pp. 206–225). Upper Saddle River, NJ: Prentice Hall.

Tiegerman-Farber, E., & Radziewicz, C. (2007d). Language differences in preschool. In E. Tiegerman-Farber & C. Radziewicz (Eds.), *Language disorders in children: Real families, real issues, and real interventions* (pp. 160–187). Upper Saddle River, NJ: Prentice Hall.

Tiegerman-Farber, E., & Radziewicz, C. (2007e). Language interventions for infants and toddlers. In E. Tiegerman-Farber & C. Radziewicz (Eds.), *Language disorders in children: Real families, real issues, and real interventions* (pp. 111–127). Upper Saddle River, NJ: Prentice Hall.

Tiegerman-Farber, E., & Radziewicz, C. (2007f). Language interventions and professional collaboration in preschool. In E. Tiegerman-Farber & C. Radziewicz (Eds.), *Language disorders in children: Real families, real issues, and real interventions* (pp. 226–256). Upper Saddle River, NJ: Prentice Hall.

Tiegerman-Farber, E., & Radziewicz, C. (2007g). Language disorders in elementary school. In E. Tiegerman-Farber & C. Radziewicz (Eds.), *Language disorders in children: Real families, real issues, and real interventions* (pp. 285–315). Upper Saddle River, NJ: Prentice Hall.

Volkmar, F. R., Chawarska, K., & Klin, A., (2005). Autism in infancy and early childhood. *Journal of the Annual Review of Psychology, 56,* 315–336.

Volkmar, F. R., Lord, C., Bailey, A., Schultz, R. T., & Klin, A. (2004). Autism and pervasive developmental disorders. *Journal of Child Psychology and Psychiatry, 45,* 135–170.

Wetherby, A., & Gaines, B. (1982). Cognition and language development in autism. *Journal of Speech and Hearing Research, 47,* 63–71.

Williams, J. G., Higgins, J. P. T., & Brayne, C. E. G. (2006). Systematic review of prevalence studies of autism spectrum disorders. *Archives of Disease in Childhood, 91*(1), 8–15.

Wimpory, D. C., Hobson, R. P., Williams, J. M., & Nash, S. (2000). Are infants with autism socially engaged? A study of recent retrospective parental reports. *Journal of Autism and Developmental Disorders, 30,* 525–536.

Windsor, J., & Doyle, S. (1994). Language acquisition after mutism: A longitudinal case study of autism. *Journal of Speech and Hearing Research, 37*(1), 96.

Wing, L. (1997). The autistic spectrum. *Lancet, 350,* 1761.

Wing, L., & Potter, D. (2002). The epidemiology of autistic spectrum disorders: Is the prevalence rising? *Mental Retardation and Developmental Disabilities Research Reviews, 8*(3), 151–161.

Wolery, M., & Winterling, V. (1997). Curricular approaches to controlling severe behavior problems. In N. N. Singh (Ed.), *Prevention and treatment of severe behavior problems: Models and methods in developmental disabilities* (pp. 87–120). Pacific Grove, CA: Brooks/Cole.

Wolk, L., & Edwards, M. (1993). The emerging phonological system of an autistic child. *Journal of Communication Disorders, 26,* 161–177.

Yell, M., & Drasgow, E. (2000). Litigating a free appropriate public education: The Lovaas hearings and cases. *Journal of Special Education, 33*(4), 205.

Yoder, P., & Stone, W. L. (2006). A randomized comparison of the effect of two prelinguistic communication interventions on the acquisition of spoken communication in preschoolers with ASD. *Journal of Speech, Language and Hearing Research, 49*(4), 698–711.

Zhang, J., & Griffin, A. I. (2007). Including children with autism in general physical education: Eight possible solutions. *JOPERD: The Journal of Physical Education, Recreation and Dance, 78*(3), 33–50.

Zwaigenbaum, L., Thurm, A., Stone, W., Baranek, G., Bryson, S., Iverson, J., Kau, A., Klin, A., Lord, C., Landa, R., Rogers, S., & Sigman, M. (2007). Studying the emergence of autism spectrum disorders in high-risk infants: Methodological and practical issues. *Journal of Autism and Developmental Disorders, 37*(3), 466–480.

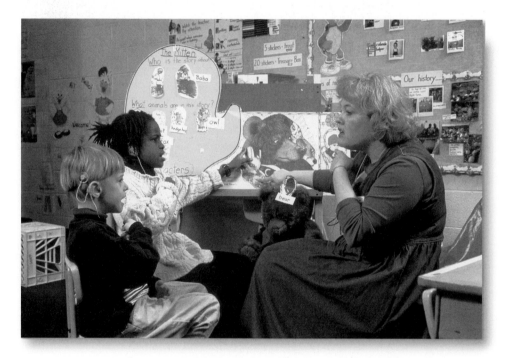

CHAPTER 8

Children with Hearing Loss

Considerations and Implications

Christine Radziewicz
School for Language and Communication Development

Susan Antonellis
St. John's University

When you finish this chapter, you will be able to

- Define and explore the type, classification, and degree of hearing loss.
- Discuss the efforts of the government and professionals toward early identification of hearing loss, and understand parents' role in this cause.
- Explore the intricate details of an audiological evaluation, and discuss each parameter that encompasses it, including otoacoustic emission testing.
- Consider the adjustments and special tests needed to prepare for the pediatric evaluation.
- Identify the proper management, including cochlear implants, needed after diagnosis of hearing loss.

- Discuss various assistive listening devices used by children with hearing loss.
- Understand the educational needs of children with hearing loss regarding reading, written language, sign language, and bilingualism.
- Discuss the inclusion option and its impact on children with a hearing loss.
- Identify several techniques that facilitate successful inclusion of preschool and school-age children with hearing loss with their normal hearing peers.
- Identify those factors that put children with hearing loss at educational risk.

The identification and rehabilitation of a child with a hearing loss is an enormous and important task. Rehabilitating these children encompasses instrumentation, methods, and follow-up. Technology has miniaturized the amplification systems available and opened up fitting choices. Technology has evolved from the bulky body aid to the completely-in-the-canal aid to cochlear implants, from the hardwire induction loop to the personal FM unit to other assistive devices, and from preschool screenings to otoacoustic emissions and testing on neonates.

The educational setting has also changed for children with hearing loss. In the past, education routinely took place in residential schools for the deaf. Today, children with hearing loss are more often educated in regular classrooms, exercising the inclusion option.

Educating children with hearing loss has been accomplished through either an aural/oral approach or an approach incorporating manually coded English. A tremendous body of research has been accumulated highlighting the advantages of each. An aural/oral approach incorporates speech and speechreading as the primary communication channels, whereas the total communication approach incorporates manual communication or sign language with speech and speechreading.

Children with hearing loss are also being identified earlier and cochlear implants are more widely available. Cochlear implants are biomedical prostheses that increase hearing sensitivity in persons who cannot benefit from conventional amplification (Estabrooks, 2000). Once a child has been implanted, it is imperative that intensive auditory therapy be initiated. Some children are implanted before the age of 1, although later implantation through the adult years is also possible. The implant provides for direct cochlear stimulation via electrodes that are inserted intracochlearly. Typically, programming of the cochlear device begins four to six weeks after implantation. Programming of the cochlear device is done by an audiologist. To achieve positive postimplant results, a strong collaborative relationship must exist among the surgeon, audiologist, and speech language pathologist.

A recent study (Eisenberg, Fink & Niparko, 2006) has examined language development in normal hearing children and children who had cochlear implants. Still in progress, this study longitudinally tracks children implanted at six implant centers in the United States. Early results of forty-two pairs of children after a one-year follow up showed that a proportion of them had achieved scores comparable to normal hearing peers on some measures of speech perception and speech intelligibility.

Today, there is a definite trend for children with implants to be included in regular education settings. A study by Damen and colleagues (2006) concluded that the academic performance of children with cochlear implants correlated negatively with duration of deafness and age at implantation. Mukari, Ling, and Ghani (2007) have suggested that the educational performance of children with cochlear implants varies. Even though many thrive in a full-time mainstream setting, a significant percentage of these students still perform at below-average level. The researchers have also emphasized that even though the cochlear implant provides children with good hearing potential, they still need solid educational supports to function well in the mainstream educational setting.

Type, Classification, and Degree of Hearing Loss

Hearing loss should be considered in terms of type, classification, and degree. There are three types of hearing loss: conductive hearing loss, sensorineural hearing loss, and mixed hearing loss. This section describes all three types and then presents a classification system used to define degree of loss.

CONDUCTIVE HEARING LOSS

Conductive hearing loss results from any barrier to sound present in the outer ear or middle ear; the inner ear functions normally (Martin & Clark, 2005). Conductive hearing loss never exceeds a hearing threshold of 70 decibels (dB) (hearing thresholds will be discussed shortly) and is generally medically treatable.

A common disorder found in children that is associated with conductive impairment is *otitis media*. It is defined as inflammation of the middle ear resulting predominantly from eustachian tube dysfunction (Stach, 1997). Chronic otitis media affects individuals in the early childhood years, most often during the critical years of speech and language development. It is linked with fluctuating hearing loss ranging anywhere from 10 to 40 dB. Presumably, hearing will return to normal after the episode is over. Because otitis media occurs most frequently during the first three years of life, it can have a dramatic effect on children's speech and language development.

Conductive hearing loss can also occur as a result of a totally blocked air conductive pathway, as in atresia, stenosis, complete stapes fixation, and ossicular discontinuity.

SENSORINEURAL HEARING LOSS

Sensorineural hearing loss results from damage to the sensory end organ, the cochlear hair cells, or the auditory nerve. Damage may have occurred during development of the ear, from an injury or infection, from the individual's environment, or from the degenerative effects of aging.

Sensorineural hearing loss may easily be overlooked during a physical examination, because the external auditory canal and tympanic membrane will appear normal. This type of hearing loss is not medically treatable and is almost always irreversible.

MIXED HEARING LOSS

Mixed hearing loss, which can occur in both children and adults, occurs simultaneously in both the conductive and sensorineural mechanisms. This results in a loss via bone conduction due to the sensorineural component and an even greater loss of sensitivity by air conduction.

CLASSIFICATION SYSTEM

Hearing loss can be defined using the following audiometric scale, suggested by Martin and Clark (2005). This scale also can be used to describe the degree of hearing loss and refers to the ANSI-1996 scale. The American National Standards Institute (ANSI, 1996) oversees the creation and use of thousands of norms and guidelines that directly impact business in various sectors, including acoustical devices.

Pure Tone Average	Degree
−10 to 15 dB	None
16 to 25 dB	Slight
26 to 40 dB	Mild
41 to 55 dB	Moderate
56 to 70 dB	Moderately severe
71 to 90 dB	Severe
91 dB+	Profound

Intensity of sound is measured in decibels (dB). Hearing is also affected by the frequency of the sound wave, which is measured in hertz (Hz). Higher-pitched sounds have higher frequencies. The classification system above is based on a *pure tone average*—that is, the average of the thresholds of 500, 1,000, and 2,000 Hz, respectively. These frequencies, commonly known as *speech frequencies,* are known to be important for hearing speech. Pure tone thresholds are discussed more fully later in this chapter.

Hearing Loss and Language Development

Various factors influence the development of language in the presence of hearing loss (Quigley & Kretschmer, 1982), including the following

- degree of hearing loss
- age of onset of loss
- slope of hearing loss
- age at identification of hearing loss
- age of habilitation (intervention)
- amount of habilitation
- type of habilitation

As noted, degree of hearing loss refers to the severity of the hearing loss and is easily measured. In the past, it was generally assumed that the greater the hearing loss, the greater the impact on speech and language development. Although a severe hearing loss of 71 to 90 or 95 dB does have a devastating effect on speech and language development, it cannot be assumed that a mild hearing loss of 26 to 40 dB will always have a minimal effect or that a profound loss of 96 dB or above will have the most detrimental effect.

To emphasize this point, Northern and Downs (1984) referred to the case study of a 13-year-old patient who had had frequent bouts of otitis media. Over seven years, from age 6 to age 13, the air conduction thresholds fluctuated from normal to mild to moderate levels. During this period, five myringotomies were performed. However, the child's repeated attacks of serous otitis media resulted in a progressive sensorineural hearing loss, with bone conduction thresholds of 25 dB at 4,000 Hz in one ear and 30 and 45 dB at 2,000 Hz and 4,000 Hz in the other ear. In this case, not only the degree of hearing loss but also the age of onset, age of identification, and type of habilitation had a critical effect on the severity of the language deficit. Although this child's loss was not discovered until age 6, he probably had experienced chronic otitis media earlier in life. The age of onset could have occurred more than five years before the age of identification and therefore could have included the critical language learning years. Furthermore, habilitation involved surgical myringotomies without speech and language therapy. Northern and Downs (1984) concluded his description of this case by stating that when the 13-year-old was given a hearing aid for habilitation, it was already thirteen years too late. The delay in the child's speech and language development was irreversible.

Although the degree of hearing loss is the most obvious variable, it is not necessarily the most critical. The combination of all the aforementioned variables determines the effect of hearing loss on speech and language development. Because of the interdependency of variables, one can never predict with certainty the detrimental effects of hearing loss on speech and language from degree of impairment alone. The only certainty is that hearing loss in any form (conductive, sensorineural, or mixed) and of any degree (mild to profound) can have a devastating effect on speech and language development.

Identification and Habilitation

Early identification of hearing loss and delivery of appropriate services are critical factors in the habilitation of children with hearing loss. Language development begins at the time a child is born, which means there is an urgent need for organized infant screening to identify those children who may have hearing loss. Identification of infants with hearing loss can be facilitated through neonatal (i.e., during the first month of life) screening of infants with a high risk of hearing loss. Early hearing detection and intervention is a public health issue. The goal is to screen all infants at 1 month, to have a diagnosis by 3 months, and to implement early intervention by 6 months.

Today, the current screening rate in the United States is 95 percent. Forty states have early hearing detection and intervention laws, and five have voluntary screening. However, there is still work to be done. It has been reported by state program coordinators that 34 percent of the babies who failed newborn hearing screenings did not receive a confirmation of diagnosis after the initial screening, and 23 percent of the babies who did receive a confirmed diagnosis were not referred to early intervention services (Shafer, 2007). If infants do not receive a hearing screening shortly after birth (while still in the hospital), there is a good likelihood that if they have a hearing loss, it will not be identified until long after 6 months of age. Some children are not identified until their second year of life or even later. This delay in identification results in a significant negative impact on spoken language, academic performance, and vocational choices.

Yoshinaga-Itano and Apuzzo (1998b) conducted a study in Colorado and found that language development was significantly delayed when a hearing loss was not identified until after a child was 6 months of age.

Another study by Yoshinaga-Itano and Apuzzo (1998a) found that children who were identified with a hearing loss before 6 months of age and who received early home intervention performed significantly better in measurements of expressive language, comprehension of language, and development of concepts than children who were identified after 6 months of age.

EARLY PARENT–INFANT INTERACTION

Researchers have shown great interest in the early language development of infants with normal hearing. Their investigations have shown that normal-hearing children have a basic capacity for perceiving speech behaviors in the environment and are sensitive to the social and affective aspects of the context of language (Eimas, 1974; Miller & Morse, 1976; Miller, Morse, & Dorman, 1977; Morse, 1972).

Bloom and Lahey (1978) stated that one of the precursors of language use occurs when infants begin to exchange gazes and vocalizations with their mothers. Bateson (1975) also described this mutual gaze or eye contact between mother and infant and called it *protoconversation*. Jaffe, Stern, and Peery (1973) studied the infant–mother dyad and found mother–infant gazing to be analogous to the rhythms of adult dialogue. Behaviors such as these are all continuous and lead to eventual development of speech and language, which begins in the second year of life. Although infants with hearing loss do not have the perceptual capabilities to receive and discriminate speech sounds as well as children with normal hearing, they do have a residual amount of hearing that allows for some discrimination when amplification is used. In addition, these infants are able to extract the social and affective aspects of the context of language (Bloom & Lahey, 1978).

Brown (1975) stated that the most important form of concept learning for the infant is probably socially mediated. The infant's first social contact is the parents. They are most responsible for the development of the behaviors that lead to language growth in the normally developing child, and they are the major forces in the habilitation of the child with hearing loss. Because studies have demonstrated that mothers of normal-hearing children play a vital role in the development in speech and language, it is obvious that mothers of infants with hearing loss play an even more crucial role.

Greenstein, Bush, McConville, and Stellini (1977) examined the mother–infant communication dyad and its effect on language acquisition in infants with hearing loss. They found that affective aspects of mother–infant interaction were central to the language acquisition of the child with hearing loss. All other aspects of the mother's language input to the child were far less significant than the existence of a good mother–infant bond. This bond frequently was broken by the mother's discovery of the child's hearing loss, however. Vorce (1974) suggested that the social relationship that exists between the mother and child stimulates the child's early vocalizations and therefore should be emphasized.

Because speech and language development begins with the earliest social exchanges between mother and infant and because the affective aspects of mother–infant interaction are crucial to future language acquisition, programs that enhance mother–infant communication are invaluable in effective intervention for children with hearing loss. First developed during the 1970s, parent–infant programs educate parents about their critical role in the development of their children. Parents are taught to make everyday experiences language-enhancing experiences. They learn to understand the implications of hearing loss on speech and language development and how to deal with their feelings about the hearing loss in their child. Furthermore, they are taught how to incorporate auditory training into the child's daily life and how to employ language learning strategies when interacting with their child. The parents and infant come to the parent–infant center at least once a week for training, and the teacher/speech-language pathologist (SLP) makes weekly visits to the home. The parents frequently meet with other professionals, such as psychologists and audiologists, for additional training and support.

The teacher/SLP can employ a variety of training techniques. For example, videotapes have been used in many ways to enhance communication between parents and infants with hearing loss. Cole and St. Clair-Stokes (1984) analyzed videotaped caregiver–child interactions to identify interactive behaviors that promote development of early language. Radziewicz (1985) used videotapes as a technique to train parents to incorporate more effective communicative behaviors in their interactions with their infants. The use of videotapes has resulted in a clearer understanding of hearing loss and more appropriate communicative interactions.

When a child with hearing loss and his or her parents enroll in a parent–infant program, that child's education begins during the critical speech and language learning years. Intervention during the first year increases the child's chances of developing more typical speech and language. Through such a program, parents can gain insights into management and effective communication behaviors that will facilitate language development in their child. They can be trained to model and develop interactive language learning opportunities during all their parent–child interactions.

Research has emphasized the degree to which parents and infants respond to and influence each other's behavior (Koester & Meadow-Orlans, 1999). Parents and children have individual patterns of temperament, which can have either a positive or negative impact on the child's development (Chess & Thomas, 1996). Early infant behavioral characteristics, such as repetitive motor activity and eye gaze behaviors, demonstrate how an infant communicates. Parents need to be trained early to interpret behaviors as well as shape them into communicative interactions. As the child grows and develops, the parents learn how to make every activity a language learning experience for him or her. As the parents become more skilled in enhancing language development, their child develops more language.

In today's multicultural society, children from diverse communities are frequently identified as having language disorders. It is important that bilingual evaluators and interpreters be used when evaluating these children. And once these children have beeen identified, it is imperative that the parents and professionals participate when developing the individualized education plan (IEP) and individualized family service plan (IFSP). When large differences, such as socioeconomic status and differences in values and beliefs, exist between families and professionals, this collaborative partnership becomes more fragile and poses challenges to all team members. For early intervention to be successful, the focus must be to work on everyday activities that are part of the family's cultural customs, and the family must view it as appropriate.

The extent to which the family has been exposed to the customs of the dominant society will determine the level of conflict that may occur between them and the professionals working with them (Hanson, Lynch, & Wayman, 1990). A study by De-Gangi and colleagues (1994) identified the challenges to family–professional collaboration related to cultural diversity and socioeconomic status. It found that families from lower SES and educational backgrounds often (1) were concerned with basic survival needs and deferred to professional judgments when setting goals; (2) had difficulty identifying their child's needs; and (3) were reluctant to share information. With all this in mind, it is imperative that professionals working collaboratively with families recognize the impact of culture and socioeconomic status on the collaborative process.

Audiological Assessment

The routine audiological evaluation consists of pure tone findings, speech audiometry (yielding speech recognition thresholds and speech recognition scores), aural acoustic immittance testing, and some form of otoacoustic emission testing. Since not all testing procedures can be used with very young children, pediatric evaluation is considered separately.

PURE TONE FINDINGS

Before the options and procedures for finding pure tone thresholds are discussed, it is necessary to define *threshold*. A pure tone threshold is the level at which the tone is so soft that it can be perceived only 50 percent of the time it is presented (Stach, 1997). Two techniques are used to measure threshold. In the *ascending method,* the person being tested is exposed to stimuli that range from inaudible to audible. In the *descending method,* the stimuli go from audible to inaudible.

In determining pure tone threshold by air conduction, proper earphone placement is essential. The diaphragm of the earphone must be placed directly over the opening of the external canal. If placement is not secure, the test results may be invalid. Specific earphones are used for the right and left ears. The better ear should be tested first. The patient should be instructed to respond when a tone is heard, even if the tone is very soft.

The test begins with a 1,000 Hz tone and allows the patient to hear what it sounds like; that is, the tone is presented at an audible level for the patient. The threshold at 1,000 Hz is found by presenting the signal using an "up 5, down 10" method. This procedure is continued for the other audiometric frequencies following this order: 2,000, 4,000, 8,000, 500, and 250 Hz. The same procedure is followed for the second ear. Each threshold obtained is plotted on the audiogram (see Figure 8.1). Then the pure tone average of each ear is determined (average 500, 1,000, and 2,000 Hz).

Bone conduction testing is conducted in the same manner, using the bone oscillator. Proper placement of the oscillator on the mastoid process is important for accuracy.

SPEECH AUDIOMETRY

The speech audiometry portion of the audiological evaluation consists primarily of determining the speech recognition threshold, speech detection threshold, and word recognition score. The *speech recognition threshold (SRT)* typically refers to the threshold level of speech, which is the lowest level (in decibels) at which the listener is able to identify approximately 50 percent of spondaic words (Stach, 1997). The SRT is administered by having the patient hear examples of test words through earphones. This test can be performed with a live voice or recorded speech signal. The pure tone average of each ear allows the technician to choose an audible level to begin the test procedure.

Speech audiometry has been used in pediatric audiological assessment for many purposes. As a stimulus, speech has been found useful with infants and young children because it has high interest value and a complex spectrum (Gravel & Hood, 1999).

The second portion of speech testing is the evaluation of the word recognition score. This test is significant because a common complaint from children is "I hear, but I don't understand." Word recognition is a measure of the ability to perceive and identify a word, or word discrimination and word intelligibility (Stach, 1997).

AURAL ACOUSTIC IMMITTANCE TESTING

In view of the major role the middle ear plays in audiological diagnosis, aural acoustic immittance testing must be considered an essential part of the audiological assessment.

Figure 8.1 **Pure Tone Thresholds Plotted on an Audiogram**

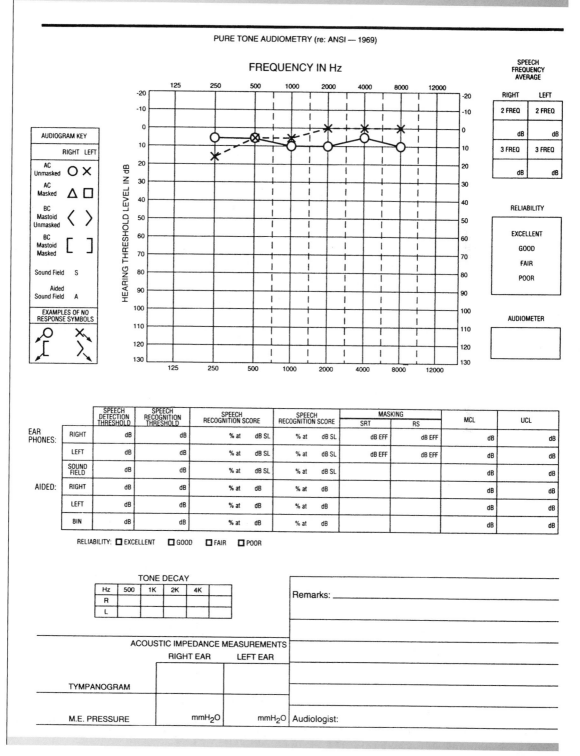

It consists of tympanometry, acoustic reflexes, and eustachian tube evaluation. (This chapter will not discuss eustachian tube evaluation.)

Tympanometry is the procedure used in the assessment of middle ear function in which the immittance of the tympanic membrane and middle ear is measured as air pressure delivered to the ear canal is varied (Stach, 1997). Tympanometry testing produces a chart of results called a *tympanogram*. Figure 8.2 illustrates several possible tympanogram results:

1. Type A tympanogram—normal tympanic membrane
2. Type B tympanogram—middle ear effusion, patent ventilating tubes, or perforation
3. Type C tympanogram—eustachian tube dysfunction, retracted tympanic membrane; effusion may be present
4. Type A_s tympanogram—stiff tympanic membrane
5. Type A_d tympanogram—flaccid tympanic membrane or ossicular discontinuity

It is important when looking at a tympanogram to observe three parameters: pressure (*x* axis), amplitude (*y* axis), and shape. Pressure is measured in milliliters of H_2O, which creates either positive or negative pressure within the canal (see Figure 8.2).

The *acoustic reflex* is the reflexive contraction of the intra-aural muscles (tensor tympani and stapedius) in response to loud sound, dominated by the stapedius muscle in humans (Stach, 1998). The diagnostic significance of the acoustic reflex lies in helping detect the presence or absence of pathology. Middle ear pathology is most common in young children. Others are central pathology and nonorganic hearing loss.

In sum, the audiological evaluation consists of a network of intricate assessments—pure tone findings, speech audiometry, and aural acoustic immittance testing—that produces a holistic picture of the child's auditory system.

AUDITORY PROCESSING TESTING

Another possibility that needs to be considered is the existence of an auditory processing disorder, which can exist without a related hearing loss. *Auditory processing* refers to the perceptual processing of auditory information. In simplified terms, it refers to how the brain recognizes and interprets the sounds around the individual.

Auditory processing disorder is most often seen in the pediatric population. Children with this disorder often are unable to recognize subtle differences between sounds in words and may demonstrate difficulty in one or more of the following areas: phonological awareness, attention to and memory for auditory information, auditory synthesis, and auditory comprehension. Today, the term *central auditory processing* is used to refer to what occurs to an auditory signal above the eighth auditory nerve, along the brain stem and the brain (Richard, 2001).

Several tests can be used to determine the presence of an auditory processing disorder:

- Staggered Spondaic Word Test (SSW) (Katz, 1986)
- Test for Auditory Processing in Adolescents and Adults (SCAN-A) (Keith, 1994)
- Test for Auditory Processing in Children (SCAN-C) (Keith, 2000)

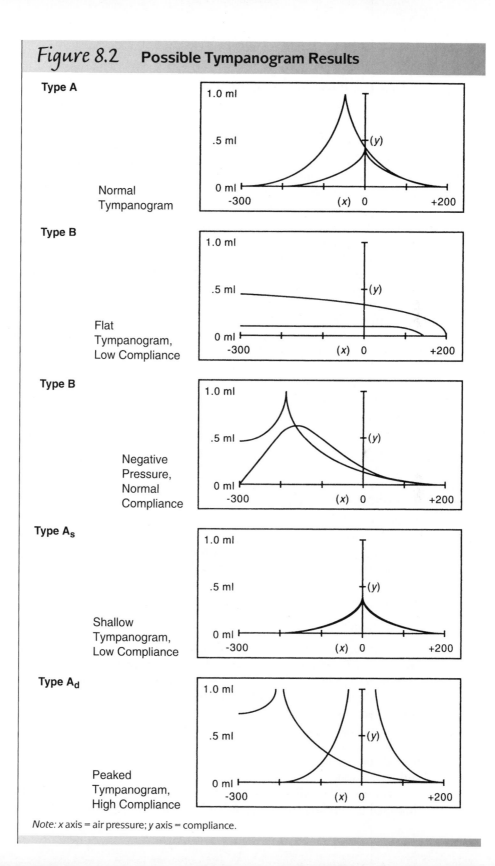

Figure 8.2 Possible Tympanogram Results

Note: x axis = air pressure; y axis = compliance.

- Auditory Processing Abilities Test (APAT) (Ross-Swain & Long, 2004)
- Test of Auditory Processing Skills (TAPS–3) (Martin & Brownell, 2005)

PEDIATRIC EVALUATION

Early detection of hearing loss in an infant is imperative, yet it is not an easy task. Although the audiological evaluation can yield a wealth of information about an individual's auditory system, many of the tests described cannot be successfully administered to an infant or preschooler. In view of this, it is necessary to discuss evaluation options for the young pediatric population.

First and foremost, it is important for the clinician to have a discussion with the parents and people closely associated with the child before actual testing. As the degree of diagnostic difficulty increases, having input from these individuals is important. Parents, care providers, teachers, and therapists can provide valuable insights (Gravel & Hood, 1999). Second, the clinician needs to establish a pleasant relationship with the child.

The *cross-check principle* has worked in this profession over the years, evolving from the work of Jerger and Hayes in 1976. This principle states that the results of any single audiometric test cannot be considered valid without independent verification from another test (Gravel & Hood, 1999). Technology has certainly added a new dimension to the pediatric evaluation, but one measure alone should not be used to assess a child's hearing.

Many factors can affect pediatric assessment, including otitis media. As stated previously, the tympanometry portion of the evaluation must be considered when interpreting audiological findings.

BEHAVIORAL ASSESSMENT

According to Gravel and Hood (1999), behavioral assessment is useful for two purposes. When used for audiometric purposes, behavioral methods provide a means for quantifying hearing sensitivity—determining thresholds across the speech range (500 to 4,000 Hz). When used for functional purposes, the auditory assessment is used to examine the child's auditory behaviors qualitatively, determining whether they are typical for his or her age.

Infants (Birth to Age 2)

Testing of infants requires having an adequate sound room, a quiet state, and measured stimuli (Northern & Downs, 1984). It is appropriate to seat the mother with the baby in her lap in the middle of the sound room. The audiologist should draw the baby's attention straight ahead by moving a toy back and forth. Next, a noisemaker is introduced without the baby seeing it. Responses to watch for are eyes widening, eyes turning, a rapid eye blink, and, if the child is at least 4 months old, a rudimentary head turn. At about 5 to 7 months, the infant will turn his or her head toward the side of a signal. The audiologist continues this procedure using speech stimuli and warble tones.

As the child reaches 9 months, the audiologist can obtain a speech awareness threshold by repeating a phrase such as "Bye-bye Amy," slowly reducing the level of presentation until the child ceases to respond. As the child's age increases, additions are made to the evaluation process. For example, the child may be asked to recognize or point to familiar pictures.

Children (Ages 2 to 5)

The procedure known as *play conditioning* can be used for children 2 to 5 years old. The 2-year-old will probably need to sit in his mother's lap for the procedure, but the 4- or 5-year-old most likely can sit alone. The audiologist introduces the procedure as a game, using motivational toys such as pegs and building blocks. The peg or block is placed in the child's hand, and the child is instructed to listen for a little sound (presented in the sound field). When a sound is heard, the child is guided in putting the peg into a bucket or box. Once the child can do the task alone, the sounds can be presented to him or her through earphones. This procedure is followed for pure tones (as discussed in the Audiological Assessment section of this chapter). It is necessary to move rapidly with small children, because their attention span is generally short. Speech audiometry also can be accomplished through various picture-pointing tasks.

OBJECTIVE ASSESSMENT

Otoacoustic Emissions (OAE)

In 1978, Kemp made an extraordinary discovery using the simple technique of coupling a small microphone to the external ear canal and recording the sound present in it during and after the presentation of click stimuli. Using a microphone system similar to that used in clinical immittance instruments, Kemp discovered that low-intensity sounds could be detected in the ear canal for several milliseconds after the presentation of each click. (The procedure is similar to the way auditory brainstem responses are obtained). These sounds provided a quick view of the cochlea's active response to sound, a response that involves the addition of energy to that provided by the stimulus arriving at the ear. Outer hair cells are thought to play a major role.

Kemp's (1978) recordings represent one form of emission of acoustic energy from the cochlea. Collectively, these sounds are known as *otoacoustic emissions* (OAE) (Glattke & Kujawa, 1991). Otoacoustic emissions are particularly important in evaluating infants who are free of external and/or middle ear pathology (Lafreniere, Smurzynski, Jung, Leonard, & Kim, 1993). Measurement of OAE in the external ear canal, regardless of the type of OAE, depends on the integrity of the middle ear system as well as the cochlea. The emissions amplitude increases from birth to the age of 1 to 9 months, and decreases in amplitude have been observed in children ages 4 to 13 years (Widen, 1997).

OAE testing is a very sensitive measure of cochlea function and plays an important role in the early identification and diagnosis of dysfunction in the pediatric population. However, it is not a test of hearing and cannot replace the audiogram (Hall, 2000).

Auditory Brainstem Response (ABR)

Auditory brainstem response (ABR) audiometry is most useful in diagnosing the difficult-to-test child. This testing evaluates responses observed by way of electrical impulses of the cerebral cortex; responses are recorded on a graph. The ABR is a test of neural synchrony. It measures the ability of the central nervous system to respond to external stimulation in a synchronous manner.

ABR provides a safe, noninvasive approach to assessing auditory function in infants and children. It can also be used to validate or invalidate the findings of behavioral audiometry. The ABR test can be useful when it is important to know the sensitivity of each cochlea separately.

Audiological Management

Diagnosing the child with a hearing loss is only the beginning. To be successful educationally, psychologically, and socially, the child with a hearing loss must have adequate audiological management.

AMPLIFICATION DEVICES

When a family first learns that their child has a hearing loss, the primary concerns are What can be done? and What physician do we see? The child first must be seen by an otolaryngologist to provide medical clearance for amplification. The audiologist then conducts an ongoing evaluation to find the appropriate type of amplification for the child. In the young child, deciding on a final fitting can take anywhere from 6 months to 1 year. In the interim, the child may be fitted with a loaner hearing aid.

A hearing aid is an electronic amplifier that has three main components: a microphone, an amplifier, and a receiver (Stach, 1998). All hearing aids are powered by a battery. There are various types of amplification, ranging from the body aid to the canal aid and from the linear circuit to the digital signal-processing circuit:

- *Body aid.* About the size of a pocket radio, the body aid is connected to an earmold in the ear by a receiver wire. In the past, only a body aid could provide adequate power to benefit someone with more than a moderate hearing loss. Today, amplifiers with high power can be fit into a small space and the body aid is rarely used. However, due to its large size, it still provides more power than other types of hearing aids and offers more flexibility in terms of circuitry and controls. Most people who use a body aid are fitted monaurally (i.e., one ear).
- *Behind-the-ear aid.* The behind-the-ear (BTE) hearing aid is also known as a *postauricular hearing aid.* This type of aid rests over and behind the pinna and has a plastic earhook at one end, near the receiver. A small piece of plastic tubing connects the hook to the earmold. The BTE hearing aid also provides flexibility as far as circuitry and control options.
- *CROS (contralateral routing of signal) aid.* This type of hearing aid is designed for unilateral loss. A microphone is placed on the poor ear, and the signal is routed to a hearing aid on the better ear (Stach, 1997). The CROS aid can be obtained as an in-the-ear aid or a behind-the-ear aid. This type of instrument is recommended for someone who has an ear that is unaidable. A variation of this aid is the BiCROS (bilateral contralateral routing of signal).

- *In-the-ear/canal aid.* The in-the-ear aid became the most popular form in the 1990s, after modern technology and miniaturization allowed for more power in a small space. This type of hearing aid holds all the components in one shell. Many people choose this type of hearing aid for cosmetic reasons. In-the-ear instruments are not always the best choice for small children, however, because the ear grows rapidly and modifications are needed more often.
- *Completely-in-the canal (CIC) aid.* The CIC hearing aid is one of the newest and most cosmetic types. It requires a deep ear impression and is placed completely in the canal; it is virtually invisible.
- *Open-ear aid.* The open-ear aid is used primarily for those who exhibit a hearing loss in the high frequencies. It consists of a miniature BTE hearing aid with a small thin tube attached with an ear bud. Essentially, the ear is open. This type of aid could be beneficial to children with fluctuating hearing loss caused by conductive pathology.

With increased miniaturization have come sophisticated new circuitry options. The basic types are known as programmable and digital hearing aid technology. *Programmable technology* gives the user flexible control of hearing aid characteristics and multiple memories for programming various conditions for different situations—for example, the child at home doing homework in a quiet room versus the child listening for directions in a noisy lunchroom. *Digital technology* provides more exact and flexible frequency shaping, better feedback reduction, more complex compression parameters, and enhanced noise reduction. The most recent digital technology comes equipped with dynamic feedback circuitry, almost eliminating the common problem of feedback.

Using a hearing aid opens a new world to the child with a hearing loss, but some problems can occur with its use. Common problems are acoustic feedback, a distorted or intermittent signal, a noisy sound, and dysfunction. Given these problems, audiological follow-up is important.

COCHLEAR IMPLANTS

Children who cannot benefit from conventional amplification are good candidates for a cochlear implant. The first reports on this technology were not promising; the most encouraging results were that speech signals were perceived as speech but were not intelligible. As research progressed, however, and as the sophistication of signal processing increased, there were reports of patients with good and sometimes markedly improved speech recognition abilities.

When damage to the cochlea is too severe, the information sent to the auditory nerve may reach the brain as sound, but it may not be enough for the understanding of a speech signal. The person may respond to tones or noise but not understand words. In this case, a cochlear implant should be considered. A cochlear implant is basically a neural stimulator. It bypasses the mechanical, bioelectric, and biochemical processes of the auditory system and directly stimulates the ganglion cells of the auditory nerve with small electrical currents. No sound passes through the outer or middle ear.

Each cochlear implant has five components, including both external and internal components:

External Components	Internal Components
Microphone	Receiver stimulator
Transmitting coil	Electrode array
Speech processor	

The criteria for candidacy of a cochlear implant have changed over the years. Initially the criteria were more restrictive. However, with the gathering of more data, criteria have loosened, and more children and adults are being implanted. The following are the current guidelines set by the U.S. Food and Drug Administration (FDA) for implant candidates:

- can be implanted as early as 12 months or earlier, if cochlea is ossified
- can have pre, peri, congenital, or acquired hearing loss
- can have bilateral severe to profound hearing loss
- receive marginal to no benefit from hearing aids
- appropriate for partially sighted and blind adults and children
- appropriate for people who are cognitively impaired with appropriate expectations (still need to be emotionally appropriate)
- appropriate for all types of cochlear abnormalities; only ruled out by no auditory nerve
- must have family support
- must have appropriate expectations and motivation

The primary reason the selection criteria have changed is that patients with implants are obtaining increasing amounts of open-set speech recognition with available devices. Although this increased performance is mainly due to the advanced technology in the field of cochlear implants, it is also due in part to the fact that patients with greater amounts of residual speech recognition skills are receiving cochlear implants (Zwolan, 2000).

When making a decision on a cochlear implant for a child, two important questions need to be answered:

1. Who decides for the child?
2. On which standards should the decision be based?

In answering the question of who decides for the child, the interests of self-interest groups should be excluded. These groups can interfere with the child's decision and right of privacy. Only the child's parents or legal guardian has the authority for all aspects of the child's life and can provide continuity and accountability. Parents will usually do the best job of deciding what is best for their child.

Answering the second question about what standards should be used to make the decision involves looking at ethical values in deciding for others. The two ethical values that become involved in this decision are respect for self-determination and concern for well-being. Children need to maintain their functional abilities. The ability to hear not only has significant communicative value but also provides auditory enjoyment and is important for personal safety. Deciding to proceed with a cochlear implant will also influence the child's opportunities for future education, employment, and interpersonal relationships (Balkany et al., 1996).

The emergence of the cochlear implant and improvements to its technology have changed the way children with hearing loss are educated.

ASSISTIVE LISTENING DEVICES (ALD)

In addition to hearing aids and cochlear implants, various other assistive listening devices (ALD) can provide extra help to a child with a hearing loss, particularly in the educational setting. Auditory trainers operate like hearing aids and are used in the classroom or at particular sites as training devices. Because they are used collectively on site, size and appearance are not important considerations. Their large size enables them to be equipped with larger components and special circuitry that produce better fidelity. ALD's can overcome background noise, bring the signal closer to the listener's ear/microphone, and overcome negative effects of reverberation, resulting in an improved signal-to-noise ratio (i.e., the ratio between the intensity of the signal and the intensity of the noise present).

There are four basic types of auditory trainer systems:

- *Desk trainers.* The components of a desk trainer are built into a case. This device is usually found on the student's desk, and he or she can carry it from one location to another. A disadvantage of this device is that its signal-to-noise ratio is poor if there is a distance between the teacher and the student. This device is useful in training sessions with one child but is not particularly recommended in a classroom of hearing-impaired children.
- *Hardwire units.* Hardwire units are also placed on children's desks, and each child has an individual volume control. The signal-to-noise ratio is good because the teacher speaks directly into a microphone. A disadvantage of hardwire units is that they are not portable.
- *Induction loop unit.* The loop system involves a wire loop around the room, installed under the carpeting or under the floor. It conducts electrical energy from an amplifier and then creates a magnetic field; current flow from the loop is induced in the induction coil at the hearing aid telecoil (Stach, 1997). Each child in the room wears a hearing aid in the telephone position. The telephone coil in the hearing aid will pick up the signal and present it to the ear. The signal-to-noise ratio is excellent, but children can hear only the teacher and not the other children or themselves. New hearing aids are available with a switch in which the microphone and telephone setting can be used simultaneously. The loop system is flexible within the room itself.
- *FM units.* A wireless unit, the FM auditory trainer is the most widely used trainer. The teacher wears a microphone transmitter, and the child wears an FM receiver with the hearing aid. The teacher transmits directly to the child's unit on an FM radio carrier wave.

Several more assistive devices are also available for the child with hearing loss:

- *Telephone solutions* amplify the telephone itself via a coil or in isolation. Many such devices are available to suit individual needs. Another method is using the TTY and/or telephone relay services.
- *Visual display devices* include systems that facilitate face-to-face communication and the reception of electronic media. These devices are appropriate for use in classroom settings. One example is *communication access REALtime translation (CART),* which involves trained reporters using a stenotype machine. A computer and real-time translation software create the text, which can be read on a computer screen or monitor, a television set or monitor, or via an overhead projection screen.
- *Signal and alerting devices* can be used for alerting children with hearing loss who are participating in competitive sports, such as track and swimming competitions. These devices may also be used to alert the child with hearing loss to smoke, a siren or alarm, a door bell, a telephone, or an alarm clock at home or in school. Hearing ear dogs also fall into this category; they are trained to alert the child with hearing loss to a doorbell or door knock, car horn, or name call, to mention a few possibilities.
- *Waterproof hearing aids* may be beneficial for children who participate in competitive swimming. They should not be submerged in water but can be used during practices. A hard-wired FM system would be appropriate for most children with hearing loss who participate in athletic events.

OTHER CONSIDERATIONS IN AUDIOLOGICAL MANAGEMENT

A child's receptive communication needs may require more than a hearing aid. Assistive technology must be provided that fits the child's lifestyle, hearing level, speech recognition, and other factors. To determine the needs of a child with hearing loss, an assessment must be performed in addition to the audiological data obtained. The Pediatric Hearing Demand, Ability and Need Profile (Healey & Palmer, 1992) helps parents and their children to determine what, when, and where they would need the use of assistive technology (see Figure 8.3).

Another consideration is the cost of technology. Very little technology is covered by third-party payers. School-related devices are provided by schools and funded by IDEA. Private-use devices, such as alerting systems, are mainly paid for by the user. Several funding sources can be investigated, including the Disabled Children's Relief Fund, the scholarship Trust for the Deaf and Near Deaf, funds for Hard of Hearing (HOH)/Deaf Children, and charitable organizations and federal programs that are locally administered.

Education is also a consideration in managing the child with hearing loss. Workshops for staff and teachers are an essential part of managing the child with hearing loss. Follow-up and maintenance of amplification and assistive devices is also a primary concern in ensuring the success of a child with hearing loss. Children's hearing should be monitored on a routine basis and at an annual assessment.

Figure 8.3 **Pediatric Hearing Demand, Ability, and Need Profile**

Name:

Age	Description of Communication Milestone/Activity	Communication Problem is Present ... With Hearing Aid:						The Problem is Due to...				Current Compensation
		HOME on / off	SCHOOL on / off	TRAVEL on / off				Hearing	Noise	Distance	Visibility	(describe)
	ALERTING											
	telephone bell											
	doorbell											
	door knock											
	alarm clock											
	smoke alarm											
	siren											
	turn signal											
	personal pager											
	PERSONAL COMMUNICATION											
	telephone											
	tv/stereo/radio											
	one-to-one (planned)											
	one-to-one (unplanned)											
	group											
	large room											
	OTHER ACTIVITIES											
	clubs/games:											
	lessons:											
	sports:											

Further information (e.g., status of hearing aids, telecoil, DAI, communication environment):

Recommendations (Assistive Technology, Communication Strategies, Environmental Manipulation):

Adapted from Healey and Palmer, 1992.

Education of Children with Hearing Loss

The educational performance of children with hearing loss in the United States has concerned educators for some time. In 1921, Reamer reported on the educational achievement of 2,500 deaf students. He found that they were academically delayed an average of four to five years when compared with hearing peers. A 1968–1970 annual survey (Gentile & DiFrancesca, 1969) gathered statistical information on the educational performance of children with hearing loss in preschool through college. This survey revealed that, on the whole, these children and youth had an average educational lag of four years. Their highest levels of performance were in the areas of spelling and arithmetic computation (Martin & Clark, 2005). However, it must be noted that arithmetic concepts and performance on word problems still presented much difficulty, as completing them inherently included the ability to decode written language.

The area of greatest lag in achievement was reading, with the average reading comprehension for 15- to 16-year-olds at the 3.5 grade level. Studies by the Office of Demographic Studies at Gallaudet University confirmed this delay in reading achievement (King & Quigley, 1985). In 1994, Allen calculated the average reading achievement of deaf students completing school to be at the fourth-grade level. Thus, the majority of students who are deaf or hard of hearing exhibit English language and reading difficulties (Paul, 1998; Paul & Jackson, 1993). This is even more troubling now that 80 percent or more of all students with hearing loss attend public schools (Luetke-Stahlman, Griffiths, & Montgomery, 1999).

Even children with unilateral hearing loss are at risk for academic failure. A 1999 study by English and Church concluded that the overall academic performance of children with unilateral hearing loss had not changed in ten years. Twenty-four percent of the 406 children in their study functioned below average when compared to their peers—the same percentage observed in the mid-1980s.

For children with bilateral hearing loss, the effects may be even greater. English and Church (1999) estimated that 8 million schoolchildren in the United States have some type and degree of hearing loss. For many of these children, classroom modifications will be necessary, as the acoustics of the learning environment are a major barrier to auditory learning. Noise from open windows and classroom doors, chairs scraping the floor, and classroom "buzz" all interfere with hearing. For children with hearing loss, this interference has a greater negative impact than for normal hearing peers. Only an enhanced signal-to-noise ratio can provide children with clear, consistent access to spoken instruction in the classroom.

Poor performance in academic subjects by children with hearing loss is not surprising, considering that reading comprehension plays a major role in academic learning and that understanding written language relates directly to understanding spoken language. From about the third or fourth grade, students are expected to read to learn; this task becomes extremely difficult for the child with a hearing loss who does not have an adequate language base. In fact, the majority of children with severe hearing loss do not develop the language skills needed to make them efficient decoders of written language. Because of this, their comprehension of written language is significantly delayed when compared with that of normal hearing children (Robbins, 1986).

This finding is probably related to the fact that children with hearing loss take longer to reach the final stage of comprehension development of spoken language, in which they attend to syntactic and morphological aspects of sentences rather than paralinguistic cues (Robbins, 1986). Furthermore, it has been suggested that children with severe hearing loss use different strategies for comprehending verbal language (Davis & Blasdell, 1975).

READING

Learning to read is a complex task that requires the integration of syntactic, semantic, and pragmatic skills, as well as the ability to decode words. It is predicated on a strong foundation of language learning skills. Once words have been decoded, the reader must translate them into a more usable form. For the person with normal hearing, this form consists of phonetic elements. For the person who has a hearing loss, this form depends on the language input model and may be phonetic forms, signs, fingerspelling, or visual orthography. In addition, the reader must be able to abstract both explicit and implicit meaning from the text through inferencing and hypothesizing (Kretschmer, 1989). Doing so is further complicated by text variables such as vocabulary, syntax, figurative language, and discourse.

Learning how to read presents a serious challenge for children with severe to profound hearing losses. One out of five children with severe hearing loss has a reading level below second grade (Dew, 1999). Paul (1998) found that the typical high school graduate with a profound hearing loss read at the fourth-grade level. Reading requires an understanding of a language and the relationship between that language and the printed word (Golden-Meadow & Mayberry, 2001). Children and adults with profound hearing loss who have poor reading skills also have both verbal and visuospatial short-term memory deficits. This appears to be true for normal-hearing persons with reading disabilities, as well (Tractenberg, 2002). Research by Kelly (1996) and Paul (1996) found that vocabulary skills and syntactical skills were important factors in the reading process. The stronger these skills were, the better the child's reading comprehension.

One of the basic approaches to teaching reading in programs for children with hearing loss is the *language experience approach (LEA)*. In the LEA, which is used in primary grades, children use their own language to write stories; that is, a child dictates a story and the teacher writes it. The story is then used in reading instruction. The LEA has been expanded to include modifying the child's dictated story to model and incorporate English syntactical forms. Once the child has achieved some writing skills, his or her written samples are incorporated into the reading program. The stories that children either dictate or write are based on personal interaction and represent their experiences with their social environment. This approach is most interesting in that it bridges the processes of reading and writing (King & Quigley, 1985).

Computer-based instruction has also been used to facilitate development of reading skills. Unfortunately, there have been relatively few studies that clearly support using this approach with children with hearing loss. However, a study by Prinz, Nelson, and Stedt (1982) highlighted improvement in word recognition and identification for 3- to 6-year-old children who were deaf trained to use the ALPHA

Program, a sight-word computer program. This program used words, pictures, and manual sign representations and therefore could be used by children whose primary form of communication was sign language. Further studies (Nelson, Prinz, & Dalke, 1989; Prinz & Nelson, 1985) on children 3 and 11 years old who are deaf supported the use of computer-based instruction for reading and writing. More recently Prinz and colleagues (1993) have supported computer-based instruction with elementary-age children. Basically, all of these studies have recommended the use of multimodality and multimedia reading programs for young children who are deaf.

Before formal training in reading begins, children with hearing loss must have developed language skills. An excellent way to develop these skills is through storytelling, which exposes children to story structure, print, and common cultural themes (Snow, 1983; Wells, 1985). A study by Schick and Gale (1995) examined storytelling with preschool children who were deaf and hard-of-hearing who used some form of manually coded English during three different language conditions: using pure ASL, using pure SEE2 (Anthony, 1971; Gustason, Pfetzing, Zawolkow, 1972), and using SEE2 with ASL features and ASL structures. SEE2 is a form of manually coded English, and ASL (American Sign Language) is the sign language typically used by adults who are deaf. Interestingly, the researchers found that children participated more and initiated more interactions when stories contained ASL signing. This study is important when considering educational approaches for children using manually coded English.

A study by Strong and Prinz (1997) also highlighted the strong positive impact that learning ASL has on reading achievement. It found that students who are deaf who use ASL as a primary mode of communication achieved higher levels of English literacy skills than their peers who do not utilize ASL.

EDUCATIONAL APPROACHES AND COMMUNICATION OPTIONS

Several educational options and placements are available for children who are deaf or hard of hearing. Generally, children can be educated using either an aural/oral approach or an approach that uses sign language. If the child's family chooses an aural/oral approach, three communication methods are available:

1. The *auditory verbal unisensory* method emphasizes auditory skills. The child is taught to develop auditory listening skills through one-on-one therapy using hearing with the aid of amplification (e.g., hearing aid, cochlear implant). There is no use of sign language, nor is the child taught to rely on visual cues (speechreading).
2. The *oral auditory oral* method also emphasizes maximum use of hearing through amplification (e.g., hearing aid, cochlear implant). Speechreading training is also included. Natural gestures are encouraged but no sign language is used.
3. *Cued speech* is a visual communication system that uses eight handshapes (cues) that go in one of four places around the face and are used with speaking. These cues help the child to distinguish between sounds that look the same on the lips. The child uses auditory, speechreading, and hand cues to understand spoken language (Rhode Island Department of Health, 2006).

Total communication is a philosophy that embraces all means of communication to communicate with the child who is deaf: signs, speechreading, body language, fingerspelling, natural gestures, oral speech, and amplification (Med-El Corporation, n.d.).

Bilingual/Bicultural Education

The bilingual/bicultural (ASL/ESL) method uses ASL to educate children who are deaf. ASL becomes the child's primary language. A variety of other sign systems have been used to educate children who are deaf. For example, Signing Essential English (Anthony, 1971) and Signing Exact English (Gustason et al., 1972) consist of manual productions of spoken English and adhere to the syntactical and grammatical forms of the spoken language. Educators who use this type of sign system are actually attempting to teach English as a first language through the use of a visual system.

During the 1970s, a body of research evolved around ASL, which is a language in its own right, with its own syntax and idioms (Bellugi & Fischer, 1972; Bellugi & Klima, 1975; Bellugi, Klima, & Siple, 1974; Wilbur, 1979). Researchers suggested that children with deafness born to parents with deafness who used ASL at home should be taught spoken and written English in a different manner than children who are deaf born to parents with normal hearing. The premise was that the children exposed to ASL had already achieved a primary language base—ASL. When they were exposed to English at school, it was their second language; therefore, the educational approach had to be a bilingual one. In addition, these children who were deaf had also been exposed to the deaf culture, with its traditions and customs. This made them bicultural and strengthened the position for teaching them with an ASL/ESL (English-as-a-second language) approach.

The idea of taking a bilingual approach to educating children who are deaf was based on the work of Cummins (1981), who hypothesized that if a child was proficient in one language, he or she would have more success in developing a second language. Thus, if a child who was deaf was proficient in ASL, then he or she would more easily acquire English literacy skills.

Today, the bilingual approach to educating children who are deaf has not been implemented to any great extent. Reasons for this include the following (Strong, 1988):

1. ASL is not the native language of the majority of children who are deaf.
2. ASL has no written form.
3. There are few trained teachers who know ASL.
4. Bilingual education in general is controversial.
5. Few ASL curricula have been published.
6. Some educators question the true language status of ASL.

In spite of these obstacles, attempts have been made to document and justify the use of a bilingual approach in education. An experimental curriculum described by Strong (1988) uses a storytelling format to introduce ASL into the classroom setting. English is then taught via ASL. This program is particularly interesting because it emphasizes metalinguistic awareness.

More recently, Prinz and Strong (1998) developed an ASL proficiency and English literacy within a bilingual deaf education model of instruction. They found a positive correlation between ASL and reading and writing in English and emphasized the need for more research and curriculum development in this area. The national Council on Education of the Deaf (CED) and the National Association of the Deaf (NAD) support the idea of a bilingual educational approach when educating students who are deaf.

Considering the difficulty with which deaf children acquire language and the poor academic performance common among many of them, it seems both possible and practical to adopt a second-language acquisition approach in the educational setting. Much more careful and systematic research is needed, however, before extensive use of such an approach can be recommended.

Inclusionary Education

Today, many educational options are available for the young child with a hearing loss. Whereas the choice was once limited to segregated settings, such as residential schools for the deaf and day schools for the hearing impaired, changes in federal legislation have brought forth new options, including day classes, resource rooms, itinerant programs, and team teaching.

Full inclusion is an educational placement in which the student with hearing loss attends all classes with hearing peers, generally in his or her home school district. Various support services are provided and may include speech and language therapy, assistive listening systems, interpreters, curriculum and test-taking accommodations, occupational therapy, and physical therapy. The full inclusion model implies that the regular education teacher provides academic instruction.

For the child who relies on speechreading, amplification, or sign language, a modification of the model is required—namely, the use of a sign language interpreter in the classroom. In 1982, this type of educational support option was challenged by the Hendrick Hudson Board of Education in New York. The case was heard by the U.S. Supreme Court in *Hendrick Hudson Board of Education v. Rowley* (1982). The court ruled that Amy Rowley did not need an interpreter; however, it upheld the argument that Public Law 94-142 entitled students with disabilities to personalized instruction such as interpreter services.

In addition to full inclusion, there are other possible modifications of inclusion placements. In the *partial inclusion model,* the child spends part of the school day in a self-contained class with other children with hearing loss that is taught by a teacher of the deaf. The other part of the day is spent in a class with hearing peers that is taught by a regular education teacher. Another variation is a *team-teaching model,* in which a classroom comprised of students who are hard-of-hearing/deaf and typical-hearing peers is taught together by a regular education teacher and a teacher of the deaf. A third variation that is more restrictive is a model in which the child who is deaf/hard-of-hearing is placed in a self-contained classroom made up entirely of children with hearing loss that is taught by a teacher of the deaf. The classroom is within a public school with typically hearing children.

Early inclusion of children who are deaf and hard-of-hearing with normal-hearing peers provides considerable educational benefits for the child with a hearing loss. Three types of preschool integration placement options are available (Luetke-Stahlman, 1994):

1. Normal-hearing preschoolers are enrolled in early childhood programs specifically set up for children who are deaf or hard of hearing (i.e., reverse mainstreaming).
2. Children who are deaf or hard of hearing are placed in a self-contained early intervention program for part of the day and then in a child care center for additional socialization experiences.
3. Children who are deaf or hard of hearing are placed in preschool classes comprised of normal-hearing peers with sufficient support services to enable the children with hearing loss to participate fully in all activities with the other preschoolers throughout the day.

Clearly, integrating preschoolers with hearing loss into mainstreamed environments poses considerable challenges. Peer interaction between children with hearing loss and normal-hearing children is generally limited, because the communication attempts of the child with a hearing loss are often inadequate and ineffective (Vendell & George, 1981). Children with hearing loss learn language by participating in conversational exchanges (Kretschmer & Kretschmer, 1989). If their conversational attempts are not reinforced because of unresponsive peers, placement in an inclusive setting will have little benefit unless specific strategies are used to facilitate rich reciprocal conversations. Such conversations will result not only in language learning but also in socially interactive complex play. Strategies for facilitating good interactions between children with hearing loss and their normal-hearing peers include encouraging children with hearing loss to articulate more clearly, encouraging hearing peers to increase their communicative interactions with the children with hearing loss, and, if the children with hearing loss sign, to insist that they use simultaneous speech and sign (Luetke-Stahlman, 1991).

Once an inclusion option has been selected for a child, it is necessary to consider what factors will lead to his or her success. Reynolds and Birch (1977) identified the following components as necessary for inclusion success:

1. The regular classroom teacher is allowed to choose whether to have a child with hearing loss in his or her class.
2. Inclusion begins early, at the preschool level.
3. A teacher of the hearing impaired is on staff.
4. In-service training is provided for all staff who work with the child with hearing loss.
5. The classroom environment is well equipped with necessary amplification units.
6. The child with hearing loss is rarely separated from the regular educational setting.
7. All the professionals who work with the child meet regularly to review his or her progress and make modifications as needed.

In its purest form, inclusion is the meaningful involvement of all students in their neighborhood, school, and community (Progorzelski & Kelly, 1995). For the most severely disabled students, the emphasis of inclusion is on socialization, not academics, and academics are modified to meet their special needs. For children with hearing loss who are capable of age-appropriate academic achievement, the concept of inclusion must not erode the integrity of academic programming and expectations. If students require the presentation of academic material via sign language, such as ASL, then full inclusion means that both a regular education teacher and an ASL-proficient teacher of the deaf collaborate within the regular education classroom.

With this in mind, consider the advantages of inclusionary programming for children who are hard of hearing/deaf (Brackett, 1997):

1. It is stimulating, and the highly verbal setting provides models of language use and social interaction for children with hearing loss.
2. The inclusion setting includes interaction with typical peers, thereby exposing the child with hearing loss to social, academic, and communicative behaviors of typical peers.
3. There are many opportunities for technological support, peer-to-peer instruction, high expectations, and exposure to varied ideas and experiences.

Summary

The acquisition of literacy, reading and writing, involves the complex integration of many areas of learning, including speaking, listening, and critical thinking. An oral or manual language system must be intact if the child with a hearing loss is to learn to read and write. Learning to read and write requires being able to store up word meanings, remember vocabulary, and make abstract judgments about causal relationships (Streng, 1964). A solid language foundation is a prerequisite for the development of literacy skills.

Individuals with hearing loss have the same innate abilities to develop speech and language as persons in the normal-hearing population. Often, however, because of the severity of their hearing loss, they cannot acquire language through auditory channels alone. Consequently, overall delays in language development can result, putting children with hearing loss at a great educational disadvantage. Only through the application of normal language development theory can educators devise more effective methodologies for educating students with hearing loss. Current federal legislation, including the mandate for the least restrictive environment (LRE), further challenges professionals working with children with hearing loss. Children with hearing loss should be educated in the LRE with normal-hearing peers. It is up to the educator to ensure that these children benefit from instruction in the regular education setting. Only through careful planning, monitoring, and a team approach can that occur. Even children with unilateral hearing loss are at risk for academic failure. Although many of these children do not always use amplification systems (hearing aids, auditory trainers) they still need to be monitored for academic difficulties.

In diagnosing hearing loss in the pediatric population, the clinician needs to remember the importance of early detection and intervention. A complete audiological assessment must include pure tone findings, speech findings, and aural acoustic emmittance testing. Otoacoustic emission testing and possible ABR testing should also be used in conjunction with behavioral testing. Appropriate test parameters must be based on the age of the child. Accuracy and reliability are significant variables. Using available objective tests as screening tools will help ensure early detection.

Each child with a hearing loss has unique management needs. He or she must be fitted properly with amplification, appropriate assistive devices must be selected, and an appropriate educational setting must be considered. Implantation of a cochlear device should be considered and utilized if appropriate. Since the introduction of the device, performance continues to improve. Not all implant users derive the same level of benefit, however; the largest benefit is demonstrated when the implant user also uses speechreading to support communication. Use of the cochlear implant does not dictate educational placement, and children will continue to need speech language services and audiological management and monitoring throughout their educational years.

Major changes have taken place in the education of children with hearing loss. Continual research and application of effective rehabilitative and educational theory will ensure that professionals can continue to meet the challenges of educating these children.

Study Questions

1. What are the three types of hearing loss?
2. What are the benefits of using assistive listening devices?
3. For what reasons is a bilingual educational approach not routinely used when educating children with severe hearing impairments?
4. Who are good candidates for cochlear implants?
5. How has hearing aid technology changed in the last twenty or so years?
6. How has widespread availability of the cochlear implant affected children in the educational setting?

References

Allen, T. E. (1994). *Who are the deaf and hard of hearing students leaving high school and entering postsecondary education?* Unpublished manuscript, Gallaudet University, Center for Assessment and Demographic Studies, Washington, DC.

Anthony, D. (1971). *Signing essential English* (vols. 1 and 2). Anaheim, CA: Educational Division, Anaheim Union School District.

Balkany, T., Hodges, A., & Goldman, K. (1996). Ethics of cochlear implantation in young children. *Archives of Otolaryngology—Head and Neck Surgery, 114,* 748–755.

Bateson, M. C. (1975). Mother–infant exchanges: The epigenesis of conversational interaction. In D. Aaronson & R. W. Reiber (Eds.), *Annals of the New York Academy of Sciences: Vol. 263,*

Developmental psycholinguistics and communication disorders (pp. 101–113). New York: New York Academy of Sciences.

Bellugi, U., & Fischer, S. (1972). A comparison of sign language and spoken language. *Cognition, 1,* 173–200.

Bellugi, U., & Klima, E. (1975). Aspects of sign language and its structure. In J. Kavanagh & J. Cutting (Eds.), *The role of speech in language* (pp. 171–203). Cambridge, MA: MIT Press.

Bellugi, U., Klima, E., & Siple, P. (1974). Remembering in signs. *Cognition, 3,* 93–125.

Bloom, L., & Lahey, M. (1978). *Language development and language disorders.* New York: Wiley.

Brackett, D. (1997). Intervention for children with hearing impairment in general education settings. *Language, Speech, and Hearing Services in Schools, 28*(4), 355–371.

Brown, R. (1975). *Social psychology.* New York: Free Press.

Chess, S., & Thomas, A. (1996). *Temperament: Theory and practice.* New York: Brunner/Mazel.

Cole, E. B., & St. Clair-Stokes, J. (1984). Caregiver–child interactive behaviors: A videotape analysis procedure. *Volta Review, 86,* 200–216.

Cummins, J. (1981). The role of primary language development in promoting educational success for language minority students. In California State Department of Education, *Schooling and language minority students: A theoretical framework.* Los Angeles: Evaluation, Assessment and Dissemination Center.

Damen, G., van der Oever-Goltsten, M., Langeris, M., Chute, P., Mylanus, E. (2006). Educational performance of pediatric cochlear implant recipients in mainstream classes. *Annals of Otology, Rhinolology, and Laryngology, 115*(7), 542–552.

Davis, J. M., & Blasdell, R. (1975). Perceptual strategies by normal hearing and hearing-impaired children in the comprehension of sentences containing relative clauses. *Journal of Speech and Hearing Research, 18,* 281–295.

DeGangi, G., Wietlisbach, S., Poisson, S., Stein, E., & Royeen, C. (1994). The impact of culture and socioeconomic status on family–professional collaboration: Challenges and solutions. *Topics in Early Childhood Special Education, 14*(4), 503–520.

Dew, D. (Ed.) (1999). *Serving individuals who are low-functioning deaf: Report of the Twenty-Fifth Institute on Rehabilitation Issues.* Washington, DC: George Washington University.

Eimas, P. (1974). Auditory and linguistic processing cues for place of articulation by infants. *Perceptual Psychology, 16,* 513–521.

Eisenberg, L. S., Fink, N. E., & Niparko, J. K. (2006). Childhood development after cochlear implantation: Multicenter study examines language development. *The ASHA Leader, 11*(16), 5, 28–29.

English, K., & Church, G. (1999). Unilateral hearing loss in children: An update for the 1990s. *Language, Speech, and Hearing Services in Schools, 30,* 26–31.

Estabrooks, W. (2000). Auditory verbal practices. In S. Waltzman & N. Cohen (Eds.), *Cochlear implants* (pp. 225–316). New York: Thieme Medical.

Geers, A., Moog, J., & Schick, B. (1984). Acquisition of spoken and signed English by profoundly deaf children. *Journal of Speech and Hearing Disorders, 49,* 378–388.

Gentile, A., & DiFrancesca, S. (1969, Spring). *Academic achievement test performance of hearing impaired students: United States* (Series D, no. 1). Washington, DC: Gallaudet College, Office of Demographic Studies.

Glattke, T. J., & Kujawa, S. (1991). Otoacoustic emissions. *American Journal of Audiology, 1*, 29–40.

Golden-Meadow, S., & Mayberry, R. (2001). How do profoundly deaf children learn to read? *Learning Disabilities Research and Practice, 16*(4), 222–229.

Gravel, J., & Hood, L. (1999). Pediatric audiologic assessment. In F. Musiek & W. Rintelmann (Eds.), *Contemporary perspectives in hearing assessment* (pp. 305–323). Boston: Allyn & Bacon.

Greenstein, J. M., Bush, B., McConville, K., & Stellini, L. (1977). *Mother–infant communication and language acquisition in deaf infants.* New York: Lexington School for the Deaf.

Gustason, G., Pfetzing, D., & Zawolkow, E. (1972). *Signing exact English.* Rossmoor, CA: Modern Sign Press.

Hall, J., III (2000). *Handbook of otoacoustic emissions.* San Diego, CA: Singular.

Hanson, M., Lynch, E. W., & Wayman, K. L. (1990). Honoring the culture diversity of families when gathering data. *Topics in Early Childhood Education, 10*(1), 112–131.

Jaffe, J., Stern, D., & Peery, J. (1973). "Conversational" coupling of gaze behaviors in prelinguistic human development. *Journal of Psycholinguistic Research, 2*, 321–328.

Jerger, J., & Hayes, D. (1976). The cross-check principle in pediatric audiometry. *Archives of Otolaryngology, 702*, 614–620.

Katz, J. (1986). *Staggered Spondaic Word Test (SSW).* Vancouver, WA: Precision Acoustics.

Keith, R. (1994). *Test for Auditory Processing in Adolescents and Adults (SCAN-A).* San Antonio, TX: Psychological Corporation.

Keith, R. (2000). *Test for Auditory Processing Skills in Children (SCAN-C).* San Antonio, TX: Psychological Corporation.

Kelly, L. (1996). The interaction of syntactic competence and vocabulary during reading by deaf students. *Journal of Deaf Studies and Deaf Education, 1*, 75–90.

Kemp, D. T. (1978). Stimulated acoustic emissions from within the human auditory system. *Journal of the Acoustic Society of America, 64*, 1386–1391.

King, C. M., & Quigley, S. P. (1985). *Reading and deafness.* San Diego, CA: College-Hill.

Koester, L. S., & Meadow-Orlans, K. P. (1999). Responses to interactive stress: Infants who are deaf or hearing. *American Annals of the Deaf, 144*, 295–403.

Kretschmer, R. (1989). Pragmatics, reading, and writing. *Topics in Language Disorders, 9*(4), 17–32.

Kretschmer, R., & Kretschmer, L. (1989). Communication competence: Impact of the pragmatics revolution on education of hearing impaired individuals. *Topics in Language Disorders, 9*(4), 1–16.

Lafreniere, O., Smurzynski, J., Jung, M. D., Leonard, G., & Kim, D. O. (1993). Otoacoustic emissions in full-term newborns at risk for hearing loss. *Laryngoscope, 103*, 1334–1341.

Luetke-Stahlman, B. (1991). Hearing impaired students in integrated child care. *Perspectives, 9*(1), 8–11.

Luetke-Stahlman, B. (1994). Procedures for socially integrating preschoolers who are hearing, deaf, and hard of hearing. *Topics in Early Childhood Special Education, 14*(4), 472–487.

Luetke-Stahlman, B., Griffiths, C., & Montgomery, N. (1999). A deaf child's language acquisition verified through text retelling. *American Annals of the Deaf, 144*(3), 270–280.

Martin, F., & Clark, J. (2005). *Introduction to audiology.* Boston: Allyn & Bacon.

Martin, N. A., & Brownell, R. (2005). *Test of Auditory Processing Skills (TAPS–3)* (3rd ed.). Austin, TX: Pro-Ed.

Med-El Corporation. (n.d.) *Communication options and educational placements: A guidebook for parents.* Durham, NC: Author. Retrieved February, 2007, from www.implants@edelus.com.

Miller, C., & Morse, P. (1976). The "heart" of categorical speech discrimination in young infants. *Journal of Speech and Hearing Research, 19,* 578–589.

Miller, C., Morse, P., & Dorman, N. (1977). Cardiac indices of infants' speech perception: Orienting and burst discrimination. *Quarterly Journal of Experimental Psychology, 29,* 533–545.

Morse, P. (1972). The discrimination of speech and speech stimuli in early infancy. *Journal of Experimental Psychology, 14,* 477–492.

Mukari, S., Ling, L., & Ghani, H. (2007). Educational performance of pediatric cochlear implant recipients in mainstream classes. *International Journal of Pediatric Otorhinolaryngology, 71*(2), 231–240.

Nelson, K., Prinz, P., & Dalke, D. (1989). Transitions from sign language to text via an interactive microcomputer system. In B. Woll (Ed.), *Papers from the Seminar on Language Development and Sign Language* (Monograph 1, International Sign Linguistics Association). Bristol, England: Centre for Deaf Studies, University of Bristol.

Northern, J., & Downs, M. (1984). *Hearing in children.* Baltimore, MD: Williams & Wilkins.

Palmer, C., & Mormer, E. (1999). Goals and expectations of the child, family and educator: Proceedings from the International Pediatric Symposium: Remediating Pediatric Hearing Loss through Amplification: Taking Science into the Clinic. *Trends in Amplification, 4,* 6–71.

Paul, P. (1996). Reading, vocabulary knowledge, and deafness. *Journal of Deaf Studies and Deaf Education, 1,* 3–15.

Paul, P. (1998). *Literacy and deafness: The development of reading, writing, and literate thought.* Boston: Allyn & Bacon.

Paul, P., & Jackson, D. (1993). *Toward a psychology of deafness: Theoretical and empirical perspectives.* Boston: Allyn & Bacon.

Prinz, P., & Nelson, K. (1985). Alligator eats cookie: Acquisition of writing and reading skills by deaf children using the microcomputer. *Applied Psycholinguistics, 6,* 283–306.

Prinz, P., Nelson, K., Loncki, F., Geysels, G., & Willems, C. (1993). A multimodality and multimedia approach to language, discourse and literacy development. In F. Coninx & B. Elsendoorn (Eds.), *Interactive learning technology for the deaf.* New York: Springer-Verlag.

Prinz, P., Nelson, K. A., & Stedt, J. (1982). Early reading in young deaf children using microcomputer technology. *American Annals of the Deaf, 127,* 529–535.

Prinz, P., & Strong, M. (1998). ASL proficiency and English literacy within a bilingual deaf education model of instruction. *Topics in Language Disorders, 18*(4), 47–60.

Progorzelski, G., & Kelly, B. (1995). *Inclusion: The collaborative process.* Buffalo, NY: United Educational Services.

Quigley, S. P., & Kretschmer, R. E. (1982). *The education of deaf children.* Baltimore, MD: University Park Press.

Radziewicz, C. (1985). *The use of videotapes as a means of parent training for parents of hearing-impaired infants.* Unpublished doctoral dissertation, Adelphi University, Garden City, NY.

Reamer, J. C. (1921). Mental and educational measurement of the deaf. *Psychological Monographs, 132.*

Reynolds, M. C., & Birch, J. W. (1977). *Teaching exceptional children in all America's schools.* Reston, VA: Council for Exceptional Children.

Rhode Island Department of Health. (2006, April). *Rhode Island resource guide for families of children who are deaf or hard of hearing.* Office of Families Raising Children with Special Needs. Retrieved June, 2006, from www.health.state.ri.us/family/specialneeds/hearinglossguideFinal.pdf.

Richard, G. (2001). *The source for processing disorders.* East Moline, IL: LinguiSystems.

Robbins, A. M. (1986). Language comprehension in young children. *Topics in Language Disorders, 6,* 12–23.

Ross-Swain, D., & Long, N. (2004). *Auditory Processing Abilities Test (APAT).* Novato, CA: Academy Therapy.

Schick, B., & Gale, E. (1995). Preschool deaf and hard of hearing students' interactions during ASL and English storytelling. *American Annals of the Deaf, 140,* 363–370.

Shafer, D. (2007, June 19). Infant screening gains media spotlight. *ASHA Leader,* pp. 1, 7.

Snow, C. (1983). Literacy and language relationships during the preschool years. *Harvard Educational Review, 53,* 165–189.

Stach, B. A. (1997). *Comprehensive dictionary of audiology.* Baltimore, MD: Williams & Wilkins.

Stach, B. A. (1998). *Clinical audiology.* San Diego, CA: Singular.

Streng, A. (1964). *Reading for deaf children.* Washington, DC: Alexander Graham Bell Association for the Deaf.

Strong, M. (Ed.). (1988). *Language learning and deafness.* New York: Cambridge University Press.

Strong, M., & Prinz, P. (1997). A study of the relationship between ASL and English literacy. *Journal of Deaf Studies and Deaf Education, 2*(1), 37–46.

Tractenberg, R. (2002). Exploring hypotheses about phonological awareness, memory and reading achievement. *Learning Disabilities, 35*(5), 407–424.

Vendell, D. L., & George, L. B. (1981). Social interaction in hearing and deaf students: Success and failures in initiations. *Child Development, 52,* 627–635.

Vorce, E. (1974). *Teaching speech to deaf children.* Washington, DC: Alexander Graham Bell Association for the Deaf.

Wells, G. (1985). Preschool literacy related activities and success in school. In D. Olson, N. Torrance, & A. Hildyard (Eds.), *Literacy, language and learning: The nature and consequences of reading and writing* (pp. 229–255). New York: Cambridge University Press.

Widen, J. E. (1997). Evoked otoacoustic emission in evaluating children. In M. S. Robinette & T. J. Glattke (Eds.), *Otoacoustic emissions: Clinical applications* (pp. 271–306). New York: Thieme Medical.

Wilbur, R. B. (1979). *American Sign Language and sign systems.* Baltimore, MD: University Park Press.

Yoshinaga-Itano, C., & Apuzzo, M. R. (1998a). The development of deaf and hard of hearing children identified early through the high-risk registry. *American Annals of the Deaf, 143,* 416–424.

Yoshinaga-Itano, C., & Apuzzo, M. R. (1998b). Identification of hearing loss after 18 months is not early enough. *American Annals of the Deaf, 143,* 380–387.

Zwolan, T., (2000). *Selection criteria and evaluation.* New York: Thieme Medical.

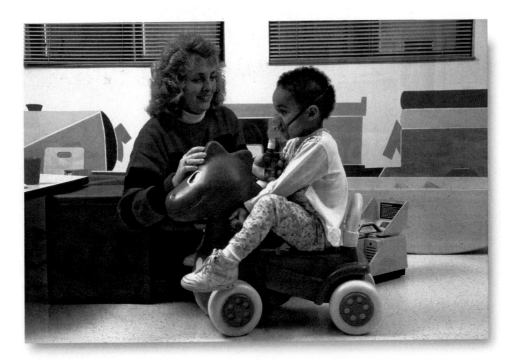

CHAPTER 9

The Role of the SLP

Ellenmorris Tiegerman-Farber
Adelphi University

When you finish this chapter, you will be able to

- Discuss why parents need to become part of the collaborative decision-making process.
- Explain why inclusion requires individualized programming.
- List the barriers to successful collaboration.
- Discuss how the makeup of the collaborative team determines the role that it plays in educational reform.

- Explain why collaborative teaming requires that speech-language pathologists, parents, and teachers change their roles and responsibilities.
- Articulate the difference between consultation and collaboration as service delivery models.

Because the Individuals with Disabilities Education Act (IDEA) of 1986 (Public Law 99-457) introduced programming for infants and preschoolers, language development has become a critical component in the evaluation and treatment of young children with disabilities. In fact, language and communication disorders (LCD) are present in most children with developmental disabilities (Tiegerman-Farber & Radziewicz, 2007d). No other professional has the knowledge, training, and expertise of the speech-language pathologist to meet this educational challenge. The importance of language in early childhood development has shifted the role of the speech-language pathologist from related service provider to classroom teacher in some programs. It is a very exciting time for the field of speech-language pathology as our professional skills become more important to all aspects of educational programming. The chapters that follow in this part present much more detail about the changing role of the speech-language pathologist (SLP) as a teacher consultant, parent trainer, and collaborative team member. This chapter explains the interactive teaming service delivery models of consultation and collaboration used to provide services for children with disabilities. The difference between the two models relates to the way that parents and professionals interact with each other to solve child-based learning problems. Interactive teaming in its various forms has become a part of the school reform movement in many schools nationwide. The interactive models take into consideration a number of issues that occur in special education.

1. Public Law 99-457 emphasizes the importance of early intervention.
2. With the reauthorization of the Individuals with Disabilities Education Act (IDEA) there is an increased focus on the provision of services within inclusive environments and natural settings.
3. To maximize the efficiency and effectiveness of service provision, professionals need to use models that facilitate the coordination of multiple services provided to children with disabilities.

4. Special education has become family focused, which requires the inclusion of parents within the decision-making process. Consultation and collaboration are used during assessment, educational/clinical programming, and annual review of the child's progress.

5. Cultural and linguistic differences between professionals and families require the use of models that facilitate and enhance effective communication.

The increased emphasis on inclusive programming in schools and natural settings requires the speech-language pathologist to use both of the consultation and collaboration models to meet the needs of culturally and linguistically diverse children and families. The dynamic interface between professionals and parents must be learned "on the job," because few teacher-training internships facilitate this type of professional interaction (Ogletree, 1999). The speech-language pathologist will also be working more frequently with children, teachers, and parents in special and regular education classrooms; this change in responsibilities requires the development of new professional competencies. Because the speech-language pathologist and the classroom teacher have different academic training experiences and professional perceptions of their roles (Nungesser & Watkins, 2005), they must be proactive in learning to work together cooperatively to identify child-based learning problems and to develop appropriate intervention strategies. This chapter will discuss how interactive teaming provides a mechanism for professionals to share their expertise with each other and with parents to maximize opportunities for parents and children in more diverse settings (Crais, Roy, & Free, 2006).

Changes in Special Education Law

EDUCATION FOR ALL HANDICAPPED CHILDREN ACT (EAHCA)

The Education for All Handicapped Children Act, Public Law 94-142, was passed in 1975 after many years of advocacy from parents and service organizations. Up until this point most children with disabilities were not being educated in local public schools. P.L. 94-142 guaranteed children with disabilities a free and appropriate public education (FAPE) to the maximum extent possible with peers without disabilities. P.L. 94-142 established national procedures and safeguards for parents to ensure that children with disabilities had the same educational opportunities as children without disabilities.

After the passage of P.L. 94-142, many researchers and educators argued that the law did not mandate services for children from birth to 5 years and therefore did not go far enough. Technological advancements enabled the earlier diagnosis of many disorders; however, with no provision for educational intervention to meet the dramatic needs of infants and preschoolers with disabilities, voluntary agencies (e.g., United Cerebral Palsy, the Association for Children with Down's Syndrome, and the Association for Children with Learning Disabilities) developed and expanded to address this need. However, the types and levels of services varied from community to community across the United States; some communities provided extensive services and some provided none for children below the age of 5 years. Clearly, identification required intervention, but it was not until 1986 that P.L. 99-457 was passed.

Essentially, P.L. 99-457 addresses two groups of children with disabilities: preschoolers and infants. It extends to the first group—preschool children ages 3 and 4—all federal requirements, rights, and protections currently applicable to school-aged children with disabilities (5 to 21 years of age). Such requirements include an Individualized Education Plan (IEP), adherence to least restrictive environment (LRE) guidelines, and due process provisions including educational committees (Committee on Special Education, Committee on Preschool Special Education/Individual Family Service Plan) that allow parents the right to challenge educational decisions. In addition, P.L. 99-457 amended the Education for All Handicapped Children Act to develop and implement comprehensive, coordinated, multidisciplinary, interagency programs of early intervention services for infants and toddlers and their families. This policy explanation is based on the recognized need

- to enhance the development of infants and toddlers with disabilities and to minimize their potential for developmental delay
- to reduce the educational costs to our society, including our nation's schools, by minimizing the need for special education and related services after infants and toddlers reach school age
- to minimize the likelihood of institutionalization of individuals with disabilities and to maximize their potential for independent living in society
- to enhance the capacity of families to meet the special needs of their infants and toddlers with disabilities

Since the passage of P.L. 94-142, programs were developed nationally to provide educational and therapeutic services to children who were either not receiving an education or were not receiving adequate services. In the 1986 reauthorization of P.L. 94-142, the 101st Congress changed the name of the Education for All Handicapped Children Act (EAHCA) to the Individuals with Disabilities Education Act (IDEA). In addition, the term "handicap" was replaced by "disability." Although the development of public education programs for children with disabilities addressed a critical need, it simultaneously presented a range of related challenges that now require attention and resolution. One of these issues relates to *how* decisions are made about a child's developmental needs.

The 2004 reauthorization of the Individuals with Disabilities Education Act, retitled the Individuals with Disabilities Education Improvement Act (IDEA 2004), shifted the "balance of power" back to school districts, holding them less accountable and weakening parental due process rights (Vitello, 2007, p. 66). IDEA 2004 describes a "shared responsibility" in the decision-making process as well as "new accountability" and "personal responsibility" for parents and students with disabilities by emphasizing dispute resolution procedures such as mediation (Turnbull, 2007).

NO CHILD LEFT BEHIND (NCLB) ACT OF 2001

NCLB holds schools that receive Title 1 federal funding accountable by requiring them to meet performance standards based on annual assessments. Statewide tests of student performance are used to evaluate schools with consequences ranging from school improvement plans to restructuring and eventual state "takeover." NCLB requires a disaggregation of school assessment scores by subgroups of students (i.e., racial minorities and children with disabilities), transparently highlighting achievement gaps across student groups in test scores. Student achievement has become the measure of student learning and school success, resulting in increasing pressures on teachers to teach to the statewide assessments and limiting curriculum content to material that appears on the exam. With the emphasis on standardized assessments and the substantial time required to prepare students to take the exam (Toch, 2006), reading and math abilities have become the primary focus of schools across the country (Guilfoyle, 2006). Although the raised standards and performance expectations have focused attention on teaching curriculum content, U.S. students still do not perform as well as their peers in other industrialized countries (Haycock, 2006). At the high school level, the National Assessment of Educational Progress (NAEP) data do not show significant change in student performance; one reason is that the emphasis on increasing student performance has not been accompanied by better methods of instruction, particularly for children with disabilities (Tiegerman-Farber & Radziewicz, 2007e). SLPs can help fill this void as well as assist in making progress to reduce achievement gaps among various groups of students by embracing collaborative opportunities in general education classrooms.

EARLY INTERVENTION

The implementation of P.L. 99-457 has dramatically changed how services are provided, where they are provided, and by whom (Bailey, Aytch, Odom, Symons, & Wolery, 1999). Part H of P.L. 99-457 requires an Individual Family Service Plan (IFSP) for children with developmental disabilities from birth through 2 years. Families receive a comprehensive range of services, including direct therapeutic and developmental services in school-based programs, and early childhood nursery school programs as well as home settings. The IFSP focuses on the needs of the *family* as well as the needs of the child. For instance, if a parent needs counseling in order to function more appropriately with the infant or toddler, the IFSP includes such counseling services. If a parent has economic hardships and has no means of getting to the counseling services, the IFSP will provide for transportation. Because the early intervention system emphasizes the role of the parent as the front-line service provider and educator for the child, these services require a collaborative relationship between family members and professionals within this system (Dinnebeil & Hale, 1999). The early intervention system that has evolved presents a change in focus from the needs and strengths of the child to the needs and strengths of the child within the family, which reflects an ecological view of the child as part of a family system (Dunst, 2002). Bronfenbrenner (1977) conceptualized this ecological view of child development as one that considers the child a member of a family unit which in turn is a member of a larger interactive community. The philosophy that generated P.L. 99-457 supports a family-centered approach that emphasizes that the needs of the child and the needs of the family are intertwined and interdependent (Dunst & Bruder, 2002; Summers, Hoffman, Marquis, Turnbull, & Poston, 2005). Within this early intervention system, the role of the speech-language pathologist has changed dramatically; differences in speech and language skills were often the first warning signs recognized by parents (McConachie, Le Couteur, & Honey, 2005; Paul-Brown & Ricker, 2003). The speech-language pathologist is the primary professional to teach parents, teachers, and peers how to facilitate the language learning process.

In the context of the program extension to younger children and the more encompassing ecological perspective that became necessary, P.L. 99-457 also requires an Individualized Education Plan (IEP) for preschool children as they transition from early intervention to the preschool system. Federal law emphasizes the need for states to develop a seamless system for children and families. As a result, transition planning and programming must be detailed within the child's IFSP and (pre-school) IEP. As stated, parental involvement is a significant part of the early intervention and preschool process. States have different designations for the school district committees that evaluate preschool and school-age children with disabilities. In New York, the Committee on Preschool Special Education (CPSE) generates a plan (IEP) collaboratively with the family. The speech-language pathologist is skilled in assessing the speech and language behaviors of the child as well as the communicative interactions of parents and caregivers and can provide insights into enhancing and developing these skills within the family. For the young child, most early learning is mediated through language; therefore, it is vital that families participate in an intervention program along with the speech-language pathologist. It is interesting to note that the majority—83 percent—of children in New York state identified with a developmental disability in 1998–1999 received speech-language services. With the early intervention system shifting to a family-centered approach, the speech-language pathologist needs to interact with parents and teachers on a more interpersonal basis in school and home (Friehe, Bloedow, & Hesse, 2003; Troia, 2005).

CHANGING ROLE OF THE SLP

SLPs along with other school professionals such as school counselors are being required to change from a pull-out model of therapeutic service provision to a collaborative model of classroom inclusion. SLPs need to be better prepared at the academic and preservice training levels to meet the needs of students with disabilities in more naturalized environments (Barnes, Friehe, & Radd, 2003). Several questions within this chapter are raised as the collaborative model is discussed:

1. Are SLPs being trained adequately to work within collaborative settings?
2. Are SLPs trained appropriately to counsel families of students with disabilities? Do SLPs understand the difference between counseling services provided by an SLP and a psychologist or school counselor?
3. Are SLPs trained to modify the general education curriculum content?

There has been an explosion of information regarding the communication behaviors of children below the age of 5 years. The American Speech-Language-Hearing Association (ASHA) published a position statement in 1990 on the role of the speech-language pathologist in service delivery to infants, toddlers, and their families. This position statement clarifies the changing roles and responsibilities of the speech-language pathologist as including:

- screening and identification
- assessment and evaluation
- design, planning, direct delivery, and monitoring of treatment programs
- case management
- consultation with and referral to agencies and other professionals that provide services to this young population and their families

These roles should be assumed as part of a comprehensive family-centered program that is coordinated with other services that families and their children may need or receive (Figure 9.1). The speech-language pathologist has become an integral member of the multidisciplinary team serving families and their infants or toddlers (ASHA, 1990). The SLP provides services to children, teachers, and parents across a continuum of settings from therapy room to classroom (Beatson, 2006; Tiegerman-Farber & Radziewicz, 2007c). In addition, diversity has been introduced into the required competencies and professional competencies of the speech-language pathologist. The issue of diversity has become a part of who we are as professionals and not just what we do. The complex needs of culturally and linguistically diverse families has required the development of specialized courses and training for speech-language pathologists and other professionals. Many academic programs are just now including courses on early

Figure 9.1 The Role of the Speech-Language Pathologist

Children	Team	Document	Settings	Role/Responsibility/Model
5–12 years	CSE	IEP	Therapy room/school/center	Evaluation team (collaboration)
			Special education classroom	Teacher (consultation)
			Regular education classroom	Co-teacher (collaboration)
			Job training site	Parent–trainer (consultation)
			Camp/Home	Private therapist–related service provider
3–5 years	CPSE	IEP	Therapy room/school/center	Teacher (consultation)
			Special education classroom	Co-teacher (collaboration/consultation)
			Camp/Home	Private therapist–related service provider
			Day care/nursery school	Co-teacher (collaboration/consultation)
3 years	IFSP	IFSP	Home/school/center	Related service provider
			Developmental group	Evaluation team (collaboration)
			Day care	Teacher (consultation)

intervention and cultural diversity within the graduate curriculum (Jones & Blendinger, 1994). For professionals already in the field, these new competencies and skills will have to be learned "on the job," causing significant difficulties for schools and clinics attempting to integrate children with disabilities. As a result, the educational field will require several years to create staff development programs to "teach" speech-language pathologists and other professionals the necessary competencies to assist schoolwide reform programs (Midkiff & Lawler-Prince, 1992). At the present time the speech-language pathologist is being encouraged to work closely with other professionals in diverse settings outside the traditional therapy room (Bopp, Brown, & Mirenda, 2004; Rogers-Adkinson & Stuart, 2007), such as within schools, early childhood programs, and camps attempting to integrate children with disabilities.

The Process Begins

Although this chapter discusses consultation and collaboration as service delivery models, it is important to make a distinction between them at this point for the sake of clarity.

Consultation can be defined as a structured series of interactions between two individuals to bring about changes in a target person. For example, when a speech-language pathologist works with a special education teacher to identify strategies that will facilitate the generalization of language learning goals for a specific child with language and communication disorders, consultation provides the mechanism for the SLP to give support and instructional advice within either special education or regular classrooms. In consultation, the professionals communicate, cooperate, and coordinate their instruction to facilitate the evaluation, planning, and implementation of learning goals, but the speech-language pathologist functions as an advisor (Tiegerman-Farber & Radziewicz, 2007a).

Collaboration is defined by joint decision making. Members of the team function as equal contributors and share the responsibility for decision making. "Collaboration is an interactive process that enables people with diverse expertise to generate creative solutions to mutually defined problems. The outcome is enhanced, altered and produces solutions that are different from those that the individual team members would produce independently" (Idole, Paolucci-Whitecomb, & Nevin, 1986). The collaboration team may include the regular education teacher, the special education teacher, the occupational therapist, the parents, the psychologist, and the speech-language pathologist.

Interactive teaming that includes consultation and collaboration is used at all stages of educational and clinical decision making, from evaluation to intervention to reevaluation. Figure 9.2 describes the mandated process used by schools to make decisions about the needs of a child and his or her family and whether or not they receive special education services. P.L. 94-142 describes the assessment responsibilities of a multidisciplinary team, called the Committee on Special Education (CSE) and the Committee on Preschool Special Education (CPSE) in New York state, consisting of professionals and parents in an interactive process of dialogue and decision making. The collaborative model is used by this multidisciplinary team from the initial point of assessment through the intervention process. Notice that the SLP is an integral member of the multidisciplinary team. Intervention that involves the actual provision of services to the child may include consultation or collaboration. Interpersonal

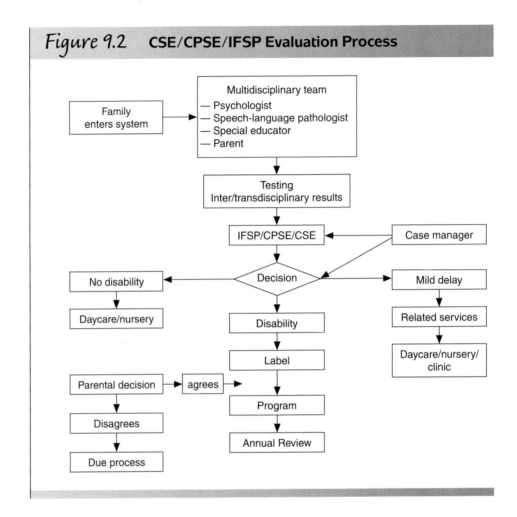

Figure 9.2   CSE/CPSE/IFSP Evaluation Process

dynamics and financial resources will often determine whether either or both models are used by professionals and parents within specific programs and schools.

As stated, P.L. 94-142 requires child assessment by means of a **multidisciplinary** team consisting of several different professionals. In the **interdisciplinary team model**, different professionals work independently to assess and then exchange information. Although treatment goals may be planned jointly, the delivery of services is often isolated. With a **transdisciplinary team model**, different professionals work together across discipline boundaries with the purpose of integrating their findings into a transdisciplinary treatment plan. This model of assessment and intervention is considered most appropriate for families and children. The needs of the family and the child determine the necessary members of the team. Cooperation among all team members is of paramount importance. Inherent within the interactive team is interdependence among team members; each member can attain individual goals only if the other team members achieve theirs. In addition, team members should have knowledge of early child development, assessment procedures, and intervention techniques (Crais, Roy, & Free, 2006; Nungesser & Watkins, 2005). Although parents have a knowledge base different from professionals, they must also become members of the team and participate in the process; this issue will be discussed further in the latter part of the chapter.

FAMILY ASSESSMENT

In order for an assessment to be complete, the team must acknowledge the importance of the family and conduct a family-focused assessment, in which both family and professionals consider the child within the context of the family. Traditionally only the needs and strengths of the child were considered; now the needs and strengths of the family must be brought to the forefront. When family strengths are considered, parents feel competent; when family needs are met, they feel empowered. The family-oriented assessment is inclusive of the child's strengths and needs, but there also needs to be an ecobehavioral focus that provides a community context to the provision of services. The family of a child with an autism spectrum disorder living in an urban area requires very different support services from a family in a rural area. Consider the following scenarios presented by parents.

> I live in a very rural area of Alabama and the closest school is 50 miles away. It is impossible to find specialists such as a speech-language pathologist, occupational therapist and physical therapist to provide services in my home on a regular basis. In addition, given my son's adaptive/physical requirements I want him to be with other children who have special needs. I have agreed to place my child on a bus for an hour so that he can attend a full-day self-contained program which I try to visit on a weekly basis.

> I live in an apartment building in Los Angeles. I am just learning English along with my child. My husband and I work several jobs during the week. I do not want social workers and professionals coming to my home; it is intrusive to my family. Besides my parents do not speak any English and I do not want to explain myself here. I want my daughter to receive her services in a half-day special education program and then be bussed to a day center in the afternoon so I can pick her up at 7 p.m. It has been difficult to find a good day care program to accept my daughter since she has a disability.

The family assessment approach interfaces community institutions with parents in order to enhance a family's ability to function well and to facilitate development of the child with a disability (Briggs-Gowan, Carter, Bosson-Heenan, Guyer, & Horowitz, 2006; Maniadaki, Sonuga-Barke, Kakouros, & Karaba, 2007). The family assessment model also meets the challenge of Part H of P.L. 99-457, which directs agencies to support and enable parents to be aware of and choose from a wide range of creative intervention options for families.

Several factors must be considered when shifting the focus from child-centered assessment to family assessment. One must remember that although assessment of the infant is ensured through law, it is up to the family to decide *if* they want an assessment to be performed. If the family understands that they are respected by the professional team and that their needs as well as their child's needs are considered important, they are more likely to be committed to the assessment process. The assessment must be conducted by personnel trained to utilize appropriate methods and procedures and is based on information provided by the family through a personal interview. The assessment must incorporate the family's description of its resources, priorities, and concerns (Dunst, 2002; Summers, Hoffman, Marquis, Turnbull, & Poston, 2005).

Several important questions need to be considered before the assessment process begins. What strategies should be used in this assessment process? When is the best time for a family assessment to be done? How can the team prevent the family from viewing the assessment process as intrusive? Who should perform the family assessment? What if the team identifies a family need that the family does not recognize? Why is an assessment of family strengths important? Figure 9.2 indicates that the multidisciplinary team may consist of a school psychologist, a speech-language pathologist, a special education teacher, and a parent. Professional members of the team need to explain to the parent not only the results of their particular assessment but also how their results fit in with the total picture of the child within the context of the family and its needs. If effective family assessment is to be achieved:

1. The child needs to be evaluated by a multidisciplinary team with the parents as members of the team—in the child's primary or natural language.
2. Professionals should use a range of multicultural assessment instruments after the child has been in an experimental/diagnostic classroom and has had an opportunity to interact with members of the evaluation team, including the parents.
3. There should be multiple observations of the child. Observational analysis and discussion will facilitate a product that reinforces common goals across discipline areas. In the school setting, the classroom represents the most natural context.
4. Parent–child analyses should be part of the diagnostic protocol. The diagnostic team might observe the child with the family, enabling the team to acquire information for a family assessment, as well as information on the quantity and quality of family–child interactions.

WHAT IS COLLABORATION?

Coufal (1993) notes that interactive teaming defines how participants interact with each other as equal contributors in a decision-making process to generate common or shared goals. This suggests that all of the stakeholders—psychologist, speech-language pathologist, special education teacher, and parent—share goals, decision making, status, accountability, and resources in an ongoing working relationship (Knackendoffel, 2005). This may initially be difficult for the psychologist, speech-language pathologist, special educator, and parent, given traditional professional expectations. The process of coming together requires a reevaluation and re-creation of roles, responsibilities, and relationships, which means that interactive teams must pay close attention to interactional variables such as communication skills, problem-solving skills, and conflict-resolution strategies. The formation and development of an interactive team involves a learning process that includes the following communicative competency skills (Crais, 1993):

- willingness to listen to others
- being supportive of someone else's ideas
- being receptive to input
- managing differences of opinion and conflict

- accepting and integrating suggestions of others
- expressing opinions and ideas without criticism
- acknowledging and using the ideas of others
- being flexible

These interactive behaviors contribute to the effectiveness and efficiency of decision making. By developing these behaviors and adopting a collaborative style, the participants ultimately create and generate an effective working relationship that will benefit the child. In addition, as schools and clinics attempt to develop inclusive programming, the need to identify an effective process for decision making becomes more important (Hunt, Soto, Maier, & Doering, 2003; Hunt, Soto, Maier, Liboiron, & Bae, 2004). Parents, teachers, and speech-language pathologists must believe that a shared effort will result in a better outcome than an individual effort. The social and psychological dynamics of contributing to group decision making create a premium on maintaining positive communicative relationships (Friend & Bursuck, 1996).

In order to achieve inclusive programming for children with language and communication disorders, a school must engage in levels of collaborative teaming (Figure 9.3). Before implementing inclusion within any classroom, there need to be

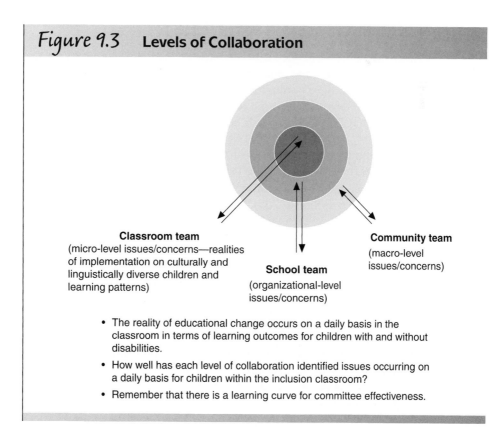

Figure 9.3   **Levels of Collaboration**

Classroom team
(micro-level issues/concerns—realities of implementation on culturally and linguistically diverse children and learning patterns)

School team
(organizational-level issues/concerns)

Community team
(macro-level issues/concerns)

- The reality of educational change occurs on a daily basis in the classroom in terms of learning outcomes for children with and without disabilities.
- How well has each level of collaboration identified issues occurring on a daily basis for children within the inclusion classroom?
- Remember that there is a learning curve for committee effectiveness.

school as well as community-based discussions (Farrell, Dyson, Polat, Hutcheson, & Gallannaugh, 2007; Knackendoffel, 2005). Part of the challenge in the development of inclusive programming within a school involves supportive networking before, during, and after changes are made within the classroom. Collaborative teams consisting of representatives from the various stakeholder groups must be provided with the opportunity to discuss the significant issues related to inclusion and general school changes that will occur (Hodkinson, 2005, 2006, 2007; Pirrie & Head, 2007).

Each level of teaming provides direction and scaffolding for the next. A decision-making hierarchy allows for a more focused analysis of issues from a macro to a micro level: community to school to classroom. As a result, decisions are based on the recommendations of the prior level. This ensures continuity as well as a progression in decision making as issues and problems become the pragmatic realities of individual teachers, parents, and children. Successful educational reform requires partnerships and alliances sharing ideas and problem solving about changes that will affect the personal lives of and interpersonal relationships between professionals, parents, and children (Tiegerman-Farber & Radziewicz, 2007b). Figure 9.3 indicates that collaborative teams must be developed to address community-based, school-based, and classroom-based reforms. These teams solve problems not only within their group, but also across groups.

COLLABORATIVE TEAMING: COMMUNITY

This community-based team should have a broad representation consisting of community leaders, regular education teachers, special education teachers, speech-language pathologists, administrators, and parents of children with and without disabilities. The purpose of the team is to develop a clear mission statement about inclusion that will be discussed, negotiated, and formulated with multicultural issues in mind. Because the school exists within a specific multicultural environment, the community as a whole needs to understand the mission of inclusion as well as the reforms that will result from this new program model. This team needs to identify cultural issues that may present as barriers to educational reform (Driscoll, 2001; Hammer, 2003; Kinnaman, 2000; Loder, 2005; Whitcomb, Borko, & Liston, 2006). If the community does not support the mission and goals of inclusion programming, the school will have a difficult time achieving physical, social, and instructional interactions between children with and without disabilities. In any collaborative team the process of resolving philosophical differences and conflicts is of critical importance, and collaborative decision making should include the following steps:

1. Identify the beliefs, attitudes, and perceptions of various cultural groups.
2. Identify ways to deal with the problem.
3. Think about the possible results of each recommendation.
4. Generate responsible proactive decision.
5. Evaluate the decision and its results.
6. Reconsider the decision.
7. Be flexible.

COLLABORATIVE TEAMING: SCHOOL

The collaborative team within a school must take into consideration the concerns and issues of the community in order to implement the goals related to the mission statement (Clough & Garner, 2003; Hanko, 2003; Nind, 2005). Will the community support the school's mission? How will the community support the school? The school-based collaborative team should consist of an administrator, a special education teacher, a speech-language pathologist, a regular teacher, and parents of children with and without disabilities. The school-based collaborative team needs to consider

- the requirements necessary to implement the mission statement within the school as an educational environment, wherein the collaborative challenge involves supportive networking between the school and community before, during, and after inclusive programming has been developed
- a timeline for programmatic development that includes community updates on progress
- a proposal for procedural changes reflecting the educational reforms that must take place
- the process of change and how long-range changes will be accomplished by classroom-based collaborative teams

Also, the strategies to achieve classroom inclusion require school modifications and problem solving regarding

- financial costs of programming changes
- hiring of new staff
- the number of children with and without disabilities in the inclusion classroom
- organizational changes within the classroom
- space allocation problems
- necessary classroom resources, such as supplies and materials
- fears and concerns of parents, teachers, and children

COLLABORATIVE TEAMING: CLASSROOM

The classroom-based collaborative team should consist of the special education teacher, regular education teacher, speech-language pathologist, and parents of children with and without disabilities. This team has the most complicated responsibilities because there are short-term as well as long-term problems that will require discussion, negotiation, and resolution within the parameters of the classroom. Successful inclusion will not be accomplished if the stakeholders cannot come to consensus about the educational benefit of inclusion for children with and without disabilities (Woolfson, Grant, & Campbell, 2007). This collaborative team will attempt to achieve physical, social, and instructional interactions between children with and without disabilities. Inclusion requires the identification and removal of barriers, including personal and instructional concerns (Gable & Hendrickson, 1997). The collaborative classroom team must learn how to make decisions by means of a group process; this involves a major reevaluation of interpersonal relationships, responsibilities, and educational decision making.

HOW COLLABORATION IS ACHIEVED

The inclusion classroom as an ecological environment is different from the traditional classroom. The goals are different, the teachers are different, the instructional process is different, learning is different, child outcomes are different, and the curriculum is different. The inclusion process stimulates a synergy of change focused within one small space—the classroom. The agents of change, the collaborators, must all share a common focus and commitment to create the necessary changes.

The purpose of a collaborative model is to provide the interactive team with a representational structure that can be used to highlight why specific interactions operate or do not operate effectively. Chess (1986) described a "goodness of fit concept" that can be used as a starting point by a collaborative team to make decisions about assessment, language goals, instructional procedures, and placement needs within the least restrictive setting. Tiegerman-Farber & Radziewicz (2007b) described decision making as an interactional process among individuals that helps the regular and special education teachers and the speech-language pathologist to understand the characteristics and behaviors of effective collaboration (Figure 9.4). If we look more closely at the "goodness of fit" model, we realize that members of the collaborative team—teachers and speech-language pathologists—need to be aware of the other person's perception of the child. Once these baseline perceptions are discussed and agreed on, joint expectations arise, manifested in mutual goals, parity, shared participation, and accountability, all of which are inherent in collaboration. A consequence of this collaborative spirit is the natural inclusion of families from the beginning of the referral process through the placement of the child with a disability in the least restrictive environment. The stakeholders develop a common focus and commitment to engage in interactive dialogue to set the ground rules. To facilitate this, several operating principles or guidelines for group decision making can be highlighted by using the "goodness of fit" model:

- co-equality and co-participation
- reciprocity
- commonality in goals

The Changing Role of the Speech-Language Pathologist

CO-EQUALITY AND CO-PARTICIPATION

In the collaborative process, the roles of the teacher (regular or special education) and the speech-language pathologist will be different within the inclusion classroom; the two professionals will have to learn to work as partners.

1. A regular education teacher and a special education teacher may spend all of their time together when schools utilize a full inclusion model and children with disabilities receive their related services in the classroom.

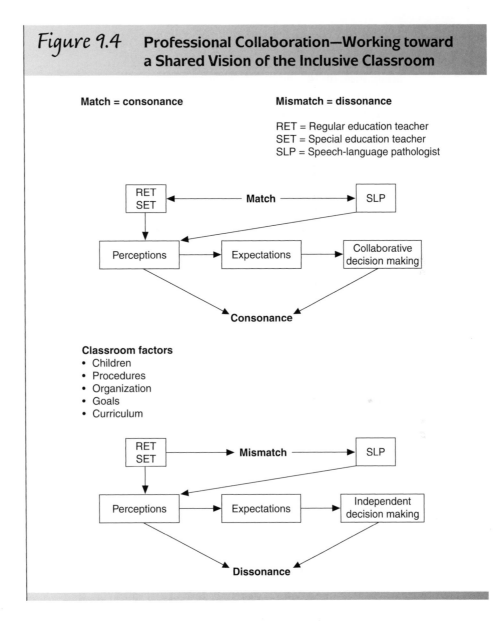

Figure 9.4   **Professional Collaboration—Working toward a Shared Vision of the Inclusive Classroom**

2. A special (or regular) education teacher and a speech-language pathologist may spend part of their time working together in the classroom when schools utilize a modified inclusion or push-in model. The speech-language pathologist provides individual speech-language services to children from the class and also works with these same children in class to generalize their language skills to a more natural setting with peers.

3. The teacher and the speech-language pathologist need to spend time together brainstorming about (a) classroom space, (b) the number of regular education students and children with disabilities, (c) the specialty needs of the children with disabilities, (d) the individual learning needs of all of the children, (e) strategies to facilitate child-to-child learning experiences. The teaching team needs to develop an educational plan for the classroom as a whole, as well as for each child individually.

4. The learning process in an inclusion classroom using the collaborative model will have distinctive features.
   a. The teacher and the speech-language pathologist will have a dynamic working relationship based on their consensus about individual and group learning, team teaching, and consultation, as well as their roles in direct intervention in the classroom.
   b. The speech-language pathologist will use instructional techniques to facilitate language for the child with a disability in a group setting.
   c. The child with a disability will have the opportunity to interact with typical peers in a variety of academic and social activities, which will change the structure and the organization of classroom learning.
   d. The physical classroom environment will be organized differently.
   e. Parents of children with and without disabilities will have more opportunities to meet, to socialize, and to learn from each other.
   f. The process for and content of learning will be based on a curriculum that includes language and communication goals.
   g. Children teaching children will become an important means of implementing the general curriculum.

Who the teachers are and how each professional functions within the inclusion classroom often present many challenges to the previous methodologies used by professionals. The teacher and the speech-language pathologist need to be provided with intensive in-service instruction and support over a long period of time. As children with language/communication disorders (LCD) are introduced into the general education classroom, the regular education teacher and the speech-language pathologist need to receive formal instructional training on the possible organizational changes that need to occur within their classrooms (O'Shea, Williams, & Sattler, 1999). They also need time to discuss their concerns and feelings about changes in their roles and responsibilities. The teacher needs to know about children with developmental disabilities and what the educational and behavioral implications are for integrating them within the classroom. She needs to know what to expect from the child with LCD in terms of communication and social skills. She also needs to know about management strategies, about the kinds of procedures and techniques that can be used to integrate the child with LCD into ongoing classroom activities (Diehl, Ford, & Federico, 2005; Ehren, 2006; Nungesser & Watkins, 2005).

CO-TEACHING

Co-teaching or team teaching is a collaborative process that may provide one educational mechanism for beginning the inclusion process (Beck & Dennis, 1997). This would mean that the relationship between the speech-language pathologist and the special education or regular education teacher would change immediately. The role of the speech-language pathologist would change from that of providing direct services to children with LCD in a separate room to providing services to *all* children in the same classroom. The fact that there will be two professionals within the inclusion classroom presents instructional and interpersonal challenges for professionals who have been trained in different discipline areas (Austin, 2001; Creese, 2006). The regular education teacher, the special education teacher, and the speech-language pathologist have highly specialized and divergently different foundations for knowledge. They approach the teaching experience from different vantage points; their academic coursework has been different, their teaching experiences have been different, and the settings within which they have worked are different. Perhaps the first and most immediate problem involves an understanding of the new working relationship that must be created (Keefe, Moore, & Duff, 2004; Murray, 2004).

In addition to assisting the classroom teacher to develop an understanding of the individual needs of children with LCD within the classroom, the speech-language pathologist—by using specialty skills that include management techniques, task analysis skills, and instructional procedures—can facilitate language learning for *all* of the children in the inclusion classroom. Children who have been classified with LCD are not the only ones with individual needs. The speech-language pathologist can also assist in facilitating interactions between the classroom teacher and the children with LCD, as well as between child peer groups (Tiegerman-Farber & Radziewicz, 2007c).

The classroom teacher can contribute to the inclusion classroom by providing instructional techniques and activities for the speech-language pathologist with the typical children in the classroom. The classroom teacher is uniquely skilled in developing academic curriculum goals that provide a level of motivation and skill development for typical children. Each professional has something to share with her or his colleagues. Each professional has something to contribute to the transdisciplinary curriculum and to the integration of students within the classroom. The professional differences create a strength in the inclusion classroom when each contributes expertise to an educational curriculum that could not have been developed by either separately. Figure 9.4 indicates that co-equality and co-participation will enhance collaborative decision making. Co-teachers need to acknowledge their academic and professional differences as a starting point as they work side by side in the classroom. Dynamic collaborative decision making through dialogue exchange creates a new classroom product and exciting interpersonal experiences (Austin, 2001; Creese, 2006; Keefe, Moore, & Duff, 2004). When there is a mismatch between professionals, collaborative decisions cannot be generated; co-teachers need to analyze the interactional dialogue by evaluating their perceptions and expectations concerning classroom factors. From these shared perceptions come a set of shared expectations. If the collaborative process is operating correctly, these expectations are based on clear communication, active listening and responding, effective brainstorming, and creative integration of ideas. Consequently, good decision making results in consonance between professionals (Goldstein, 2004; Pritchard Dodge, 2004; Smith & Dillenbeck, 2006). If, on the other hand, the two professionals do not communicate clearly and listen to each other, maintaining a good rapport, there will be no attainment of shared perceptions or expectations. When a state of dissonance arises, the result will be independent decision making rather than shared problem solving.

CONSULTATION

Consultation within the classroom provides a different interactive relationship between the speech-language pathologist and the special or regular education teacher. The speech-language pathologist provides related services either within the classroom or within a separate setting, but her relationship with the teacher is different than the one she would have within a collaborative model. By means of teacher consultation, the speech-language pathologist provides instructional advice about procedures and techniques to facilitate the generalization of language goals for a specific child from an individual therapeutic setting to a more natural social setting with classroom peers. In both collaboration and consultation, the speech-language pathologist has a caseload of children who require speech-language therapy (Figure 9.5). One

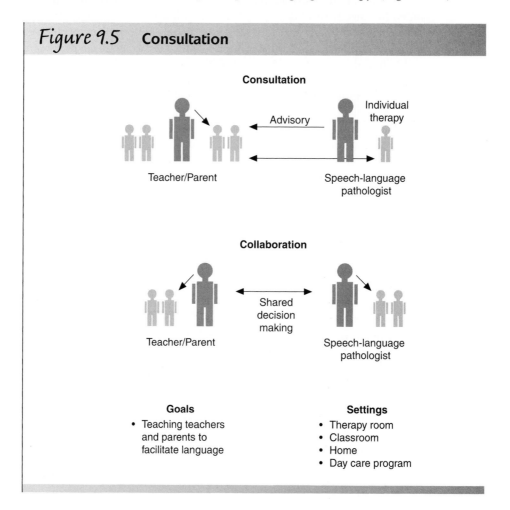

Figure 9.5   Consultation

Consultation

Advisory

Individual therapy

Teacher/Parent

Speech-language pathologist

Collaboration

Shared decision making

Teacher/Parent

Speech-language pathologist

Goals
- Teaching teachers and parents to facilitate language

Settings
- Therapy room
- Classroom
- Home
- Day care program

difference between the models is that in collaboration the decision-making process is developed together and shared for use in the primary setting of the classroom. In consultation, the speech-language pathologist assumes a different role and has a different relationship with the teacher, assuming an advisory position while the classroom teacher remains the primary facilitator within the classroom.

RECIPROCITY

Many special education teachers are concerned that with the development of inclusive classrooms, they will lose their jobs, expressing the frustration that their skills and training are being phased out of the educational system. Many regular education teachers, on the other hand, describe an inability to meet the challenge of inclusive instruction, claiming that they are poorly prepared to work with children with LCD in a regular classroom. Some regular education teachers express negative attitudes about children with LCD because of the necessary changes that must occur as these students are integrated, fearing that behavioral disruptions and other demands imposed by children with LCD will take away valuable instructional time from the other children. Most teachers express feelings of incompetence, fear, anger, and frustration about being coerced into inclusion classrooms (Hyter, 2003; Nungesser & Watkins, 2005). Professional change must include a process of personal growth, in which professionals need to talk about their feelings, their fears, and their concerns (Shaughnessy & Sanger, 2005).

If teachers do not have control over their classrooms, what do they have control over? Professionals need to speak to each other and see themselves within a supportive environment. The inclusion classroom must be supportive of professional change for the speech-language pathologist, the special education teacher, and the regular education teacher. The reciprocity of interpersonal exchange allows the regular teacher, the special education teacher, and the speech-language pathologist to work toward recognizing how they can support each other in their personal and professional growth. They must each come to realize that they have an investment in the classroom. Co-teaching and teacher consultation cannot occur without the commitment of each professional; in fact, the movement to provide services within the least restrictive environment (LRE) will never be successfully achieved unless all professionals are working together (Pritchard Dodge, 2004). Professionals must learn how to talk to each other about children, curriculum, and management issues. They must learn that co-teaching and teacher consultation cannot succeed with "territorial" thinking.

Co-teaching and teacher consultation require mutual support and respect, as well as an understanding that professionals will work as interdependent partners within the classroom (Sonnenmeier, McSheehan, & Jorgensen, 2005; Tiegerman-Farber & Radziewicz, 2007c; Troia, 2005). Reciprocal exchange between professionals suggests that the classroom is really a bridge that spans across a professional divide: each professional from his or her side builds towards and reaches a common meeting place in the middle. Ultimately, inclusion within the regular classroom can only be achieved when the bridge between professionals provides a firm foundation for all children, with and without LCD, to walk across.

The Changing Role of the Parent

The inclusion classroom leads to a recognition of the unique characteristics of families and the role of parents as members of the collaborative team. The inclusion classroom encourages a culturally sensitive, family-centered process of educational decision making (Beatson, 2006; Summers, Hoffman, Marquis, Turnbull, & Poston, 2005; Whitmire, 2000). The collaborative team must include the parent as an equal decision maker, with the goal that developmental information, knowledge, and input concerning the child can be effectively shared by parents. Information networking across discipline boundaries should include parent input to develop an appropriate common focus to understanding the needs of the family. The parent as caregiver has highly specialized concerns, insights, and priorities regarding his or her child. Historically, the role of parents has changed within the educational system as children receiving services have become younger; it is now not only desirable but necessary to incorporate parents into the decision-making process.

CO-EQUALITY AND CO-PARTICIPATION

Parents provide critical information about family issues and cultural concerns (Beatson, 2006; Smith & Dillenbeck, 2006). As the primary caregiver and mediator of change in the child's home environment, the parent can contribute to child learning and educational generalization. Parents play a role in the identification of the child's communication needs and of events that critically affect developmental changes within the child. Although the parent may not have clinical knowledge, a parent's insights and knowledge provide valuable information that can be used by professionals to determine educational objectives and priorities (Steckbeck, 2004).

As a member of the collaborative team, the parent participates as a respected *equal* contributor in the decision-making process, providing information that is helpful in prioritizing and organizing IEP goals (Hess, Molina, & Kozleski, 2006). The collaborative team needs to incorporate the feelings and concerns of the parent when establishing short-term and long-term classroom goals. By being a member of the team, parents in turn become supportive of the educational process, investing in the outcome and success of the inclusion experience (see Figure 9.6). Having contributed to the goals and decisions related to the child and the classroom, the parent can continue to plan and collaborate on the daily educational changes required for inclusion. School reform can only be achieved if the parent is recognized as a partner in classroom learning and generalization (Briggs, 1998). However, specific modifications are required to create successful collaborative relationships with parents (Tiegerman-Farber & Radziewicz, 2007b):

1. Successful collaboration in which parents become part of school teams develops a process for parent advocacy by changing
   - how parents and teachers interact
   - how parents contribute to decision making in the classroom
   - how parent input is incorporated into problem-solving solutions to influence child outcomes

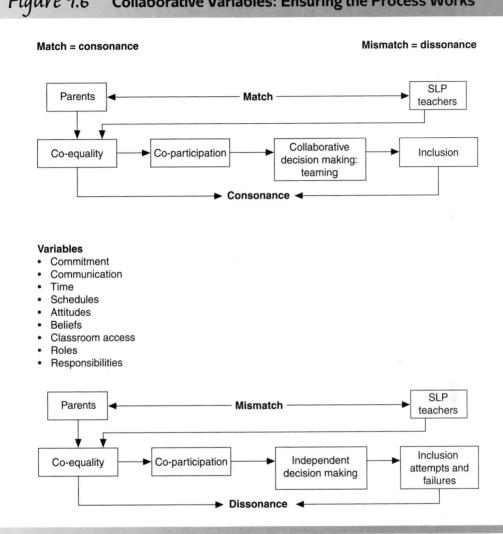

Figure 9.6   Collaborative Variables: Ensuring the Process Works

Match = consonance

Mismatch = dissonance

Parents ◄——— **Match** ———► SLP teachers

Co-equality ——► Co-participation ——► Collaborative decision making: teaming ——► Inclusion

Consonance ◄——

Variables
- Commitment
- Communication
- Time
- Schedules
- Attitudes
- Beliefs
- Classroom access
- Roles
- Responsibilities

Parents ◄——— **Mismatch** ———► SLP teachers

Co-equality ——► Co-participation ——► Independent decision making ——► Inclusion attempts and failures

Dissonance ◄——

2. Successful collaboration involves teaching parents about educational issues, scheduled with working parents in mind, such as
   - laws and procedures
   - advocacy skills
   - child development and disorders
   - instructional techniques and procedures
3. Successful collaboration establishes parent–teacher teams for each classroom.
4. Successful collaboration acknowledges the primary role of parents in inclusive classrooms.

5. Successful collaboration requires educational modifications and accommodations for parents to participate in their child's learning (observing in the classroom, videotapes, etc.).

The inclusion of parents in team decision making is an investment ensuring that parents will maintain a working relationship with professionals and successful transition planning can be achieved (Geenen, Powers, & Lopez-Vasquez, 2001; Stoner, Angell, House, & Jones Bock, 2007). Parental empowerment requires that parents be recognized as decision makers and, therefore, serve as acknowledged members of their child's learning. It is not enough for parents to participate if they cannot contribute substantively as decision makers to the process.

RECIPROCITY

The term *reciprocal exchange* suggests an ongoing relationship that involves modification over time. Equal partners—parent and professional—exchange information, working together to make decisions about child change and educational needs. A mutual respect for each other and differences in perspectives create a healthy tension between parent and professional (Lazar & Slostad, 1999). Reciprocal exchange does not mean that the speech-language pathologist or teacher simply "hears what the parent has to say." Reciprocal exchange does mean that the speech-language pathologist and teacher listen and incorporate what the parent has to say into the ongoing educational programming provided for the child (Hess, Molina, & Kozleski, 2006).

It is interesting to note that, historically, the issue of parent participation has related specifically to parents of children with disabilities. The legal cases concerning advocacy, least restrictive environment, and educational placement all involved families of children with disabilities (Connor & Ferri, 2007; Rogers, 2007; Trotter, 2006). Collaboration provides the opportunity to change traditional relationships and ideas within the classroom by presenting a benefit for parents of regular education students as well. Because the classroom will include an integration of children with and without LCD, parents of regular education students may also seek to expand their relationships with professionals. Just as the inclusion classroom provides a commingling of experiences for children, it could also provide a collaborative experience for parents of children with and without LCD (Arllen, Gable, & Hendrickson, 1996).

PARENT–TEACHER–SPEECH-LANGUAGE PATHOLOGIST TEAMING

Inclusion cannot be successfully achieved without collaborative interaction between parent, teacher, and speech-language pathologist. It was noted earlier that collaboration requires co-equality and co-participation among members of the team. This suggests that the parent has as much to say as professionals about the process of learning, the procedural aspects of instruction, and the academic components of curriculum development. A great deal of parent–teacher–speech-language pathologist planning and programming must occur prior to the establishment and during the implementation of the inclusion classroom (Clarke, 2006; Whitmire, 2000). This suggests that parent–teacher–speech-language pathologist teaming requires an innovative working relationship; the collaborative variables of time and communication must be addressed if the team outcomes are to be successful (see Figure 9.6).

Parent–teacher–speech-language pathologist teams need to delineate their roles, rules, and responsibilities during their meetings. Teams also need to establish specific times and goals for all of their meetings by means of a formalized process. This will obviously have an effect on scheduling, because it may be difficult for teams to meet during the day. The school should make a clear commitment to flexible hours and after-school meetings to facilitate interactions among the parent, teacher, and speech-language pathologist. The goals of collaboration require changes in schedules, working hours, and commitments from all of the collaborators involved with the process. Perhaps the greatest benefit will be a break from traditional ideas and notions about roles, rules, and responsibilities to expand the workscope of the SLP to include evidence-based practice (EBP), response to intervention (RtI) approaches, and literacy development in school settings (Ehren & Nelson, 2005; Johnson, 2006; Kamhi, 2003). The more flexibility that parents and professionals have for creative solutions, the greater will be the probability that the goals of inclusion will be accomplished through the collaborative process.

EVIDENCE-BASED PRACTICE (EBP)

Many professions including speech-language pathology have acknowledged the significance of evidence-based practice in clinical decision making (Horner, Carr, Halle, McGee, Odom, & Wolery, 2005; Johnson, 2006; Ratner, 2006; Reilly, 2004). Evidence-based practice involves a process of questioning and investigation that challenges traditional procedures when they are not substantiated by validated scientific evidence. Similar to the collaborative process, the changes required to implement EBP within the field of speech-language pathology and various clinical/educational settings will require systemic as well as personal reforms. Graduate school programs training the next generations of professionals must change their preprofessional curricula to begin the process. Cascella and Colella (2004) noted that graduate programs had not changed how SLPs were being trained over the past 30 years to meet the needs of students with autism spectrum disorders (ASD). The attention paid to evidence-based practice probably has the same status.

There is always a dilemma for university training programs as new clinical issues appear within the professional field. How much time should be designated to teaching graduate students about, for example, specific disorders, collaborative teaming, and evidence-based practices? Do these issues require additional courses? The reality of educational accountability within IDEA 2004 and school settings leaves the field of speech-language pathology with little choice—SLPs must "get on board." We will have to substantiate clinical decisions and practices by means of scientifically validated investigations along with psychologists and special educators (Johnson, 2006).

The problem for speech-language pathologists who are presently working within various clinical practice settings is much more complicated. Zipoli and Kennedy (2005) described a "window in professional training" that determined SLPs' positive attitudes toward research and EBP. Without such exposure, clinical decision making tends to be based on traditional practice patterns, personal experiences, and the professional recommendations of other clinicians. For the majority of SLPs now in clinical practice the barriers to implementing EBP are both personal and institutional. Meline and Paradiso (2003) noted that "EBP requires the conscientious use of current theories, current research, and empirical data to guide practice" (p. 274). The clinician–researcher relationship may be facilitated in most professional settings by collaborative teaming. Working within educational settings presents many barriers to the requirements of EBP. By striving for collaborative teaming, EBP may become an important by-product achieved more easily by psychologists, special educators, and SLPs working together rather than by SLPs alone.

Collaborative Teaming: Evidence-Based Practice

Collaborative teaming requires a change in thinking about how professionals interact with one another to solve specific problems. Evidence-based practice requires a change in thinking about how professionals solve student learning problems and other educational issues. EBP requires that the basis for decision making must be substantiated by scientifically validated studies. School practitioners have a very limited amount of time within their schedules to meet and discuss their students, let alone examine research-based methodologies. However, there may be several educational and clinical approaches that might be utilized by collaborative teams to begin the EBP process within school settings. The assumption here is that a group of professionals (i.e., SLPs or multidisciplinary professionals) who are interested in EBP commit to meeting on some regular basis before school, after school, or during lunch.

Clinical Initiation to EBP

For most school-based practitioners the investigatory approach to the EBP process might be simpler. The collaborative team should identify an educational issue, student-based problem, or specific instructional methodology that affects their educational work in school. Then each should perform a search to find published research about the targeted issue (i.e., ASHA archives, Google, ERIC, and PubMed). The collaborative team then meets to evaluate the scientific and clinical significance of the published studies (Gillam & Gillam, 2006; Meline & Paradiso, 2003; Nail-Chiwetalu & Ratner, 2006; Ratner, 2006; Zipoli & Kennedy, 2005). Next the collaborative team needs to discuss the targeted problem given the scope of the research and clinical studies identified. This investigatory process may be quite illuminating when professionals recognize that evidence-based research and clinical practice vary across professions (Nail-Chiwetalu & Ratner, 2006). Collaborative discussions about research may lead to changes in an instructional method being used or support for continuing a specific clinical practice. Presently in school settings there is a developing emphasis on using scientifically validated practices and programs in students' IEPs. The flexibility to change procedures and programs during the course of a schoolyear is an administrative barrier that will need to be addressed if EBP is to continue at an institutional level. Going forward, the collaborative team may not be able to implement an immediate change but utilize the resulting EBP recommendations for planning the next schoolyear. The discussions within our profession are extensive but the realities of implementation will be directly related to the creativity, motivation, and persistence of SLPs in the field.

CONSULTATION

Consultation provides the mechanism for the speech-language pathologist to assume an advisory role with parents in school or in the home (see Figure 9.5). Here, the decision making is not shared but advisory and supervisory in nature. The primary function of consultation is for the speech-language pathologist to teach the techniques and procedures so that the parent can become an agent of change for the child to generalize language skills to natural settings. The starting point for parent education begins with formalized instructional programming (Tiegerman-Farber & Radziewicz, 2007c). If parents are going to be taught to facilitate their children, they must receive some kind of educational instruction. Schools must assume the responsibility of developing parent-training programs. Schools must also determine how to teach and what to teach parents; again, the speech-language pathologist can assume the role of the consultant with school educators to develop parent-training programs and goals that are culturally and linguistically sensitive to the needs of diverse families (Harry, 2002; Whitbread, Bruder, Fleming, & Park, 2007). Parent training provides a knowledge base that empowers parents to advocate effectively. The child with LCD presents a constellation of problems. Early intervention, parent education, respite services, therapeutic programs, and counseling underscore the need for a broad-based comprehensive approach to facilitating family involvement. Many children with LCD continue to have language learning problems as they grow older. Although many children with LCD are eventually mainstreamed or included within regular classrooms, parent educators need to help families address their fears and concerns about a life-cycle continuum of services and a lifelong commitment to advocacy (Matuszny, Banda, & Coleman, 2007).

Summary

There is general agreement that parent involvement is critical to the success of school reform and the successful achievement of inclusion (Matuszny, Banda, & Coleman, 2007). The reality, however, is that few public schools have committed time and resources to developing and implementing programs for parents although the Individuals with Disabilities Education Improvement Act (2004) does emphasize "shared responsibility," which includes more parent and student responsibility (Turnbull, 2007; Vitello, 2007). Whereas children with LCD have entered the "schoolhouse doors," parents of children with and without LCD have not. One reason that parents nationally have advocated for school reform and vouchers is the growing frustration that they do not have access to classrooms and educational decision making. Few schools have incorporated the clear results of many research investigations emphasizing that parents must be equal partners. Interestingly enough, this appears to be less of a problem for speech-language pathologists, given our historically close working relationship with parents. Speech-language pathologists, like parents, have never been acknowledged as significant facilitators to classroom learning, because "language" was taught in a therapy room by a related service provider. However, speech-language pathologists are no longer *just* related service providers, because language has finally been recognized as critical to all aspects of educational learning. The speech-language pathologist may be the key professional to the successful integration of parents and children with LCD into the regular classroom (Tiegerman-Farber & Radziewicz, 2007b).

This chapter has discussed some of the issues underlying decision making and interactive teaming. Interactive teaming provides the mechanism for diverse individuals to come together to develop inclusive programming within a learning process for all of the members who embark on the inclusion mission. Parents and professionals who have had the opportunity to be part of an interactive process have indicated the remarkable changes that have occurred as members of a team working together to develop a mission and a program. Eventually, the team has a life force of its own and proceeds through a series of changes as each member learns about the process and commits to the mission. The diversity and the difference of each individual contribute to the collective creativity of the team. The resulting creative product reflects a synergy that could not have been achieved by members individually. Interactive teaming reflects what the inclusive process is all about; differences can be a force for creative change when they are focused to accomplish a mission or goal. We all learn together and from each other. The "inclusion whole" becomes greater than the sum of its parts. Each stakeholder contributes to the creation of the inclusion classroom. It is important to stress that inclusion, although an opportunity for all, remains the final step in an educational journey. The speech-language pathologist has a significant role to play in the child-based decision making that will ultimately benefit each and every child within the classroom. It is important to caution that inclusion is an option for every child but not necessarily an academic or social benefit. This is a controversial issue in education; many professionals do not support a full-inclusion model that does not allow for a continuum of educational options for children with LCD. The interactive team must also discuss who will benefit and how each child will benefit from an inclusive classroom experience. Clearly, though, interactive teaming provides the pathway to educational reform.

Study Questions

1. Describe the changing role of the speech-language pathologist in educational decision making.
2. Discuss why parents should be advocates for their children.
3. Explain the difference between consultation and collaboration in terms of the provision of services for children with developmental disabilities.
4. Discuss the educational problems related to inclusion of children with disabilities within the regular educational classroom for teachers and parents.
5. What does responsible decision making mean?
6. Co-equality and co-participation are part of the collaborative process; explain what these terms mean.

References

American Speech-Language-Hearing Association (ASHA). (1990). The roles of speech-language pathologists in service delivery to infants, toddlers, and their families. *ASHA, 32* (suppl. 2), 4.

Arllen, N., Gable, R. A., & Hendrickson, J. M. (1996). Accommodating students with special needs in general education classrooms. *Preventing School Failure, 41*, 7–13.

Austin, V. L. (2001). Teachers' beliefs about co-teaching. *Remedial & Special Education, 22*(4), 245–255.

Bailey, D. B., Aytch, L. S., Odom, S. L., Symons, F., & Wolery, M. (1999). Early intervention as we know it. *Mental Retardation and Development Disabilities, 5*, 11–20.

Barnes, P. E., Friehe, M. J., & Radd, T. R. (2003). Collaboration between speech-language pathologists and school counselors. *Communication Disorders Quarterly, 24*(3), 137–142.

Beatson, J. E. (2006). Preparing speech-language pathologists as family-centered practitioners in assessment and program planning for children with autism spectrum disorder. *Seminars in Speech & Language, 27*(1), 1–9.

Beck, A., & Dennis, M. (1997). Speech-language pathologists' and teachers' perceptions of classroom-based interventions. *Language, Speech, and Hearing Services in Schools, 2*, 146–153.

Bopp, K., Brown, K., & Mirenda, P. (2004). Speech-language pathologists' roles in the delivery of positive behavior support for individuals with developmental disabilities. *American Journal of Speech-Language Pathology, 13*, 5–19.

Briggs, M. H. (1998). Families talk: Building partnerships for communicative change. *Topics in Language Disorders, 18*(3), 71–84.

Briggs-Gowan, M. J., Carter, A. S., Bosson-Heenan, J., Guyer, A. E., & Horowitz, S. M. (2006). Are infant-toddler social-emotional and behavioral problems transient? *Journal of the American Academy of Child & Adolescent Psychiatry, 45*(7), 849–858.

Bronfenbrenner, U. (1977). Toward an experimental ecology of human development. *American Psychologist, 32*, 512–531.

Cascella, P. W., & Colella, C. S. (2004). Knowledge of autism spectrum disorders among Connecticut school speech-language pathologists. *Focus on Autism and Other Developmental Disabilities, 19*(4), 245–252.

Chess, S. (1986). Early childhood development and its implications for analytical theory and practice. *American Journal of Psychoanalysis, 46*, 122–148.

Clarke, C. (2006). IDEA Part B Final Regulations Released: ED Sidesteps Federal Role, Sends Many Issues to States. *The ASHA Leader*, pp. 30–31.

Clough, P., & Garner, G. (2003). Special educational needs and inclusive education: Origins and current issues. In S. Bartlett & D. Burton (Eds.), *Education studies: Essential issues.* London: Sage.

Connor, D. J., & Ferri, B. A. (2007). The conflict within: Resistance to inclusion and other paradoxes in special education. *Disability & Society, 22*(1), 63–77.

Coufal, K. (1993). Collaborative consultation for speech/language pathologists. *Topics in Language Disorders, 14*(1), 1–14.

Crais, E. R., Roy, V. P., & Free, K. (2006). Parents' and professionals' perceptions of the implementation of family-centered practices in child assessments. *American Journal of Speech-Language Pathology, 15*, 365–377.

Crais, K. (1993). Families and professionals as collaborators in assessment. *Topics in Language Disorders, 14*(1), 29–40.

Creese, A. (2006). Supporting talk? Partnership teachers in classroom interaction. *International Journal of Bilingual Education & Bilingualism, 9*(4), 434–453.

Diehl, S., Ford, C., & Federico, J. (2005). The communication journey of a fully included child with autism spectrum disorder. *Topics of Language Disorders, 25*(4), 375–387.

Dinnebeil, L. A., & Hale, L. (1999). Early intervention program practices that support collaboration. *Topics in Early Childhood Special Education, 19*(4), 225.

Driscoll, J. P. (2001). Charter schools. *Georgetown Journal on Poverty Law & Policy, 8*(2), 505–511.

Dunst, C. (2002). Family-centered practices: Birth through high school. *Journal of Special Education, 36,* 139–147.

Dunst, C., & Bruder, M. (2002). Valued outcomes of service coordination, early intervention, and natural environments. *Exceptional Children, 68,* 361–375.

Ehren, B. (2006). Partnerships to support reading comprehension for students with language impairment. *Topics in Language Disorders, 26*(1), 42–54.

Ehren, B. J., & Nelson, N. W. (2005). The responsiveness to intervention approach and language impairment. *Topics in Language Disorders, 25*(2), 120–131.

Farrell, P., Dyson, A., Polat, F., Hutcheson, G., & Gallannaugh, F. (2007). Inclusion and achievement in mainstream schools. *European Journal of Special Needs Education, 22*(2), 131–145.

Friehe, M. J., Bloedow, A., & Hesse, S. (2003). Counseling families of children with communication disorders. *Communication Disorders Quarterly, 24*(4), 211–220.

Friend, M., & Bursuck, W. D. (1996). *Including students with special needs.* Boston: Allyn & Bacon.

Gable, R. A., & Hendrickson, J. M. (1997). Teaching all the students: A mandate for educators. In J. Choate (Ed.), *Successful inclusive teaching: Detecting and correcting special needs* (2nd ed., pp. 2–17). Boston: Allyn & Bacon.

Geenen, S., Powers, L. E., & Lopez-Vasquez, A. (2001). Multicultural aspects of parent involvement in transition planning. *Exceptional Children, 67,* 265–282.

Gillam, S. L., & Gillam, R. B. (2006). Making evidence-based decisions about child language intervention in schools. *Language, Speech, and Hearing Services in Schools, 37,* 304–315.

Goldstein, L. (2004). Tandem teaching. *Teacher Magazine, 15*(5), 48.

Guilfoyle, C. (2006). NCLB: Is there life beyond testing? *Association for Supervision and Curriculum Development Educational Leadership, 64*(3), 8–13.

Hammer, B. (2003). Public school reform would close racial gap in education, authors say. *Black Issues in Higher Education, 20*(20), 14–15.

Hanko, G. (2003). Towards an inclusive school culture—But what happened to Elton's 'affective curriculum'? *British Journal of Special Education, 30*(3), 125–131.

Harry, B. (2002). Trends and issues in serving culturally diverse families of children with disabilities. *Journal of Special Education, 36*(3), 131–138.

Haycock, K. (2006). No more invisible kids. *Association for Supervision and Curriculum Development Educational Leadership, 64*(3), 38–42.

Hess, R. S., Molina, A. M., & Kozleski, E. B. (2006). Until somebody hears me: Parent voice and advocacy in special educational decision making. *British Journal of Special Education, 33*(3), 148–157.

Hodkinson, A. J. (2005). Conceptions and misconceptions of inclusive education: A critical examination of final-year teacher trainees' knowledge and understanding of inclusion. *Research in Education, 73,* 15–28.

Hodkinson, A. J. (2006). Conceptions and misconceptions of inclusive education—one year on: A critical analysis of newly qualified teachers' knowledge and understanding of inclusion. *Research in Education, 76,* 43–55.

Hodkinson, A. J. (2007). Conceptions and misconceptions of inclusive education—one year on: A critical analysis of newly qualified teachers' knowledge and understanding of inclusion. *Research in Education, 76,* 43–55.

Horner, R. H., Carr, E. G., Halle, J., McGee, G., Odom, S., & Wolery, M. (2005). The use of single-subject research to identify evidence-based practice in special education. *Exceptional Children, 71.*

Hunt, P., Soto, G., Maier, J., & Doering, K. (2003). Collaborative teaming to support students at risk and students with severe disabilities in general education classrooms. *Exceptional Children, 69*(3), 315–332.

Hunt, P., Soto, G., Maier, J., Liboiron, N., & Bae, S. (2004). Collaborative teaming to support preschoolers with severe disabilities who are placed in general education early childhood programs. *Topics in Early Childhood Special Education, 24*(3), 123–142.

Hyter, Y. D. (2003). Language intervention for children with emotional or behavioral disorders. *Behavioral Disorders, 29*(1), 65–76.

Idole, L., Paolucci-Whitecomb, P., & Nevin, A. (1986). *Collaborative consultation.* Rockville, MD: Aspen.

Individuals with Disabilities Education Improvement Act of 2004, 20 U.S.C. 1400 Etseq. (2004) (reauthorization of the Individuals with Disabilities Education Act of 1990).

Johnson, C. J. (2006). Getting started in evidence-based practice for childhood speech-language disorders. *American Journal of Speech-Language Pathology, 15,* 20–35.

Jones, L. T., & Blendinger, J. (1994). New beginnings: Preparing future teachers to work with diverse families. *Action in Teacher Education, 16,* 79–88.

Kamhi, A. G. (2003). The role of the SLP in improving reading fluency. *ASHA Leader, 8*(7), 6–8.

Keefe, E. B., Moore, V., & Duff, F. (2004). The four "knows" of collaborative teaching. *Teaching Exceptional Children, 36*(5), 36–42.

Kinnaman, D. E. (2000). New momentum for school choice. *Curriculum Administrator, 36*(3), 104.

Knackendoffel, E. A. (2005). Collaborative teaming in the secondary school. *Focus on Exceptional Children, 37*(5), 1–16.

Lazar, A., & Slostad, F. (1999). How to overcome obstacles to parent-teacher partnerships. *The Clearing House, 72*(4), 206–210.

Loder, T. L. (2005). African American women principals' reflections on social change, community othermothering, and Chicago public school reform. *Urban Education, 40*(3), 298–320.

Maniadaki, K., Sonuga-Barke, E., Kakouros, E., & Karaba, R. (2007). Parental beliefs about the nature of ADHD behaviours and their relationship to referral intentions in preschool children. *Child: Care, Health & Development, 33*(2), 188–195.

Matuszny, R. M., Banda, D. R., & Coleman, T. J. (2007). A progressive plan for building collaborative relationships with parents from diverse backgrounds. *Teaching Exceptional Children, 39*(4), 24–31.

McConachie, H., Le Couteur, A., & Honey, E. (2005). Can a diagnosis of Asperger syndrome be made in very young children with suspected autism spectrum disorder? *Journal of Autism and Developmental Disorders, 35*(2), 167–176.

Meline, T., & Paradiso, T. (2003). Evidence-based practice in schools. *Language, Speech, and Hearing Services in Schools, 34,* 273–283.

Midkiff, R. B., & Lawler-Prince, D. (1992). Preparing tomorrow's teachers: Meeting the challenge of diverse family structures. *Action in Teacher Education, 14,* 1–5.

Murray, C. (2004). Clarifying collaborative roles in urban high schools. *Teaching Exceptional Children, 36*(5), 44–51.

Nail-Chiwetalu, B. J., & Ratner, N. B. (2006). Information literacy for speech-language pathologists: a key to evidence-based practice. *Language, Speech, and Hearing Services in Schools, 37,* 157–167.

Nind, M. (2005). Introduction: Models and practice in inclusive curricula. In M. Nind, J. Rix, K. Sheehy, & K. Simmons (Eds.), *Curriculum and pedagogy in inclusive education: Values into practice.* London: Routledge Falmer.

Nungesser, N. R., & Watkins, R. V. (2005). Preschool teachers' perceptions and reactions to challenging classroom behavior: Implications for speech-language pathologists. *Language, Speech, and Hearing Services in Schools, 36,* 139–151.

O'Shea, D. J., Williams, A. L., & Sattler, R. O. (1999). Collaboration across special education and general education: Preservice teachers' view. *Journal of Teacher Education, 50,* 147–157.

Ogletree, B. T. (1999). Practical solutions to the challenges of changing professional roles: Introduction to the special issue. *Intervention in School & Clinic, 34*(3), 131.

Paul-Brown, D., & Ricker, J. H. (2003). Evaluating and treating communication and cognitive disorders: Approaches to referral and collaboration for speech-language pathology and clinical neuropsychology. Technical Report. *ASHA Supplement, 23,* 47–57.

Pirrie, A., & Head, G. (2007). Martians in the playground: Researching special education needs. *Oxford Review of Education, 33*(1), 19–31.

Pritchard Dodge, E. P. (2004). Communication skills: The foundation for meaningful group intervention in school-based programs. *Topics in Language Disorders, 24*(2), 141–150.

Ratner, N. B. (2006). Evidence-based practice: An examination of its ramifications for the practice of speech-language pathology. *Language, Speech, and Hearing Services in Schools, 37,* 257–267.

Reilly, S. (2004). The challenges in making speech pathology practice evidence based. *Advances in Speech-Language Pathology, 6*(2), 113–124.

Rogers, C. (2007). Experiencing an 'inclusive' education: Parents and their children with 'special educational needs.' *British Journal of Sociology of Education, 28*(1), 55–68.

Rogers-Adkinson, D. L., & Stuart, S. K. (2007). Language, speech, and hearing services in schools. *American Speech-Language-Hearing Association, 38,* 149–156.

Shaughnessy, A., & Sanger, D. (2005). Kindergarten teachers' perceptions of language and literacy development, speech-language pathologists, and language interventions. *Communication Disorders Quarterly, 26*(2), 67–84.

Smith, V. K., & Dillenbeck, A. (2006). Developing and implementing early intervention plans for children with autism spectrum disorders. *Seminars in Speech & Language, 27*(1), 10–20.

Sonnenmeier, R. M., McSheehan, M., & Jorgensen, C. M. (2005). A case study of team supports for a student with autism's communication and engagement within the general education curriculum: Preliminary report of the beyond access model. *AAC: Augmentative & Alternative Communication, 21*(2), 101–115.

Steckbeck, P. (2004, November 2). Early literacy and language identification and intervention: A team approach. *The ASHA Leader*, 6–7.

Stoner, J. B., Angell, M. E., House, J., & Jones Bock, S. (2007). Transitions: Perspectives from parents of young children with autism spectrum disorder (ASD). *Journal of Developmental & Physical Disabilities, 19*(1), 23–39.

Summers, J., Hoffman, L., Marquis, J., Turnbull, A., & Poston, D. (2005). Relationship between parent satisfaction regarding partnerships with professionals and age of child. *Topics in Early Childhood Special Education, 25*, 48–58.

Tiegerman-Farber, E., & Radziewicz, C. (2007a). Collaborative language assessment and decision making for infants and toddlers. In *Language disorders in children: Real families, real issues, and real interventions* (pp. 75–110). Upper Saddle River, NJ: Pearson Prentice Hall.

Tiegerman-Farber, E., & Radziewicz, C. (2007b). Collaborative language assessment and decision making in elementary school. In *Language disorders in children: Real families, real issues, and real interventions* (pp. 316–341). Upper Saddle River, NJ: Pearson Prentice Hall.

Tiegerman-Farber, E., & Radziewicz, C. (2007c). Collaborative language assessment and decision making in preschool. In *Language disorders in children: Real families, real issues, and real interventions* (pp. 206–225). Upper Saddle River, NJ: Pearson Prentice Hall.

Tiegerman-Farber, E., & Radziewicz, C. (2007d). Language disorders in infants and toddlers. In *Language disorders in children: Real families, real issues, and real interventions* (pp. 37–74). Upper Saddle River, NJ: Pearson Prentice Hall.

Tiegerman-Farber, E., & Radziewicz, C. (2007e). Understanding elementary schools. In *Language disorders in children: Real families, real issues, and real interventions* (pp. 260–284). Upper Saddle River, NJ: Pearson Prentice Hall.

Toch, T. (2006). Turmoil in the testing industry. *Association for Supervision and Curriculum Development Educational Leadership, 64*(3), 53–57.

Troia, G. A. (2005). Responsiveness to intervention roles for speech-language pathologists in the prevention and identification of learning disabilities. *Topics in Language Disorders, 25*(2), 106–119.

Trotter, A. (2006). IDEA issues getting ear of high court. *Education Week, 26*(11), 1–23.

Turnbull, H. R. (2007). A response to Professor Vitello. *Remedial and Special Education, 28*(2), 69–71.

Vitello, S. J. (2007). Shared responsibility reconsidered: A responsibility to Professor Turnbull on IDEIA 2004 accountability and personal responsibility. *Remedial and Special Education, 28*(2), 66–68.

Whitbread, K. M., Bruder, M. B., Fleming, G., & Park, H. J. (2007). Collaboration in special education. *Teaching Exceptional Children, 39*(4), 6–14.

Whitcomb, J., Borko, H., & Liston, D. (2006). Living in the tension—Living with the heat. *Journal of Teacher Education, 57*(5), 447–453.

Whitmire, K. (2000). Action: School services. *Language, Speech and Hearing Services in Schools, 31*, 194–199.

Woolfson, L., Grant, E., & Campbell, L. (2007). A comparison of special, general and support teachers' controllability and stability attributions for children's difficulties in learning. *Educational Psychology, 27*(2), 295–306.

Zipoli, R. P., Jr., & Kennedy, M. (2005). Evidence-based practice among speech-language pathologists: Attitudes, utilization, and barriers. *American Journal of Speech-Language Pathology, 14*, 208–220.

CHAPTER 10

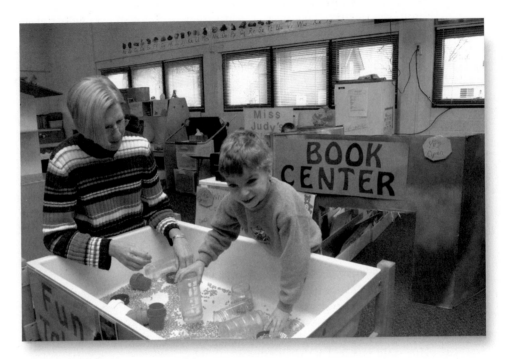

Planning Language Intervention for Young Children

Amy L. Weiss
University of Rhode Island

When you finish this chapter, you will be able to

- Discuss how SLPs develop language intervention programs for preschool-age children.
- Understand the changes in federal legislation that have mandated provision of services for young children with disabilities and how they have affected the role and responsibilities of SLPs, including prevention and literacy learning, in designing service delivery programs for children of preschool age.
- Select goal attack strategies and appropriate goals for intervention programs with preschool-age children.

- Identify a series of intervention techniques that can be used to teach new language forms and functions to preschool-age children.
- Facilitate generalization of language goals from therapeutic contexts to nontreatment settings.
- Understand the basic principles of evidence-based practice as applied to defining best practices for treatment of preschool-age children with language disorders.

In this chapter, readers will be challenged to think about language intervention planning and implementation with young children as dynamic processes that are driven by a young client's changing abilities, temperament, and needs, as well as the clinical skills and experience of speech-language pathologists (SLPs) and those of additional support personnel, not to mention the less easily measured environmental factors that impinge on language development and use, such as caregiver input and the child's opportunities for social interaction with peers. In addition, the alternatives for intervention contexts will be explored, including suggestions for choosing among those alternatives. A case will also be made for the importance of thorough generalization planning when first designing treatment protocols; the reader will be introduced to several methods useful for increasing the likelihood that generalization and maintenance of competencies will occur as a result of the language intervention provided. It will also be made obvious to the reader that many of the general principles of working with young children who have language disorders are really the same general principles used with any population with a communication disorder (e.g., promotion of generalization, increasing task difficulty with client progress).

What Is Language Intervention?

THE DEMOGRAPHICS OF EARLY LANGUAGE DISORDER

According to research findings compiled by the American Speech-Language-Hearing Association (ASHA, 2000b), language disorders are found in approximately 8 to 12 percent of the preschool population. Estimates of the occurrence of specific language impairment (SLI), where other developmental systems (e.g., cognitive, socioemotional, and physical) appear to be intact and functioning within normal limits, average around 7.4 percent of the kindergarten-age population (Tomblin, Records, Buckwalter, Zhang, Smith, & O'Brien, 1997). Additional studies that have examined the development of speech and language in late talkers have reported that a significant proportion of these children, identified prior to their second birthdays and delayed in both expressive and receptive language, remained delayed in language development when 3 years of age (Thal, 1999), thus having a higher risk for a later diagnosis of a learning disability (Catts, Fey, Zhang, & Tomblin, 2002; Stothard, Snowling, Bishop, Chipchase, & Kaplan, 1998). This latter finding is particularly important because it supports the need for aggressive and comprehensive programs for early identification of and intervention for communication problems.

In addition to the challenges posed by the numbers of service recipients, SLPs have increasingly seen changes over the last couple of decades in cultural diversity of the national caseload (Battle, 1998; Cole, 1989). More than 10 years ago, Cole (1989) noted that SLPs need to be aware of the multicultural issues they face:

1. More individuals representing minorities require assistance.
2. More minority children are born at risk for communication disorders.
3. Non-European service recipients present with different etiologies and prevalences for disorders.
4. Less normative data is available for nonmajority populations.
5. Perspectives on the concepts of health and disorder may vary in different cultures.
6. Conflicts in the intervention context may increase based on cultural differences.
7. Service delivery preferences may differ from the mainstream of different cultural groups.
8. Linguistic differences are greater within nonmajority populations.

The difficulties of these challenges are enhanced by the demographic stability of the ASHA membership. As of 2006, only 5.8 percent of over 127,000 ASHA members described themselves as belonging to a racial or ethnic minority group (information was not available for more than 54,000 members, however). This number remains low when compared with the proportion of racial and ethnic minorities in the United States, and it represents no appreciable increase in the racial or ethnic makeup of the ASHA membership over the past several years (Janota, 1999). Besides identifying themselves as members of the majority culture, the vast majority of ASHA members are also monolingual (Screen & Anderson, 1994), which adds to the difficulty of providing appropriate services to all children with language disorders (ASHA, 1985). As will be discussed later in this chapter, the issue of cultural differences is a critical one in the development of appropriate intervention programming for young children, as it is for all clients of SLPs.

The difficulty of providing appropriate service delivery to children who are culturally and linguistically different is national in scope (Goldstein, 2000). Roseberry-McKibben and Eicholtz (1994) reported findings from their national survey investigating how children diagnosed as limited English proficient (LEP) were serviced in the schools. They found that although treatment focusing on language was most often provided by the more than 1,100 SLPs who replied to the survey, more than 90 percent did not speak the language (most often Spanish) spoken by their clients well enough to provide treatment in that language. In addition, the authors noted that more than three-quarters of their respondents indicated that they had not completed any coursework designed to prepare them for working with children who were LEP (now referred to as ELL: English language learners). Clearly, our profession needs to continue to emphasize ways of infusing multicultural information into the curricula of our graduate programs and providing adequate continuing education opportunities so that practitioners can better meet the needs of their diverse clientele.

WHY EARLY LANGUAGE INTERVENTION IS NEEDED

Several investigators have studied young children with language disorders over time and determined that disorders of language first identified in childhood often continue to be a part of the social and communicative life of the individual and are not easily outgrown (Aram, Ekelman, & Nation, 1984; Hall & Tomblin, 1978; Records, Tomblin, & Freese, 1992; Stothard et al., 1998). Thus, language disorders in children not only exist, they have the potential to be a long-standing problem for the children themselves, their families, school personnel, SLPs charged with the responsibility of teaching them, and perhaps society as a whole. Longevity of language disorders has encouraged SLPs to focus on prevention.

Moreover, because the needs for competent language use are pervasive in our daily lives, if a person's language abilities are just functional, that person will likely lead a life that is compromised in some respect. Consider the role played by language in establishing and maintaining relationships between friends, colleagues, and loved ones, or in functioning as a productive member of a society through one's career, civic, and social activities. Language is such an integral part of our lives that the development of techniques to augment the language learning abilities of young children who exhibit language disorders is a very important charge to SLPs, caregivers, and others who work with this population.

Ramey and Ramey (1998, pp. 115–117) delineated six principles—mostly intuitive—for enhancing success that emerged from their review of the research literature describing the effectiveness of early intervention provided for children identified as at risk for developmental disorders. These principles provide good rationales for early initiation of SLPs' work with families who have children with developmental language disorders. These investigators were struck by the converging data that clearly suggested the following:

1. A "principle of developmental timing" suggests that the earlier an intervention is begun and the longer it continues, the more benefit it will have versus intervention programs that are begun later and are of shorter duration.

2. A "principle of program intensity" suggests that programs designed to be more intensive in nature, in terms of the amount of contact between the intervention-ist(s) as well as the degree to which the family participates in the designated program, will be more successful.

3. A "principle of direct versus intermediary provision of learning experiences" suggests that programs focusing directly on delivery of services to children rather than on training parents or other caregivers to provide the treatment are more successful.

4. A "principle of program breadth and flexibility" suggests that comprehensive programs addressing the needs of the child and family in multiple ways are more likely to yield positive results than programs that take a more limited perspective of intervention services.

5. A "principle of individual differences in program benefits" suggests that not all children will benefit equally from the services provided and that one strong predictor of successful intervention is probably the child's status at the beginning of treatment.

6. A "principle of ecological domain and environmental maintenance of development" suggests that unless there is an environmental support system in place to help maintain the skills learned by the child through the intervention program, it is unlikely that the gains made by the child will be maintained over time.

Taken together, these principles provide SLPs with a great deal of direction for programming recommendations when young children with diagnosed language disorders or those at risk for developing language disorders are being considered.

A DEFINITION OF LANGUAGE INTERVENTION AND INTERVENTIONISTS

According to the 2003 omnibus survey conducted by ASHA, the majority of this sample's SLPs who worked full time in either schools or nonresidential health care settings regularly served children diagnosed with language disorders. Taking the diagnoses of autism/PDD, ADHD, learning disabilities, pragmatics/social communcation, literacy, articulation/phonological disorders, and specific language impairment into account and considering SLPs employed full time in the schools, 70 percent on average regularly serve clients with these diagnoses, according to the ASHA 2006 Schools Survey (ASHA, 2006). This percentage was as high as 91 percent for children with articulation/phonological disorders.

There have been several recent changes in how we perceive and enact our roles with young children having language disorders. With the refining of collaborative models, the responsibility for language facilitation is often shared with classroom teachers. (See Chapter 3 for more information on this topic.)

In a second and related change, transdisciplinary teaming models are becoming more frequently instituted than the more traditional multidisciplinary and interdisciplinary team approaches, where multiple professionals are involved in planning and providing young children's treatment programs. The concept of "role release," essential to the transdisciplinary teaming model, allows team members to transcend the typical boundaries of their disciplinary training, where necessary, to provide clients with comprehensive service delivery. For example, an SLP working to facilitate accurate articulatory productions in a child with cerebral palsy may work to reduce the child's hypertonicity before beginning speech activities, a goal usually reserved for the physical therapist. The roles and responsibilities of SLPs have shifted to meet the demands posed by changes in service delivery models.

The third major change to the role of SLPs in their treatment of language disorders in young children is the renewed effort—mandated by the reauthorization of the Individuals with Disabilities Education Act (IDEA 2004)—to provide family-focused intervention, where the functioning of the child's family unit is viewed as being inextricably tied to the child's treatment and the appropriate context for intervention (Pletcher, 1995). The family systems approach acknowledges that the family's strengths and needs must be accounted for and addressed by the intervention program. Federal law requires that families be included in planning the intervention program for their young children, assisting professionals in choosing among possible treatment plans and helping to prioritize goals in treatment, after their prior involvement in the assessment procedures that yielded the data for intervention planning. (See Chapter 3 for a more comprehensive accounting of how federal legislation has affected service delivery options for the preschool population.)

IDEA 2004 along with the No Child Left Behind Act (NCLB) of 2002 also mandated SLPs to be involved in the prevention of speech and language disorders in children. NCLB also specifically focused educators on identifying and utilizing teaching methods that have been shown to work. Thus, the increasing research literature in the field of speech-language pathology addressing evidence-based practice (EBP) is a response, at least in part, to federal legislation. There will be a more in-depth discussion of EBP below.

For the purposes of this chapter, language intervention is defined as the careful planning, manipulation, and implementation of instructional contexts designed to facilitate language learning. Depending on the needs and abilities of the client and his or her family, programs of language intervention will differ in terms of *who* is involved in the intervention, *where* the intervention takes place, *what* the specific goals of the treatment are, and the *degree of structure* imposed on the client within the instructional context.

It is important for student SLPs to recognize that the goal of language intervention, or any type of intervention, is to make itself and the job of the clinician obsolete. That is, the objective of any language intervention program is to eliminate its rationale for existence by demonstrating that the client is ready for dismissal. This can be done in at least two ways. One is to help the client become his or her own clinician through the development of accurate self-monitoring skills. The client must therefore learn strategies to facilitate new learning for examples not specifically taught in a therapeutic setting, which would be a demonstration of generalization. Once the client has demonstrated correct discrimination between acceptable and unacceptable language productions (or effective and ineffective communication), an essential competency for achieving generalization to new, untrained contexts has been acquired. Once self-monitoring is established, the client can consistently extend learning without the clinician's input.

The second way to achieve "planned obsolescence" involves demonstrating that the client has the language competencies typically observed in normally developing individuals similar to the client in age, education, and culture. Here, techniques for future learning are less important than showing that the client is presently a successful communicator in all settings in which language is used. For some of our clients, particularly those considered to be culturally or linguistically different, this may involve the use of code-switching or changing from one language or dialect system to another as called for by changing communication contexts.

Appropriate dismissal criteria indicate that treatment services can be removed without an appreciable loss of the gains made by the client through therapy and that additional intervention services are not likely to be needed in the future (Fey, 1988; Olswang & Bain, 1985). Therefore, although it is very important to demonstrate generalization, the child's ability to maintain the gains made in treatment over time once treatment is withdrawn is equally critical. Dismissal from treatment is never an irrevocable decision (Fey, 1988), however. Should a client demonstrate an inability to maintain the new competencies learned in treatment, reinstatement into treatment is a possible avenue. The 1997 revision of the Individuals with Disabilities Education Act defined dismissal criteria from speech and language intervention as when one or more of the following conditions are met (ASHA, 2000a):

- The child's parents request that the child no longer receive services.
- All objectives set for the child have been met and no further errors require intervention.
- Measurable benefits from treatment can no longer be documented although attempts have been made to modify strategies used.
- The child's educational performance is no longer affected by his or her language disorder.
- Lack of motivation on the part of the child to participate in treatment cannot be remedied.
- Circumstances that may be transient or permanent in nature prevent the child from benefiting from treatment.
- Special education or other related services are no longer necessary for this child to receive educational services in the mainstream.

This chapter now addresses some of the decision-making processes of SLPs engaged in formulating therapy plans for a young child with a language disorder.

The Role of Speech-Language Clinicians in Early Language Intervention

THE EFFICACY OF EARLY LANGUAGE INTERVENTION

As already noted (Ramey & Ramey, 1998), it is generally agreed that earlier is better for identifying communication and language disorders, whether the etiology of the problem is genetic or due to environmental agents (Warren & Kaiser, 1988). Bricker (1986) noted the general acceptance that the child's early learning is needed to support the more sophisticated learning that will follow and that early intervention allows SLPs and other professionals to set up "proper support systems for families and children to inhibit the development of secondary or associated disabilities" (p. 30). Because speech-language disorders have been shown to have both a pervasive and cumulative effect on children's growth and development, waiting to begin intervention may mean that the problem will be significantly greater by the time a program is instituted. Although sometimes unavoidable—either because of lack of availability of services or the need to convince families that language intervention is the best approach—most children stand to lose valuable time in the language learning process when lengthy delays occur.

Support for the efficacy of early intervention also comes from research studies demonstrating that development during the prelinguistic period is crucial to the acquisition of linguistic competence (Leonard, 1991). In addition, advanced research technologies have allowed investigators to determine that infants know much more about the world around them by the end of the first year of life than had been previously suspected (Rovee-Collier, Lipsitt, & Hayne, 1998). Thus, delays in beginning intervention have the potential effect of putting young children with language disorders even further behind their normally developing peers than had been previously thought.

There has also been continued interest in the topic of the "late talker" (Kelly, 1998), the child who is delayed in the development of vocabulary and word combinations, sometimes identified as early as 18 months of age but more often identified at about age 2 (Rescorla, 1989). Although many children identified as "late talkers" go on to catch up with their peers by age 3 or 4, a substantial proportion of children thus identified still continue to demonstrate delays in language development, with most studies pointing to proportions ranging from 25 to 50 percent of these children (Leonard 1998). When we look carefully at the studies completed, some factors clearly tend to place the child labeled as a "late talker" at higher risk for ongoing problems, with one of the most common being demonstrated delays in development of *both* receptive and expressive language skills (Olswang, Rodriguez, & Timler, 1998). Capone and MacGregor (2004) more recently reported that children designated as "late talkers" who show no other symptoms of language disorder than delayed expressive language (e.g., receptive language within normal limits, normal nonverbal communication skills) are likely to catch up to their age-matched peers.

Leonard (1998) cautioned that it may not yet be possible to make a highly reliable prognosis of which late talkers will go on to demonstrate language disorders throughout childhood before the child reaches the age of 3, given all of the variability inherent in early language learning. However, he maintained that this should not be interpreted as suggesting that intervention for these at-risk children before age 3 is inappropriate. On the contrary, he suggested that given the potential for some of these children to fall increasingly behind their peers, early intervention is warranted.

Some language intervention programs for this young population are centered around teaching parents how to interact communicatively with their at-risk or disordered infants and toddlers to capitalize on what the infants are capable of doing (Klein & Briggs, 1987; MacDonald & Carroll, 1992a; Sparks, 1989). Although SLPs must carefully evaluate the infant or toddler in order to carry out this type of program, the focus of direct training will often be primarily on the parents, who will be trained to become the primary therapeutic agents in classroom programs for preschool-age children designed to teach families how best to work with their children to carry over classroom learning into the home environment.

A CONTINUUM OF LANGUAGE DIFFICULTIES

Another reason for the burgeoning interest in early language intervention probably comes from the recognition that individuals identified in the preschool years as having language disorders are often the same students diagnosed as language learning disabled later in their academic careers (Aram, Ekelman, & Nation, 1984; King, Jones, & Lasky, 1982). The problem may persist despite the fact that language intervention is provided to many of these children. Findings from follow-up studies of young children who were identified as speech-language disordered consistently demonstrated that the majority of these children were still showing signs of language disorders or additional problems with learning many years after their initial diagnoses. As noted by Maxwell and Wallach (1984), "one myth, that the majority of children 'outgrow' their early language disabilities, is dispelled by this research" (p. 20). Studies of young children identified as language delayed (Rescorla & Schwartz, 1990; Scarborough & Dobrich, 1990) have indicated that catching up to their peers may take longer than once expected.

If language learning difficulties are resistant to change in the long term, how are the lives of our clients affected? Records et al. (1992) studied the quality of life experienced by young adults with lifelong language learning disorders. Interestingly, these investigators found that when they were asked about their perceptions of their own life quality, including issues of personal happiness, satisfaction with their lives, and perceived status with regard to education, their occupations, and their families, the subjects' responses were not significantly different from those of a matched control group of young adults with no history of language learning disorders. However, when these two groups of subjects were compared objectively according to income levels and educational achievement, they were clearly different, with the language-disordered group having achieved to a significantly lesser degree. The authors noted that this result led them to conclude that "language impairment seems to be associated with the objective aspects of life, but not with the subjective aspects" (p. 49).

One reason for the long-term effects of language learning difficulties undoubtedly is related to the connection between a child's oral language competencies and acquisition of literacy skills. The connections between the two systems are complicated and are not the same all the way through the developmental process (Wallach & Butler, 1994), so at times spoken language exerts an influence on literacy learning and at other points in the process the development of literacy competencies influences production of spoken language. An example of this takes place when a young child, having become familiarized with literate storytelling style through book reading at school, begins to generalize it to accounts of school activities when she is at home. Even when assembling language intervention programs for young children, which are usually focused on expressive oral language production, the SLP should probably keep in mind that she should be purposefully setting the stage for literacy learning at the same time (Catts & Kamhi, 1998).

Snyder (1980) put some of the blame for the long-standing nature of language disorders on the type of intervention services provided. She suggested that the language intervention provided to school-age children diagnosed as language disordered had little effect on making the children sufficiently "mobilized for reading" (p. 40). Specifically, she noted that the ability to make syntactic predictions and inferences were two skills necessary for reading success and that these were not usually addressed in language intervention programs for young children. The author acknowledged that some of the more specific competencies needed to learn reading and writing have been neglected by SLPs who work with preschoolers. Fey, Catts, and Larrivee (1995) discussed the academic and social demands placed on children in school and suggested ways to prepare preschool-age children with language impairments for meeting those demands.

Further, because many preschool-age children with language disorders go on to exhibit difficulties with reading and writing even though their oral language competencies appear to have been resolved (Stothard et al., 1998), a number of investigators have specifically recommended that SLPs incorporate the specific teaching of emergent literacy skills (Justice & Ezell, 2004; Kaderavek & Justice, 2004). Specifically, although exposure to books and print are helpful, a more comprehensive and explicit curriculum including the teaching of book and print conventions, phonological awareness, and alphabet recognition and naming, as well as writing practice are better for preparing young children to read and write.

DETERMINING THE "WHERES" AND "HOWS" OF LANGUAGE INTERVENTION

As already noted, attitudes and "fashion" with regard to what SLPs call themselves and the clinical services they perform have changed over time (Miller, 1989). Similarly, the settings where speech-language clinicians most commonly perform language intervention have changed. In fact, the changes in typical settings for clinical service have been dramatic over the past several years, in large part due to the substantive changes mandated through federal legislation. This should not be surprising, given that the changes are in keeping with a more general shift in the perception of the role of SLPs as well as increases in the demand for their services. Table 10.1 presents the benefits and drawbacks inherent in three different language intervention settings: (1) the pull-out model, (2) the classroom model, and (3) the combined collaborative-consultation model. Professionals in the field of speech-language pathology have attempted to address weaknesses in each of the models by developing new models or revising present models, as shown in Figure 10.1.

The Pull-Out Model

Traditionally, SLPs engaged in the "pull-out" model of service delivery for children attending school programs. With classroom programs for preschoolers with disabilities becoming more commonplace, it is likely that this approach has also been used with very young children. In the pull-out model, students are removed from their classrooms or the home environment to work with SLPs either individually or in groups, usually consisting of other children who exhibit similar problems. Pull-out

Table 10.1 Benefits and Drawbacks of Service Delivery Models

Model	Benefits	Drawbacks
Pull-out	Child less distracted by classroom activities	Setting for language learning is decontextualized
	Child given opportunities to learn/practice in a less threatening, less competitive atmosphere	May be stigmatizing to child to be withdrawn from class Child misses important class time
Classroom	Clinician experiences child's language difficulties as they happen	May be distracting to other students or the teacher
	"Where the action is"	May be stigmatizing to the child to be observed receiving special assistance
Collaborative consultation	Intervention strategies taught to the teacher by the clinician Teacher is primary intervention agent <div align="center">OR</div>Teacher and clinician share mutual respect and mutual responsibility for the child's program	Teacher may perceive clinician as language expert to deliver intervention services Teacher may perceive self as too busy

therapy has typically been performed in small rooms or areas away from the child's classmates and can be used for either individual or group therapy sessions. The rationale for this model probably stemmed from the belief that separating the child(ren) from the rest of the class would provide a quiet location where the specific goals of therapy could be addressed. Not only should there be less opportunity for the child to become distracted, but the therapy provided would not disrupt the classroom program of classmates who do not have language disorders.

Figure 10.1 Relationships among Models of Language Intervention Service Delivery

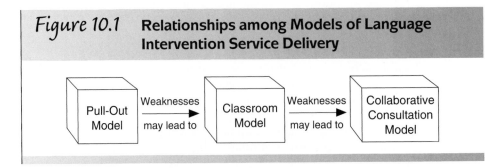

One potential down side to this approach is that it singles out a child for having a problem and possibly stigmatizes the child as being different from the classmates who stay behind (Brush, 1987). Furthermore, the child is removed from the very setting in which he or she is likely to use the language features being taught. Through the pull-out model, language is often taught without context or at least taught in a rather contrived, unrealistic context. One very important way to ensure generalization—context validity—is eliminated. It should also be noted that for the child receiving therapy in a community clinic or private practice, language intervention can also resemble the decontextualized setting of the pull-out model. Unless steps are taken by SLPs to help the young child recognize that the clinical setting and other frequently experienced settings (e.g., home, school) have some communicative similarities, there is no reason to expect the child to apply the structures and strategies learned in therapy outside of the clinic.

Despite the philosophical move away from the pull-out model that was accelerated by legislation mandating that children with disabilities receive appropriate services in the least restrictive environment possible, the 2003 Omnibus Survey Caseload Report for SLPs (ASHA, 2003) revealed that on average, school-based clinicians were spending almost 20 hours per week providing traditional pull-out services. In comparison, these SLPs reported spending an average of just over 90 minutes per week in collaborative consultation.

Specifically, federal law has mandated that early intervention services be provided as often as possible in the same natural environments where children without disabilities can be found. Sequestering a child from his or her classmates for language intervention may represent a too restrictive environment, justified only if it is shown to be essential for the success of an individual child's treatment. Thus, the context of therapy should promote normalization.

Intervention in the Classroom

An appreciation for the social foundations of language development and the need for context support in language learning has led to attempts to remedy the problems that may be posed by the pull-out model. One solution has been to provide speech-language intervention in the classroom itself. Whether a preschool, a kindergarten, or a grade-school classroom, it is the classroom context where language problems, if they exist, are likely to manifest themselves, because it is here that the educational as well as social demands involving language are placed on the child. The classroom is also likely to offer more natural opportunities for conversational exchanges between teachers and students and between students and their peers. SLPs who provide treatment in the classroom will have a better chance to observe problem situations as they unfold for the child and to provide "on-line" assistance or suggestions for remedying communication breakdowns. This is the perfect opportunity for curriculum-based therapy.

One of the difficulties with a classroom-based approach is that the classroom routine could be affected by the presence of another adult who may be working at cross-purposes with the classroom teacher. That is, the classroom teacher presents information for all of the children, whereas SLPs usually present information that is relevant for just one or maybe a few students. The SLP's interactions with the child may draw attention to themselves and away from the classroom teacher when attention paid to the classroom teacher would be beneficial for completing class projects. Further, the child with a language disorder is still the recipient of extra assistance in the classroom, and the child or the child's classmates may see this difference in a negative light (Jenkins & Heinen, 1989). So, although working in the classroom eliminates some of the problems presented by the pull-out approach, it may create others for the clients being served.

Collaborative Consultation

A third option is the collaborative consultation model for service delivery (Frasinelli, Superior, & Meyers, 1983). Actually, when we use the term *consultation,* we are referring to a family of possible models for interaction between the SLP and school personnel (Marvin, 1987). By serving as consultants to classrooms, SLPs can eliminate some of the drawbacks to the pull-out and in-class models. In addition, both professionals end up learning more about the other's area of expertise; the classroom teacher should end up learning more about how communication can be facilitated, and the SLPs should learn more about the classroom curriculum and its demands (Prelock, Miller, & Reed, 1995). (See Chapter 3 for a more detailed accounting of the collaborative consultation model of service delivery.)

There is probably an endless variety of ways in which the collaborative consultation model can be implemented. Prelock et al. (1995) described a Language in the Classroom (LIC) program involving collaborative partnerships between speech-language clinicians and classroom teachers. In this particular program, collaborative efforts include assessment, "goal setting, planning, and implementation of intervention for students with communication disorders as well as for those students who are at risk for language and learning problems" (p. 286). In another approach to service delivery, Farber, Denenberg, Klyman, and Lachman (1992) described what they call the Language Resource Room Level of Service, incorporating aspects of "the classroom, a team teaching model, itinerant support, and consultative services" (p. 293). Farber et al. (1992) suggested that with SLPs potentially assuming roles of co-teacher, consultant, or direct service provider depending on programming needs, a greater number of treatment options was possible (p. 293).

No discussion of speech and language services in the classroom would be complete without an acknowledgment of the "bigger picture" of the regular education initiative (REI), more commonly referred to as *inclusion* or *full inclusion* (Wolery & Wilbers, 1994). Following federal legislation mandating the provision of appropriate education to all children in the "least restrictive environment" (P.L. 94-142, 1975; P.L. 99-457, 1986; P.L. 101-576, 1990; P.L. 105-17, 1997; and the reauthorization of IDEA, 2004), many state departments of education and individual school districts have interpreted these laws in ways that more or less conform to the notion of the REI, whereby special education and regular education are melded into one (Stainback & Stainback, 1990).

By definition, supporters of full inclusion believe that the "least restrictive environment" is a mainstreamed classroom for all children, regardless of level of ability. That is, as promoters of the full-inclusion standpoint, Stainback, Stainback, and Forest (1989) view the concept of "inclusion" as the logical outcome of the practice of providing children with the least restrictive educational environment; there should be no differentiated, segregated, special education classrooms. However, these authors believe that inclusion is more than just mainstreaming. They note that "an inclusive school is a place where everyone belongs, is accepted, supports, and is supported by his or her peers and other members of the school community in the course of having his or her educational needs met" (p. 3). Within an inclusive classroom model, "the focus is on how to operate supportive classrooms and schools that include and meet the needs of everyone" (p. 4). A more comprehensive discussion of the scope of inclusion theory and practice is provided in Chapter 3.

Another and more recent intervention initiative has been the Response to Intervention or RtI model (Ehren & Nelson, 2005). RtI is innovative in that intervention provided by SLPs to children in regular classrooms who are showing signs of communication failure precedes their assessment and diagnosis as language disordered. A more complete description of RtI will be provided elsewhere in this text. Let it suffice to mention here that RtI represents an exciting way to be certain that misdiagnosis related to cultural and/or linguistic differences is kept to a minimum.

SLPs' Responsibilities for Language Intervention

A SYSTEMS APPROACH TO EVALUATING TREATMENT OUTCOME

If you take a comprehensive point of view, the responsibility for language facilitation and remediation falls to some extent on everyone who has contact with the child diagnosed with a language disorder. This section presents a synopsis of what parents, classroom teachers, and SLPs are most typically expected to bring to the language intervention table. Obviously, SLPs are trained to provide intervention services. Therefore, it is important for them to have a strong background in language development as well as in the latest procedures for the assessment of young language-disordered individuals (Weiss, Tomblin, & Robin, 2000). An appreciation for the fact that language development represents only one aspect of the growing child's development is also important, as is an understanding of normal cognitive, social-emotional, and physical development patterns. An understanding of learning theory is also essential, along with more specific knowledge of language treatment programs, techniques, and their rationales. Because the study of treatment efficacy is a burgeoning area of research, SLPs should be prepared to continuously update their internalized databases with regard to which strategies for language facilitation have been shown to be both effective and efficient for which types of clients.

Success in language intervention takes more than a wealth of background knowledge, however. There is a clinical art that tempers clinical science. Goldberg (1993) suggests that lists of desirable clinical characteristics typically describe an individual who is "a non-defensive, confident, and accepting individual" (p. 40).

In addition, because the demographics of our nation are changing in substantive ways, along with these changes have come changes to the distribution of our clients in terms of cultural backgrounds. Recognizing this pattern, Hanson (2004) suggested that "an appreciation and respect for cultural variations, as well as group and individual differences, is crucial for the interventionist" (p. 5). Lynch (2004) added that interventionists working with families from cultures other than their own will enhance their communicative effectiveness by focusing on the other culture as a potential learning experience and remaining open to the different perspectives that will be shared by virtue of working together to develop a workable treatment program.

Along with having basic knowledge about language development and disorders, SLPs should know how to use that information to decide which young children are developing language normally and which ones are not. Once the decision has been made that a problem exists, it must be decided whether language intervention is warranted. Olswang and Bain (1991) described three methods: profiling, the static determination of what a client knows at a particular point in time; dynamic assessment, an analysis of the extent to which a client can benefit from cues and support in the environment; and monitoring (or tracking), a systematic evaluation of progress over time that allows for a prediction of future development, which can be incorporated into the decision-making process to facilitate appropriate recommendations for treatment (p. 255). According to the authors, the two critical determinants for treatment readiness are significant differences between competencies of different language components or between linguistic and cognitive competencies and evidence that the client is ready to make changes in language performance. Specifically, profiling and dynamic assessment are most useful in providing clues as to when to begin intervention, and tracking or monitoring can be used retrospectively to evaluate whether the decision to intervene was a good one. See also Bain and Olswang (1995), Long and Olswang (1996), and Olswang and Bain (1996) for additional uses of a dynamic assessment approach to determine when young children are ready to tackle specific expressive language objectives.

If the SLP believes that intervention is warranted, then decisions must be made about a specific plan of action. Many variables must be considered to develop a plan of action for a child. Of course, how communicative the child is, how much language the child already has, and how much of it is typically used will need to be considered. The clinician must also consider how the child best learns, as well as the degree to which the parents and others who have significant contact with the child and the treatment program can be called on to carry over what is learned in treatment into the home environment. A listing of additional questions that should yield useful information for decision-making purposes is presented in Table 10.2.

CLINICAL JUDGMENT

Information derived from answers to the questions listed in Table 10.2 alone will not be sufficient to develop an appropriate intervention program. Skilled SLPs recognize that good decision making and intervention planning result from a blend of objective information and good clinical "feel" for the therapeutic situation. There is an art to clinical practice that is difficult to specify but that is most likely a product of clinical experience melded with the facts of clinical science (Records & Weiss, 1990). Given

Table 10.2   Selected Information Needed to Develop a Language Intervention Plan

1. Is the child cooperative and able to comply with structured tasks?
2. Is the child willing to separate from the parent or caregiver to work with the clinician?
3. Are pictures meaningful to the child, or should three-dimensional objects be used?
4. Does the child exhibit both receptive and expressive language disorders?
5. Do any members of the child's immediate family also have a language disorder?
6. Have the parents expressed interest in participating in their child's language intervention program?
    (a) If so, how much time could they reasonably devote to specific activities?
    (b) If so, how knowledgeable are the parents regarding language development milestones?
    (c) If so, is their typical interaction style with their child directive? egalitarian?
7. Does the child show any awareness of the language disorder?
8. Has the child been reported to become frustrated in attempting to communicate?
9. Will intervention activities hold the child's attention for 5 minutes? 10 minutes? 15 minutes?
10. Is the child involved in a classroom program?
    (a) If so, what is the focus of the classroom (e.g., academic, preacademic, daycare)?
    (b) If so, does the child's language disorder compromise the child's interactions with classmates?
    (c) If so, does the child appear to enjoy the classroom experience?
    (d) If so, are there other children in the child's class with language difficulties? other developmental problems?
    (e) If so, has the child's teacher(s) expressed concern about the child's language abilities? willingness to participate in language intervention?

this subjective portion of clinical judgment, clinicians must guard against falling victim to unsubstantiated biases as they make decisions. Despite gains in efficacy research, there is still not enough conclusive information to indicate which intervention programs are best suited to which children. Thus, there is a danger in assuming that an intervention plan that apparently worked well with one child will necessarily work well with all children.

One way to help overcome a tendency toward bias in selecting intervention approaches is to focus on our rationales for choosing certain clinical methods and to maintain a healthy skepticism until supporting data become available (Newhoff, 1995). Continuing to collect objective data to substantiate client progress or lack of progress helps prevent clinicians from becoming too complacent with one or another therapeutic technique.

EVIDENCE-BASED PRACTICE

Probably the biggest change in thinking within the field of speech-language pathology over the last five to ten years has been a concentrated shift to consideration of evidence-based practice (EBP) data in clinical decision making. The term EBP is defined by Dollaghan (2007) as including the "best available *external* evidence from systematic research" (p. 2) along with the "best available evidence *internal* to clinical practice" (p. 2) as well as the "best available evidence concerning the preferences of a fully informed patient" (p. 2). Thus, EBP is more than just research findings but includes carefully weighted clinical expertise and client preferences and values. The goal of utilizing an EBP orientation is to provide best practices in terms of service delivery to all of our clients, young and old alike. Readers are encouraged to visit the website of the American Speech-Language-Hearing Association, www.asha.org, for tutorials and resource information about EBP.

FLOWCHARTS AND DECISION TREES FACILITATE DECISION MAKING

Some clinicians use flowcharts or decision trees with an "if X, then Y" format to assist in the decision-making process. Several years ago, Yoder and Kent (1988) edited a collection of these decision-making tools covering a vast range of clinical case types (e.g., child language disorders, adult neurogenic disorders), and situations (e.g., dismissal from treatment, eligibility for treatment). Many SLPs find these particularly helpful to "view" the thinking process that expert clinicians go through as they work through a case step by step. This approach tends to reduce the cognitive load on the individual clinician and allows him or her to benefit indirectly from the experience of SLPs and other professionals who have established themselves as experts in a particular clinical area. For example, in a flowchart designed for SLPs planning an intervention program for a child with difficulties in language learning in the absence of detectable problems with the child's hearing, motor, cognitive, or social-emotional development, we would probably want to view a decision-making tree designed by Ellis Weismer (1988), as well as decision-making information suggested by Paul (2007) and Nelson (1998).

What steps are critical in thinking through a clinical case in terms of planning for intervention? SLPs must take into consideration all the intake information gleaned from the case history collected from the primary caregiver(s) and additional test data collected from other professionals such as audiologists, psychologists, and developmental specialists, including results from a "comprehensive communication profile" (Weismer, 1988, p. 42) to determine what language and other communicative demands are placed on the child in the activities of daily living and the degree to which the child is capable of meeting those demands. This profile is likely to yield a relative priority for each language need in terms of the functional communicative weighting it carries. In addition, as part of the input information, the SLP should include the family in helping prioritize concerns about the child's communication performance. They can provide essential information regarding the context-based nature of the communication problem. Is the deficit in communication skills also observed in the home environment?

Note that having the child's hearing assessed is a crucial prerequisite to language testing whenever a language disorder is suspected in a young child. This is nonnegotiable. Remember that having psychological testing also serves to determine whether the child can be considered "specifically language impaired." This diagnosis is important because it will likely lead to different intervention planning and at least to different information being transmitted to the family with regard to prognosis and need for additional support services.

The information provided by the intake data will allow SLPs to make the most appropriate choices concerning selection of a test battery that will determine whether a language disorder is present. SLPs should consider the presence of both standardized and nonstandardized test formats, with some observation of the child in as naturalistic a setting as possible included so that a more complete picture of the child's communicative competencies can be formulated.

Following analysis of the results from the test instruments chosen by the SLP, a determination is made, whether by comparison with normative data or in reference to age-appropriate demands on the child's language, about whether the child is capable of meeting expectations for performance. If not, and it is believed that the results of the testing are a fair representation of the child's abilities, the diagnosis of a language disorder is made. It will be important at this time to determine whether the problem is present in both comprehension and production of language—or in one or the other. This information will have a bearing on prognosis as well as on treatment selection.

Following goal selection and the selection of a goal attack strategy, it is critical to gather new information or use what is already known about how the child responds to support in a teaching environment to best facilitate changes in communication behavior. This can be viewed as diagnostic therapy or the dynamic assessment that must precede our first "best guesses" about what will work best in treatment. Included in this step of the flowchart is the determination of ways we can help the child adequately make use of language input provided during intervention. For example, if the child is demonstrating a language problem and has been unable to learn the rule structures of language, then maybe the language input presented has not been sufficiently structured for that purpose. Specific suggestions can be provided about how linguistic input might be altered to achieve greater success. Any alterations of the input signal (e.g., timing, slowed rate of presentation) or emphasis of important language forms or structures and other prosodic cues (Bedore & Leonard, 1995; Robertson & Ellis Weismer, 1999) could make the difference between the child's understanding or misunderstanding of language both in and out of intervention.

It is also important for the clinician to determine the best setting for intervention. Certainly the settings selected will differ according to each child's special circumstances as well as the availability of intervention services. SLPs may be fortunate enough to have many alternatives to choose from or may be relegated to only one option. Obviously, the caregivers are a critical element in the final selection of a placement for the child; it is a good idea for SLPs to remember that working toward consensus with the child's caregivers is an important part of a clinician's role in a family-centered service delivery model.

Once the initial methods for language input and intervention context have been determined, the clinician must then choose the specific training technique to be used. Ellis Weismer (1988) cautioned that clinicians must select the technique carefully, depending on the area of language targeted for intervention. Decisions concerning use of reinforcers, how feedback will be provided, and how generalization and maintenance will be promoted also should be considered at this early point in planning. Remember that although these are not arbitrary decisions, they represent a best guess on the part of the SLPs from observation of this specific client, the SLP's own past clinical experiences, and input from the caregivers; they may change in time as new data are collected.

The SLP's role as a decision maker does not end with the actual implementation of the intervention program. To determine whether the early decisions have been appropriate, it is critical for SLPs to systematically collect data that support or refute the contention that progress has been made. If the data show that progress has been made, the intervention program has likely been effective and should be continued. If no measurable progress has been demonstrated, then the clinician will need to return to the beginning steps of the program where goals are selected and procedures developed to troubleshoot the program for errors. Sometimes major changes in the program need to be made, and at other times relatively minor changes will get the client's learning trajectory back on track. That is, assessment is ongoing. Fey (1988) discusses a decision-making tree devoted specifically to dismissal decisions. He systematically addresses the troubleshooting of an intervention program complete with carefully delineated criteria for dismissal where no decision to dismiss is ever irrevocable.

Others Who Share in the Provision of Language Intervention

It has already been mentioned that, to some extent, anyone in contact with a child in need of language intervention can share in the responsibility for intervention. Most individuals who come in contact with the child provide incidental language modeling (input) or opportunities for interaction where language can be used and learned. Because all interactions can potentially provide positive language learning experiences, a challenge for student clinicians is to start viewing every interaction with a client in terms of its particular language facilitation possibilities. Given the pervasiveness of language learning contexts, children's parents, other caregivers, classroom teachers, siblings, and peers can and should share in the intervention process to a greater or lesser extent depending on the specifics of the client's needs, abilities, and circumstances. SLPs can play a role in teaching these potential language partners how best to serve this function.

Two aspects of the intervention process with which these "others" are most closely associated are first in promoting generalization, either stimulus or response generalization to untrained contexts (Hughes, 1985), and second in the facilitation of language learning itself, where these more knowledgeable language users consider what the child already knows in creating low-risk language learning experiences (van

Kleeck & Richardson, 1988). This is sometimes called scaffolding (Bruner, 1985) and is closely related to the concept of dynamic assessment, already referred to as a technique to determine readiness for intervention (Olswang & Bain, 1991).

THE ROLE OF PARENTS: DECISION MAKING AND SERVICE DELIVERY

As first mandated by the Education of the Handicapped Amendments of 1986 (P.L. 99-457) and substantiated with subsequent legislation, parents are viewed as integral members of the team for both planning and executing an Individualized Family Service Plan (IFSP) or Individual Educational Plan (IEP), to be drawn up with substantive assistance from professionals representing various disciplines. This legislation deemed that parents are highly responsible parties in intervention planning, although of the team's members they probably do not possess the most information about enhancing the efficacy of language intervention. The need to bring parents into the circle of service providers in a manner that builds mutual respect and consensus for the duration of service delivery has led to a substantial literature on the best ways to accomplish this (Crais, 1991; Pletcher, 1995). Crais (1991) noted that the involvement of parents in service delivery has shifted the focus of intervention, which is apparent in the changing terminology used, where terms referring to the family-focused or family-centered nature of treatment are commonplace. She further suggested "that families are equal partners in assessment and intervention, that families will be encouraged and allowed to choose their own level of involvement in decision making and implementation of both assessment and intervention practices, and that supporting the family in the ways they consider useful is a primary goal of intervention services" (Crais, 1991, p. 2).

SLPs should note that the notion of incorporating parents into the decision-making process, while implemented as a means to empower family members and acknowledge their important role in service delivery, operates as a culturally sensitive phenomenon. That is, when a practitioner from the majority culture is working with families from some nonmajority cultures (e.g., Asian, Hispanic), he or she may be viewed as the expert to whom the child has been brought for the express purpose of deciding on a course of action. If the parents are then asked to take part in the decision-making process by giving and setting priorities, this may signal that the so-called experts are less than competent and the professionals' credibility is diminished. In a general sense, when the speech-language clinician is a member of a different culture from that of the family, it is important to be cognizant of potential misunderstandings brought on by differences in belief systems surrounding health care, child care routines, wellness management, and so on. Hanson (2004) refers to these misunderstandings as potentials for "cultural clashes" (pp. 4–5).

Lynch (2004) noted that cultures differ in terms of their preferred mode of information transfer, with some cultures exhibiting a preference for explicit transfer through oral language and others preferring to transmit information implicitly by means of the contextual cues inherent in a situation, the relationship that holds between the participants, and nonlinguistic cues. This difference in style translates into two culture types, according to the author. There is a "high-context" culture that is observed to be more formal than the "low-context" culture type, which is more informal and demonstrates a tendency toward more egalitarian interaction (Lynch, 2004). The assumption by SLPs that a family adheres to a particular style of childrearing, for example, which does not actually match the family's set of beliefs and practices, may result in unintended communications of insensitivity, which are likely to impede the working relationships of the participants. Therefore, it is worthwhile for SLPs to attempt to determine, as early in their interactions as possible, the level of context-based communication that will be comfortable for the family in question. In her paper describing the assumptions made by mainstream SLPs about how families work that make themselves apparent in the suggestions provided to parents for their role in the intervention process, van Kleeck (1994) warns us to remember that there is much cross-cultural variation in terms of the quality and quantity of family routines, or viewpoints regarding who is an appropriate conversation partner for a young child, to give two examples. SLPs who recommend that the family spend fifteen minutes each night during their dinner time having the child talk about his or her day may meet with resistance not because the family is disinterested in helping but because the assumption of a routine dinner time and discourse focusing on the child are both foreign concepts.

The amount of time that parents spend with their children will vary from family to family, but it is very likely that they spend more time with the child than do SLPs. That means that in addition to their legal role as decision makers for their child, they also are likely to have a great deal of influence over their child's language intervention by virtue of their language input and their frequent presence as language interactants. SLPs should find some way to use the parents' proximity and interest in helping their child with a language disorder. The parental role in intervention will also vary from parent to parent depending on facility, willingness, or availability to learn intervention techniques, reporting skills for monitoring the child's language use at home; and ability to follow through at home with the therapeutic contingencies used in the clinic. Techniques for making the home environment more like the intervention setting and the intervention setting more like home have been suggested by Hughes (1985) and others to promote generalization outside the treatment setting. Parents are the perfect consultants for putting these suggestions into practice.

It is also important for speech-language clinicians to remember that, as important as the development of speech-language competence is, it may be considered a lower priority than some of the other concerns parents may have. In families where having sufficient food and shelter are daily worries, or catastrophic health issues are present, following through on a language intervention program may take a backseat. Just as it is important not to set children up to fail by instituting impossible goals, it is also important when incorporating parents into an intervention plan not to ask them to do more than can be reasonably expected. Asking a parent to spend a half hour per night engaged in a specific language task is often too much to ask. Most parents want to be as helpful as possible, but for many such a request would seriously compromise other familial duties, and noncompliance may result.

One approach that might solve this problem is to work with parents on ways to facilitate their child's participation in naturally occurring language "happenings," perhaps during quiet times when the child and parent are the only participants, or when several family members can participate in some group activity. Promoting conversations at mealtimes—when the family does have routine mealtimes—is one suggestion that parents frequently say works well. Here the family members can all serve to reinforce the child's attempts to communicate. Better still, the parents do not have to be put in a position of doling out performance-based rewards or punishments.

Several investigators have studied the effects of having parents serve as conveyers of treatment programs. In one study, Fey, Cleave, Long, and Hughes (1993) compared two techniques for facilitating grammatical productions in children with language impairments, one of which utilized the child's parents for service delivery. The authors noted that although both the parent-administered technique and a more traditional clinician-administered technique appeared to yield positive results, it was the clinician-administered approach that provided more consistently positive treatment effects. This led the authors to caution their readers that parent-administered programs may require clinicians to monitor change more closely over time and to institute changes to the program if the child's progress falls below what is expected. This conclusion by Fey and colleagues (1993) may provide support for the notion that although parents are generally highly useful resources for implementing some language programs, they do not take the place of trained SLPs. In a similar vein, results reported by Girolametto, Tannock, and Siegel (1993) revealed that parents' subjective judgments of posttherapeutic improvements by their children bore little relationship to objective data chronicling pre- to posttherapy changes in the same children's performances. This again suggests that parents are very interested in their children's successes but are unlikely, because of the bias in wanting to see progress as well as their lack of specialized training in speech-language pathology, to take the place of the SLP's eyes, ears, and expertise. When Cleave and Fey (1997) compared the progress made by children who had received clinician-directed treatment versus intervention administered by their parents, they concluded that probably the best treatment would have been a combination of the two, in which the parent program was administered at the same time as the clinic-based treatment.

Other investigators have suggested that parents be given rather specific goals for providing their children with language learning experiences. Pierce and McWilliams (1993) noted that the parents of children with severe speech and physical impairments who indicated willingness to participate can be given specific suggestions for increasing the literacy and preliteracy experiences of their young children. In a study by van Kleeck, Gillam, Hamilton, and McGrath (1997), a direct link was noted between middle-class parents' different methods of reading and discussing books with their preschoolers and the children's later demonstration of more or less abstract language formulation.

THE ROLE OF CLASSROOM TEACHERS IN FACILITATING LANGUAGE LEARNING

Classroom teachers can play an important role in a young child's language intervention program. By understanding their young student's language deficiencies, and usually with some assistance from the speech-language clinician, the teacher can provide frequent language learning experiences in the classroom and make these experiences more relevant to the child's ongoing classroom curriculum (Fujiki & Brinton, 1984).

As the expert on the classroom curriculum, the classroom teacher is a valuable resource for the clinician who is working in the classroom itself or serving as a classroom consultant. Classroom teachers can help to pinpoint the situational demands on language that occur during the classroom routine, and they are in a good position to monitor the child's successes and failures in generalizing the language features targeted in intervention. Teachers also have the knowledge and expertise to facilitate success in the classroom. For example, by periodically changing the child's seating arrangement to promote interactions with a variety of classmates (some of whom may be more willing to interact with a child who has a language disorder than others), the child may have more opportunities to practice and perfect new communication skills. The classroom teacher should have expert understanding of the client's and his or her classmates' social dynamics, and this information can be used to advantage by those planning language intervention. Ehren (2002) encourages utilizing the classroom teacher's insight in therapy planning.

THE ROLE OF CLASSMATES IN FACILITATING LANGUAGE LEARNING

Normally developing young children seem to learn quickly which of their classmates have difficulties with communicating. This has been demonstrated by their ability and willingness to accommodate their own language to the less-sophisticated abilities of their classmates (Guralnick & Paul-Brown, 1977). It is also clear that normally developing children are preferred when a peer wants to initiate contact or when children in a classroom are asked to indicate with whom in the classroom they would prefer to play (Craig & Washington, 1993; Rice, 1993; Rice, Sell, & Hadley, 1991). Further, when children with language difficulties do communicate, they tend to do so with adults, perhaps because historically they have found more acceptance in such interactions.

Rice, Hadley, and Alexander (1993) suggested that data describing the interactions of preschool-age children with different abilities within classroom settings point to a pattern of social consequences for children with language impairment or limitations in language use. That is, if a child demonstrates limited language abilities, he or she will be less likely to be involved in experiences that will facilitate peer initiation abilities or to practice the language competencies that are needed to develop friendships. Furthermore, when a child discovers that he or she is not a likely candidate for friendships with classmates, there is probably less motivation for the child to work to develop those needed language skills. After a short period of time in classrooms where young children with disabilities are mainstreamed, it is not unusual for the normally developing children to ignore their classmates with language impairments in favor of interacting with their normally developing peers (Snyder, Apolloni, & Cooke, 1977). With very young children, some of this behavior results from immature socialization skills, but with older children it seems that the children are being ignored because of their poor language skills. As Craig (1993) noted with reference to children with specific language impairment, "it appears that the amount of their peer interaction is limited and that, when it does occur, it probably is reduced in quality compared to that of children with normal language development" (p. 214).

Children from nonmajority cultures may present both language and socialization challenges to the speech-language clinician (Damico & Damico, 1993). Given that so much important language learning is closely tied with the development of children's social skills, it is important for SLPs (as well as the classroom teacher) to learn how to assist the culturally different children in their classrooms "in becoming more empowered in their social and educational contexts" (p. 241).

These findings lead us to believe that SLPs and classroom teachers must not assume that beneficial language learning interactions take place between all children in classrooms; instead, they need to figure out ways to facilitate the opportunities for interaction both inside and outside of the classroom. Rice (1993) additionally suggested that teachers and others not only redirect the requests and statements made to adults by children with language difficulties to classmates, but also teach the children specific strategies to do so. This technique makes it less likely that the child with limited language abilities will use the adults in the classroom as the "default" interactant. Schuele, Rice, and Wilcox (1995) described a method of redirection training that they found enabled a higher degree of successful and generalized interactions between normally developing preschoolers and their classmates diagnosed with SLI. Hadley and Schuele (1998) also discussed ways in which SLPs could set treatment objectives to utilize the social structure of the classroom to encourage peer interactions between children of different language abilities. A number of programs have used storybook reading as the central activity to facilitate not only interactions between classmates but also preliteracy skill learning (Cole, Maddox, & Kim, 2006).

In another approach to capitalizing on the benefits of peer interaction, Goldstein, English, Shafer, and Kaczmarek (1997) developed what they called a "peer-mediated" treatment program. Here the goal was to focus on increasing the abilities of the normally developing children to determine when their classmates with language impairments were attempting to communicate with them so that they could be more helpful in making those communicative interactions successful ones. As a result of this program, the investigators observed an increase in the amount of social integration between the groups of children who were normally developing and those with disabilities. Furthermore, generalization of these skills across children was observed.

Even in classroom situations where language "models" are employed, it cannot be taken for granted that these children, by virtue of their normal language status and presence in the classroom, are providing adequate language modeling for their classmates with limited language. Weiss and Nakamura (1992) investigated the extent to which normally developing children serving as "model" children in a class of language-disordered children interacted with their classmates. They found that two of the three model children spent minimal time with their peers who had language disorders. Unfortunately, the underlying purpose of this classroom's reverse mainstreaming plan was to promote interactions between the models and their classmates so that those with language disorders would benefit from competent language input provided by the models. The authors recommended that teachers should take the lead in putting groups of child conversants together and give them less opportunity to form their own interactant groups based on language competencies.

Taking this thought one step further, Venn, Wolery, Fleming, DeCesare, Morris, and Cuffs (1993) reported on the use of a mand-model procedure to teach normal classroom peers to interact with their classmates who had language disorders. In a mand-model procedure, a clinician requests a response from a child, taking into consideration the child's focus. If the child fails to provide a relevant comment, one is modeled by the clinician. Not only did the normal classmates easily learn to incorporate the mand-model appropriately, but the children with disabilities with whom they were paired increased both the frequency of their responses to their peers and the production of their own unprompted requests.

Facilitating Language Change

THE CONNECTION OF THEORIES TO TREATMENT

SLPs need methods for critically assessing and choosing among the many approaches to language intervention that are possible. Johnston (1983) proposed that, to develop efficacious intervention procedures, SLPs must determine their own theory of language development as well as disorders and design treatment approaches or select from among those already available ideas that are consistent with their beliefs. This is really the clinical expertise portion of EBP. The development of intervention strategies for children demonstrating disorders in language have paralleled the changes in theories proposed to explain child language acquisition. Although changes in therapeutic approaches have lagged somewhat behind major shifts in perspectives on language acquisition theory, a review of the history of language intervention reveals strong connections between the two (McLean, 1983).

For example, SLPs who adhere to a social-interactionist viewpoint typically have placed emphasis on early intervention services by suggesting that children begin to learn important pieces of the language puzzle long before they produce their first words. Sometimes medical or social problems upset the possibility for natural caregiver–child interactions, as may be the case with prolonged hospitalizations following premature birth or other birth complications. SLPs may be asked to analyze infant behaviors and abilities to develop a program demonstrating to family members how to capitalize on their infant's limited capabilities for early communication (Ensher, 1989; Sparks, 1989). Similarly, the importance of early-childhood special programs for children developing more slowly than their peers has received support due to the popularity of the social-interaction approach. The passage of P.L. 99-457, which first mandated services to children ages 3 to 5 who have disabilities, was probably an outcome of the interest in the language learning that goes on during the preschool years and the recognition that the presence of language-based activities in the child's social milieu can provide opportunities for learning and practicing of language in context.

In addition, transition of service delivery to a collaborative consultation model or at least to a classroom-based model from the more traditional pull-out model of therapy can also be traced to adherence to the social-interaction approach. The language milieu in the classroom has been shown to be quite different from that in the home environment. To be successful conversationalists in school, children need to learn the rule systems of both, determining where they are similar and where they are different. For example, there are constraints to turn taking in the classroom that may not exist in the child's home speaking environment. Instead of learning discourse conventions of the classroom in a third setting, the therapy room, treatment in the classroom itself provides immediate occasions for using the new structures and strategies targeted in therapy.

GETTING STARTED

The role of SLPs in facilitating language change with young children proceeds from a series of decisions, and these decisions follow a logical, scientific progression not unlike those made by SLPs working with other populations of individuals presenting with communication disorders. The three aspects of EBP mentioned above (i.e., clinical expertise, data from systematic research, and the preferences of a well-informed client/family) are all taken into consideration.

The first major decision involves a "best guess" about where to begin in therapy; this will come from the results of both standardized and nonstandardized tests and measures completed during the child's diagnostic evaluation. Added to this will be the observations of parents and other caregivers able to contribute information relevant to how well the child can use the language he or she does have to best advantage and also able to provide input with regard to the language demands in the child's life. Along with determining whether a problem exists, the clinician should determine the scope of the problem and how the child can best learn language. Often these last two features of the case are not determined until after a period of diagnostic therapy or within the framework of dynamic assessment procedures (Goldberg, 1993; Olswang & Bain, 1991; Weiss et al., 2000).

During diagnostic therapy, a variety of materials can be employed, and different combinations of input stimuli are emphasized while the child's performance is carefully monitored for changes. Questions concerning the breadth of the problem and most useful methods for remediation are important and need to be answered by the clinician because their answers will furnish useful insights for designing treatment plans that have a greater chance of success. Answers to these questions supply the "how" of the therapy plan's implementation. Here are four examples:

1. *What presentation methods facilitate the child's ability to demonstrate new language targets?* That is, should the targets be embedded in a story retelling task, or should sentence contexts be used? If the child is supplied with opportunities to produce targeted structures in natural conversation exchanges, will the child tend to take advantage of these with little prompting?

2. *How much stimulus support does the child need to be successful?* For example, are auditory cues alone sufficient to result in production of the targeted language structures, or are combinations of auditory and visual cues necessary? Does the child benefit from orthographic cues (letter symbols) or are these confusing? For some young children, orthographic cues may not be meaningful and may present more of a hindrance than a help.

3. *Is the child willing to risk being wrong?* Does the child refuse to incorporate newly targeted structures and forms unless provided with imitative prompts leaving little guesswork when formulating language? Or is this young child willing to try to incorporate new language targets into spontaneous language? If the latter is true, under what circumstances is spontaneous usage more likely to occur?

4. *What motivates the child to improve language performance?* Does the child demonstrate any awareness of difficulties in being understood or in understanding others? When placed in a situation where a communication breakdown is likely to occur, does the child exhibit any understanding of what happened when the breakdown occurs? What strategies does the child use, if any, to remedy a breakdown in communication?

Obviously, along with the "hows," the "whats" of the therapy plan also need to be determined. Goals that emerged from formal testing and therefore appear to be appropriate should be targeted in baseline testing before their final selection. That is, several trials containing a number of examples of the potential structure or forms to be targeted for therapy should be administered so that the clinician can determine whether test results were artifacts of the testing process, of the test itself, or truly represent the child's specific deficits. Sometimes baseline trials are administered in one session; sometimes they are administered over the course of several days. The point is that a stable baseline of the child's performance should be established so the clinician knows the child's level of competence before therapy begins. Failure to have this information leaves open the possibility that time will be wasted either by targeting "goals" already established and leaving other appropriate goals untargeted, or by incorrectly crediting the child's miraculous progress to the therapy program. See Hegde (1993) for a detailed discussion of the implementation of baseline testing.

SELECTING GOAL ATTACK STRATEGIES

If the goals are shown to be appropriate, the SLP's next step is to designate a goal attack strategy (Fey, 1986; Paul, 2007) that will provide a framework for the intervention program. A **goal attack strategy** is a pattern of goal sequencing and emphasis used in treatment programs. Fey (1986) noted that selecting a goal attack strategy is an important decision worthy of careful consideration because different types of clients, different types of goals, and different philosophies fit better into different goal attack strategy types. To make this selection, SLPs need to answer several pertinent questions in light of the goal attack strategies available:

1. What characteristics of the language learner may render one or another of the strategies more or less successful?
2. Will the specific goals selected for the child have a particular impact on attack strategy chosen?
3. What is the theory of the clinician with regard to language learning?

Fey (1986) described three different goal attack strategies: vertical, horizontal, and cyclical. In the **vertical goal attack strategy,** one goal is worked on until a predetermined criterion level of performance is reached. This criterion may have been set by the clinician at 80, 90, or 100 percent correct. Percentage level criteria are arbitrary but typically are set at a level the clinician believes will ensure adequate learning by the child for generalization of that goal, maintenance of that skill without further treatment, or success at the next higher level of difficulty. When the criterion performance level is met, the next goal becomes the focus of treatment. Entire sessions are often devoted to the teaching of one goal, and it is likely that this goal will remain the focus of intervention for a considerable period of time. Because of the intensive nature of the vertical strategy, some children are less likely to become distracted or confused when it does come time to change goals. This approach is believed to be less cognitively demanding and ensures concentrated practice on one goal, which the child learns well before moving on to the next. A potential negative feature of the vertical strategy is that the child may become bored during a session due to its narrow focus. Another is that the child may have more difficulty seeing generalities across different speech-language behaviors. The child may not recognize the shared features of goals 1 and 2 because work on these goals is separated in time. Because generalization may thus be impeded, some clinicians suggest that the vertical approach is the least time efficient of the three for many children in certain clinical situations.

The **horizontal goal attack strategy** prescribes work on more than one goal in the same session. These goals may be closely related to each other (e.g., all conversation act types) or quite dissimilar (e.g., plural morpheme -*s*, tag questions, and responses to clarification requests). The underlying principle is that this strategy better reflects normal language learning because many different language forms and structures are experienced and learned at the same time. The horizontal strategy may be more time efficient because general insights and skills in language learning gained from working on goal 1, such as learning to monitor self-performance, may benefit progress on goal 3. Children known to be distractible may not be considered good candidates for this strategy, because they might not recognize when a different goal, with different expectations for acceptability, is being targeted. It will also take more time for individual goals to become well learned or to become routine, because less time is devoted to each. For children who have particular problems with language learning, overlearning may be necessary for success, and for them the vertical goal attack strategy may be a wiser selection.

In the **cyclical goal attack strategy**, a number of different goals are worked on with a particular time unit of treatment (e.g., month, semester, or school year), but unlike the horizontal goal attack approach, each goal is presented individually, in its own session. After each of the goals has been worked on sequentially over the time frame of interest, the targets in the cycle are reevaluated and the cycle is revised (goals may be added or subtracted) or repeated if need be. Cyclical approaches suggest that much of the child's learning takes place when the clinician is not present. The child takes what is learned in the therapy setting, considers it, and practices it when outside of therapy. Therefore, intensive ongoing client–clinician contact often duplicates effort or wastes time because its benefits may be easily derived by the child alone, provided that the clinician has successfully taught the necessary tools for learning language. According to proponents of the cyclical goal attack strategy, true changes in language competencies occur only after the child has figured out how to incorporate new language targets into his repertoire over time. Hodson and Paden (1991) popularized this strategy working with highly unintelligible children. Figure 10.2 lists some of the variables a clinician must consider when selecting a goal attack strategy. Also, see Weiss (2001) for a comparison of how the three goal attack strategies can be used to target goals typical to the young child with a language impairment.

SELECTING INTERVENTION SETTINGS

Beginning SLPs often fail to recognize that many decisions dealing with the disposition of a treatment plan need to be *tentatively* made at the beginning stages of treatment. That is, the clinician needs to know where the young child with a language

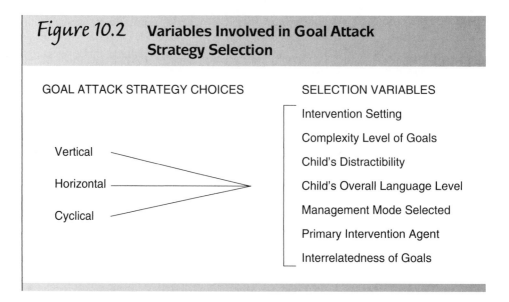

Figure 10.2   **Variables Involved in Goal Attack Strategy Selection**

GOAL ATTACK STRATEGY CHOICES   SELECTION VARIABLES

Vertical   Intervention Setting

Horizontal   Complexity Level of Goals

Cyclical   Child's Distractibility

                                     Child's Overall Language Level

                                     Management Mode Selected

                                     Primary Intervention Agent

                                     Interrelatedness of Goals

disorder uses language and then plan treatment so that the child's new language competencies will be incorporated in an ever-widening set of daily circumstances. In short, the clinician should start therapy having already made some decisions concerning where therapy should take place, with whom, and the amount of structure to be imposed. In addition, there should be some general plan for increasing the "degree of difficulty" for the child as progress is made. One conceptualization for making these sorts of decisions was described by Fey (1986) as a "naturalness continuum" (Figure 10.3).

Common sense dictates that for language intervention to be considered successful, the goals targeted for intervention must be apparent in the child's spontaneous language repertoire. Therefore, at some point in the intervention process, SLPs will need to ensure that the therapeutic environment bears some resemblance to the child's natural environment, or vice versa (Hughes, 1985), or else generalization of newly learned language competencies to the child's activities of daily living may not be easy. Some SLPs wait until the closing stages of intervention before introducing activities aimed specifically at promoting generalization. Others develop intervention programs that account for the generalization of language goals from the very start of treatment. Growing sentiment in the field of speech-language pathology supports the latter approach.

As shown in Figure 10.3, Fey (1986) delineated three features on his naturalness continuum: the activity by the clinician, the physical context used for intervention, and the social context in which the intervention transpires. For each parameter, he suggested that a continuum exists, ranging from more to less naturalness. Taken together, the relative naturalness of the therapy plan can be estimated. A treatment program that incorporates daily activities in the child's home with parents would be perceived as possessing a very high degree of naturalness. That means that the therapeutic setting closely resembles a *non*therapeutic setting. When the child achieves

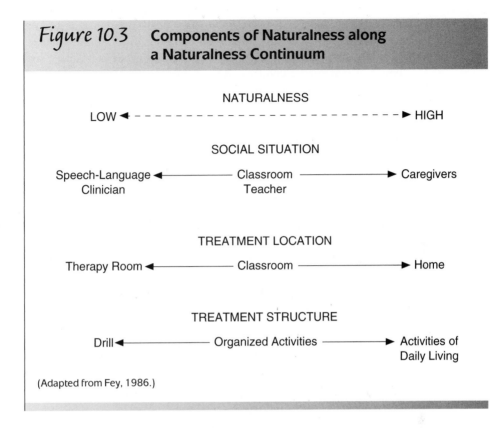

Figure 10.3 **Components of Naturalness along a Naturalness Continuum**

NATURALNESS

LOW ◄ – – – – – – – – – – – – – – – – – – – ► HIGH

SOCIAL SITUATION

Speech-Language ◄——————— Classroom ———————► Caregivers
Clinician   Teacher

TREATMENT LOCATION

Therapy Room ◄——————— Classroom ———————► Home

TREATMENT STRUCTURE

Drill ◄——————— Organized Activities ———————► Activities of
Daily Living

(Adapted from Fey, 1986.)

success in this type of a treatment milieu, the clinician can be more comfortable that the transition to generalization will be accomplished with less directed effort. If the child already views the two settings as similar, he or she should view the opportunities and requirements for language use as similar as well.

Just because a highly natural treatment setting appears to have a major advantage for generalization purposes does not mean that all intervention programs should be designed in the same way. As with selecting the most appropriate goal attack strategy for a particular child, there are client characteristics that may steer the clinician to one or another location along the naturalness continuum at one time in treatment or another. Imposing more structure and very little naturalness in the therapy setting on some children early on may better ensure that they learn new structures. However, generalization will eventually need to be addressed in the therapy program for these children as well. That is, to some degree, an increase in naturalness will have to be incorporated.

SELECTING MANAGEMENT MODES: ONE EXAMPLE

One way for SLPs to arrive at a general framework for intervention planning is by looking carefully at the essential component parts of therapy and assembling them logically and creatively according to the child's needs and the clinician's own philosophy of management. Most SLPs can tell you that "drill" is more structured than "play," but the specifics of how the two treatment methods differ and in what ways they are similar are less widely understood. By understanding these specifics, we have a better chance of matching a child to an appropriate treatment approach and knowing which components may need to be altered when and if a change in our initial therapy plan becomes necessary.

In their germinal article discussing therapy modes useful in the management of young children with phonological disorders, Shriberg and Kwiatkowski (1982) described four categories of treatment components:

1. *Target responses:* the clinicians intended target responses compared to the client's actual responses
2. *Training stimuli:* the stimuli that will be used to elicit responses from clients, presented individually or in sets, and the termination criterion for moving on to high degrees of difficulty in the treatment plan
3. *Instructional events:* the clinical teaching we do, referred to as **antecedent instructional events**, and the feedback we provide to clients following their responses, referred to as **subsequent instructional events**
4. *Motivational events:* events employed to "accelerate learning by heightening a child's receptivity to all instructional events" (Shriberg & Kwiatkowski, 1982, p. 245), possibly incorporated as antecedent motivational events prior to the client's attempts at a response or as subsequent motivational events, also referred to as **reinforcement**

The authors arranged these component parts into four different management modes, called **drill, drill play, structured play,** and **play.** The modes exist along a continuum from "most structured" (drill) to "least structured" (play). It should also be noted that as one moves from the more structured end of the management mode continuum to the less structured end, the treatment focus moves from being clinician centered to being client centered (which in this case is also child centered). That is, on the less-structured end of the continuum, the child exerts more influence on the pace and focal point of therapy, whereas on the more-structured end of the continuum, clinicians are in control of therapeutic focus and pace.

By incorporating the components described by Shriberg and Kwiatkowski (1982) as the entire set of options for the four modes, we can observe the ways in which the four management modes are related to one another, as illustrated in Figure 10.4. Note that structured play and play are quite similar, as are drill play and drill. For example, drill and drill play are identical with one exception. In drill play there is an antecedent motivational event that is missing in drill. That is, something is added to the drill play approach to increase the likelihood that the child will comply with the task. The antecedent motivational event, then, represents a small shift away from the most structured end of the continuum. In both of these modes, drill and drill play, there is a subsequent motivational event (a reinforcer), but this will be presented only in cases where the child's actual response is equivalent to the response definition delineated. Said another way, the child is not being reinforced for willingness to participate; the reinforcer is tied directly to the adequacy of the response.

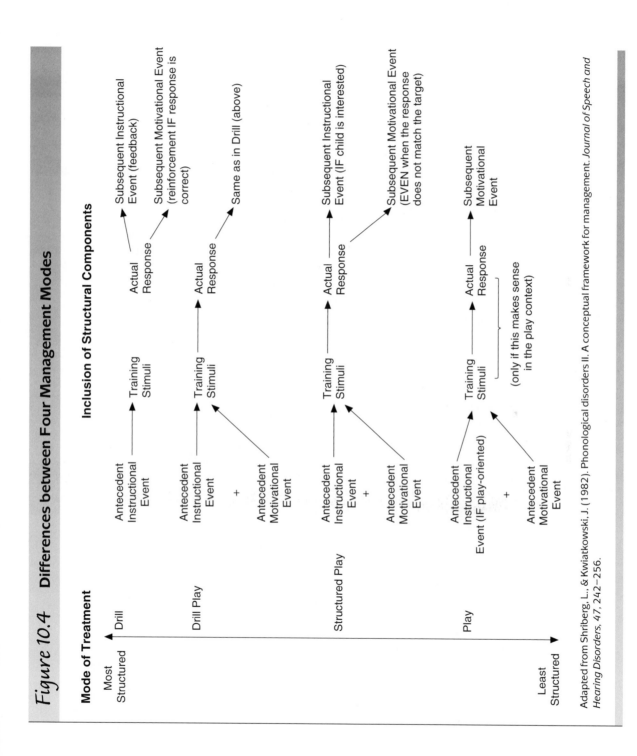

Figure 10.4 **Differences between Four Management Modes**

Adapted from Shriberg, L., & Kwiatkowski, J. (1982). Phonological disorders II. A conceptual framework for management. *Journal of Speech and Hearing Disorders, 47,* 242–256.

As the structured nature of the management mode decreases, there is less emphasis on the antecedent instructional event. This means that formalized teaching of the target becomes a less important part of the treatment. For example, in the play management mode, the definition of an acceptable response and the criterion needed for terminating therapy are not even brought to the child's attention in therapy. This is quite a contrast to the way proponents of drill view therapy, but this management mode is considered equally viable and more appropriate than drill for certain children in certain therapeutic situations. In structured play, which is closer to the clinician-centered end of the continuum than play, the child is presented with information about response definition if he is interested in that information. What is more important in structured play is that the clinician will spend time emphasizing the enjoyableness of the therapy activity.

In follow-up work with this model, Shriberg and Kwiatkowski (1982) reported the results of studies that incorporated their taxonomy in the treatment of twenty-two children with phonological disorders. Their findings indicated that the drill and drill play modes were more effective and efficient than were the structured play and play modes. SLPs who had participated in the studies reported that they believed drill play was the most effective and efficient mode, and not surprisingly they preferred to use the drill play approach; they believed that their clients preferred drill play, structured play, or play over drill. One small study focused on determining the specific client characteristics that would better match with one or another management mode, but unfortunately this investigation yielded inconclusive results.

USING INFORMATION ABOUT CAREGIVER–CHILD INTERACTIONS IN THERAPY

Once the goals for therapy have been selected and arranged according to the chosen goal attack strategy, and the management mode has been developed, the clinician must decide how interactions with the child will teach or facilitate the learning of these goals. Research on how caregivers and young children interact serves as a basis for some language therapy techniques; these techniques are sometimes called **experiential language intervention techniques.** Researchers have noted recurring patterns of language use, usually from research with mother–child dyads, and have hypothesized that these play an important role in facilitating infants' developing linguistic competence. It has been suggested that these patterns should have a similar effect on the child who is not learning language normally. Therefore, patterns such as expansion, expatiation, modeling, and scaffolding have been discussed in the literature of language development as well as that of language intervention (Connell, 1982; Leonard, 1981; Paul, 2007; Ratner & Bruner, 1978; Snow, 1986; Weiss, 1981). In terms of management mode, most of the natural caregiver–child techniques fit most closely with the less structured modes—structured play and play—because they are usually embedded within conversation contexts.

This is probably an appropriate point for a cautionary note on the cultural biases inherent in the caregiver–child research used as a basis for much of this branch of language intervention. The vast majority of research done on caregiver–child interventions has been done with families from the mainstream culture. As a result, it is very likely (and in fact we know this to be true) that there are enough significant differences from one culture to another in terms of childrearing practices, view of children's talking with adults, and so on, that the techniques described may not be typical for many of the clients an SLP sees professionally (Hammer, 2004).

Research by van Kleeck (1994) reported on a number of cultural differences that could lead to misunderstandings when SLPs attempt to teach caregivers how to interact "appropriately" with their children for therapeutic purposes. For example, in some cultures in which young children are not encouraged to initiate conversations with their elders, teaching parents strategies for responding to their child's initiations probably would not be a particularly fruitful approach. Even the assumption that the mother—or father—is the child's primary caregiver and thus primary language partner may be erroneous. In cultures where large extended families tend to be the rule rather than the nuclear family, it may be a grandmother, aunt, or older sibling who has the role of primary caregiver.

Adopting caregiver–child interaction techniques in therapy has also been challenged by some SLPs, who think that because most caregivers engage their young children in similar types of language interaction, the language-disordered child has probably already been exposed to these techniques. If the usual type of caregiver–child interaction patterns had been sufficient to effect language development for the child, they would have done so. Opponents to using natural caregiver–child interaction techniques suggest instead that more directive bombardment with examples of acceptable structures in natural conversation contexts is needed such as focused stimulation (Ellis Weismer & Robertson, 2006). They believe that, by definition, the child diagnosed as having a language disorder probably possesses some sort of deficit that makes it more difficult to benefit from natural interaction patterns. Thus, reliance on these natural intervention techniques alone has no reasonable chance for success. Despite this controversy, experiential language intervention techniques have been widely used and deserve consideration.

Remember that experiential language intervention techniques have their roots in natural caregiver–child interactions for mainstream populations and that their use in therapy should not compromise the naturalness of the treatment. Although the manner in which they are presented by the clinician is prescribed, in practice they are supposed to sound less like a contrived script and more like the normal course of conversational events. The following techniques are commonly used in programs that emphasize conversation development in children who are severely limited in their ability to express themselves (MacDonald & Gillette, 1984; Weiss, 1981; Wetherby, Warren, & Reichle, 1998).

Imitation

The clinician's use of imitation appears to accomplish several things. First, it has been hypothesized that it validates the acceptability of the child's own production. It also gives the child an opportunity to imitate for emphasis by copying what the clinician said. That is, the child may believe that if the clinician repeated what he said first, it must be acceptable. When the child is expected to imitate the clinician, it represents a less risky attempt at contributing to a conversation. Remember that children with language impairments often know that language is not their strong suit and so being a risk taker in terms of language use is not a typical pattern. Although imitation has been used widely in operant programs as the main means for eliciting decontextualized responses from clients, the discussion here refers to a less-structured use. Imitation occurs frequently in language samples collected from normally developing children and their caregivers (Cross, 1978).

Definitions of what constitutes an imitation differ. Imitations may refer to a verbatim reiteration of what was said or only part of it (a partial imitation). An imitation called for by the clinician may require an immediate imitation or a delayed imitation, where either a pause or some intervening dialogue is imposed. Imitation by the clinician also serves as a topic maintainer, letting the child know that the clinician acknowledges the topic established by the child.

Expansion

Expansion refers to the clinician's embellishment of a young child's immature production so that it reflects the adult version of what the child was attempting to produce. Sometimes this is tricky because it is not always clear what the child's intention was. The clinician is not supposed to extend the boundaries of the child's original production, so if the child produced "kitty go," for example, an appropriate expansion would be "The kitty goes." To extend beyond the verb (e.g., "The kitty goes in the car") would constitute the use of expatiation, a slightly different experiential language intervention technique.

The clinical assumption is that expansion, like imitation, provides some useful feedback to the child. Here the message is not necessarily that the child's contribution was acceptable, but that its value as a contribution to the conversation structure has been acknowledged. That is, the clinician has accepted the child's contribution as a turn that served to initiate, maintain, or bring to a close an already established topic. Furthermore, the clinician has modeled a more acceptable version of the child's production, possessing the same communicative intention but with a different surface structure.

As to the "tricky part" of expansion use, unless the clinician carefully uses the linguistic and nonlinguistic information available from the context of the ongoing conversation—for example, what was happening at the time of the child's utterance, what constituted the clinician's linguistic turn just before the child spoke—the clinician may misinterpret what the child was attempting to convey and the child may not have the ability or willingness to correct the adult.

Expatiation

Expatiation is closely related to expansion in that the clinician produces an adult-appropriate version of what the child was attempting to produce. However, in expatiation, the clinician's version of the child's utterance extends beyond the apparent limits of the child's original utterance. Again, the clinician must carefully consider the context of the child's utterance to produce something reflecting the child's intent. If the main goal of expressive language development is to enable the child to encode the relationships among the people, places, things, and events in the world, then what is said must match closely the child's own perceptions. This is not always easy to do, especially when SLPs operate in situations where contextual information can be compromised, as in a therapy room.

Recasting

Recasting is a technique for providing new linguistic information to a child by producing a "new linguistic structure embedded within a partial repetition of the child's own prior utterance" (Camarata, 1995, p. 72). Similar to the description of expansions and expatiations provided above, recasts are required to be produced immediately after production of an incorrect (or incomplete) child utterance and they must provide the child with added linguistic information relative to how the child can more accurately use the language structure he or she attempted. So, for example, if the child said, "More cookie," the adult might recast that utterance by saying, "You want more cookies." According to Nelson and his colleagues (Nelson, Camarata, Welsh, Butkovsky, & Camarata, 1996), recasts represent "rare events" in child–caregiver conversations, but when they do occur with sufficient frequency, they can facilitate the development of new language structures in a child's repertoire.

More recently, Camarata and Nelson (2006) have reported that recasts appear to have been differentially effective in facilitating language development depending on the language level of the child and the specific grammatical feature targeted. More specifically, recasts appear to have a greater positive impact with children who typically produce utterances of more than two words in length.

Modeling

Definitions of the modeling technique abound. For our purposes, a very broad definition has been adopted. Modeling can be thought of as an utterance that attempts to demonstrate one viable linguistic option that could be used in that situation. Unlike imitation, expansion, and expatiation, the basis for the modeled utterance does not have to be something said by the child.

Sometimes the clinical expectation in modeling is that the child will imitate the clinician's production. In other clinical applications, modeling provides the child with examples of the acceptable target structure, either in a structured setting or within quasi-natural conversation, and no response from the child is expected. What is expected is that the child will listen carefully and observe how the clinician's utterances "work" in the situation. In still others, reinforcers are given to the speaker-model for acceptably modeled utterances. Sometimes the speaker is a third participant (Leonard, 1975), and the client is asked to consider all of the examples provided and then determine what made some of the modeled utterances acceptable and others unacceptable. In this way, the child is led along a path of rule induction.

In some language intervention programs, self-talk and parallel talk are described as separate techniques, but under the broad definition used here, they are both more specific types of modeling. **Self-talk** refers to the clinician's monologue about what she is doing. **Parallel talk** refers to the clinician's running commentary describing what the child is doing. Neither situation necessitates that the child says anything in response. Instead, it is hypothesized that the client is being provided with opportunities to match ongoing activity with appropriate linguistic encoding in a nonthreatening manner.

Scaffolding

Bruner (1985) and others have used the term *scaffolding* to describe a pattern of interaction noted in mother–child dyads. It is a description of what Vygotsky may have been referring to when he suggested that children learn through the assistance of competent confederates (Bruner, 1985). Caregivers become well versed in their children's abilities, whether language or motor skills, so that when they request action or information from their children they can predict whether their child will be able to comply successfully. It has been generally observed that most parents want to see their children succeed. Knowing their child's capabilities is useful not only because caregivers like to have their children "show off," but also because they want to be able to *reasonably* increase the degree of difficulty in the tasks they request of their children. In this way, they can maintain the challenge of the interaction (and thus their child's attention) and promote success at the same time. These two characteristics of a language task will help to ensure their child's continued participation and learning (Kirchner, 1991).

This sort of scaffolding interaction has been demonstrated in repetitions of storybook readings observed between young children and their caregivers (Crain-Thoreson & Dale, 1999; Dale, Crain-Thoreson, Notari-Syverson, & Cole, 1996). Often children request readings of the same book night after night. When examples of these separate readings were analyzed in a controlled study, Snow and Goldfield (1983) found that the dialogue between caregiver and child changed as the child became more familiar with the book. Specifically, the mother in the study was asking new and more challenging questions of her child when she was reasonably sure the child would be able to answer correctly.

Scaffolding also serves as a useful metaphor for speech-language intervention. That is, treatment goals should always represent achievements still beyond the child's easy grasp. If they are too easily achieved or cannot be achieved, the goals are inappropriate. Reaching an easily achieved goal does not represent true growth, and improbably difficult goals only frustrate the child. Prerequisite skills for achieving selected goals should be in place, making the eventual reaching of the goal reasonable with sufficient teaching and practice. Competent SLPs constantly monitor their clients' performances for evidence that tasks and goals have been chosen appropriately.

S.O.U.L.

S.O.U.L (Silence, Observation, Understanding, and Listening) is a technique developed in conjunction with the INREAL (Inclass Reactive Language Therapy) program (Weiss, 1981) to establish an empathetic relationship with the child. The four portions of S.O.U.L. are part of the general reactive approach espoused by INREAL proponents, who are taught to "follow the child's lead" rather than impose structure on the client. Remaining silent at least initially in your dealings with a young child, observing what the child is able to do and is interested in, attempting to make sense of the observations you have made, and listening to what the child says whether or not you are involved in the conversation should permit you and the young child to get to know each other. According to the INREAL approach, that is the way an adult earns the right to enter into a therapeutic relationship with a child (Weiss, 1981).

Note that although the acronym is particular to the INREAL approach, the Hanen program, with its focus on teaching parents language facilitating interaction strategies, has similar goals (Giralometto & Weitzman, 2006).

See Table 10.3 for examples of these six techniques carried out in context.

Table 10.3 **Dialogue Excerpts Illustrating Language Intervention Techniques**

Setting: A preschool classroom at snacktime. A speech-language clinician and a child with a language disorder are seated next to each other. They talk while consuming grape juice and celery sticks spread with peanut butter.

S.O.U.L.: Before joining the child at the snack table and engaging the child in conversation, the clinician spent several minutes silently observing the child. Listening carefully, the clinician realized that the child had some concerns about the snack. He had never eaten celery before and was told by his teacher that he had to at least try some. The child appeared to be quite apprehensive as the clinician approached.

Imitation

CHILD: Don't want more juice.

CLINICIAN: Don't want more juice?

Expansion

CHILD: That crunchy one. (*referring to celery*)

CLINICIAN: You're right. That's a crunchy one.

Expatiation

CHILD: Gimme more uh that.

CLINICIAN: Give me some more of that celery because it's *good.*

Modeling (parallel talk)

CLINICIAN: You've licked all the peanut butter out of that celery stalk. Now you're chewing that celery very carefully. Oh, you're done with it.

Scaffolding

CLINICIAN: That peanut butter is crunchy.

That celery is crunchy.

That snack is crunchy. That peanut butter is _____.

CHILD: Crunchy.

CLINICIAN: Yeah. It sure is. Tell me about that celery.

CHILD: Celery is crunchy.

Recasting

CHILD: Celery is crunchy.

CLINICIAN: Yes, celery is crunchy and healthy.

Current Intervention Approaches

This section is divided into four parts, each of which reflects an aspect of the current intervention literature for treating language disorders in young children. To begin with, indirect therapy approaches that focus on parent training will be addressed. In particular, one popular approach to providing caregivers with the tools to facilitate their young children's language learning within a conversation framework, It Takes Two to Talk—The Hanen Program for Parents (Giralometto & Weitzman, 2006) will be summarized. Note that the Hanen Program is one of several parent-focused programs available. Next, recent findings in intervention research focusing on three questions will be tackled: Does therapy setting matter? Do we have evidence that our treatment approaches work? More specifically, do programs focused on temporal processing work? Note that many entire texts deal with the topic of language intervention for children so the information presented in this section is necessarily limited.

A PARENT-FOCUSED INTERVENTION APPROACH: USE OF CONVERSATIONAL FRAMEWORKS

To begin with, The Hanen Program for Parents has been on the language intervention scene for more than 30 years, although the It Takes Two to Talk portion of the program has been developed more recently (Manolson, 1992). Considered an indirect intervention program because parents and other caregivers are the ones who learn the language facilitation strategies, there are actually four programs disseminated by the Hanen Centre in Toronto that vary in terms of the population of children for whom the parent strategies are intended. It Takes Two to Talk is a systematic program for teaching caregivers to use experiential language techniques many of which have been described above (e.g., modeling, parallel talking) to maximize the language learning of their children with receptive and/or expressive language disorders. Similar to the INREAL program (Weiss, 1981), parents are taught to adopt a social-interactionist perspective when communicating with their children. That is, in order to facilitate conversation with less linguistically sophisticated children, it is important for parents to practice being reactive rather than proactive during communication exchange, allowing their children to participate in conversation regardless of their language competencies. Note that in its original form, It Takes Two to Talk followed a general stimulation approach, meaning that specific language goals were not selected for children. Rather, through use of language facilitation techniques by the caregivers, any increases in conversational turn taking was viewed as successful. The more recent version of It Takes Two to Talk, however, has adopted a focused stimulation approach that requires selecting specific language goals for the children. According to a review of efficacy studies provided by Girolametto and Weitzman (2006), the focused stimulation version of It Takes Two to Talk yielded more compelling evidence of facilitation of language development, particularly for "late talkers" (Girolametto, Pearce, & Weitzman, 1996), as well as more carry-over into play settings than did the general stimulation version of the program. Both programs, however, demonstrated an impact on increasing the children's participation in conversation routines.

As noted earlier in this chapter, incorporating parents into treatment programs is not a new focus for language interventionists working with young children. Caregivers presumably spend a significant amount of time with their children, involved in daily routine activities that can be used as context for a program of language learning opportunities. MacDonald and Carroll (1992a, 1992b) have also delineated a systematic approach for teaching parents, as well as whoever else typically interacts with children, how to facilitate conversational exchanges with young partners who are very limited in how they can make conversational contributions. Their overriding rationale for this program is that when a child with a language disorder can communicate successfully with adults, all developmental areas will benefit, not just the development of the child's communication skills (p. 47).

MacDonald and Carroll (1992a) refer to their approach as the ECO model, signifying that when involving young children with language deficits in conversations it is important also to involve "their social ecology, including the relationships and play contexts" and to remember the framework supplied by the scaffolding technique, discussed above, where a more knowledgeable interactant provides assistance to the degree needed to ensure the less competent participant's success. In this case, all potential language-competent conversation partners can serve as supportive, enabling participants for the child with language disorders. Notice how the heart of the intervention is in the most social of venues: conversation.

These authors suggest that it is important to teach children to be initiators in their conversational interactions as well as to be adequate responders. Note that Rice and colleagues (1993) reported that children with language deficits rarely initiate and are only infrequently selected to receive the social/conversational bids of their peers. It was this finding that led Rice and her colleagues to suggest that classroom teachers intervene directly to redirect the children's adult-directed conversation turns to their classmates. MacDonald and Carroll's (1992a, 1992b) program may represent a prerequisite step in this process inasmuch as it focuses more directly on adult–child communications.

As with It Takes Two to Talk and other versions of the Hanen Program, the ECO model provides guidance for adults who want to increase the likelihood that children with limited language will be successful communicators in these interactions. Part of the battle may first involve increasing the likelihood that the child will be willing to communicate with the adult.

The following five interactive styles of communication are suggested by MacDonald and Carroll (1992a) as effective for facilitating communication with young children. Adults are told that *balance,* as it relates to the egalitarian nature of sharing the responsibility for conversation, should be a goal. That is, neither partner should be expected to carry the burden of the conversation; similarly, no one participant should dominate the conversation. Adults are also told to promote *responsiveness,* meaning that as rudimentary as a child's early attempts at conversation turn taking are, efforts should be made by the adult to fit these turns within a meaningful conversation framework. It is also important for the adults to *match* the child's current linguistic repertoire with the expectations for conversation participation. This should ensure a maximum of participation on the part of the child because he or she will be less likely to feel overwhelmed with the conversation task and more likely to risk participation. Another interactive style is that of *nondirectiveness,* meaning that the child's lead is followed by the adult where the former clearly has a topic or focus. In addition, nondirectiveness has to do with the adult's demonstrated willingness to allow the child to direct the interaction (i.e., changing or shading topics). Finally, *emotional* attachment refers to the stage of participation in the dyad when the adult begins to converse with the child because the activity is rewarding in and of itself, rather than because the particular conversation serves as a means to an end.

Note that the Hanen program as well as the INREAL program developed by Weiss and her colleagues take much the same tack. That is, the child with a language disorder is viewed as part of a communication dyad, most often with a primary caregiver, that needs repair to function optimally. With conversation as its basis, participants—both child and adult—are taught how to communicate more successfully within the limitations imposed by the child's deficient language repertoire. In all cases, caregivers are trained to become more reactive to their children's language attempts.

DO THERAPY SETTINGS MATTER?

Wilcox, Khouri, and Caswell (1991) reported the results from a study of twenty children roughly between a 1½ and 4 years of age who were learning their first vocabularies. All of the children had been diagnosed with language delays; half received treatment within a classroom setting and half received individual treatment. Treatment measures of vocabulary growth indicated that neither service delivery situation had yielded superior results until the investigators looked at the children's abilities as measured by generalization to their home environments. Specifically, the children taught the new targeted vocabulary items in the classroom were significantly more likely to generalize these vocabulary words to the home environment than were the children who had received individual (pull-out) instruction. Therefore, the researchers concluded that for the purpose of early vocabulary training, the classroom environment is not only a viable location for service delivery but is also superior.

In another study that looked at differences between service delivered within the classroom and outside of the classroom setting, Roberts, Prizant, and McWilliam (1995) focused on the communication dynamics of the clinician–client dyads in both venues. Although they looked carefully at a number of potential differences in conversation behaviors, only two reached significance. Their findings revealed that during the within-class interactions, children were less responsive to the clinicians, showing a significantly greater degree of compliance during the out-of-class sessions. On the other hand, their SLPs tended to contribute more turns to conversations conducted during out-of-class sessions than those held within the classroom. Given that only these two differences were discovered, the authors suggested that decisions concerning selection of in-class versus out-of-class service delivery should be made on the basis of more than just these differences in communication dynamics. They argued that their findings did not allow them to conclude that a higher degree of treatment efficacy could necessarily be related to a particular service delivery model.

There are other sources of data. The National Outcomes Measurement System, developed by ASHA in 1997, represents an attempt to systematically demonstrate the impact of therapy services provided by SLPs and audiologists. Using a standard set of functional outcome measures (FCMs) that were developed to be specific to different communication disorders, participating SLPs measured their clients' baselines and posttherapy performances and could intuit that the degree of change observed was related to the therapy provided. Compilations of data submitted by the participating clinicians revealed, for example, that where improvement of language production and comprehension competencies in preschoolers is the goal, participation in an individual versus a group therapy setting does not appear to matter. However, for preschoolers with articulation goals only or goals dealing with pragmatics, individual sessions yielded more progress. If children with articulation goals had other language needs, group versus individual session did not appear to matter. Not too surprising was the finding that as the amount of therapy time increased (in the aggregate, not per session), preschoolers were more likely to exhibit greater achievement of both articulation and language production goals. The most progress with articulation goals was achieved by preschoolers who not only had accrued more than ten hours of therapy time but had also successfully completed a home program specified by the clinician.

DO WE HAVE EVIDENCE THAT OUR TREATMENT APPROACHES WORK?

Ellis Weismer, Murray-Branch, and Miller (1994) attempted to determine the effects of two procedures—modeling only and modeling with an evoked production—on teaching new vocabulary items to three young children identified as late talkers. Two of the three subjects demonstrated learning that could be attributed to the treatment procedures, but interestingly, one of the two children appeared to benefit from one of the techniques and the other benefited from the other technique. Unfortunately, attempts to use dynamic assessment methods to determine whether it might have been possible to predict ahead of time which subject would do better with which treatment technique failed to yield helpful results. The third subject did not appear to make gains from implementation of either treatment method.

Studies by Camarata, Nelson, and Camarata (1994) and Nelson et al. (1996) demonstrated differential effects when two methods, one employing imitation and one employing conversational recasting, were employed to teach a number of different grammatical structures to young children diagnosed with specific language impairment. Although both of the techniques appeared to be effective in facilitating the subjects' productions of the majority of the targeted structures, the conversational recasting procedure was more facilitative when both spontaneous productions of the trained targets and generalized, spontaneous productions of untrained structures were considered. These findings suggest that a method that is less structured and more naturalistic may be better able to foster generalization, specifically to conversational settings.

In a study utilizing the techniques of verbal routines and expansions, Yoder, Spruytenburg, Edwards, and Davies (1995) found that their four subjects, who ranged in age from two years to four and a half years, made gains as measured by mean length of utterance (MLU) over the duration of the treatment. However, looking retrospectively at the results, which included assessing generalization across trainers, interaction styles, and modalities, the authors noted that the children in the earlier stages of language development appeared to make greater gains than those subjects who were in the later stages, which may have had to do with the measure of progress chosen (MLU), which is less sensitive to gains in language development after the MLU reaches 3.0.

Remember that we already discussed Fey and his colleagues' work comparing the performance of parents and clinicians in providing treatment (Cleave & Fey, 1997) and the differences in recasting production by parents of children with language impairments versus the recasting production of parents with normally developing children (Fey, Krulik, Loeb, & Proctor-Williams, 1999). Both studies yielded useful clinical implications. In the first study, both parents and clinicians were trained to provide treatment using focused stimulation and cyclical goal attack strategies. Although both groups of children improved, the authors concluded that a combination of clinic-based services and parent programs would have gleaned the most positive results. In the latter study, Fey et al. (1999) observed no appreciable differences between the quality and quantity of recasting provided by the two groups of parents to their differently abled children which led the investigators to conclude that their language-impaired subjects probably needed the benefit not only of more recasting but recasting that was more focused on their language needs. This finding was also substantiated by the results of a study by Proctor-Williams, Fey, and Loeb (2001). The authors interpreted their findings as evidence that if children with specific language impairment are to benefit from recast use, they must be greatly increased from what may be available in the natural environment with parent interaction. Parents as well as the child's clinician and perhaps classroom teachers will have to purposefully increase the number of recasts provided. In a more recent study Fey and Loeb (2002) interpreted the findings from their treatment study as indicating that the success of recasts may be in part determined by the grammatical marker targeted. Note that what we are really addressing is individual differences in treatment effectiveness. This is an exciting topic in and of itself but much too broad for a discussion here.

Several groups of investigators have been interested in the connections between phonological and language treatment. Fey, Cleave, Ravida, Long, Dejmal, and Easton (1994) were interested in examining the effects of two grammar-focused treatment programs on the phonological abilities of their group of subjects, all of whom were diagnosed with deficits in both grammatical and phonological development. Given that phonology is a bona fide component of language, exploring the potential connectedness for treatment purposes between syntax and phonology makes sense but represents an area where there is little information for clinicians. Despite the fact that both treatment procedures were shown to have had a positive effect on facilitation of the subjects' grammar performance, there were no obvious effects on the children's phonological skills. The authors concluded that their results do not support a shared effect between language treatment focused on grammar and phonological gains and that difficulties with the speech sound system should be addressed directly with preschool-age children.

In a study similar in focus, Tyler and Sandoval (1994) reported the findings of their treatment study from preschool-age subjects who were diagnosed with both language and phonological deficits. There were three possible treatment methods received by the subjects, and they yielded significantly different results. Specifically, subjects who were recipients of direct intervention on their phonology targets ended up demonstrating moderate gains for both their phonology and language goals; those who were recipients of language treatment only showed some small language gains but little improvement in their phonology targets. Those subjects who were the recipients of a combined program focusing on both language and phonology demonstrated appreciable positive gains in both areas. The authors suggested that in most cases, if you can only focus on one of the two treatment areas, treating phonology is more likely to provide you with carryover effects to language than the other way around. However, when children are observed to have deficits in both areas, the most efficacious route would probably be to treat both phonology and language at the same time. Tyler and Sandoval (1994) noted that it was their least severely involved subjects who benefited the most from combined speech and language treatments.

In an update of this important work, Tyler, Lewis, Haskill, and Tolbert (2002, 2003) found that their young participants with both phonological and morphosyntactic deficits achieved more "cross-domain" benefit from intervention focused on morphosyntax goals, especially when the work on morphosyntax preceded work on phonological goals and not in the opposite order.

DOES LANGUAGE INTERVENTION FOCUSING ON TEMPORAL PROCESSING WORK? FAST FORWORD (FFW)

One of the proposed etiologies for the language problems experienced by children with the diagnosis of specific language impairment is the presence of an auditory/perceptual deficit that renders the child at a disadvantage for processing rapidly changing auditory information such as the acoustic parameters that signal sound transitions in speech (Watkins, 1994). The Fast ForWord (FFW) training program (Scientific Learning Corporation, 1998), as developed by Tallal, Merzenich, and their colleagues, is an attempt by the authors to retrain the child's brain so that the rapid temporal processing necessary for decoding linguistic input can be accomplished in a normal manner. This computer-based program is a series of games that includes acoustically altered stimuli where speech signal duration is lengthened and speech sound transitions are amplified; these alterations of stimuli are gradually diminished as the child demonstrates more success with the more rapidly presented acoustic information (Veale, 1999). This training methodology has received a great deal of publicity due to the claims made by the publisher and the authors regarding the overwhelming success experienced by children who have used the program. In fact, the authors claim that FFW is an appropriate treatment for reading disorders as well as language learning disorders (Tallal, 2004). For a recent review of FFW and its supportive documentation, the reader is encouraged to read Agocs, Burns, DeLey, Miller, and Calhoun (2006).

According to Gillam (1999), however, there are a number of reasons why SLPs should approach a recommendation to adopt this program with caution. He noted that despite their reported successes with children in a couple of smaller studies (with twenty-two and seven children, respectively) and one larger field study (with data collected from 500 children who had received their training from more than fifty different professionals who had been trained in the FFW procedure), there are many questions about the efficacy of this approach. First and foremost, Gillam questions the basic assumptions of the program, that language impairment is caused by temporal processing deficits and the claim that the FFW program can actually change brain structure and functioning. Further, although he reports that there are some children who have apparently made significant gains as judged by pre- and posttesting on the instruments selected by the program's authors, he wonders to what extent these children also demonstrate truly different and improved communicative use of language in activities of daily living. Veale (1999) provides readers with her own critical assessment of FFW, with an emphasis on the subject selection criteria that have been employed and probably should be employed when deciding whether this is an appropriate program to try with a particular client. Both authors are hesitant to endorse this approach in view of the obvious lack of scientific data to support its basic claims.

More recent research on the efficacy of FFW has brought into question whether this program does more than increase children's performance on specific, structured language tasks (Loeb, Stoke, & Fey, 2001). That is, the children who participated in the FFW did not demonstrate improvement in their functional language competencies. Further, in a three-way comparison of FFW, comparable intensity of traditional therapy, and another computer-based language therapy program not specifically focused on improving temporal processing, Gillam, Loeb, and Friel-Patti (2001) failed to demonstrate a significant correlation between their participants' language skill gains and their performance on the FFW program. Results reported by Agnew, Dorn, and Eden (2004) and Pokorni, Worthington, and Jamison (2004) also did not support the use of FFW for improvement of reading abilities or expressive language competencies. Clearly the utility of this program remains controversial. Clinicians are encouraged to look for the appearance of more definitive EBP information.

Intervention with Children from Multicultural Populations

Providing language intervention services to children from nonmajority populations can represent a challenge to the speech-language clinician, who may not share the same cultural background or first language with the client. Wyatt (1997) noted that SLPs should think carefully about the potential points of bias in the construction of intervention programs or selection of appropriate assessment tools to ensure quality service delivery for all of their clients—even those with whom they share cultural background and language.

For example, as Terrell and Hale (1992) noted, cultural differences may be manifested as differences in individual learning styles. It is important for SLPs to determine what that learning style difference is and how it can be best utilized for language learning purposes. Certainly it is true that paying attention to how our clients learn best should always be of paramount concern to speech-language clinicians. One major difference in learning style that SLPs should be aware of is that of low- versus high-context learning styles (Paul, 2007). Children raised in the majority culture tend to adopt a **low-context learning style,** meaning that they rely a great deal on explicit, verbal messages to learn new material, and often the teaching that occurs is decontextualized. On the other hand, the child who adopts a **high-context learning style**—and many of these children are from nonmajority populations—depends more on observation of the teacher and other nonlinguistic information than on the verbal information provided.

When interacting with children from cultures other than one's own, it is critical that the clinician convey both "respect for and appreciation of the child's L1 and culture" (Roseberry-McKibben, 1994, p. 84). (L1 represents the child's first or native language.) Given a family system's approach to treatment management for young children, it is very likely that the parents or the extended family will be involved with the treatment program. Therefore, it will be necessary to determine the family's attitude toward intervention provided by someone from outside their cultural milieu—because statistically this is likely to be the case, given ASHA's membership demographics—and more generally, how the family approaches the notion of a disorder of communication and treatment for same. Knowing something of the family's cultural beliefs and attitudes about childrearing, family members' roles and responsibilities, and illness and disease, will facilitate appropriate communication exchanges between the clinician and the family.

We will assume that the readers of this chapter are well aware of the language difference versus language disorder issue: the SLP should not be providing speech-language therapy for children demonstrating normal development in their first language although they may not be competent English language speakers (ASHA, 1983).

For children with bona fide language disorders in their first language, treatment should be provided in that first language. Unfortunately, most SLPs are not bilingually competent to do so (ASHA, 1985), which means that provision of services may need to rely on the teaming of monolingual SLPs with someone who does possess linguistic competence in the child's first language. This person may already be a member of the child's treatment team (e.g., a resource room specialist), or may be a paraprofessional person hired because of bilingual competence. When the speech-language clinician works "through" another person, the type of working relationship that develops may range from one similar to the collaborative consultation model discussed to one that is very directive, as in the case of the paraprofessional.

Facilitating Generalization

Generalization is such an important topic in the consideration of language intervention that it deserves its own section for discussion. Generalization is the hallmark of a successful intervention program and serves as one of the best ways, if not the best way, for SLPs to demonstrate the benefits of the programs they execute. As already mentioned, the seasoned clinician will develop a language intervention program with generalization in mind and not "train and hope" (Hughes, 1985, p. 1) that it will occur. If generalization did not occur, language intervention programs would be interminably long because clinicians would have to teach every possible occurrence of every goal.

Generalization is usually described as the use of trained responses in untrained situations. It is evidence that the child actually learned something in intervention that is transferable beyond the treatment setting, although, as will be discussed, that "something" may not always be what was intended by the clinician. Note the use of the term *response* here. Much of the work done concerning generalization has come out of the learning theory tradition, with its historical roots in behaviorism. Therefore, the child's participation in language exchanges is most often viewed as a response to the stimuli presented by the world at large, whether by the parent, teacher, peer, sibling, or speech-language clinician.

GENERALIZATION TYPES

There are two basic types of generalization: stimulus generalization and response generalization, and the possibilities for both occurring should be considered. **Stimulus**

generalization refers to the use of trained responses in (1) a new setting (e.g., at school when the intervention took place at home or in the playground at school when intervention occurred in the classroom), (2) with new people (e.g., with the classroom teacher when an SLP provided intervention, with a classmate when the classroom teacher provided intervention, or with a new clinician during the spring semester when the child had been taught the goal by last fall's clinician), and (3) with new materials (e.g., the child responds to the clinician's use of pictures when only object stimuli had previously been used in intervention or the child who was taught narrative skills in intervention using sequencing cards now displays those skills when shown a videotape). In each case, the child exhibits command over language goals that had been taught in a different situation.

Response generalization refers to learning that has transcended a language complexity level or that has extended to untrained examples at the same level of complexity. For example, if a language goal was targeted at the sentence level and the child demonstrates production (or comprehension) of that goal in text (e.g., a narrative or an expository paragraph), response generalization has been achieved. Similarly, if in spontaneous interactions with the clinician the child uses request forms that were never specifically targeted in therapy, response generalization has occurred, provided that different request types had been targeted in therapy. If the new request forms in this last example were produced in conversation with the child's classroom teacher, both response and stimulus generalization could be said to have occurred. That is, new response types were produced (response generalization), and they were produced with a new person (stimulus generalization). Table 10.4 lists some of the differences between stimulus and response generalization.

WHY ATTEMPTS TO TEACH GENERALIZATION FAIL

When generalization does not occur, there are several probable explanations. The fact that the clinician has an agenda to enhance generalization through teaching does

Table 10.4   **Example Showing Differences between Stimulus and Response Generalization**

Scenario: Child, age 5, receives language intervention at school twice weekly in individual sessions. The clinician uses picture cards with action illustrations to prompt child to form past tense of verbs. Child enters the house and announces: "Mom, I walk*ed* home with Joe."

Stimulus generalization	*Response generalization*
Use with:	Use at a different language complexity level
a new person (with mother),	(in a sentence, not a single word)
or	*or*
in a new setting (at home)	Use of an untrained example at the same
or	language complexity level (*walked* was
new materials (spontaneous production)	never targeted)

not mean that the agenda has been conveyed to the child. What may seem perfectly well connected, logical, and rule-based to a competent adult language user may not be quite as logical when perceived by a young child with a language disorder.

In the case of response generalization, what we are really hoping to convey to our young clients is that we are teaching them general rules that can be applied in multiple settings. We do this by teaching a subset of examples that are drawn from all possibilities and that we hope are good, representative examples. Sometimes we use only a few examples of the targeted rule; this has been referred to as "training deep" (Elbert & Gierut, 1985). For some children, the commonality that exists among these few examples cannot be understood. So, in some cases where generalization does not occur, training too deeply may be the problem.

At other times we may make use of too many examples, and the rule may be lost on the young child. Using a large number of exemplars has been referred to by Elbert and Gierut (1985) as "training broad." Training broad may be the problem standing in the way of generalizations for some children in some language learning situations. SLPs sometimes must struggle to find that "just right" mixture where we do not burden the child with too many examples or undercut his or her ability to find the general rule by providing too few examples. Sometimes, too, the examples are poor or nonrepresentative, and that may be another reason why generalization fails to occur.

Some empirical data have been reported to assist clinicians in making these kinds of choices. Elbert, Powell, and Swartzlander (1991) noted that the number of exemplars needed for generalization to occur varied significantly among their nineteen phonologically impaired subjects. The majority of these children needed three exemplars (59 percent), but 14 percent required ten exemplars to reach the generalization criterion specified by these investigators. It might stand to reason that the child with a language impairment who has difficulty with the manipulation of language symbols would have more difficulty discerning common patterns in words, phrases, and sentences and would need those patterns to be treated in common ways without extensive practice and using a large number of examples.

RESPONSE SETS

Another possibility for explaining generalization failure has to do with not knowing the appropriate response set for the examples taught. A **response set** is the extension of a language rule that can be reasonably expected. For example, few SLPs would expect that by targeting *-ing*, the present progressive morpheme, one could logically expect the client to then generalize to learning to correctly use nominative and objective case pronouns correctly—for example, *he* versus *him*. Because these two goals seem to be entirely unrelated, generalization between them appears to be unlikely. What about teaching the initial /s/ sound and testing for generalization to the final /s/? That seems to be logical and could be expected, although there are a number of possible mitigating variables. If it turned out that probe testing revealed generalization to final /s/, it could be said that for that child initial /s/ and final /s/ belonged to the same response set. If not, then we could conclude that at least at this point the child does not see the connection or generalizability between the two.

This discussion of response set is important because it is possible to become overzealous in the quest for generalization and to expect generalization where generalization is not likely to occur. SLPs must remember to try to take the child's perspective and to keep the expectation for generalization from exceeding what is reasonable. Children who have language disorders have already experienced too much failure. Often, their failure to generalize can be traced back to the clinician's own faulty planning. More specifically, the child's failure to generalize could be the result of expecting generalization where none should be expected; using exemplars in intervention that are poor representatives of the rule, principle, or construct being taught; using too few or too many examples; or not having spent enough time in intervention to expect generalization learning to have occurred in the first place.

PLANNING FOR GENERALIZATION

As stated throughout this chapter, SLPs must plan strategies for generalization from the very start of intervention planning. Remember that to some extent concerns about generalization and context-appropriate treatment led to the movement toward classroom-based language intervention. Providing intervention in a context (the classroom) where newly taught gains in language competencies could be utilized frequently should make it more likely that generalization to the classroom will occur *without* the presence of the clinician. Opportunities for using the new language abilities should occur whether the clinician is present or not. SLPs who want to encourage generalization will be wise to spend substantial time pointing out to the child what the identifying characteristics of these opportunities are.

Hughes's (1985) text, *Language Treatment and Generalization,* contains many thoughtful and thought-provoking suggestions for generalization planning. The author presents two sets of these suggestions, one for making therapy more like natural environments (p. 157) and one for making the natural environment more like therapy (p. 158). In each case, the clinician attempts to give the client a broader perspective of where it is appropriate to use his new language skills. For example, Hughes suggests that SLPs should experiment in the therapy setting by transferring from contrived consequences to more natural consequences or prompts that might occur in activities of daily living, as well as suggesting to the child's caregivers that they use the same prompts used in the treatment setting by the clinician when they are at home with the child.

Apropos of this last suggestion, it is not uncommon to hear a young noncompliant child tell a parent who is trying to do carry-over work in the home: "I don't do that with you. I do that with [name of child's speech-language clinician]." In these cases, the child appears to categorize language functioning according to setting. Certain language is used in one setting and not in another. If the child "knows" this, then we may have fostered it, and we will have to spend time presenting counter-evidence to *un*teach it.

SLPs should also recognize that some goals will be more easily generalized than others, due to the inherent, functional nature of the goal. These more easily generalized goals should be considered priorities in intervention, because they may assist the young child in understanding the gist of generalization. Consider, for example, the goal of demonstrating consistent production of request forms (e.g., "Can I have that?") versus the goal of spontaneously producing superlative adjective forms (e.g., fluffiest). Being able to produce a variety of request forms (e.g., "What did you say?" "Tell me another story," "Do you know where Mark is?") will permit a child to specifically request the information or action desired. Request forms are produced frequently in conversations and allow speakers to exert some control over an ongoing conversation and the immediate world. On the other hand, having a firm grasp on how to form superlative adjective forms is less functional. Superlative adjective forms are neither as common nor as critical to communication as the request form.

Last, as the child begins to grasp the specified language goal within a task or intervention structure, generalization can be facilitated if the speech-language clinician begins to systematically alter the teaching situation. Hughes (1985) referred to this as "teaching loosely" (p. 160). Within the teaching phase of intervention, the clinician adds some change to the proceedings. Perhaps this will mean that another person, maybe a parent, begins to sit in on the treatment sessions. It could mean that feedback is given on every other attempt at the teaching task made by the child, so that the intervention more closely resembles life away from the treatment setting. Outside the therapy room, it is rare indeed to receive a pat on the back for a well-constructed sentence! Regardless of how the clinician attempts to loosen up the intervention process, the result should be the same: intervention that more closely resembles something other than intervention.

A FINAL WORD ON GENERALIZATION

These basic suggestions for promoting generalization apply whether intervention takes place in or outside a classroom and whether a teacher collaborates with the speech-language clinician or the speech-language clinician provides direct service delivery or, as in the case of the Hanen Program, parents are providing the therapy. The variables involved in enhancing generalization (e.g., settings, providers, targets for generalization) will differ from case to case depending on how the intervention was originally devised. However, no matter what the format of the language intervention, there is no excuse for not promoting generalization from the very first intervention session.

Some Remaining Issues for the Future

When considering language intervention for young children, it seems SLPs continue to leave at least two critical issues only partially answered. The first has to do with the ability as professionals to predict language learning outcomes, and the second can be best described as an issue of following through on professional commitment to promote evidence-based practice. That is, SLPs need to be better able to predict on the basis of their earliest behaviors which children who present themselves as at risk for language learning problems will actually experience difficulties and what will be the magnitude of those problems. The logical concomitant issue has to do with how SLPs then go about acquiring sufficient evidence for selecting the most efficient and most effective treatment plan for each individual client.

Note that the twin issues of enhancing the powers of predictability and promoting the evidence that supports the treatment provided both carry with them sets of underlying assumptions. The predictability question, for example, presupposes the availability of valid and reliable measures for evaluating a child's early language, social, and motor behaviors and the existence of adequate information concerning how these behaviors relate to normal developmental expectations. Questions of evidence-based practice also have several underlying assumptions. In order to develop appropriate, supportable treatment plans, preliminary studies will first have to establish that each option is efficient and effective in its own right. Additional research will then have to determine which intervention plans are best suited to individual children based on carefully constructed profiles of each child's language learning strengths and weaknesses.

Becoming reliable predictors of future speech and language performance as well as providing the most efficient and effective intervention programs for clients represents a challenge to clinicians and researchers alike. In fact, it is likely that it will take many years to be able to present a comprehensive end point to either quest. However, the answers to these questions are not luxuries. Rather, they are necessary if SLPs are to provide clients with the best possible clinical services.

Summary

This chapter described the speech-language pathologist's role in the development of language intervention programs for young children. It is important to understand the challenging nature of the decisions the clinician must make along the way, the different options available for selection, and the rationales behind those selections. Given the changing demographics of the young clients served by speech-language clinicians, it is additionally important that SLPs acknowledge the ways in which cultural differences should affect the treatment choices made.

Further, an understanding of the different and dynamic theories of language acquisition allows the speech-language clinician to appreciate the evolution of the speech-language clinician's role in the therapeutic process itself. Specifically, many SLPs have moved from viewing themselves as language "trainers" to language "facilitators." This change can be credited directly to the belief that in most cases the child is an active participant in the language development process and the view that learning language involves the learning of a generative rule system.

Language intervention may be accomplished in many different settings. SLPs should acknowledge the benefits and drawbacks to each service delivery model in terms of client progress, keeping an eye out for EBP updates. In addition, the roles of the classroom teacher and the child's parents in the successful completion of the language intervention program should be considered. It is rarely the case that language intervention for a child can afford to be viewed as the responsibility of SLPs alone. The child in therapy also plays an important role in the forward progress of intervention thorough motivation displayed and ability to self-monitor, for example.

Finally, the concept of generalization is one of the most essential to the development of appropriate language intervention procedures. Because language is generalizable, we are able to assume that a small and carefully chosen subset of all of the possible examples of a goal form or structure will be sufficient to teach a more general rule. For language intervention programs to work, SLPs must pay close attention to how they expect the children to generalize their learning from the first intervention contact. Troubleshooting the expected course of generalization from the very first planning stages will allow SLPs a greater chance for succeeding in increasing the language competence of the young child with a language disorder.

Study Questions

1. How do parents, SLPs, and preschool classroom teachers serve indispensable functions in the success of language intervention programs developed for young children and their families?
2. Assume that SLPs have the luxury of determining which service delivery model will be used with each client in their caseloads. Delineate the pros and cons of choosing a pull-out, classroom-based, or collaborative consultation service delivery model.
3. If generalization is essential to the success of any language intervention program, SLPs should account for it as early as possible in their planning. List five general strategies for enhancing the generalization observed in a young child with a language disorder. Indicate the child's age, a particular goal for consideration, and the service delivery model through which the child receives language intervention.
4. You are planning a language intervention program for a young child from a culture other than your own. What information would you want to have before developing a plan that will assist you in designing an appropriate program? What information would you be able to collect during a diagnostic therapy phase that would help you to fine tune your treatment approach?
5. What is the nature of the information collected during the evaluation/assessment phase of service delivery to a young child with language needs that would help you to develop an appropriate beginning treatment plan for this child?

References

Agocs, M., Burns, M., DeLey, L., Miller, S., & Calhoun, B. (2006). Fast ForWord Language (pp. 471–508). In R. McCauley & M. Fey (Eds.), *Treatment of language disorders in children.* Baltimore: Paul H. Brookes.

Agnew, J., Dorn, C., & Eden, G. (2004). Effect of intensive training on auditory processing and reading skills. *Brain and Language, 88*(1), 21–25.

American Speech and Hearing Association. (1983). Social dialects: A position paper. *ASHA, 25*(1), 23–24.

American Speech and Hearing Association. (1985). Clinical management of communicatively handicapped minority language populations. *ASHA, 27*, 29–32.

American Speech-Language-Hearing Association. (2000a). *IDEA and your caseload: A template for eligibility and dismissal criteria for students ages 3 to 21.* Rockville, MD: ASHA Action Center.

American Speech-Language-Hearing Association. (2000b). *Prevalence of communication disorders in the United States*. Rockville, MD: ASHA Science and Research Department.

American Speech-Language-Hearing Association. (2003). *ASHA 2003 Omnibus Survey*. Rockville, MD: Author.

American Speech-Language-Hearing Association. (2006). *2006 Schools Survey report: Caseload characteristics*. Rockville, MD: Author.

Aram, D., Ekelman, B., & Nation, J. (1984). Preschoolers with language disorders: 10 years later. *Journal of Speech and Hearing Research, 27*, 232–244.

Bain, B., & Olswang, L. (1995). Examining readiness for learning two-word utterances by children with specific expressive language impairment: Dynamic assessment validation. *American Journal of Speech-Language Pathology, 4*(1), 81–91.

Battle, D. (1998). Communication disorders in a multicultural society. In D. Battle (Ed.), *Communication disorders in multicultural populations* (2nd ed., pp. 3–29). Boston: Butterworth-Heinemann.

Bedore, L., & Leonard, L. (1995). Prosodic and syntactic bootstrapping and their clinical applications: A tutorial. *American Journal of Speech-Language Pathology, 4*(1), 66–72.

Bricker, D. (1986). An analysis of early intervention programs: Attendant issues and future directions. In R. Morris and B. Blatt (Eds.), *Special education: Research and trends* (pp. 28–65). New York: Pergamon.

Bruner, J. (1985). Vygotsky: A historical and conceptual perspective. In J. Wertsch (Ed.), *Culture, communication, and cognition: Vygotskian perspectives*. Cambridge, UK: Cambridge University Press.

Brush, E. (1987, November). Public school language, speech and hearing services in the 1990s. Paper presented to the annual convention of the American Speech-Language-Hearing Association, New Orleans.

Camarata, S. (1995). A rationale for naturalistic speech intelligibility intervention. In M. Fey, J. Windsor, & S. Warren (Eds.), *Language intervention: Preschool through the elementary years* (pp. 63–84). Baltimore: Paul H. Brookes.

Camarata, S., & Nelson, K. (2006). Conversational recast intervention with preschool and older children (pp. 237–264). In R. McCauley & M. Fey (Eds.), *Treatment of language disorders in children*. Baltimore: Paul H. Brookes.

Camarata, S., Nelson, K., & Camarata, M. (1994). Comparison of conversational-recasting and imitative procedures for training grammatical structures in children with specific language impairment. *Journal of Speech and Hearing Research, 37*, 1414–1423.

Capone, N., & MacGregor, K. (2004). Gesture development: A review for clinical and research practices. *Journal of Speech, Language, and Hearing Research, 47*, 173–187.

Catts, H., & Kamhi, A. (Eds.). (1998). *Language and reading disabilities*. Boston: Allyn & Bacon.

Catts, H., Fey, M., Zhang, X., & Tomblin, J. (2002). A longitudinal investigation of reading outcomes in children with language impairments. *Journal of Speech, Language, and Hearing Research, 45*, 1142–1157.

Cleave, P., & Fey, M. (1997). Two approaches to the facilitation of grammar in children with language impairments: Rationale and description. *American Journal of Speech-Language Pathology, 6*(1), 22–32.

Cole, L. (1989). E pluribus pluribus: Multicultural imperatives and the 1990s and beyond. *ASHA, 31*, 65–70.

Cole, K., Maddox, M., & Kim, Y. (2006). Language is the key: Constructive interactions around books and play. In R. McCauley & M. Fey (Eds.), *Treatment of language disorders in children* (pp. 149—173), Baltimore: Paul H. Brookes.

Connell, P. (1982). On training language rules. *Language, Speech and Hearing Services in Schools, 13,* 231–248.

Craig, H. (1993). Clinical forum: Language and social skills in the school-age population, social skills of children with specific language impairment: Peer relationships. *Language, Speech, and Hearing Services in Schools, 24,* 206–215.

Craig, H., & Washington, J. (1993). Access behaviors of children with specific language impairment. *Journal of Speech and Hearing Research, 36,* 311–321.

Crain-Thoreson, C., & Dale, P. (1999). Enhancing linguistic performance: Parents and teachers as book reading partners for children with language delays. *Topics in Early Childhood Special Education, 19*(1), 28–40.

Crais, E. (1991). *A practical guide to embedding family-centered content into existing speech language pathology course work.* Chapel Hill, NC: Carolina Institute for Research in Infant Personnel Preparation.

Cross, T. (1978). Mothers' speech adjustments: The contribution of selected child listener variables. In C. Snow & C. Ferguson (Eds.), *Talking to children: Language input and acquisition.* Cambridge, UK: Cambridge University Press.

Dale, P., Crain-Thoreson, C., Notari-Syverson, A., & Cole, K. (1996). Parent-child story-book reading as an intervention technique for young children with language delays. *Topics in Early Childhood Special Education, 16,* 213–235.

Damico, J., & Damico, S. (1993). Language and social skills from a diversity perspective: Considerations for the speech-language pathologist. *Language, Speech, and Hearing Services in Schools, 24,* 236–243.

Dollaghan, C. (2007). *The handbook for evidence-based practice in communication disorders.* Baltimore: Paul H. Brookes.

Ehren, B. (2002). Maintaining a therapeutic focus and sharing responsibility for student success: Keys to in-classroom speech-language services. *Language, Speech, and Hearing Services in Schools, 31,* 219–229.

Ehren, B., & Nelson, N. (2005). The responsiveness to intervention approach and language impairment. *Topics in Language Disorders, 25*(2), 120–131.

Elbert, M., & Gierut, J. (1985). *Handbook of clinical phonology.* San Diego, CA: College-Hill.

Elbert, M., Powell, T., & Swartzlander, P. (1991). Toward a technology of generalization. How many exemplars are sufficient? *Journal of Speech and Hearing Research, 34*(1), 81–87.

Ellis Weismer, S. (1988). Specific language learning problems. In D. Yoder & R. Kent (Eds.), *Decision making in speech-language pathology.* Toronto: B. C. Decker.

Ellis Weismer, S., Murray-Branch, J., & Miller, J. (1994). A prospective longitudinal study of language development in late talkers. *Journal of Speech and Hearing Research, 37,* 852–867.

Ellis Weismer, S., & Robertson, S. (2006). Focused stimulation approach to language intervention. In R. McCauley & M. Fey (Eds.), *Treatment of language disorders in children* (pp. 175–201). Baltimore: Paul H. Brookes.

Ensher, G. (1989). The first three years: Special education perspectives on assessment and intervention. *Topics in Language Disorders, 10*(1), 80–90.

Farber, J., Denenberg, M., Klyman, S., & Lachman, P. (1992). Language resource room level of service: An urban school district approach to integrative treatment. *Language, Speech, & Hearing Services in Schools, 23,* 293–299.

Fey, M. (1986). *Language intervention with young children.* Boston: Allyn & Bacon.

Fey, M. (1988). Dismissal criteria for the language-impaired child. In D. Yoder & R. Kent (Eds.), *Decision making in speech-language pathology.* Toronto: B. C. Decker.

Fey, M., Catts, H., & Larrivee, L. (1995). Preparing preschoolers for the academic and social challenges of school. In M. Fey, J. Windsor, & S. Warren (Eds.), *Language intervention: Preschool through the elementary years* (pp. 3–34). Baltimore: Paul H. Brookes.

Fey, M., Cleave, P., Long, S., & Hughes, D. (1993). Two approaches to the facilitation of grammar in children with language impairment: An experimental evaluation. *Journal of Speech and Hearing Research, 36,* 141–157.

Fey, M., Cleave, P., Ravida, A., Long, S., Dejmal, A., & Easton, D. (1994). Effects of grammar facilitation on the phonological performance of children with speech and language impairments. *Journal of Speech and Hearing Research, 57,* 594–607.

Fey, M., Krulik, T., Loeb, D., & Proctor-Williams, K. (1999). Sentence recast use by parents of children with typical language and children with specific language impairment. *American Journal of Speech-Language Pathology, 8*(3), 273–286.

Fey, M., & Loeb, D. (2002). An evaluation of the facilitative effects of inverted yes-no questions on the acquisition of auxiliary verbs. *Journal of Speech, Language, and Hearing Research, 45,* 160–174.

Fujiki, M., & Brinton, B. (1984). Supplementing language therapy: Working with the classroom teacher. *Language, Speech and Hearing Services in Schools, 15,* 98–109.

Gillam, R. (1999). Computer-assisted language intervention using Fast ForWord: Theoretical and empirical considerations for clinical decision making. *Language, Speech, and Hearing Services in Schools, 30*(4), 363–370.

Gillam, R., Loeb, D., & Friel-Patti, S. (2001). Looking back: A summary of five exploratory studies of Fast ForWord. *American Journal of Speech-Language Pathology, 10,* 269–273.

Giralometto, L., & Weitzman, E. (2006). It takes two to talk—The Hanen Program for Parents: Early language intervention through caregiver training. In R. McCauley & M. Fey (Eds.), *Treatment of language disorders in children* (pp. 77–103). Baltimore: Paul H. Brookes.

Giralometto, L., Pearce, P., & Weitzman, E. (1996). Effects of lexical intervention on the phonology of late talkers. *Journal of Speech, Language, and Hearing Research, 40,* 338–348.

Girolametto, L. Tannock, R., & Siegel, L. (1993). Consumer-merited evaluation of interactive language intervention. *American Journal of Speech-Language Pathology, 2,* 41–51.

Goldberg, S. (1993). *Clinical intervention: A philosophy and methodology for clinical practice.* New York: Macmillan.

Goldstein, B. (2000). *Cultural and linguistic diversity resource guide for speech-language pathologists.* San Diego, CA: Singular/Thomson Learning.

Goldstein, H., English, K., Shafer, K., & Kaczmarek, L. (1997). Interaction among preschoolers without disabilities: Effects of across-the-day peer intervention. *Journal of Speech, Language, and Hearing Research, 40*(1), 33–48.

Guralnick, M., & Paul-Brown, D. (1977). The nature of verbal interactions among handicapped and non-handicapped preschool children. *Child Development, 48,* 254–260.

Hadley, P., & Schuele, M. (1998). Facilitating peer interaction: Socially relevant objectives for preschool language intervention. *American Journal of Speech-Language Pathology, 7*(4), 25–36.

Hall, P., & Tomblin, J. (1978). A follow-up study of children with articulation and language disorders. *Journal of Speech and Hearing Disorders, 43,* 227–241.

Hammer, C. (2004). Parental beliefs about literacy learning in non-majority households: Information relevant for the speech-language pathologist. *Perspectives on Language Learning and Education, 11*(3), 17–21.

Hanson, M. (2004). Ethnic, cultural, and language diversity in intervention settings. In E. Lynch & M. Hanson (Eds.), *Developing cross cultural competence: A guide for working with young children and their families* (3rd ed., pp. 3–18). Baltimore: Paul H. Brookes.

Hegde, M. (1993). *Treatment procedures in communicative disorders* (2nd ed.). San Diego, CA: College-Hill.

Hodson, B., & Paden, E. (1991). *Targeting intelligible speech: A phonological approach to remediation* (2nd ed.). Austin, TX: Pro-Ed.

Hughes, D. (1985). *Language treatment and generalization: A clinician's handbook.* San Diego, CA: College-Hill.

Jenkins, J., & Heinen, A. (1989). Students' preferences for service delivery: Pull-out, in-class, or integrated models. *Exceptional Children, 55*(6), 516–523.

Johnston, J. (1983). What is language intervention? The role of theory. In J. Miller, D. Yoder, & R. Schiefelbusch (Eds.), *Contemporary issues in language intervention* (ASHA Reports No. 12). Rockville, MD: American Speech-Language-Hearing Association.

Justice, L., & Ezell, H. (2004). Print referencing: An emergent literacy enhancement strategy and its clinical applications. *Language, Speech, and Hearing Services in Schools, 35,* 185–193.

Kelly, D. (1998). A clinical synthesis of the "late talker" literature: Implications for service delivery. *Language, Speech, and Hearing Services in Schools, 29*(2), 76–84.

King, R., Jones, C., & Lasky, E. (1982). In retrospect: A fifteen-year follow-up report of speech-language disorders in children. *Language, Speech and Hearing Services in Schools, 13,* 24–32.

Kaderavek, J., & Justice, L. (2004). Embedded-explicit emergent literacy intervention II: Goal selection and implementation in the early childhood classroom. *Language, Speech, and Hearing Services in Schools, 35,* 212–228.

Kirchner, D. (1991). Using verbal scaffolding to facilitate conversational participation and language acquisition in children with developmental disorders. *Journal of Childhood Communicative Disorders, 14,* 81–98.

Klein, M., & Briggs, M. (1987). Facilitating mother–infant communicative interaction in mothers of high-risk infants. *Journal of Childhood Communicative Disorders, 14,* 81–98.

Leonard, L. (1975). Modeling as a clinical procedure in language training. *Language, Speech, and Hearing Services in Schools, 6,* 72–85.

Leonard, L. (1981). Facilitating linguistic skills in children with specific language impairment: A review. *Applied Psycholinguistics, 2,* 89–118.

Leonard, L. (1991). New trends in the study of early language acquisition. *American Speech-Language-Hearing Association, 33*(4), 43–44.

Leonard, L. (1998). *Children with specific language impairment.* Cambridge, MA: MIT Press.

Loeb, D., Stoke, C., & Fey, M. (2001). Language changes associated with Fast ForWord-Language: Evidence from case studies. *American Journal of Speech-Language Pathology, 10,* 216–230.

Long, S., & Olswang, L. (1996). Readiness and patterns of growth in children with SELI. *American Journal of Speech-Language Pathology, 5*(1), 79–85.

Lynch, E. (2004). Developing cross-cultural competence. In E. Lynch & M. Hanson (Eds.), *Developing cross-cultural competence* (3rd ed., pp. 41–77). Baltimore: Paul H. Brookes.

MacDonald, J., & Carroll, J. (1992a). Communicating with young children: An ecological model for clinicians, parents and collaborative professionals. *American Journal of Speech-Language Pathology, 1*(4), 39–48.

MacDonald, J., & Carroll, J. (1992b). A social partnership model for assessing early communication development: An intervention model for preconversational children. *Language, Speech, & Hearing Services in Schools, 23,* 113–124.

MacDonald, J., & Gillette, Y. (1984). Conversation engineering: A pragmatic approach to early social competence. *Seminars in Speech and Language, 5,* 171–183.

Manolson, A. (1992). *It takes two to talk.* Toronto: The Hanen Centre.

Marvin, C. (1987). Consultation services: Changing roles for SLPs. *Journal of Childhood Communication Disorders, 11,* 1–15.

Maxwell, S., & Wallach, G. (1984). The language learning disabilities connection: Symptoms of early language disability change over time. In G. Wallach & K. Butler (Eds.), *Language learning disabilities in school-age children.* Baltimore: Williams & Wilkins.

McLean, J. (1983). Historical perspectives on the content of child language programs. In J. Miller, D. Yoder, & R. Schiefelbusch (Eds.), *Contemporary issues in language intervention* (ASHA Reports No. 12). Rockville, MD: American Speech-Language-Hearing Association.

Miller, L. (1989). Classroom-based language intervention. *Language, Speech and Hearing Services in Schools, 20,* 153–169.

Nelson, K., Camarata, S., Welsh, J., Butkovsky, L., & Camarata, M. (1996). Effects of imitative and conversational recasting treatment on the acquisition of grammar in children with specific language impairment and younger language-normal children. *Journal of Speech and Hearing Research, 39,* 850–859.

Nelson, N. (1998). Childhood language disorders in context: Infancy through adolescence (2nd ed.). Boston: Allyn & Bacon.

Newhoff, M. (1995). So many fads, so little data. *Clinical Connection, 8*(3), 1–5.

Olswang, L., & Bain, B. (1985). Monitoring phoneme acquisition for making treatment withdrawal decisions. *Applied Psycholinguistics, 6,* 17–37.

Olswang, L., & Bain, B. (1991). Clinical Forum: Treatment efficacy: When to recommend intervention. *Language, Speech, and Hearing Services in Schools, 22,* 255–263.

Olswang, L., & Bain, B. (1996). Assessment information for predicting upcoming changes in language production. *Journal of Speech and Hearing Research, 39*(2), 414–423.

Olswang, L., Rodriguez, B., & Timler, G. (1998). Recommending intervention for toddlers with specific language learning difficulties: We may not have all the answers, but we know a lot. *American Journal of Speech-Language Pathology, 7*(1), 23–32.

Paul, R. (2007). *Language disorders from infancy through adolescence: Assessment and intervention.* St. Louis, MO: Mosby-Year Book.

Pierce, R., & McWilliams, P. (1993). Emerging literacy and children with severe speech and physical impairments (SSPI): Issues and possible intervention strategies. *Topics in Language Disorders, 1*(2), 47–57.

Pletcher, L. (1995). *Family-centered practices: A training guide.* Raleigh, NC: ARCH National Resource Center.

Pokorni, J., Worthington, C., & Jamison, P. (2004). Phonological awareness intervention: Comparison of Fast ForWord, Earobics, and LIPS. *Journal of Educational Research, 97*(3), 147–157.

Prelock, P., Miller, B., & Reed, N. (1995). Collaborative partnerships in a language in the classroom program. *Language, Speech, and Hearing Services in Schools, 26,* 286–292.

Proctor-Williams, K., Fey, M., & Loeb, D. (2001). Parental recasts and production of copulas and articles by children with specific language impairment and typical development. *American Journal of Speech-Language Pathology, 10,* 155–168.

Ramey, C., & Ramey, S. (1998). Early intervention and early experience. *American Psychologist, 53,* 109–120.

Ratner, N., & Bruner, J. (1978). Games, social exchange and the acquisition of language. *Journal of Child Language, 5,* 392–401.

Records, N., Tomblin, J., & Freese, P. (1992). The quality of life among young adults with histories of Specific Language Impairment. *American Journal of Speech-Language Pathology, 1*(2), 44–53.

Records, N., & Weiss, A. (1990). Clinical judgment: An overview. *Journal of Childhood Communication Disorders, 13*(2), 153–165.

Rescorla, L. (1989). The Language Development Survey: A screening tool for delayed language in toddlers. *Journal of Speech and Hearing Disorders, 54,* 587–589.

Rescorla, L., & Schwartz, E. (1990). Outcome of toddlers with specific expressive language delay. *Applied Psycholinguistics, 11,* 393–407.

Rice, M. (1993). Social consequences of specific language impairment. In H. Grimm & H. Skowranek (Eds.), *Language acquisition problems and reading disorders: Aspects of diagnosis and intervention* (pp. 111–128). New York: de Gruyter.

Rice, M., Hadley, P., & Alexander, A. (1993). Social biases toward children with speech and language impairments: A correlative causal model of language limitation. *Applied Psycholinguistics, 14,* 445–471.

Rice, M., Sell, M., & Hadley, P. (1991). Social interactions of speech and language impaired children. *Journal of Speech and Hearing Research, 34,* 1299–1307.

Roberts, J., Prizant, B., & McWilliam, R. (1995). Out-of-class versus in-class service delivery in language intervention: Effects on communication interaction with young children. *American Journal of Speech-Language Pathology, 4*(2), 87–94.

Robertson, S., & Ellis Weismer, S. (1999). Effects of treatment on linguistic and social skills in toddlers with delayed language development. *Journal of Speech, Language and Hearing Research, 42,* 1234–1248.

Roseberry-McKibben, C. (1994). Assessment and intervention for children with limited English proficiency and language disorders. *American Journal of Speech-Language Pathology, 3*(3), 77–88.

Roseberry-McKibben, C., & Eicholtz, G. (1994). Serving children with limited English proficiency in the schools: A national survey. *Language, Speech, & Hearing Services in Schools, 25,* 156–164.

Rovee-Collier, C., Lipsitt, L., & Hayne, H. (Eds.). (1998). *Advances in infancy research 12.* Stamford, CT: Ablex.

Scarborough, H., & Dorbrich, W. (1990). Development of children with early language delay. *Journal of Speech and Hearing Research, 33,* 70–83.

Schuele, M., Rice, M., & Wilcox, K. (1995). Redirects: A strategy to increase peer initiations. *Journal of Speech and Hearing Research, 38*(6), 1319–1333.

Screen, R., & Anderson, N. (1994). *Multicultural perspectives in communication disorders.* San Diego, CA: Singular.

Shriberg, L., & Kwiatkowski, J. (1982). Phonological disorders II: A conceptual framework for management. *Journal of Speech and Hearing Disorders, 47,* 242–256.

Snow, C. (1986). Conversations with children. In P. Fletcher & M. Garman (Eds.), *Language acquisition* (2nd ed.). New York: Cambridge University Press.

Snow, C., & Goldfield, B. (1983). Turn the page please: Situation-specific language acquisition. *Journal of Child Language, 10,* 551–569.

Snyder, L. (1980). Have we prepared the language disordered child for school? *Topics in Language Disorders, 1*(1), 29–45.

Snyder, L., Apolloni, T., & Cooke, T. (1977). Integrated settings at the early childhood level: The role of non-retarded peers. *Exceptional Children, 43,* 262–266.

Sparks, S. (1989). Assessment and intervention with at risk infants and toddlers: Guidelines for the speech-language pathologist. *Topics in Language Disorders, 10*(1), 43–56.

Stainback, S., Stainback, W., & Forest, M. (Eds.). (1989). *Educating all students in the mainstream of regular education.* Baltimore: Paul H. Brookes.

Stainback, W., & Stainback, S. (1990). *Support networks for inclusive schooling: Independent integrated education.* Baltimore: Paul H. Brookes.

Stothard, S., Snowling, M., Bishop, D., Chipchase, B., & Kaplan, C. (1998). Language impaired preschoolers: A follow-up into adolescence. *Journal of Speech, Language, and Hearing Research, 41*(2), 407–418.

Tallal, P. (2004). Improving language and literacy is a matter of time. *Nature Reviews Neuriscience, 5,* 721–728.

Terrell, B., & Hale, J. (1992). Serving a multicultural population: Different learning styles. *American Journal of Speech-Language Pathology, 1*(2), 5–8.

Thal, D. (1999, November). Early identification of risk for language impairment: Challenges for the profession. A seminar presented at the annual convention of the American Speech-Language-Hearing Association, San Francisco.

Tomblin, J. B., Records, N., Buckwalter, P., Zhang, X., Smith, E., & O'Brien, M. (1997). Prevalence of specific language impairment in kindergarten children. *Journal of Speech, Language, and Hearing Research, 40,* 1245–1260.

Tyler, A., & Sandoval, K. (1994). Preschoolers with phonological and language disorders: Treating different linguistic domains. *Language, Speech, and Hearing Services in Schools, 25,* 215–234.

Tyler, A., Lewis, K., Haskill, A., & Tolbert, L. (2002). Efficacy and cross-domain effects of a morphosyntax and a phonology intervention. *Language, Speech, and Hearing Services in Schools, 33,* 52–66.

Tyler, A., Lewis, K., Haskill, A., & Tolbert, L. (2003). Outcomes of different speech and language goal attack strategies. *Journal of Speech, Language, and Hearing Research, 46,* 1007–1094.

van Kleeck, A. (1994). Potential cultural bias in training parents as conversational partners with their children who have delays in language development. *American Journal of Speech-Language Pathology, 3,* 67–78.

van Kleeck, A., Gillam, R., Hamilton, L., & McGrath, C. (1997). The relationship between middle class parents' book-sharing discussion and their preschoolers' abstract language development. *Journal of Speech, Language, and Hearing Research, 40*(6), 1261–1271.

van Kleeck, A., & Richardson, A. (1988). Language delay in the child. In N. Lass, L. McReynolds, J. Northern, & D. Yoder (Eds.), *Handbook of speech-language pathology and audiology*. Toronto: B. C. Decker.

Veale, T. (1999). Targeting temporal processing deficits through Fast ForWord: Language therapy with a new twist. *Language, Speech, and Hearing Services in Schools, 30*(4), 353–362.

Venn, M., Wolery, M., Fleming, L., DeCesare, L., Morris, A., & Cuffs, M. (1993). Effects of teaching preschool peers to use the mand-model procedure during snack activities. *American Journal of Speech-Language Pathology, 2*(1), 38–46.

Wallach, G., & Butler, K. (1994). Creating communication, literacy, and academic success. In G. Wallach & K. Butler (Eds.), *Language learning disabilities in school age children and adolescents: Some principles and application* (pp. 2–26). New York: Macmillan.

Warren, S., & Kaiser, A. (1988). Research in early language intervention. In S. Odom & M. Karnes (Eds.), *Early intervention for infants and children with handicaps*. Baltimore: Paul H. Brookes.

Watkins, R. (1994). Specific language impairments in children: An introduction. In R. Watkins & M. Rice (Eds.), *Specific language impairments in children* (pp. 1–15). Baltimore: Paul H. Brookes.

Weiss, A. (2001). *Preschool language disorders resource guide: Specific language impairment.* San Diego, CA: Singular/Thomson Learning.

Weiss, A., & Nakamura, M. (1992). Language-normal children in preschool classrooms for children with language impairments. *Language, Speech and Hearing Services in Schools, 23,* 64–70.

Weiss, A., Tomblin, J., & Robin, D. (2000). Language disorders. In J. Tomblin, H. Morris, & D. Spriesterbach (Eds.), *Diagnosis in speech-language pathology* (2nd ed., pp. 129–173). San Diego, CA: Singular.

Weiss, R. (1981). INREAL intervention for language handicapped and bilingual children. *Journal of the Division of Early Childhood, 4,* 40–51.

Wetherby, A., Warren, S., & Reichle, J. (Vol. Eds.). (1998). In S. Warren & J. Reichle (Series Eds.), *Communication and language intervention series: Vol. 7. Transitions in prelinguistic communication.* Baltimore: Paul H. Brookes.

Wilcox, M., Kouri, T., & Caswell, S. (1991). Early language intervention: A comparison of classroom and individual treatment. *American Journal of Speech-Language Pathology, 1*(1), 49–62.

Wolery, M., & Wilbers, J. (Eds.). (1994). Including children with special needs in early childhood programs. *Research Monograph of the National Association for the Education of Young Children, 6,* Washington, DC: NAEYC.

Wyatt, T. (1997). Assessment issues with multicultural populations. In D. Battle (Ed.), *Communication disorders in multicultural populations* (2nd ed., pp. 379–425). Boston: Butterworth-Heinemann.

Yoder, D., & Kent, R. (1988). *Decision making in speech-language pathology.* Philadelphia: B. C. Decker.

Yoder, P., Spruytenburg, H., Edwards, A., & Davies, B. (1995). Effect of verbal routine contexts and expansions on gains in the mean length of utterance in children with developmental delays. *Language, Speech, and Hearing Services in Schools, 26,* 21–32.

CHAPTER 11

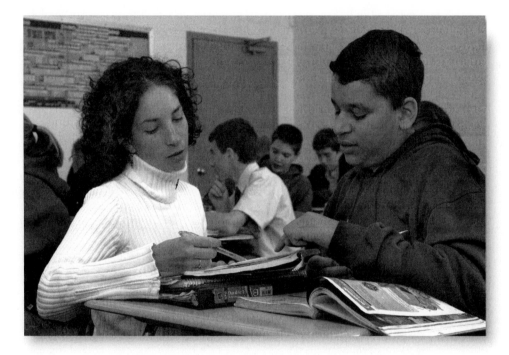

Making Sense of Language Learning Disability

Assessment and Support for Academic Success

Sylvia F. Diehl
University of South Florida
Elaine R. Silliman
University of South Florida

When you finish this chapter, you will be able to

- Understand the effect of federal legislation on assessment and intervention practices and the impact of providing tiered support models.
- Comprehend the synergistic relationship needed between professionals to provide a tiered continuum of support in basic literacy and content area instruction.
- Evaluate system patterns for individual children and interpret their possible meanings as these patterns of performance relate to classrooms.

- Determine the focus of assessment and intervention based on current scientific evidence about relationships between aspects of spoken language knowledge and learning to read, write, and spell.
- Establish appropriate programming to support literacy that is responsive to the adolescent learner.
- Utilize a consistent process to evaluate treatment outcomes on an ongoing basis.

The No Child Left Behind (NCLB) Act, passed in 2001, is a federal law requiring standards-based accountability at the school level for educational outcomes. A major impetus for NCLB was to increase the quality of reading education for students from cultural and linguistic minority groups so that referrals for specific learning disabilities would decrease. In 2004 African American and Hispanic students represented 17.3 and 19.2 percent, respectively, of the total school-age population. However, in terms of special education services, both groups, as well as students of Asian/Pacific Islander and American Indian/Alaskan Native heritages, were significantly overrepresented in the specific learning disabilities category (U.S. Department of Education, 2003). In the 2005–2006 school year, 40.7 percent of students receiving special education services were classified with specific learning disabilities (NCES, 2007). Usually, this classification means that a student is struggling with learning to read.

The 2004 reauthorization by the United States Congress of the Individuals with Disabilities Education Act (IDEA) significantly changed the role of school-based speech-language pathologists. Consistent with NCLB goals, new provisions required that beginning reading instruction for all children should be based on scientific evidence gathered during the 1990s. Furthermore, how a student responded over time to scientifically-based instruction provided by qualified teachers was a preferred approach to decision making about the need for a special education referral. Although speech-language pathologists (SLPs) have always used scientific evidence to inform their oral language assessments and interventions, they have not been typically involved in interventions that connect components of oral language to literacy learning. This chapter's purpose is to illuminate what SLPs must know to successfully assume new roles in language and literacy learning. At the broadest level, SLPs must understand that successful literacy learning is interconnected with spoken language abilities. For example, the SLP must be prepared to (1) recognize that the oral language basis of learning is essential for children's academic success, (2) view both language and literacy learning as central components of assessment, (3) use the general education curriculum as a guide for the development of more authentic assessment approaches, and (4) develop skill as a collaborative partner in the educational process.

In order to provide prospective SLPs with a framework for curriculum-related assessment within a response to intervention approach, this chapter is divided in two sections, with each segment highlighting a case example of a child with language learning disabilities. The first case is a kindergarten-age student struggling to read. Featured in the second section is a middle school student who is having significant problems with reading comprehension and writing. For both cases, readers will learn how to use evidence-based practices to build an integrated approach to language and literacy intervention that is interconnected with the academic language expectations of the classroom.

Response to Intervention: Prevention of Initial Reading Problems

Response to intervention (RtI) is a method of service delivery that encompasses both general and special education. The 2004 reauthorization of IDEA allowed school districts with significant overidentification of specific learning disabilities in minority students to implement a prereferral process, termed RtI (Foorman & Nixon, 2006), and allocated up to 15 percent of IDEA funds for the prevention of reading problems by improving reading instruction in the general education classroom (Foorman, 2007). RtI shifts the focus from assessment and identification to intervention for prevention with children who are not as responsive as their peers to early literacy instruction. In other words, RtI alters the concept of evaluation from "Test and treat [to] treat and test" (Fletcher, Lyon, Fuchs, & Barnes, 2007, p. 64). For the SLP, this is a strong shift of priorities from a "wait to fail" perspective to a "supporting success" orientation in services provided to children who may be at risk for reading failure. RtI also allows SLPs to become "central players" (Ehren, 2007, p. 10) in literacy programs in two ways: making their knowledge about the language foundations of literacy more visible to the school community and actively participating in the design of RtI programs.

There are two kinds of RtI models (Fuchs, Mock, Morgan, & Young, 2003): the problem-solving model, which is based on a multidisciplinary approach to tailoring more individualized instruction, and the standard-protocol approach in which the same treatment approach is used for all children. Both models have strengths and limitations (Fuchs et al., 2003); however, both emphasize decision making in the context of how students actually respond to instruction. In the following section focusing on the lower elementary level, we show how the SLP can become a major member of an RtI literacy team charged with assisting a 6-year-old child struggling with beginning reading and spelling. The question is whether this child's strenuous efforts to break the alphabetic code is constrained by an underlying language learning disability, a combination of experiential factors, or both.

RtI Tiers: The Roles of the Speech-Language Pathologist

The RtI model is similar in some ways to the concept of dynamic assessment. In both RtI and dynamic assessment, the goal is to determine how a child benefits from supported intervention in a specific area. However, there are differences in how both approaches are implemented (Ehren & Nelson, 2005).

In RtI, teaching takes place first. If, after a period of time, the child does not evidence an expected rate of learning, then specific measures are administered to determine a baseline—for example, the child's rate and accuracy of oral reading. Then modified instruction, which is always curriculum related, is directed to help the child to progress, followed by periodic assessment of increases in the rate and accuracy of oral reading.

In contrast, with dynamic assessment, the child's baseline is determined first, such as assessing facility with narrative structure. Next, the child is engaged in challenging activities related to narrative structure with varying degrees of SLP support (the teaching phase). The objective is to assess how quickly the child can learn and apply newly taught information in an increasingly independent way. Intervention may or may not be curriculum related.

Another dimension along which RtI and dynamic assessment differ is that most RtI designs feature a continuum of tiered services, whose scope and intensity depend on the tier level. All of the tiers include activities that address both assessment and intervention. In implementing an RtI approach, an essential step is districtwide agreement on its purpose, which may be to identify those children who

- are candidates for early reading intervention
- have a language or learning disability
- qualify for both early reading intervention and identification of a disability (Fuchs & Deshler, 2007)

Consensus on purpose is essential for decision making on the number of prevention tiers. As shown in Figure 11.1, a three-tier prevention system is considered most efficient when the plan is to separate general and special education in only a minimal way (Fuchs & Fuchs, 2007). Regardless of the number of tiers, RtI must be accompanied by (a) the frequent monitoring of progress, preferably connected to a curriculum-based measure; (b) evaluation of implementation consistency in the delivery of instruction (or intervention); and (c) specific criteria for identifying when children are not responding to instruction in expected ways (Fletcher et al., 2007).

An additional point is that, for any tier, practices should be selected that have a strong scientific evidence base. SLPs should become familiar with meta-analyses of intervention studies (for guidance, see Johnson, 2006). A meta-analysis is the highest standard of evidence for evaluating treatment outcomes. It involves the independent synthesis of peer-reviewed articles in a particular practice area according to specific criteria. The purpose is to estimate whether the results from multiple intervention

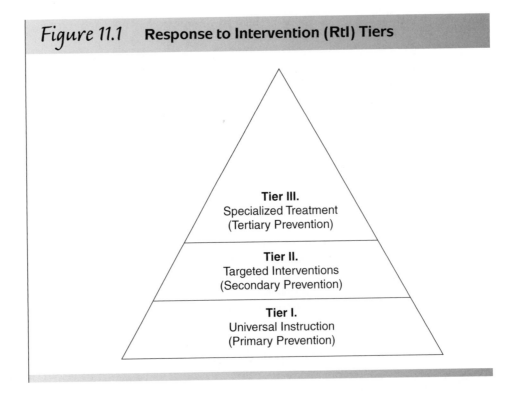

Figure 11.1   **Response to Intervention (RtI) Tiers**

Tier III.
Specialized Treatment
(Tertiary Prevention)

Tier II.
Targeted Interventions
(Secondary Prevention)

Tier I.
Universal Instruction
(Primary Prevention)

studies with different research designs have sufficient impact to warrant a claim for a causal relationship between the intervention and its outcomes. To date, no meta-analysis has been conducted for language intervention with school-age children and adolescents because of the emphasis on preschool language intervention (Silliman & Scott, in press). In contrast, there have been several meta-analyses of instructional practices in reading and writing. These include (a) dialogic book reading, which will be discussed shortly (van Kleeck & Littlewood, in press), (b) reading interventions in kindergarten to grade 3 (Scammacca, Roberts, Vaughn, Wanzek, & Torgesen, 2007), (c) strategy instruction in general reading comprehension (Scammacca, Roberts, Vaughn, Edwards, Wexler, Rentebuch, & Torgesen, 2007) as well as expository text comprehension (Gajria, Jitendra, Sood, & Sacks, 2007), and (d) writing instruction for adolescents (Graham & Perin, 2007a, 2007b).

TIER 1: PRIMARY PREVENTION

Tier 1 is aimed at primary prevention in the general education classroom. Students targeted for "preventative intervention" (Fuchs & Fuchs, 2007, p. 15) must first provide evidence of an insufficient response to the common core beginning reading program.

A basic assumption with Tier 1 is that students are receiving a "scientifically validated" (Fuchs & Deshler, 2007, p. 131) reading curriculum; however, to date, only a few reading programs have been independently evaluated.

For example, the What Works Clearinghouse of the Institute of Education Sciences (http://ies.ed.gov/ncee/wwc/reports), a federal agency charged with independent evaluation of research on literacy programs, recently released assessments on the effectiveness of seventeen beginning reading programs for kindergarten to grade 3 in four areas: alphabetic code knowledge, fluency, comprehension, and general reading achievement. Both alphabetic knowledge and fluency are part of code-related instruction. Only one of the seventeen programs met evidence standards for two of the four areas, whereas six other studies met evidence standards with reservations in at least one of the areas. As a consequence, another critical decision for primary prevention is the selection of a beginning reading curriculum that has had independent evaluation. Selection must be weighed with the knowledge that the chosen instructional program may have stronger effects on one area than another.

The Role of the SLP in Tier 1

There is no clear agreement within the profession on the nature and amount of Tier 1 participation. Some (e.g., Ukrainetz, 2006) argue that Tier 1 participation of SLPs is not practical without a significant reduction in their caseloads; without decreases, SLPs will just be asked to do more and likely will not do it well.

Others strongly recommend Tier 1 participation (Ehren & Nelson, 2005; Justice, 2006; Troia, 2005) to enhance the quality of learning in the classroom and to reduce the incidence of reading failure. For example, the SLP can collaborate with the classroom teacher and prereferral teams to make the best use of a literacy-rich reading environment. The focus of collaboration could consist of an organized examination of the space and time dedicated to literacy activities (at least 90 minutes daily) and the scheduling of various literacy activities. Scheduling might include flexible groupings for modified instruction and ongoing or intermittent measurement of students' progress. SLPs can also support younger students in their emerging literacy skills by providing assistance in the oral foundations of beginning literacy (Ehren & Nelson, 2005). See the Case Study on p. 524 for a description of how one SLP collaborated with a kindergarten teacher in Tier 1 activities.[1]

TIER 2: SECONDARY PREVENTION

Tier 2 is secondary prevention. It involves more intensive supplementary instruction and progress monitoring for children who do not respond as expected to the common core content of Tier 1 instruction. In other words, these children are making inadequate progress in their initial reading development, particularly in the area of phonological awareness. When children do not make adequate progress in Tier 1 after an appropriate period of time, the question is whether or not Tier 2 intervention is routine classroom instruction. If it is not a part of everyday classroom instruction, then parental consent under the provisions of IDEA may be necessary to undertake either Tier 2 or Tier 3 intervention and an Individualized Education Plan (IEP) might need to be developed (Zirkel, 2007). However, because of the wide range of variability in the levels of children's phonological awareness at this age, secondary intervention is still preferable to a formal assessment for determining special education eligibility (Foorman, Breier, & Fletcher, 2003).

---

[1]The SLPs, teachers, and case examples featured in this chapter are all based on real individuals. However, for confidentiality purposes, their names have been changed.

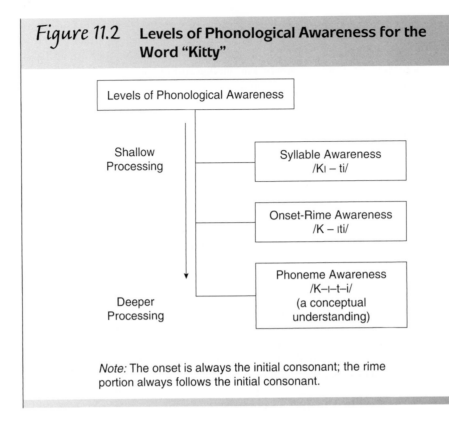

Figure 11.2 **Levels of Phonological Awareness for the Word "Kitty"**

Levels of Phonological Awareness

Shallow Processing

Syllable Awareness
/KI – ti/

Onset-Rime Awareness
/K – Iti/

Phoneme Awareness
/K–I–t–i/
(a conceptual understanding)

Deeper Processing

Note: The onset is always the initial consonant; the rime portion always follows the initial consonant.

Levels of Phonological Awareness

Figure 11.2 displays the levels of phonological awareness and the type of processing required by tasks within a particular level. A task requiring *syllabic segmentation* would have the child tap or clap out how many "parts" he or she hears as /ki-ti/ is said. A *rime* task might use pictures and provide the child with two foils plus the target match (e.g., *bucket, pretty, happy*), asking the child to select the picture that "rhymes" with *kitty*. It is evident from Figure 11.2 that a child's sensitivity to the phoneme as a *representation* of sound segments within the word requires conceptual understanding at a deeper level of processing. An example of a *phoneme segmentation* task would be "How many small parts do you hear in /k-i-t-i/?" It is important not to use these levels interchangeably. If the SLP or teacher refers to segmentation, it should be clear if the meaning is at the syllable, onset-rime, or phonemic level (for an excellent glossary, see Scarborough & Brady, 2002).

The Nonresponder

The child who is nonresponsive to code-related instruction, sometimes called the "treatment resister" (Torgesen, 2000), creates a troublesome situation. There are several reasons why children may not respond as expected in Tier 1. According to Al Otaiba and Fuchs (2002, 2006) different intervention studies define *nonresponsive* in dissimilar ways, not all studies have used the same outcome measures for monitoring progress, few longitudinal studies have been conducted to track progress over time, and even fewer studies involving teachers have documented the consistency with which teachers implemented the "scientifically validated" reading program. As a result, the finding that 8 to 80 percent of children across studies show minimal progress (Al Otaiba & Fuchs, 2002, 2006) may be an artifact of variations in research designs.

Two other factors may contribute to certain children being evaluated as nonresponsive to phonological awareness instruction. Most of the intervention studies on early reading development have been conducted by researchers in special education, psychology, or literacy education. Rarely do these researchers administer oral language measures to rule in or rule out a language learning disability. A second issue is children's motivation to read and sense of confidence in knowing what to do when they encounter difficulty. Although these are hard concepts to measure, some researchers conduct interviews of children asking questions like "About how long did it take you to read this book? Was this book so good that you couldn't stop reading it? What did you do when you came to (hard) parts?" (Guthrie, Hoa, Wigfield, Tanks, Humenick, & Littles, 2007, p. 310). In addition, motivation to read is often triggered and sustained by children's interest in what they are reading (Nolen, 2007). In general, little is known about the situational factors influencing engagement in reading and writing activities in children with a language learning disability.

The SLP's Role in Tier 2

As with Tier 1, there is no clear agreement in the speech-language pathology profession about the SLP's role in Tier 2. Ukrainetz (2006) makes the strong case that the less responsive child will not benefit from more intensive code instruction. Instead, the less responsive child also needs explicit support in oral language learning. Moreover, code instruction and expanding on aspects of oral language cannot be taught at the same time. The recommendation from Ukrainetz is that two tracks should be available in Tier 2: a code track and a language track. The language track would be taught by the SLP and focus on significant oral language experiences. Ehren and Nelson (2005) take a similar position to Ukrainetz (2006). Prevention is still the goal for Tier 2, but the center of attention now needs to be on the oral language foundations of the curriculum.

In contrast, Justice (2006) views Tier 2 services as providing more intensive code instruction in small groups or even one on one. The SLP should participate in these groupings since some of these less responsive children might have an underlying language learning disability. These differences in professional opinion can only be resolved through intervention research in which the three sets of recommendations are systematically studied.

See the Case Study on page 525 for the case of a Tier 2 collaborative plan for Damon, a 6-year-old in kindergarten, who was not responding to code-related instruction as expected. The plan reflects a combination of the language-focused position (Ehren & Nelson, 2005; Ukrainetz, 2006) and the code-related perspective (Justice, 2006), as well as an integration of language learning targets with the curriculum.

Engaging Parents in Dialogic Book Sharing.   As outlined in Table 11.1, dialogic book reading is often used for parental involvement in Tier 2 plans. There is strong

Table 11.1   **Book Sharing Ideas for Parents and Teachers**

Phase	Goal	Activities
Before reading	Choose the right book	• Match the length of the book to children's attention abilities. • Check for visual attractiveness. • Match the complexity of the language to the child's ability to understand; ask for guidance from librarians, SLPs, or teachers, if uncertain. • Choose books that reflect children's interests or experience.
	Make it routine	• Make shared book reading (or read-alouds) part of a routine. It helps children pay more attention to the specific content of the book as well as to its vocabulary and syntax. (They have already learned the basic structure of the reading activity [i.e., how to establish joint attention, turn the pages, hold the book, and respond to questions].)
	Focus on prediction	• Help children make predictions from the pictures about the story or what may happen next.
During reading	Make it motivating	• Relate book content to children's interests and experiences. • Be positive and reinforcing.
	Teach vocabulary	• Select three new word meanings and define them in a child-friendly (contextualized) way as the words come up. • Focus on basic comprehension along with connecting the word with children's previous experiences.
	Use a variety of prompting during reading	• Include recall prompts related to specific vocabulary, use open-ended prompts, and ask *what, why, where,* and *how* questions about the text that require more inferencing. • Ask questions that relate to children's previous experience.
	Gradually increase participation	• Let individual children do more talking and take more responsibility for comprehending the book as their experience and knowledge grows.
	Adjust the balance of conversation	• Adults should do more talking when concepts or words are new. • Children should do more talking when they have already mastered the concepts or are familiar with the book.

Phase	Goal	Activities
After reading	Confirm predictions	• Talk about what children predicted earlier and confirm or alter the prediction.
	Encourage retellings and use of new meanings	• Help children use the book to tell you or others the story using the new vocabulary words. • Follow up with the new vocabulary words so that children will apply them to other situations outside of book sharing.
	Talk about future plans	• Talk about what books you would like to read next time.

Based on Beck, McKeown, & Kucan, 2002; van Kleeck, 2006a,b; van Kleeck & Vander Woude, 2003; Zevenbergen & Whitehurst, 2003.

evidence that, for young children from middle class homes, dialogic book reading increases the foundations of print as expressing meaning, promotes vocabulary growth, and advances the use of language to share ideas by supporting children to assume the role of a conversational partner (Bus, van Ijzendoorn, & Pellegrini, 1995; Huebner, 2000; van Kleeck & Littlewood, in press). Ms. Connor from the case study was aware of three findings from the research on dialogic book reading (van Kleeck, 2006a, 2006b): first, cultures different from the middle class culture do not necessarily emphasize oral book reading with their young children; second, how parents read or do not read with their children may reflect their basic parenting style; and, third, for storybook reading to be successful, it must be more than reading aloud. A critical piece is that *discussion* must take place around the text and pictures being read in order to support children like Damon in their inferencing (van Kleeck, 2006b). Hence, Ms. Connor discussed with Damon's parents their views on dialogic book sharing, carefully listening for any concerns they expressed about this practice and then discussing how this practice represented the kind of "school" talk that Damon needed to become more familiar with (Wilkinson & Silliman, in press). Following van Kleeck's (2006b) recommendations, the SLP guided the parents on how to choose books to share, how to make it a routine, how to increase vocabulary during book sharing, and how to increase Damon's verbal participation gradually by using *what, where, why,* and *how* questions and not *yes/no* questions.

Engaging Damon in Tier 2 Activities. In addition to shared book reading, three 30-minute small-group sessions with two other kindergartners with similar literacy learning challenges were added to Damon's weekly schedule. The SLP led one of these small-group sessions while the teacher and paraprofessional were responsible for the other two. Damon's small-group sessions were a modification of the phonological awareness program developed and validated on a preliminary basis by Gillon (2000) for children with spoken language impairment. This plan included all of the research-based components specified for children of kindergarten age (Vellutino, Scanlon, Small, & Fanuele, 2006; Vellutino, Tunmer, Jaccard, & Chen, 2007). Each session addressed emergent literacy skills and included reading by and to the children, including talk about the text content, promoting phonemic awareness, developing letter name and letter–sound knowledge, and writing. Special attention was paid to phonemic awareness, which required precise awareness of the individual phonemes in a word, because children like Damon who are at risk for reading failure require explicit instruction (Foorman & Torgesen, 2001).

When teaching phonemic awareness, four evidence-based practices should be incorporated into meaningful reading activities: (1) use engaging and motivating activities, (2) focus on one or two phoneme manipulation skills, such as blending and segmenting phonemes, (3) include letters for phoneme manipulation across materials and activities, and (4) provide intensive instruction over time, but sequence activities so that they are not more than 30 to 50 minutes long for any single session (National Reading Panel, 2000; Torgesen et al., 2001). In addition, continuant sounds, rather than stops, should be selected initially since continuants are more acoustically prominent (Troia, 2004). All of these points can be incorporated into a Tier 2, 12-week plan (a total of 30 hours). The duration of 12 weeks is based on other emerging literacy intervention programs (e.g., Gillon, 2000; Justice, 2006) in which children with speech or language problems were at risk for reading problems. Dedicated time was allocated to each session as follows:

- dialogic book reading (10 minutes) to focus on print as meaning
- promoting phonemic awareness (10 minutes) by using letter sound names (e.g., continuants such as /f/, /s/, and /z/) to generate letter–sound correspondences
- spelling and dictated writing to the teacher, SLP, or paraprofessional (10 minutes) to apply what had been learned

The classroom teacher and the paraprofessional assisted the child in continually applying new learning throughout the day by using reading and writing experiences that integrated the small-group content.

How Long Will It Take?

How long it "takes" for individual children, like Damon, to learn the necessary code-related skills so that they can then connect graphemes (letters) to phonemes fluently and develop speed and accuracy in their word recognition will vary depending on several factors. These include: (1) teacher/clinician qualifications, (2) the goals of instruction, (3) how many skills are being taught, and (4) the nature of difficulties that the child is encountering, which may require further modifications to the components of instruction (National Reading Panel, 2000; Torgesen, 2000).

Damon After 12 Weeks of Tier 2 Instruction and Parent Involvement

After 12 weeks, everyone on the team agreed that Damon was steadily improving in letter naming and ability to connect letter names with sounds, but he still was struggling with segmentation and blending activities and in applying what he was learning to simple word recognition without high levels of teacher or clinician support. This conclusion was reached according to an empirically based "dual discrepancy" criteria (Fuchs, Fuchs, McMaster, Yen, & Svenson, 2004), which combines the child's *performance level* with his or her *growth rate*. Performance level is defined as the number of correct words per minute that are read *at the end of the treatment period* (determined as the mean of the last two scores). The cut-off point between "no risk" and reading failure risk (i.e., nonresponsive to code instruction) is the oral reading of fifteen words per minute or less. The growth rate or slope of progress measures how many more correct words per minute are read *each week of treatment*. For example, a given slope of progress might mean a growth rate of one more word read correctly each week. Nonresponsiveness could then be defined as a minimum of 1 standard deviation (SD) below class peers in both performance level and rate of growth (Fuchs & Deshler, 2007). Figure 11.3 displays Damon's progress on these two dimensions. As this curriculum-based approach to progress monitoring shows, Damon made minimal progress after 12 weeks in his small group sessions, as well as in day-to-day school work.

Significant improvements were observed in his participation in dialogic book sharing. For example, the need to prompt Damon to participate decreased as he entered the book conversation more often on his own. He even began to respond appropriately to some *when* and *where* questions that required minimal inferencing. Damon's parents also reported a similar pattern. In addition, they noted that, occasionally, he would attempt to read more familiar words in the story. However, Ms. Connor, the SLP, related that Damon was still having difficulty with pronouns, tended to become confused with complex instructions, and did not appear to produce

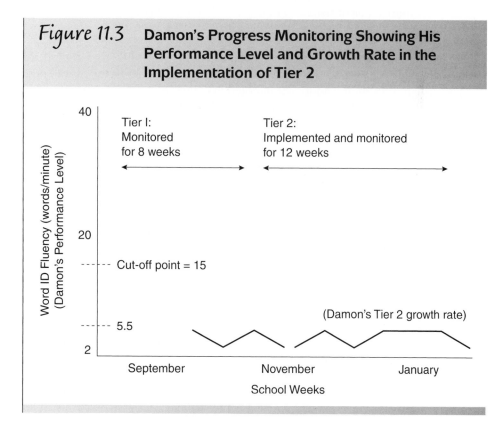

Figure 11.3 **Damon's Progress Monitoring Showing His Performance Level and Growth Rate in the Implementation of Tier 2**

Tier I:
Monitored
for 8 weeks

Tier 2:
Implemented and monitored
for 12 weeks

Cut-off point = 15

(Damon's Tier 2 growth rate)

5.5

Word ID Fluency (words/minute)
(Damon's Performance Level)

40

20

2

September   November   January

School Weeks

the semantic/syntactic complexity in his language production expected of a 6-year-old. It seemed appropriate to consider Tier 3 intervention for Damon.

TIER 3: TERTIARY PREVENTION

Tier 3 can function as a special education service. In accord with IDEA, a multidisciplinary team must be involved in further decision making once Tier 3 needs are determined. Also, key distinctions between Tiers 2 and 3 are a lower student–teacher ratio, more intensive instructional time, and flexibility in moving the student into and out of the general education classroom into Tiers 1 or 2 as "needs change in relation to the demands of the general education curriculum" (Fuchs & Fuchs, 2007, p. 20). Weekly progress monitoring remains essential in order to have an objective base of information on the rate and quality of progress.

At this point in time, evaluation may consist of a comprehensive assessment with a battery of standardized measures or an assessment of more limited scope that addresses instructional questions about a child's participation in Tiers 1 and 2 (Fuchs & Fuchs, 2007). For example, evaluation might be directed to differentiating whether a child's tier profile is more consistent with a learning (reading) disability or a language learning disability that may or may not include a reading disability. It is recommended that the multidisciplinary evaluation not be a comprehensive one, however. Instead, "a specifically tailored, instructionally focused multidisciplinary evaluation is more efficient than a full-blown evaluation" (Fuchs & Fuchs, 2007, p. 18).

The SLP's Role in Tier 3

Within the profession, there is agreement that the SLP has a central role in Tier 3. While perspectives vary on the specific focuses of Tier 3, the overall point of view is that SLPs should adopt the instructional aims advocated by Fuchs and Fuchs (2007) for Tier 3, which can be accomplished by diagnostic teaching explicitly designed to match interventions to specific learner needs.

One view on diagnostic teaching is that Tier 3 allows curriculum-relevant language intervention to be provided in collaboration with other team members before the final determination that the child is eligible for classification as language impaired (Ehren & Nelson, 2005). Another view (Ukrainetz, 2006) is that the SLP should no longer attend to code-related goals. Rather, the SLP should concentrate on providing children with repeated opportunities in a concentrated format to acquire the necessary academic language experiences consistent with the literate learning objectives of schooling. On the other hand, there is little consensus on the nature of the specialized diagnostic interventions that should characterize Tier 3 when "virtually all else has failed" (Troia, 2005, p. 115).

Damon in Tier 3

Based on his Tier 2 participation, it now appeared obvious that, from a an "inside-the-head" (cognitive) perspective, Damon was struggling with decoding because he was not yet developmentally primed to engage in the deeper levels of phonological processing that beginning decoding required, possibly because of a language learning disability. For example, Damon could not convert letters and letter patterns into their phonological representations quickly, which interfered with his ability to blend phonemes. To state this differently, although Damon was showing flickers of emerging analytical ability referred to as metaphonological awareness (Scarborough & Brady, 2002), it was still too challenging for him to deal with phonemes as a concept. The question is why. There are three possibilities that are not mutually exclusive. Any one of these possibilities singly or in combination can affect children's acquisition of a more literate vocabulary necessary for proficient reading comprehension.

1. *The phonological memory possibility.* It may be the case that Damon is experiencing problems with the efficiency of his phonological memory, a component of the working memory system where verbal information, including the decoding of print by beginning readers, is initially translated and held for temporary storage. An efficient phonological memory, which has a language processing function, "helps the beginning reader by storing sounds they retrieve from permanent storage that are associated with letters and letter patterns in the to-be-decoded word" (Wagner et al., 2003, p. 56).

2. *The lexical–phonological interaction possibility.* Even before a child can to decode, there may be a relationship between phonological memory and oral vocabulary learning. All words must have both meaning and phonological representations if they are to be pronounced. One hypothesis is that phonological memory acts as a "go-between" for new word meanings and their pronunciation, at least before age 5 in typically developing children (Gathercole, 2006). One likelihood is that Damon has yet to achieve a well-integrated set of phonological and lexical representations, which would then impact how efficiently he is able to fast map, or incidentally learn, new word meanings (Alt & Plante, 2006). It is well established that children with more robust vocabularies have an easier time learning to decode (Foorman, Anthony, Seals, & Mouzaki, 2002) since the purpose of decoding is to "get the meaning" of the word. It is also well documented that many children with a language learning disability, like Damon, have less well-developed vocabularies (see Brea-Spahn & Silliman, in press, for a review; also van Kleeck & Littlewood, in press).

3. *The frequency possibility.* A second critical factor influencing vocabulary learning is related to "outside-the-head" experiences in the social world. The phonological patterns of word meanings will vary in two intersecting ways: the frequency of occurrence of those patterns in the North American English language and the frequency with which these patterns are used in the individual's everyday verbal interaction (Brea-Spahn & Silliman, in press). Thus children who have frequent experiences with diverse word meanings in their interactions with parents or caregivers will be the ones who likely enter school with larger vocabularies. Conversely, children whose experiences with new word meanings are less frequent and less diverse will probably enter school with smaller vocabularies (Hart & Risley, 1995). Such children, like Damon, may be the ones at highest risk for beginning reading failure because of the relationship between oral vocabulary richness and decoding (word-level recognition). However, whether the oral vocabulary–word recognition relationship is direct or indirect remains unanswered (McDowell, Lonigan, & Goldstein, 2007; Ricketts, Nation, & Bishop, 2007; Wise, Sevcik, Morris, Lovett, & Wolf, 2007a,b).

Taking these three possibilities into account and considering improvements that Damon made with dialogic book sharing, Ms. Connor and the other team members made a new decision that best met Damon's current needs. They would add to the intensity of Tier 3 small-group instruction by shifting to 50-minute sessions five times a week and alter demands of code instruction from a deeper to a medium depth of processing (i.e., onset-rime; see Figure 11.2) since this level appeared to be where Damon could respond more consistently. For effective learning to take place, the evidence indicates that a minimum of 100 hours of intensive instruction is required (Scammacca, Roberts, Vaughn, Wanzek, & Torgeson, 2007).

Pronoun Focus.   In the first 25 minutes of each daily session, Ms. Connor would concentrate on the integration of pronoun referencing with expanding more literate vocabulary use in story book activities. The integration was based on the guideline that no single linguistic area should ever be targeted alone in a language intervention program (Fey, Long, & Finestack, 2003). Examination of Damon's pronoun use in narrative retellings revealed that pronoun production was always correct in gender and plurality (number). This indicated that he comprehended pronouns. In contrast, he consistently used the object form of the pronoun for marking both subjects and possession, indicating that his problem resided in the production area (Arnold, Brown-Schmidt, & Trueswell, 2007). An example is taken from a picture book retelling (pronoun violations are italicized):

> "Two kids playin' in the park. *Him* sees outer space guys. *Him* sees outer space ship guys. *Him* sees spaceship with mommy, daddy, and a dog. Grandma waves from the door of the spaceship. *Them* had octopus legs. Brother got scared."

This pattern held in 100 percent of the obligatory pronoun contexts. Pronoun referencing represents shifts in perspective (i.e., from first to third person and the reverse) as well as the coordination of "one's focus of attention with other discourse participants" (Arnold et al., 2007, p. 561). It may be the case that Damon's use of the object form was partially related to the difficulty he experienced in coordinating the rapid shifting of conceptual stances from himself to others while simultaneously coordinating his focus of attention with what his conversational (discourse) partners were saying. The use of the within-category object pronoun referent for the subject referent may be an easier strategy for him under these conditions.

The linguistic strategy selected to support Damon's accurate pronoun choices was *conversational recasts,* a procedure in which the adult responds immediately to child utterances and one that has a strong evidence base for younger children. In a recast, the adult response would repeat "some of the child's words and correct or otherwise modify the morphological or syntactic form of the child's prior utterance while maintaining the central meaning of the child's production" (Proctor-Williams & Fey, 2007, pp. 1029–1030). In effect, recasting offers a "linguistic scaffold" for the child by providing a verbal model and increasing the *input frequency* of particular linguistic items. An example of recasting from Damon's narrative might be:

Damon: *Them* had octopus legs.

Ms. Connor: *They* do have legs that look like an octopus.

Damon (expected response):   Yep. *They* got octopus legs.

However, in this case, Ms. Connor developed a plan for distributing the rate of her recast use so that competition would not be created for Damon between recasts and the dialogic structure of the storybook activity (Proctor-Williams et al., 2007). It was also decided that conversational recasting could be used in the classroom and the small-group language intervention sessions. Additionally, books were chosen that highlighted the pronoun targets for inclusion in the book-sharing sessions that the parents had already implemented (Paul, 2006).

Vocabulary Focus.   Word meaning is a continuum, from no knowledge of a meaning to situational understanding to a rich understanding of multiple meanings independent of particular situations (Nagy, 2005). Since words represent concepts, the job of "learning a new concept is more challenging than simply adding a new word to one's vocabulary" (Stahl & Nagy, 2006, p. 60). Also, fluent reading depends on the rapid retrieval of well-integrated familiar meanings (Perfetti, 2007). Explicit teaching is necessary, therefore, for most children, including children like Damon, to acquire ownership of new meanings. To complement the dialogic book reading, the approach implemented for Damon was based on text talk (read-alouds) and word levels that represent the complexity of the word meaning continuum (Beck, McKeown, & Kucan, 2002, 2005; Beck & McKeown, 2007; McKeown & Beck, 2003).

- *Level 1 words.* Everyday, high-frequency meanings that most children know and bring to school, for example, *clock, baby, happy, walk, jump.*
- *Level 2 words.* More literate or all-purpose word knowledge that results in greater precision and specificity of meanings and plays an important role in developing a more elaborated lexicon. These include meanings like *absurd, huge, fortunate, coaxed, substantive, treacherous, fascinating, pursuit, ponder, controversy, concepts, discipline.*
- *Level 3 words.* Specialized literate meanings connected with content areas, such as science (*echolocation, fission*), geography (*peninsula, tectonics, population*), and math (*quadrant, algebra, algorithm*).[2]

The focus of text talk is level 2 meanings. The story is first introduced briefly with words needed for comprehension simply explained as they occur. Open-ended questions are inserted as appropriate to encourage the child to talk about important ideas (e.g., "What's the problem with Henry wanting a pet snake?"), and then there is a summary of the story. Next, after completing the story, two to three level 2 words are selected that are likely unfamiliar to Damon and his group members but are important for the overall story theme and have intervention potential. The SLP then explains the word meaning in child friendly terms ("*Coax* means to talk in a really nice way to get what you want"), provides a typical use ("How do you *coax* Jerry to play with you?"), and asks Damon to generate his own use of the word ("I *coax* him with baseball cards"). The story is then returned to and Damon is asked questions such as "Why did Henry say he could *coax* anybody?" There are multiple strategies for progressively supporting Damon and his group peers to "own the meaning" and readers are advised to consult the appropriate resources (e.g., Beck et al., 2002, 2005; Beck & McKeown, 2007; McKeown & Beck, 2003; Stahl & Nagy, 2006).

---

[2]Prospective SLPs should be aware that no agreement exists on which literate meanings are valuable to teach according to either grade or developmental level (see Coxhead, 2000).

Phonological Awareness Focus. In the second half of each session, the resource teacher, Joe Hanson, would embed a rime unit or a word family into reading and spelling events (Hines, Speece, Walker, & DaDeppo, 2007), for example, <u>c</u>at, <u>m</u>at, <u>s</u>at (the rime segments are underlined), and follow the Hines and colleagues (2007) procedures for implementation and transfer. As Hines et al. note, transfer is a major problem for students struggling to read and needs to be emphasized in each session, not as an afterthought.

SIX CAUTIONS ABOUT THE RTI MODEL

While the RtI model has promise as a much-needed shift from the current "wait to fail" approach to a prevention philosophy for younger children like Damon with language and learning difficulties, there are six cautions that must be considered as SLPs enter this new territory.

1. Successful implementation requires strong administrative support, extensive professional development experiences over time for all educational staff, including SLPs, as well as the motivation of the educational staff to provide intervention services in this format (Fuchs & Deshler, 2007).
2. Little is known about multitiered instruction beyond early reading (Fuchs & Deshler, 2007) and even less is known at the current time about the effectiveness of the RtI model for children with a language learning disability (Troia, 2005).
3. The participation of classroom teachers versus special education specialists in Tiers 2 and 3, including the criteria used to evaluate student responsiveness through RtI, requires definition (Fuchs & Deshler, 2007).
4. Minimal information is available on how long a given student like Damon should remain in a specific tier given the possibility that progress can be illusory once learning demands become more challenging (Troia, 2005).
5. There is currently no consensus on what the cut-off point should be to document either adequate progress or a lack of responsiveness (Fletcher et al., 2007).
6. Meta-analyses have yet to be conducted on the outcomes of RtI approaches (Scammacca et al., 2007a).

Despite these concerns, a well-designed RtI program has the diagnostic power to go well beyond the one-time, snapshot approach of traditional assessment. As Fletcher and colleagues (2007) advise, the considerable resources now devoted to decision making about children from a single diagnostic session would be better spent after "proper attempts at instruction have been made" (p. 84).

Response to Intervention: What Might It Look Like at the Middle School Level?

In this section we present the second case, David, a 12-year-old with a language learning disability who had grappled with academic demands reasonably well until he entered middle school in grade 6. The focal point is how an RtI approach might function at the secondary level rather than consideration of eligibility concerns for special education services. Before presenting David, we briefly frame his situation within the larger issue of adolescent literacy achievement because prospective SLPs should understand the bigger policy picture that impacts service delivery.

MIDDLE SCHOOL AS THE TRANSITION TO STUDENTS' FUTURES

In the past several years, a national consensus has emerged to reform adolescent literacy achievement for reasons best expressed by a 2004 report, *Reading Next,* from the Carnegie Corporation of New York:

> Today young people who leave high school without excellent and flexible reading and writing skills stand at a great disadvantage. In the past, those students who dropped out of high school could count on an array of options for establishing a productive and successful life. But in a society driven by knowledge and ever-accelerating demands for reading and writing skills, very few options exist for young people lacking a high school diploma. Even with a diploma in hand, today's young people face increasing literacy demands. Yet the large number of students who struggle with reading and writing has not changed noticeably in decades. This disparity between the demands of modern life and the inadequate literacy achievement of eight million struggling readers and writers has therefore given a new urgency to the need for reform. (Biancarosa & Snow, 2004)

Based on research evidence, Biancarosa and Snow recommended fifteen elements of effective adolescent literacy programs in middle and high school, among which are the following:

- direct and explicit reading comprehension instruction that emphasizes comprehension processes and strategies
- effective instructional principles embedded in content area learning that provides practice in reading and writing specific to the content area
- intensive writing connected to the types of writing that students will have to perform well in high school and beyond
- interdisciplinary teacher teams that meet on a regular basis to talk about students and align instruction to their needs
- in-depth professional development that is long-term and ongoing
- ongoing assessments of how individual students are learning (termed *formative* assessment)
- ongoing *summative* assessments of students and programs (i.e., the assessment of outcomes) that are disseminated for the purposes of accountability and research

Different secondary programs would have varied combinations of the fifteen components. However, Biancarosa and Snow (2004) make the case that any mixture of program elements must include professional development as well as formative and summative assessments.

RTI TIERS IN MIDDLE SCHOOL: DESIGNING AN INTEGRATED PROGRAM FOR DAVID

Although a tier continuum has been suggested for the secondary level, the effectiveness of RtI models for either middle or high school currently lacks an evidence base.

The use of RtI with older students is problematic because of the underlying premise that academic problems of younger students can be prevented (or "fixed") if identified early enough and intensive and explicit intervention is applied. On the secondary level, this logic is not so easily endorsed. Students still experiencing significant difficulty in the secondary years typically have learning problems that are less responsive to short intensive interventions. However, other components of RtI, such as evidence-based instruction, consistent progress monitoring (formative assessments), intervention tied to content area curriculum, student mentoring, and collaborative practices with other professionals are as important at the secondary level as for kindergarten to grade 3.

A final point regarding implementation of RtI tiers at the middle school level is that the transition to middle school is a time when students' self-esteem is challenged in ways that can significantly influence their academic achievement. This challenge is even greater for preadolescents like David with language and learning disabilities when they enter middle school in grade 6 with less social maturity as opposed to grade 7 (Snow, Porche, Tabors, & Harris, 2007). Their background experiences in and out of school have often shaped a feeling of helplessness that frequently translates into reduced motivation and effort (Ehren, Lenz, & Deshler, 2004).

Fortunately for David, the principal and educational staff of his middle school had already incorporated many of the fifteen keystone elements proposed by Biancarosa and Snow (2004) into their academic program (see the Case Study on page 526 for descriptions of David and the school philosophy). As Ms. Connor, Damon's SLP, was a an integral member of her school's RtI team, so too was Mr. Harmody, the middle school SLP, a prominent member of the teaching team that collaborated on building tiered intervention for David. As a team, they wanted to be a positive factor in enhancing his sense of competence and self-worth and to send the message that they cared about him as a unique individual. They anticipated that their interest and high expectations would thereby increase David's motivation to sustain engagement in literacy-related activities across content areas (Alvermann, 2002).

Formative and Summative Assessment Patterns

From David's formative and summative assessments, the team identified two inter-related patterns that could explain his communicative challenges across content areas. The first obstacle was his word reading accuracy and fluency, which were also reflected in his spelling patterns and fluency limitations in writing. The second barrier was his inferencing difficulties during reading comprehension combined with his limited vocabulary of general and specialized academic meanings. The inferencing process is supported when readers first make connections among "different parts of the text [and then] fill in missing information, in order to produce a coherent overall representation [of the text]" (Oakhill & Cain, 2007, p. 23). Simply put, readers must connect the dots to achieve a unified text representation, which is the basis of comprehension. One issue may be that David was not connecting information from different linguistic sources (Cain & Oakhill, 2007). For example, when examining his writing (see Table 11.2), we note that David does not condense sentence content, which requires the ability to connect and integrate relevant information into a coherent whole. Hence, he constructed sentences such as "Irony means unexpected/And it means surprise" (versus "Irony

Table 11.2 **Excerpt from David's Essay About the Types of Irony and Examples in the Book *Time Traveler***

Sentence	David's Essay	Translation	Number of Words
The Prompt was: "Irony is found in conversations, movies, and books. Before you begin writing, think about the types of irony and different examples we discussed in class. Now explain the use of irony in *Time Traveler*."			
1	Irony means unekspekid.	Irony means unexpected.	3
2	And it means suprize.	And it means surprise.	4
3	There are three tipes.	There are three types.	4
4	The tipes are verble and sichuashun and drama.	The types are verbal and situational and dramatic.	8
5	Verble means joking.	Verbal means joking.	3
6	It means surprize in talking.	It means suprise in talking.	5
7	And you are suprizd and laugh.	And you are surprised and laugh.	6
8	It means he tells a joke and we laffd.	It means he tells a joke and we laughed.	9
9	It means a word means two things.	_____	7
10	The book has irony.	_____	4
11	He thinks a joke about Morloks.	He thinks a joke about Morlocks.	6
12	Sichuashun means suprize.	Situation means surprise.	3
13	The fire stashun is on fire.	The fire station is on fire.	6
14	It was like boom.	_____	4
15	There is a suprize and it is unedspekid.	There is a surprise and it is unexpected.	8

means an unexpected surprise"). David's team also believed that this integration process was further hampered by his inconsistent use of comprehension strategies to connect different sources of text information and his difficulties with the more advanced syntax that characterizes context area textbooks (Silliman & Scott, in press).

Oral Reading Accuracy and Fluency

David's teachers were concerned about his oral reading fluency. There are different definitions of fluency, but the one selected for David, that fluency is the rate and accuracy of oral reading (Torgesen, Rashotte, & Alexander, 2001), was a narrow one that would allow the ongoing curriculum-based (formative) assessment of his progress with word recognition (see Figure 11.3 for a comparable method of formative assessment).

One reason that assessing fluency is so important is that it "is our best known bridge to ease in comprehension" (Wolf et al., 2003, p. 371). Fluent reading is more automatic. It allows the brain to focus on text ideas and their connections to previously learned information rather than on the letter and phoneme segments of each word. The continuous integration of language and word recognition skills requires extensive reading practice and is a gradual process that continues throughout a reader's lifetime as new vocabulary is learned. By grade 3, David should have moved from word-by-word reading to reading fluently (Tomkins, 2003).

As described in the case study, David's fluency was well below expectations for a grade 6 student. David was able to apply basic decoding skills but lacked strategies for identifying complex multisyllabic words, which contributed to his problems with understanding novel words in his content area texts and impacted his ability to read fluently. There is some debate whether addressing word-level decoding and fluency is appropriate for the older student. Based on a meta-analysis, the evidence suggests that intensive and skillful instruction can still have a positive impact on both reading comprehension and fluency for older students like David (Scammacca, Roberts, Vaughn, Edwards, et al., 2007; Torgeson et al., 2007). However, it is important to target only those students whose oral reading accuracy is relatively low rather than students whose reading comprehension is low for other reasons.

Word Recognition and Fluency Focus.   The team decided that David's schedule would be amende to included one hour per day of small-group instruction with the reading specialist. The focus of the instruction would be word recognition and fluency since the words that he can automatically recognize must steadily increase for him to meet grade-level expectations (Torgesen & Hudson, 2006). Also integrated was a focus on spelling patterns that the SLP helped to develop (see Writing and Spelling later in this chapter). The team also decided to monitor David's progress weekly via formative assessments, initially using curriculum-based measures to assess his fluency. Reading practice is another important part of fluency. Although reading rates do not become significantly faster after grade 6 (Tindal, Hasbrouck, & Jones, 2005), David's team understood that reading practice was imperative for him to quickly link the phonological, orthographic, and morphological features of a word to known words in his reading vocabulary (also called the orthographic lexicon). David's parents were enlisted to help him attain the repeated practice needed for fluent reading. A popular book series was chosen that he and his parents could read together for pleasure. Audiobooks of the same book series were also checked out of the local library to provide additional models of fluent phrasing.

Inferencing, Reading Comprehension, and Vocabulary

Language and literacy skills are interdependent, crossing the curriculum from kindergarten through high school. A recent meta-analysis of general reading comprehension strategies (Scammacca, Roberts, Vaughn, Edwards et al., 2007) showed that, for meaningful outcomes to occur with middle school students struggling with reading, instructional strategies must be "well-designed [and] effectively delivered" (p. 15), meaning that instruction had to be intensive, long-term, and connected to content areas. In addition, the same meta-analysis indicated that learning new meanings through vocabulary interventions produced major effects for middle school students.

Middle school content areas depend on student understanding of expository text, which is often difficult for students like David to understand because of the focus on unfamiliar and often complex ideas. Also, the structure of expository texts is more challenging to master. Unlike the event-based sequences of narrative structure, expository texts can combine two or more structures within the same paragraph, for example, compare–contrast, problem–solution, description, and so on (Williams et al., 2005). Furthermore, there is evidence from a meta-analysis of twenty-nine studies involving students with learning disabilities that there are strategies that "work" to support student understanding of expository texts (Gajria et al., 2007).

David's content area teachers considered findings from this meta-analysis in their design and implementation of a reading comprehension intervention plan. They faced three tasks. Firstly, they defined the goal of comprehension strategy instruction as "teaching students how to learn rather than mastery of specific content information . . . so that they can become more active, deliberate, and self-regulated learners" (Gajria et al., 2007, p. 216). Next, the content area team understood that they had to promote instructional processes that encouraged strategic reading and new vocabulary learning in general. For example, multiple strategy instruction taught in an ordered way produces greater benefits than teaching only one or two strategies (Pressley & Hilden, 2004). Finally, they had to develop an inventory of strategies for supporting literacy demands, including vocabulary, specific to their discipline. The distinctive demands of the individual disciplines were addressed through content area–specific strategies in science (Creech & Hale, 2006; Fang, 2006), social studies (Massey & Heafner, 2004), and math (Barton, Heidema, & Jordan, 2002; Draper, 2002). The purpose was to ensure that reading comprehension strategies were infused throughout the school day. (See Bailey and Butler [2007] and Wilkinson and Silliman [in press] for further information on the language demands of content areas, such as science, math, and social studies).

Reading Comprehension Strategy Focus.   Two types of strategies were selected: cognitive strategies to facilitate the generation and application of content and content enhancement strategies to assist in the active and deeper processing of text (Gajria et al., 2007; National Reading Panel, 2000). Mr. Harmody, the middle school SLP, coordinated with David's content area teachers to provide more explicit instruction when oral and written language concerns might be preventing David from assuming more responsibility for applying either cognitive or content enhancement strategies.

1. Multiple cognitive strategies included teaching David and a small group of his peers, prediction, questioning, relating to prior knowledge, monitoring of comprehension, and summarizing—practiced in cooperative learning groups in which students discussed what they had read (Langer, 2001; Torgesen et al., 2007), examples of which are shown in Tables 11.3 and 11.4 (p. 520).
2. Content enhancement strategies consisted of unit organizers (see Figure 11.4, p. 521, for an example from a unit on figurative language; see also Table 11.2 for David's essay on irony from this unit). Among the kinds of organizers are Venn

Table 11.3 **Reading Comprehension Strategies That, in Combination, Can Facilitate an Active Approach to Expository Text Processing**

Strategy	Purpose	Description
Directed Reading Thinking Activity (DRTA) (Stauffer, 1969)	Encourages *prediction* during and after reading. • Makes connections to previous knowledge. • Encourages self-monitoring of comprehension. • Gives a purpose to reading to confirm predictions.	• Students read text title and brainstorm ideas about the text from the title. Their predictions are recorded. • Expansion of clues to include index, table of contents, pictures, charts, and tables. • Predictions are then revised with students providing reasons for the revisions. • Students then read a section of the text and stop to confirm, revise, or make new predictions and give reasons for them. • These steps are continued until the text sections are completed.
KWLH (I *know*, what I *want* to know, what I *learned*, *how* I learned it) (Ogle, 1986; Weaver, 1994)	Activates students' *prior knowledge* as the initial phase to the process of learning how to learn	Four steps are highlighted: • what I know about a topic via brainstorming • what I want to know through student directed discovery • what I learned via summarizing • how we can learn more via discussion
Reciprocal Teaching (Gajria et al., 2007; Palincsar & Brown, 1986)	Adult scaffolds via think-alouds how to apply four multiple cognitive strategies (one at a time) and then students take turns teaching and evaluating their strategy effectiveness.	Multiple strategies include: • summarizing • asking questions • clarification • making predictions • noting any problems with the content
QAR (Question-Answer Relationships) (Gajria et al., 2007 Raphael, 1986; Raphael & McKinney, 1983;)	Illustrates *self-questioning* relationships to increase reading comprehension. Students also assume the role of teacher and ask questions.	Four question types are taught: • right there • think and search • author and you • on my own

Strategy	Purpose	Description
Three Connections (Keene & Zimmerman, 1997)	Supports students to • activate background and text schemas • make connections to other reading material • apply these schemas to the real world	The three type of connections are • text to self (connection between reading and personal experience) • text to text (connection between reading and another story of a similar genre) • text to world (connection between reading and information about the world)
Think-Alouds (Kobayashi, 2007; Schellings, Aarnoutse, & van Leeuwe, 2006)	Increases metacognitive awareness and approach to problem solving.	Thinking aloud is used while problem solving. • Thinking process is talked through as it occurs. ("How can I figure out what this word means?") • Students allowed to hear what is going on in the mind of a teacher, SLP, or peer. ("Let's see if I can look for the root word.") • The strategies a student is using to understand text is made audible to teachers or SLPs. ("First, I need to find the key word in this sentence; then I am going to see if I know the meaning at all. Next, I will try to make a connection to the meaning I know.")

diagrams, information charts, semantic webs, multiple meaning webs, and so on. (For more information on the purposes and selection of specific unit organizers, see www.specialconnections.ku.edu.)

Vocabulary Focus. Vocabulary instruction in middle school is challenging because there are no agreed-on "best practices." It is known that having students learn isolated "vocabulary" words is no more effective in middle school than in elementary school. Although there has been little research on the quality of lexical representations in preadolescents or adolescents with language learning disability like David, Perfetti (2007) speculates that students who can make high-quality lexical representations would be able to use meanings, especially academic meanings, in a more all-purpose way and would furthermore have good reading comprehension. In contrast, students only able to make low-quality lexical representations would be more bound to situational meanings leading to effortful decoding and the frequent retrieval of inaccurate meanings during their reading of texts.

Table 11.4 **Cooperative Group Discussion Options to Support Inferencing and Text Comprehension**

Strategy	Purpose	Description
My Appointments	Access prior knowledge about a topic; review a topic after a lecture, reading, or other presentation; learn about interests of others	• Students make an "appointment" with at least two other students (whom they do not sit near). • When signaled throughout the day or week, they find their appointment and discuss a prompt that the teacher gives.
Pass a Problem (Kagan, 1989)	Brainstorm solutions to problems or challenges	• Small groups brainstorm challenges related to a specific topic or prompt. • Then, they develop a problem statement which is written on a 3 × 5 card and passed to the table group next to them. • Each table group brainstorms and lists possible solutions to the problem. • The table group sends the card back to the originating table group.
Think-Pair-Share (Bromley & Modlo, 1997; Ketch, 2005; Rao & DiCarlo, 2000)	Process or debrief information from a lecture or reading; access prior knowledge; share opinions	• Pairs are given a prompt by the teacher and "think time." • Then pairs are asked to share their thoughts with a partner for one minute each.
Sticky Note Discussions (Padak & Coman, 1999)	Gives purpose for reading; supports summarization and comprehension	• Students use sticky notes to mark text locations that they want to talk about. • Next students divide into cooperative groups. • After all students have marked their text locations, they reread, talking about the parts they have marked.
Jigsaw Matching (Cretu, 2003)	Allows students to have a purpose for discussing content learned; promotes positive sense of self as an expert; creates opportunities for students to review or share information, knowledge, and opinions with others	• Teams are assigned a general area and each student becomes an expert in a particular subtopic. • Students then leave their teams to join members of other teams who are also experts on the same subtopic. • After meeting in expert groups, students go to their home team and teach their individual subtopic to their teammates.

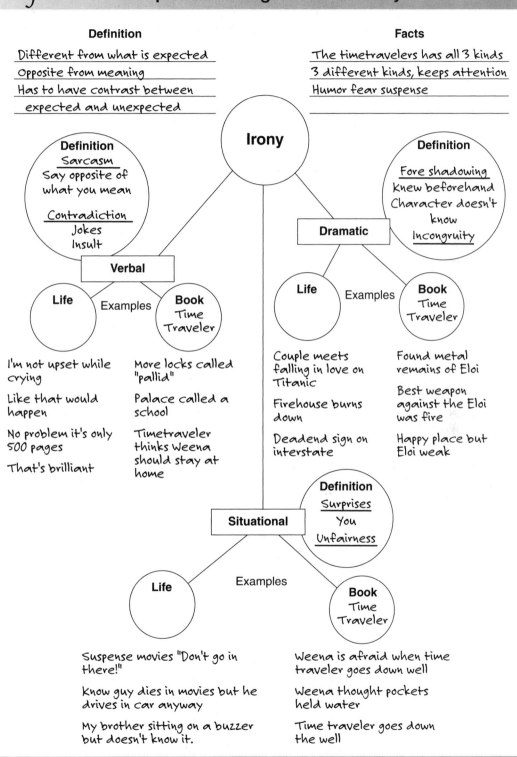

Figure 11.4   Example of a Unit Organizer for the Irony Theme

Definition
Different from what is expected
Opposite from meaning
Has to have contrast between
    expected and unexpected

Facts
The timetravelers has all 3 kinds
3 different kinds, keeps attention
Humor fear suspense

Irony

Definition
Sarcasm
Say opposite of
what you mean

Contradiction
Jokes
Insult

Verbal

Life   Examples   **Book**
Time
Traveler

I'm not upset while
crying

Like that would
happen

No problem it's only
500 pages

That's brilliant

More locks called
"pallid"

Palace called a
school

Timetraveler
thinks Weena
should stay at
home

Dramatic

Definition
Fore shadowing
Knew beforehand
Character doesn't
know
Incongruity

Life   Examples   **Book**
Time
Traveler

Couple meets
falling in love on
Titanic

Firehouse burns
down

Deadend sign on
interstate

Found metal
remains of Eloi

Best weapon
against the Eloi
was fire

Happy place but
Eloi weak

Situational

Definition
Surprises
You
Unfairness

Life   Examples   **Book**
Time
Traveler

Suspense movies "Don't go in
there!"

Know guy dies in movies but he
drives in car anyway

My brother sitting on a buzzer
but doesn't know it.

Weena is afraid when time
traveler goes down well

Weena thought pockets
held water

Time traveler goes down
the well

David's team was aware of his significant problems with vocabulary in expository texts and on tests (his summative assessments). They decided to model their vocabulary instruction on a still-experimental word study program for middle school students being developed by the Strategic Education Research Partnership Institute (SERP 2006). The guiding principle for this approach, similar to text talk for younger children (Beck et al., 2002), is that "students learn new words best [in content areas] from multiple encounters with those words within meaningful contexts" (SERP, 2006, p. 5). The program emphasizes: (1) important general purpose vocabulary, for example, in math and science, (2) reading materials that are relevant to student interests and their lives, (3) texts linked to the curriculum, and (4) mandatory 10–15 instructional minutes a day for study of the weekly words. The approach also allows for flexible and frequent progress monitoring (formative assessments) that reflects the particular curriculum and expository texts used by the Suncoast Middle School. (For further information on this word study approach, see www.serpinstitute.org.)

WRITING AND SPELLING

The patterns identified from David's writing sample on irony (see Table 11.2) led the team to focus on two interrelated issues to augment writing instruction in the classroom. Mr. Harmody agreed to take the lead in coordinating any individualized or small-group instruction that addressed the writing process.

Through his continuing education studies, Mr. Harmody was familiar with two major meta-analyses on the outcomes of writing instruction with adolescents in regular classroom settings (Graham & Perin, 2007a,b). One finding from these meta-analyses was the effectiveness of strategy instruction in writing (that is, advance planning, revising, and editing) when teachers had intensive professional development in the approach (Graham & Perin, 2007a). A second finding was that stronger effects were associated with modifying writing assignments and instruction to meet the needs of individual students while still maintaining high expectations (Graham & Perin, 2007b). Another important outcome from the meta-analyses was the value of teaching students how to combine simple independent sentences into more complex ones via sentence combining rather than concentrating on traditional grammar (Graham & Perin, 2007a,b). This last finding was critically important for David, who had been taught writing strategies. Despite his slow but steady progress with expository writing, the over-all quality of his writing was not satisfactory because of problems with sentence combining. This drawback also limited his sentence length, measured by the number of words per sentence shown in Table 11.2 (see Silliman & Scott, in press). Hence, for students like David, a focus only on writing strategies will not be sufficient.

Focusing Instruction

Combining Writing Instruction with Content Instruction.   The SLP and the language arts teacher, Mrs. Smith, jointly selected an applied academic format (Graham & Perin, 2007a) to assist David with his essay writing in language arts. In this format the classroom teacher and a specialist like Mr. Harmody use language arts themes, such as the irony theme, as the content of writing instruction. For example, David needed more support to connect his background knowledge to everyday examples in his explanatory writing about irony. Mr. Harmody and Mrs. Smith agreed on implementing the three connections strategy (see Table 11.3). Mr. Harmody then developed filled-in graphic organizers that illustrated the three connections strategy for the irony unit. In a small group in the language arts classroom, Mr. Harmody guided David and his peers on how to use these completed graphic organizers to support their explanatory essay writing.

Advancing More Complex Syntax and Explicit Referencing of Pronouns. The second focus area was to increase the complexity of David's written sentences. To increase his syntactic awareness, including his understanding of summarization and revision, David was explicitly focused on sentence combining. The SLP introduced think-alouds to model the process for combining. Then the specific procedures were organized in increasingly more complex phases (Saddler & Preschern, 2007), using David's irony essay (see Table 11.2).

1. *Cued practice.* In this first phase, David is provided with a clue word as a prompt to generate a sentence combination via *condensing.*
   Irony means unexpected.
   <u>And</u> it means surprise.
   <u>New combination</u>: Irony means unexpected and surprised.
2. *Student problem solving.* As David takes on some responsibility for revising his sentences, he moves to the next phase. He must decide what new information in a second sentence might be incorporated into a combined sentence via *expansion.*
   There are three types.
   The types are verbal, situational, and dramatic.
   <u>New combination</u>: The three types of irony are verbal, situational, and dramatic.
3. *Considering alternate constructions.* At this point, David and his peers can now discuss what combinations make a sentence more interesting to a reader.
   Irony may be verbal, situational, or dramatic
   OR
   Types of irony can vary from verbal to situational to dramatic.

It is important that students first buy into the reason for sentence combining. Saddler and Preschern (2007) recommend that students understand not only will this skill help them to write more interesting sentences but also that "good writers often work with their sentences to make them sound better" (p. 8). In addition, students should feel safe in making mistakes.

Spelling Patterns. Like sentence combining, spelling is also a linguistic process. When approached in this way, David's patterns of misspellings are understandable. His errors were distributed across phonological, orthographic, and morphological categories. At David's age, this pattern is consistent with children who have a language learning disability (Silliman, Bahr, & Peters, 2006). By grade 6, typically developing children have their misspellings primarily clustered in the orthographic and morphological categories, including derivational morphology (Bahr, Silliman, & Berninger, 2007; see also Chapter 5). For example, among David's phonological errors were the vocalic /r/ and voicing (*suprize* for *surpri<u>s</u>e*), the schwa (unstressed vowel as in *verble* for *verbal*), long vowel confusions (*tipes* for *types*), and syllable reduction (*drama* for *dramatic*). To help David further develop his word consciousness, including his realization that English spelling is patterned and not irrational, Mr. Harmody built comparison and contrast activities into the word recognition and fluency focus. For example, the *-er*, as in *mother*, was contrasted and compared with the vocalic /r/, as in *bird* and *surprise*, first at the phonological level and then at the orthographic levels.

Summary

This chapter delineates the knowledge needed by the speech-language pathologist (SLP) in language and literacy. It discusses the impact of legislation on the role of the SLP and the need for a clear bridge between an assessment, educational standards, and grade-level expectations for academic achievement. Across grade levels, standards and expectations share the attainment of critical literacy through proficiency in using the language tools of reading, writing, and spelling. The importance of oral language in achieving academic success is exemplified through a suggested framework to connect components of oral language to literacy learning within a response to intervention approach. The chapter is divided in two sections with each segment highlighting a case example of a child with language learning disabilities. The first case is a kindergarten-age student struggling to read. Featured in the second section is a middle school student who is having significant problems with reading comprehension and writing. For both cases, readers will learn how to use evidence-based practices for building an integrated approach to language and literacy intervention that is interconnected with the academic language expectations of the classroom.

Case Study   The Participation of an SLP in Primary Prevention (Tier 1) in a Kindergarten Class

Ms. Connor is an ASHA-certified SLP at Cross Country Elementary School. She is very active in promoting literacy learning in her school and actively participates in curriculum choices. Ms. Shepherd is a new kindergarten teacher in the school. Ms. Connor has offered to support Ms. Shepherd in her efforts to create effective beginning reading experiences for the children in her class both in terms of a literacy-rich environment and the selection of evidence-based instructional practices.

Focus 1: The Literacy Environment

To assess how adequately the classroom met standards as a literacy rich environment with easy access to literacy tools, Ms. Connor suggested that the *Classroom Literacy Environmental Profile* (Wolfersberger, Reutzel, Sudweeks, & Fawson, 2004) might act as an initial guide in this area. This profile seeks to identify how the classroom is provisioned with literacy tools, how classroom space is arranged, how students' interest is gained in literacy events, and how students' interactions with literacy tools are sustained. The professionals worked together to reach the *enriched* classification on this scale by ensuring that the classroom had

- books in a variety of places
- an assortment of reference sources (e.g., globes, reference books, atlases, address books, dictionaries, calendars, etc.)
- evidence of print used functionally throughout the classroom (e.g., written schedules, directions, labels, class rules, sign-up sheets, menus, charts)
- places for children to display their literacy efforts (e.g., drawings, charts, journals, poems, songs, graphs)
- dramatic play areas, along with centers for writing that included a range of writing tools, including pens, markers, pencils, crayons, magic slates, and stamps

Focus 2: Literacy Instruction

The school district's policy required that literacy instruction at the kindergarten level be targeted from 60 to 90 minutes daily. The SLP and teacher jointly planned literacy learning around thematic units (for classroom-based collaborative strategies, see DiMeo, Merritt, & Culatta, 1998; Silliman, Ford, Beasman, & Evans, 1999) and they team-taught some lessons (see Throneburg, Calvert, Sturm, Paramboukas, & Paul, 2000; Wilcox, Kouri, & Caswell, 1991). In these lessons, based on research findings, meaning and form activities were separated to avoid heavy processing demands (van Kleeck & Littlewood, in press). Meaning activities primarily involved shared book reading (or read-alouds), following the explicit strategies outlined in Table 11.1. Vocabulary learning was also incorporated into shared book reading in a contextualized way, following Beck, McKeown, and Kucan (2002). Form instruction was indirectly embedded in other activities whenever appropriate (Justice & Kaderavek, 2004). Great care was taken to incorporate print concepts, alphabet recognition, phonological awareness, grapheme–phoneme activities, and beginning writing (including invented spelling) into lessons since all are linked to achievement in print word recognition (Foorman, Anthony, Seals, & Mouzaki, 2002). Over time, form activities became more explicit—for example, discovering easier grapheme–phoneme connections in single syllable words using letter cards that children could manipulate (see Beck, 2006).

Case Study **A Secondary Prevention Collaboration for Damon, Age 6 Years**

Ms. Shepherd, the kindergarten teacher, had concerns about Damon, a 6-year-old of African American heritage who was struggling with basic code instruction. Benchmark measures used by the school district after the first eight weeks of school for assessing progress confirmed Damon's struggle. He knew that groups of words were units of meaning oriented from left to right when looking at a book, could spell his name, and identified three letters; but he knew no letter sound names (letters that have the sound in their pronunciation, such as *p, t, d,* and *m*), and only recognized rhyme patterns, like *mouse* and *house,* 10 percent of the time. Research has shown that children with more alphabetic knowledge are more successful in transitioning to decoding letters into phonemes (Muter, Hulme, Snowling, & Stevenson, 2004; Schatschneider, Fletcher, Francis, Carlson, & Foorman, 2004; Storch & Whitehurst, 2002; Vellutino et al., 1996). Also, Ms. Shepard observed that Damon often did not know the specific names of vocabulary items used in class and started sentences with "Me" instead of "I." This information was shared with Ms. Connor, the SLP, and they decided that Damon should be discussed at the next collaborative support team meeting.

At the meeting, a review of Damon's records showed that he had received speech therapy for a moderate expressive phonological disorder in Head Start and was dismissed. Ms. Connor thought that Damon's dismissal might be a sign of "false recovery" (Scarborough, 2001), where one set of symptoms seems to decrease only to be later replaced by a new set of symptoms brought on by the new demands placed on the child. It was decided that (1) Damon would be placed in a Tier 2 small group that met for 50 minutes three times a week, (2) Ms. Connor would lead one of the small-group sessions and the other two would be taught by the teacher or the paraprofessional, (3) an overture would be made to involve Damon's parents in book sharing activities at home, and (4) benchmark assessment would take place in 12 weeks to gauge his progress. Following a parent night at school on shared book reading, Damon's parents were excited about incorporating this activity into their schedule at least every evening.

Case Study   David, Age 12 Years, Grade 6: Middle School Challenges

David is a 12-year-old in grade 6 with an identified language learning disability who attends Suncoast Middle School. He has a history of learning challenges. He received special education intervention in the form of language therapy during kindergarten and grade 1. After grade 1, he made appropriate progress as measured by state standardized testing with the support of periodic, but not continuous intervention, from an SLP and a learning disabilities specialist. However, his first year of middle school proved very challenging and his teachers noticed his difficulties in daily work, performance evaluations, and content area tests.

The staff of the Suncoast Middle School believed that a number of variables should be considered in the design of learning experiences for all students, including (1) the context of learning, (2) students' background experiences, (3) social pressures prevalent in middle school, and (4) the needs of students struggling with language and literacy learning for meaningful social interactions combined with their search for personal identity (Ehren, Lenz, & Deshler, 2004). The staff divided the students into teams that formed smaller learning communities (Perks, 2006) in an effort to instill a sense of belonging in the students and to ensure that each student had adult advocacy. The teams planned together using schoolwide themes to promote connections throughout the content areas of math, science, English, and social studies.

The collaborative support team's review of David's academic records revealed the following:

- *Oral reading fluency.* David's English teacher was concerned that he still was not a fluent reader. Fluent reading was a benchmark for grade 3 (Tomkins, 2003). Although David scored at a level 3 on the grade 5 state measure of reading achievement (scored on a 1 to 5 scale), a curriculum-based assessment of oral reading administered by his English teacher found that he was only reading 42 words per minute versus a class average of 127 words per minute. David's oral reading rate placed him in the 10th percentile for grade 6 in the fall of the school year. It was noted that David was stilled "glued to print" in that he sounded out words phoneme by phoneme, which certainly impacted his reading comprehension.
- *Content area vocabulary knowledge (level 3).* On curriculum-based vocabulary probes that consisted of simple matching of definitions to words in his content areas, David's accuracy ranged from 64 to 88 percent. His teachers felt that he contributed appropriately during oral content discussions but that he did not seem to apply that knowledge in content area reading and writing.
- *Reading comprehension.* Performance on content area questions at the end of reading assignments were poor, ranging from 56 to 70 percent in accuracy. In contrast, on a standardized measure of reading comprehension that involved verbally answering literal and inferential questions, David achieved a percentile rank of 25, which placed him within 1 SD of the mean. The SLP, Mr. Harmody, explained that the disparity in achievement might be due to the facts that David's readings in content area textbooks (1) were considerably longer than the passages read on the standardized measure, (2) required more integration of ideas with his background and vocabulary knowledge, and (3) used a verbal response format on the standardized measure whereas responses from the reading assignments had to be generated in writing. In addition, Mr. Harmody pointed out that different reading comprehension measures (i.e., the questions at the end of textbook chapters versus a standardized test), consist of different items and, therefore, a student's performance will likely vary depending on the measure used (Cutting & Scarborough, 2006).
- *Writing.* An excerpt from an essay David wrote for an English unit on irony (see Table 11.2) was disseminated to the team. In the opinion of the English teacher, the essay was representative of David's writing when he gave maximum effort. In terms of organization and content, David (1) focused on the required parameters, (2) did not introduce any extraneous information, and (3) had an introduction, three main points, and a conclusion. However, the essay was not informative because the types of irony were not elaborated on and there was redundant vocabulary selected as well as an absence of diversity in sentence construction. In addition, David did not always specify his pronoun referents. His misspellings primarily involved multisyllabic words that were often derivations.

Study Questions

1. How does a tiered continuum of support respond to the intent of No Child Left Behind and IDEA 2004? How does it differ from traditional views of assessment and intervention? What are the benefits and challenges?
2. Discuss the importance of collaboration in a tiered level of support. How does it differ in supporting basic literacy and content area instruction? Focus on the role of the speech-language pathologist.
3. Consider the role of formative and summative evaluations in identifying patterns of performance in children struggling with literacy issues. How might it change as a child matures?
4. The educational team at an elementary school brings up a child who would be called a "nonresponder." How would the team recognize this child as such? Discuss the possible reasons for challenges to the child's acquisition of new more literate vocabulary. What impact would these factors have on intervention?
5. A ninth grader, who has just recently come to the high school that you serve, is still struggling with basic literacy skills. What unique characteristics does the adolescent bring to literacy learning? Develop a plan to support fluency and reading comprehension that incorporates the development of content level vocabulary. Consider whether a focus on word level decoding and fluency is appropriate.
6. A child in the sixth grade of a middle school cannot pass the state writing assessment. A writing process that included advance planning, revising, and editing was presented in his classrooms throughout elementary school. Additionally, many writing strategies had been taught to him by his previous speech language pathologists. While observing him during the writing process, you realize that he is not independently using the writing strategies taught to him and needs scaffolding to select the appropriate support. Craft a writing program that ensures the efficacy of his instruction is analyzed in an ongoing manner.

References

Al Otaiba, S., & Fuchs, D. (2002). Characteristics of children who are unresponsive to early literacy intervention: A review of the literature. *Remedial and Special Education, 23*, 300–316.

Al Otaiba, S., & Fuchs, D. (2006). Who are the young children for whom best practices in reading are ineffective? *Journal of Learning Disabilities, 39*(5), 414–431.

Alt, M., & Plante, E. (2006). Factors that influence lexical and semantic fast mapping of young children with specific language impairment. *Journal of Speech, Language, and Hearing Research, 49*(5), 941–954.

Alvermann, D. E. (2002). Effective literacy instruction for adolescents. *Journal of Literacy Research, 34*(2), 189–208.

Arnold, J. E., Brown-Schmidt, S., & Trueswell, J. (2007). Children's use of gender and order-of-mention during pronoun comprehension. *Language and Cognitive Processes, 22*(4), 527–565.

Bahr, R. H., Silliman, E. R., & Berninger, V. W. (2007, April). Spelling patterns in natural writing, grades 1–9: Implications for reading instruction. Paper presented at the Florida Reading Research Conference, Tampa, FL.

Bailey, A. L., & Butler, F. A. (2007). A conceptual framework of academic English language for broad application to education. In A. L. Bailey (Ed.), *The language demands of school: Putting academic English to the test* (pp. 68–102). Yale, CT: Yale University Press.

Barton, M. L., Heidema, C., & Jordan, D. (2002). Teaching reading in mathematics and science. *Educational Leadership, 60*(3), 24–28.

Beck, I. L. (2006). *Making sense of phonics: The hows and whys.* New York: Guilford.

Beck, I. L., & McKeown, M. G. (2007). Different ways for different goals, but keep your eye on the higher verbal goals. In R. K. Wagner, A. E. Muse, & K. R. Tannenbaum (Eds.), *Vocabulary acquisition: Implications for reading comprehension* (pp. 182–204). New York: Guilford.

Beck, I. L., McKeown, M. G., & Kucan, L. (2002). *Bringing words to life: Robust vocabulary instruction.* New York: Guilford.

Beck, I. L., McKeown, M. G., & Kucan, L. (2005). Choosing words to teach. In E. H. Hiebert & M. L. Kamil (Eds.), *Teaching and learning vocabulary: Bringing research to practice* (pp. 207–222). Mahwah, NJ: Lawrence Erlbaum.

Biancarosa, G., & Snow, C. E. (2004). *Reading next—a vision for action and research in middle and high school literacy: A report from Carnegie Corporation of New York.* Washington, DC: Alliance for Excellent Education. Retrieved September 27, 2007, from www.ncte.org.

Brea-Spahn, M. R., & Silliman, E. R. (in press). Tuning into language-specific patterns: Nonword repetition and the big picture of bilingual vocabulary learning. In A. Y. Durgunoglu & M. Gerber (Eds.), *Language learners: Their development and assessment in oral and written language.* New York: Guilford.

Bromley, K., & Modlo, M. (1997). Using cooperative learning to improve reading and writing in language arts. *Reading and Writing Quarterly: Overcoming Learning Difficulties, 13*(1), 21–35.

Bus, A. G., van Ijzendoorn, M. H., & Pellegrini, A. (1995). Joint book reading makes for success in learning to read: A meta-analysis on intergenerational transmission of literacy. *Review of Education Research, 65,* 1–21.

Cain, K., & Oakhill, J. (2007). Reading comprehension difficulties: Correlates, causes, and consequences. In K. Cain & J. Oakhill (Eds.), *Children's comprehension problems in oral and written language: A cognitive perspective* (pp. 41–75). New York: Guilford.

Coxhead, A. (2000). A new academic word list. *TESOL Quarterly, 34*(2), 213–238.

Creech, J., & Hale, G. (2006). Literacy in science: A natural fit. *Science Teacher, 73*(2), 22–27.

Cretu, D. (2003). Students' motivation in class. *Thinking Classroom, 4*(2), 21–28.

Cutting, L. E., & Scarborough, H. S. (2006). Prediction of reading comprehension: Relative contribution of word recognition, language proficiency, and other cognitive skills can depend on how comprehension is measured. *Scientific Studies of Reading, 10*(3), 277–299.

Dimeo, J. H., Merritt, D. D. & Culatta, B. (1998). Collaborative partnerships and decision making. In D. D. Merritt & B. Culatta (Eds.), *Language intervention in the classroom* (pp. 37–97). San Diego, CA: Singular.

Draper, R. J. (2002). School mathematics reform, constructivism, and literacy: A case for literacy instruction in the reform-oriented math classroom. *Journal of Adolescent and Adult Literacy, 45*(6), 520–529.

Ehren, B. J. (September 25, 2007). Responsiveness to intervention: An opportunity to reinvent speech-language services in schools. *The ASHA Leader*, 10–11, 12, 25.

Ehren, B. J., & Nelson, N. W. (2005). The responsiveness to intervention approach and language impairment. *Topics in Language Disorders, 25*, 120–131.

Ehren, B., Lenz, B., & Deshler, D. (2004). Enhancing literacy proficiency with adolescents and young adults. In C. A. Stone & E. R. Silliman (Eds.), *Handbook of language and literacy* (pp. 681–702). New York: Guilford Press.

Fang, Z. (2006). The language demands of science reading in middle school. *International Journal of Science Education, 28*(5), 491–520.

Fey, M., Long, S., & Finestack, L. (2003). Ten principles of grammatical intervention for children with specific language impairments. *American Journal of Speech-Language Pathology, 12*, 3–15.

Fletcher, J. M., Lyon, G. R., Fuchs, L. S., & Barnes, M. A. (2007). *Learning disabilities: From identification to intervention*. New York: Guilford.

Foorman, B. R. (2007). Primary prevention in classroom reading instruction. *Teaching Exceptional Children, 39*(5), 24–30.

Foorman, B. R., Anthony, J., Seals, L., & Mouzaki, A. (2002). Language development and emergent literacy in preschool. *Seminars in Pediatric Neurology, 9*(3), 173–184.

Foorman, B. R., Breier, J. I., & Fletcher, J. M. (2003). Interventions aimed at improving reading success: An evidence-based approach. *Developmental Neuropsychology, 24*, 613–639.

Foorman, B. R., & Nixon, S. M. (2006). The influence of public policy on reading research and practice. *Topics in Language Disorders, 26*(2), 157–171.

Foorman, B., & Torgesen, J. (2001). Critical elements of classroom and small-group instruction promote reading success in all children. *Learning Disabilities Research and Practice, 16*(4), 203–212.

Fuchs, D., & Deshler, D. D. (2007). What we need to know about responsiveness to intervention (and shouldn't be afraid to ask). *Learning Disabilities Research & Practice, 22*(2), 129–136.

Fuchs, D., Fuchs, L. S., McMaster, K. L., Yen, L., & Svenson, E. (2004). Nonresponders: How to find them? How to help them? What do they mean for special education? *Teaching Exceptional Children, 37*(1), 72–77.

Fuchs, D., Mock, D., Morgan, P. L., & Young, C. L. (2003). Responsiveness-to-intervention: Definitions, evidence, and implications for the learning disabilities construct. *Learning Disabilities Research & Practice, 18*(3), 157–171.

Fuchs, L. S., & Fuchs, D. (2007). A model for implementing responsiveness to intervention. *Teaching Exceptional Children, 39*(5), 14–20.

Gajria, M., Jitendra, A. K., Sood, S., & Sacks, G. (2007). Improving comprehension of expository text in students with LD: A research synthesis. *Journal of Learning Disabilities, 40*(3), 210–225.

Gathercole, S. E. (2006). Nonword repetition and word learning: The nature of the relationship. *Applied Psycholinguistics, 27*(4), 513–543.

Gillon, G. T. (2000). The efficacy of phonological awareness intervention for children with spoken language impairment. *Language, Speech, and Hearing Services in Schools, 31*, 126–141.

Graham, S., & Perin, D. (2007a). A meta-analysis of writing instruction for adolescent students. *Journal of Educational Psychology, 99*(3), 445–476.

Graham, S., & Perin, D. (2007b). What we know, what we still need to know: Teaching adolescents to write. *Scientific Studies of Reading, 11*(4), 313–335.

Guthrie, J. T., Hoa, A. L. W., Wigfield, A., Tonks, S. M., Humenick, N. M., & Littles, E. (2007). Reading motivation and reading comprehension growth in the later elementary years. *Contemporary Educational Psychology, 32*(3), 282–313.

Hart, B., & Risley, T. R. (1995). *Meaningful differences in the everyday experiences of young American children.* Baltimore: Paul H. Brookes.

Hines, S., Speece, D., Walker, C., & DaDeppo, L. (2007). Assessing more than you teach: The difficult case of transfer. *Reading and Writing, 20*(6), 539–552.

Huebner, C. E. (2000). Promoting toddlers' language development through community-based intervention. *Journal of Applied Developmental Psychology, 21*(5), 513–535.

Johnson, C. J. (2006). Getting started in evidence-based practice for childhood speech-language disorders. *American Journal of Speech-Language Pathology, 15*(1), 20–35.

Justice, L. M. (2006). Evidence-based practice, response to intervention, and the prevention of reading difficulties. *Language, Speech, and Hearing Services in Schools, 37*(4), 284–297.

Justice, L. M., & Kaderavek, J. N. (2004). Embedded-explicit emergent literacy intervention I: Background and description of approach. *Language, Speech, and Hearing Services in Schools, 35*(3), 201–211.

Kagan, S. (1989). *Cooperative learning.* San Juan Capistrano, CA: Resources for Teachers.

Keene, E. L., & Zimmerman, S. (1997). *Mosaic of thought: Teaching comprehension in a reader's workshop.* Portsmouth, NH: Heinemann.

Ketch, A. (2005). Conversation: The comprehension connection. *Reading Teacher, 59*(1), 8–13.

Kobayashi, K. (2007). The influence of critical reading orientation on external strategy use during expository text reading. *Educational Psychology, 27*(3), 363–375.

Langer, J. (2001). Beating the odds: Teaching middle and high school students to read and write well. *American Educational Research Journal, 38*, 837–880.

Massey, D. D., & Heafner, T. L. (2004). Promoting reading comprehension in social studies. *Journal of Adolescent and Adult Literacy, 48*(1), 26–40.

McDowell, K. D., Lonigan, C. J., & Goldstein, H. (2007). Relations among socioeconomic status, age, and predictors of phonological awareness. *Journal of Speech, Language, and Hearing Research, 50*(4), 1079–1092.

McKeown, M. G., & Beck, I. L. (2003). Taking advantage of read-alouds to help children make sense of decontextualized language. In A. van Kleeck, S. A. Stahl, & E. B. Bauer (Eds.), *On reading books to children: Parents and teachers* (pp. 159–176). Mahwah, NJ: Lawrence Erlbaum.

Muter, V., Hulme, C., Snowling, M. J., & Stevenson, J. (2004). Phonemes, rimes, vocabulary, and grammatical skills as foundations of early reading development: Evidence from a longitudinal study. *Developmental Psychology, 40*(5), 665–681.

Nagy, W. (2005). Why vocabulary instruction needs to be long-term and comprehensive. In E. H. Hiebert & M. L. Kamil (Eds.), *Teaching and learning vocabulary: Bringing research to practice* (pp. 27–44). Mahwah, NJ: Lawrence Erlbaum.

National Reading Panel. (2000). *Teaching children to read: An evidence based assessment of the scientific research literature on reading and its implication for reading instruction.* Washington, DC: U.S. National Institute for Literacy.

Nolen, S. B. (2007). Young children's motivation to read and write: Development in social contexts. *Cognition and Instruction, 25*(2), 219–270.

Oakhill, J., & Cain, K. (2007). Introduction to comprehension development. In K. Cain & J. Oakhill (Eds.), *Children's comprehension problems in oral and written language: A cognitive perspective* (pp. 3–40). New York: Guilford.

Ogle, D. (1986). K-W-L: A teaching model that develops active reading of expository text. *The Reading Teacher, 39,* 564–570.

Padak, N., & Coman, C. (1999). What Jamie saw. (Available from the ERIC Document Reproduction Service No. ED 435-856.)

Palincsar, A. S., & Brown, A. L. (1986). Interactive teaching to promote independent learning from text. *The Reading Teacher, 39,* 771–777.

Paul, R. (2006). *Language disorders from infancy through adolescence: Assessment and intervention.* St. Louis, MO: Mosby Elsevier.

Perfetti, C. (2007). Reading ability. Lexical quality to comprehension. *Scientific Studies in Reading, 11*(4), 357–383.

Perks, K. (2006). Reconnecting to the power of reading. *Principal Leadership, 7*(1), 16–20.

Pressley, M., & Hilden, K. (2004). Toward more ambitious comprehension instruction. In E. R. Silliman & L. C. Wilkinson (Eds.), *Language and literacy learning in schools* (pp. 151–174). New York: Guilford.

Proctor-Williams, K., & Fey, M. E. (2007). Recast density and acquisition of novel irregular past tense verbs. *Journal of Speech, Language, and Hearing Research, 50*(4), 1029–1047.

Rao, S. P., & DiCarlo, S. E. (2000). Peer instruction improves performance on quizzes. *Advances in Physiology Education, 24*(1), 51–55.

Raphael, T. (1986). Teaching question answer relationships, revisited. *Reading Teacher, 39,* 516–522.

Raphael, T. E., & McKinney, J. (1983). An examination of fifth- and eighth-grade children's question-answering behavior: An instructional study in metacognition. *Journal of Reading Behavior, 15,* 67–86.

Ricketts, J., Nation, K., & Bishop, D. V. M. (2007). Vocabulary is important for some, but not all reading skills. *Scientific Studies of Reading, 11*(3), 235–257.

Saddler, B., & Preschern, J. (2007). Improving sentence writing ability through sentence-combining practice. *Teaching Exceptional Children, 39*(3), 6–11.

Scammacca, N., Vaughn, S., Roberts, G., Wanzek, J., & Torgesen, J. K. (2007a). Extensive reading interventions in grades k-3: From research to practice. Portsmouth, NH: Research Corporation, Center on Instruction. Retrieved October 11, 2007, from www.centeroninstruction.org.

Scammacca, N., Roberts, G., Vaughn, S., Edwards, M., Wexler, J., Reutebuch, C. K., & Torgesen, J. K. (2007b). *Intervention for adolescent struggling readers: A meta-analysis with implications for practice.* Portsmouth, NH: Research Corporation, Center on Instruction. Retrieved September 29, 2007, from www.centeroninstruction.org.

Scarborough, H. S. (2001). Connecting early language and literacy to later reading (dis)abilities: Evidence, theory, and practice. In S. B. Neuman & D. K. Dickinson (Eds.), *Handbook of early literacy research* (pp. 97–125). New York: Guilford.

Scarborough, H. S., & Brady, S. A. (2002). Toward a common terminology for talking about speech and reading: A glossary of the "phon" words and some related terms. [Electronic version]. *Journal of Literacy Research, 34*(3), 299–336.

Schatschneider, C., Fletcher, J. M., Francis, D. J., Carlson, C. D., & Foorman, B. R. (2004). Kindergarten prediction of reading skills: A longitudinal comparative analysis. *Journal of Educational Psychology, 96*(2), 265–282.

Schellings, G., Aarnoutse, C., & van Leeuwe, J. (2006). Third-grader's think-aloud protocols: Types of reading activities in reading an expository text. *Learning and Instruction, 16*(6), 549–568.

Silliman, E. R., & Scott, C. M. (in press). Research-based language intervention routes to the academic language of literacy: Finding the right road. In S. Rosenfield & V. W. Berninger (Eds.), *Translating science-supported instruction into evidence-based practices: Understanding and applying the implementation process.* New York: Oxford University Press.

Silliman, E. R., Bahr, R. H., & Peters, M. L. (2006). Spelling patterns in preadolescents with atypical language skills: Phonological, morphological, and orthographic factors. *Developmental Neuropsychology, 29*(1), 93–123.

Silliman, E. R., Ford, C. S., Beasman, J., & Evans, D. (1999). An inclusion model for children with language learning disabilities. *Topics in Language Disorders, 19*(3), 1–18.

Snow, C. E., Porche, M. V., Tabors, P. O., & Harris, S. R. (2007). *Is literacy enough? Pathways to academic success for adolescents.* Baltimore: Paul H. Brookes.

Stahl, S. A., & Nagy, W. E. (2006). *Teaching word meanings.* Mahwah, NJ: Lawrence Erlbaum.

Stauffer, R. G. (1969). *Directing reading maturity as a cognitive process.* New York: Harper & Row.

Storch, S. A., & Whitehurst, G. J. (2002). Oral language and code-related precursors to reading: Evidence from a longitudinal structural model. *Developmental Psychology, 38*(6), 934–947.

Strategic Education Research Partnership Institute (2006). Word generation teacher's guide: A word study program for middle schools. Retrieved September 29, 2007, from www.serpinstitute .org.

Throneburg, R. N., Calvert, L. K., Sturm, J. J., Paramboukas, A. A., & Paul, P. J. (2000). A comparison of service delivery models: Effects on curricular vocabulary skills in the school setting. *American Journal of Speech-Language Pathology, 9*(1), 10–20.

Tindal, G., Hasbrouck, J., & Jones, C. (2005). *Oral reading fluency: 90 years of measurement. (Technical report no 33, Behavior research and teaching).* Eugene: University of Oregon.

Tomkins, G. (2003). *Literacy for the 21st century.* Upper Saddle, NJ: Pearson Education.

Torgesen, J. K., Houston, D., & Rissman, L. (2007). *Improving literacy instruction in middle and high schools: A guide for principals.* Portsmouth, NH: Research Corporation, Center on Instruction.

Torgesen, J. K., Houston, D. D., Rissman, L. M., Decker, S. M., Roberts, G., Vaughn, S., et al. (2007). *Academic literacy instruction for adolescents: A guidance document from the center on instruction.* Portsmouth, NH: RMC Research Corporation, Center on Instruction. Retrieved September 29, 2007, from www.centeroninstruction.org.

Torgesen, J. K., Rashotte, C. A., & Alexander, A. W. (2001). Principles of fluency instruction in reading: Relationships with established empirical outcomes. In M. Wolf (Ed.), *Dyslexia, fluency, and the brain* (pp. 333–355). Timonium, MD: York Press.

Torgesen, J., Alexander, A., Wagner, R., Rashotte, C., Voeller, K., & Conway, T. (2001). Intensive remedial instruction for children with severe reading disabilities: Immediate and long-term outcomes from two instructional approaches. *Journal of Learning Disabilities, 34,* 33–58.

Torgesen, J. K. (2000). Individual differences in response to early interventions in reading: The lingering problem of treatment resisters. *Learning Disabilities Research & Practice, 15*(1), 55–64.

Torgesen, J. K., & Hudson, R. (2006). Reading fluency: Critical issues for struggling readers. In S. J. Samuels, & A. Farstrup (Eds.), *Reading fluency: The forgotten dimension of reading success.* Newark, DE: International Reading Association.

Troia, G. A. (2004). Building word recognition skills through empirically validated instructional practices: Collaborative efforts of speech-language pathologists and teachers. In E. R. Silliman & L. C. Wilkinson (Eds.), *Language and literacy learning in schools* (pp. 98–129). New York: Guilford Press.

Troia, G. A. (2005). Responsiveness to intervention: Roles for speech-language pathologists in the prevention and identification of learning disabilities. *Topics in Language Disorders, 25,* 106–119.

Ukrainetz, T. A. (2006). The implications of RTI and EBP for SLPs: Commentary on L. M. Justice. *Language, Speech, and Hearing Services in Schools, 37*(4), 298–303.

U.S. Department of Education, Office of Special Education and Rehabilitation. (2003). Twenty-fifth annual report to Congress on the implementation of the Individuals with Disabilities Education Act. Available at www.ed.gov/pubs/edpubs.html.

U.S. Department of Education, National Center for Educational Statistics. (2007). The condition of education (NCES 2007-072). Washington, DC: Author.

van Kleeck, A. (2006a). Cultural issues in promoting interactive book sharing in the families of preschoolers. In A. van Kleeck (Ed.), *Sharing books and stories to promote language and literacy* (pp. 179–230). San Diego, CA: Plural.

van Kleeck, A. (2006b). Fostering inferential language during book sharing with prereaders: A foundation for later text comprehension strategies. In A. van Kleeck (Ed.), *Sharing books and stories to promote language and literacy* (pp. 269–317). San Diego, CA: Plural.

van Kleeck, A., & Littlewood, E. (in press). Fostering form and meaning in emerging literacy using evidence-based practices. In M. Mody & E. R. Silliman (Eds.), *Language and reading disabilities: Brain, behavior, and experience.* New York: Guilford.

van Kleeck, A., & Vander Woude, J. (2003). Book sharing with preschoolers with language delay. In A. van Kleeck, S. A. Stahl, & E. B. Bauer (Eds.), *On reading books to children* (pp. 58–92). Mahwah, NJ: Lawrence Erlbaum.

Vellutino, F. R., et al. (1996). Cognitive profiles of difficult-to-remediate and readily remediated poor readers: Early intervention as a vehicle for distinguishing between cognitive and experiential deficits as basic causes of specific reading disability. *Journal of Educational Psychology, 88*(4), 601–638.

Vellutino, F. R., Scanlon, D. M., Small, S., & Fanuele, D. P. (2006). Response to intervention as a vehicle for distinguishing between children with and without reading disabilities: Evidence for the role of kindergarten and first-grade interventions. *Journal of Learning Disabilities, 39*(2), 157–169.

Vellutino, F. R., Tunmer, W. E., Jaccard, J. J., & Chen, R. (2007). Components of reading ability: Multivariate evidence for a convergent skills model of reading development. *Scientific Studies of Reading, 11*(1), 3–32.

Wagner, R. K., Muse, A. E., Stein, T. L., Cukrowicz, K. C., Harrell, E. R., Rashotte, C. A., et al. (2003). How to assess reading-related phonological abilities. In B. R. Foorman (Ed.), *Preventing and remediating reading difficulties: Bringing science to scale* (pp. 51–70). Baltimore: York Press.

Weaver, C. (1994). *Reading process and practice: From socio-psycholinguistics to whole language* (2nd ed.). Portsmouth, NH: Heinemann.

What Works Clearinghouse. (2007, August 13). The beginning reading what works clearinghouse (WWC) review. Retrieved September 7, 2007, from http://ies.ed.gov/ncee/wwc/reports.

Wilcox, M. J., Kouri, T. A., & Caswell, S. B. (1991). Early language intervention: A comparison of classroom and individual treatment. *American Journal of Speech-Language Pathology, 1*(1), 49–62.

Wilkinson, L. C., & Silliman, E. R. (in press). Academic language proficiency, academic discourse requirements, and literacy instruction. In L. Wilkinson, L. Morrow, & V. Chou (Eds.), *Improving the preparation of teachers of reading in urban settings: Policy, practice, & pedagogy.* Newark, DE: International Reading Association.

Wise, J. C., Sevcik, R. A., Morris, R. D., Lovett, M. W., & Wolf, M. (2007a). The growth of phonological awareness by children with reading disabilities: A result of semantic knowledge or knowledge of grapheme-phoneme correspondences? *Scientific Studies of Reading, 11*(2), 151–164.

Wise, J. C., Sevcik, R. A., Morris, R. D., Lovett, M. W., & Wolf, M. (2007b). The relationship among receptive and expressive vocabulary, listening comprehension, pre-reading skills, word identification skills, and reading comprehension by children with reading disabilities. *Journal of Speech, Language, and Hearing Research, 50*(4), 1093–1109.

Wolf, M., O'Brien, B., Adams, K. D., Joffee, T., Jeffrey, J., Lovett, M. W., et al. (2003). Working for time: Reflections on naming speed, reading fluency, and intervention. In B. R. Foorman (Ed.), *Prevention and remediating reading difficulties: Bringing science to scale* (pp. 355–379). Timonium, MD: York Press.

Wolfersberger, M. E., Reutzel, R., Sudweeks, R., & Fawson, P. (2004). Developing and validating the classroom literacy environmental profile (CLEP): A tool for examining the "print richness" of early childhood and elementary classrooms. *Journal of Literacy Research, 36,* 211–272.

Zevenbergen, A. A., & Whitehurst, G. J. (2003). Dialogic reading: A shared picture book reading intervention for preschoolers. In A. van Kleeck, S. A. Stahl, & E. B. Bauer (Eds.), *On reading books to children: Parents and teachers* (pp. 177–200). Mahwah, NJ: Lawrence Erlbaum.

Zirkel, P. A. (2007). What does the law say? *Teaching Exceptional Children, 39*(6), 66–68.

CHAPTER 12

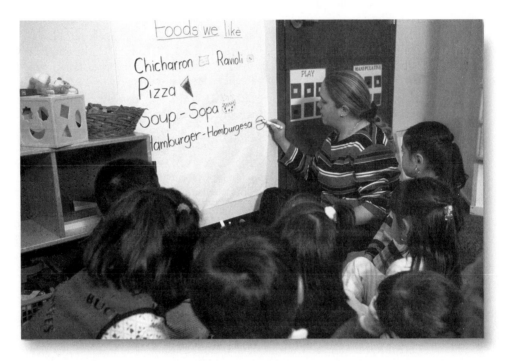

Assessment and Intervention for Culturally and Linguistically Diverse Children

Dolores E. Battle
Buffalo State College

When you finish this chapter, you will be able to

- Explain how cultural variables affect language development in children with disabilities.
- Describe the role of the speech-language pathologist in determining the difference between a dialect difference and a developmental disability in an African American child.
- Describe some of the difficulties in the assessment process as children with cultural and linguistic diversity are being evaluated in academic environments.
- Discuss the differences between norm- and criterion-referenced assessments.
- Describe the development of phonology and morphology in Spanish-speaking children.
- Discuss how linguistic diversity has changed in the past several decades and how it will continue to change in the United States in the next several decades.

Linguistic Diversity in the United States

Native Americans were the original inhabitants of what was to become the United States. Since the "discovery" of this land by Europeans in the fifteenth century until the present time, the United States has been a nation of immigrants. The early immigrants came primarily from European countries that shared a similar cultural background, seeking religious freedom and economic prosperity. These persons of European heritage adopted the culture and language of their new country in order to share economic success. Also for economic reasons, the institution of slavery brought nonvoluntary immigrants from the countries of Africa. Economic development later brought people from Asia to work in western gold mines and build railroads and more Europeans to participate in the industrial revolution. The United States became a nation of persons from many different cultures, speaking many different languages, and holding many different cultural values. The resulting diversity was unlike any found in other parts of the world. Most of these immigrants eventually adopted the language and culture of the new nation in order to participate fully in the educational and economic possibilities of their new country; this was much easier for those of European ethnicity.

In the latter part of the twentieth century, a new wave of immigration began with persons coming primarily from Central and South America, Asia and the Pacific Islands, the Middle East, and Africa. This wave of immigration was different from previous ones because the great majority of immigrants came from non-European countries. As shown in Table 12.1, the twenty-first century has seen continued immigration from around the world, with most coming from non-European countries such as Mexico and the Asian countries. In addition to immigrants, the country saw an

Table 12.1 **Leading Continents and Countries of Origin of U.S. Immigrants by Country of Birth, 2005***

Countries		Continents	
Mexico	161,400	Europe	167,600
India	84,600	Asia	400,100
China	69,900	Africa	85,100
Phillippines	60,700	North America	341,600
Cuba	36,200	South America	103,100
Vietnam	32,700		
Dominican Republic	27,500		
Korea	26,500		

*Does not account for those who enter the country as undocumented immigrants.
Source: U.S. Department of Homeland Security, Office of Immigration Statistics, *2005 Yearbook of Immigration Statistics.*

increase of refugees who came seeking refuge from political turmoil in such countries as Somalia in Africa, and Haiti in the Caribbean islands.

The increasing diversity of the United States has affected current views of language development and language disorders. No longer is the United States a nation of European immigrants with European cultural values speaking English as their primary language. Unlike earlier immigrants, the new immigrants are interested in maintaining their cultural identity and their native language while they learn the language and culture necessary to achieve success in this country.

Table 12.2 **Resident Populations of the United States by Race and Hispanic Origin (with Percentage Increase from 2002–2005)**

		% Increase 2002–2005
Total	296,410,000	5.3%
One Race		
White	237,855,000	+4.3%
Black/African American	37,909,000	+6.2%
American Indian/Alaskan Native	2,863,000	+7.5%
Asian	12,667,000	+19.8%
Two or more race	4,579,000	+17.5%
Hispanic/Latino (of any race)	42,667,000	+20.9%

As shown in Table 12.2, of the more than 280 million people in this country, nearly 31 percent identify themselves as being nonwhite. This represents a nearly 5 percent increase from the number of nonwhites in 1990. Persons of Hispanic or Latino origin make up the largest group at 12.5 percent, followed by African Americans at 12.3 percent, Asian Americans at 3.6 percent, and Native Americans at 0.1 percent. To add to the complexity of the demographics represented in the census, the 2000 census allowed persons to identify themselves as two or more races. In addition, Hispanic or Latino was considered a racial group in the 1990 census. However, in the 2000 census, Hispanic was considered an ethnic group. Persons responding to the census could identify themselves as a member of an ethnic group (i.e., Hispanic) and also as a member of a racial group (i.e., Black). Such changes make comparisons of demographic data from previous censuses difficult and conclusions about any racial or ethnic identity become more problematic.

In spite of changes in the way the census data is collected, it appears that the most significant increases racial and ethnic groups in this country are in Hispanic and Asian populations. In 2003 it was estimated that Latin American and Asian immigrants accounted for a large part of the foreign-born population, which made up 11.7 percent of the total population. Latin American immigrants made up 53.3 percent and Asian immigrants 25 percent of all immigrants to the United States (U.S. Bureau of the Census, 2007). As shown in Table 12.1, in 2005 alone nearly 161 million persons were legal immigrants from Mexico, 84.6 million were from India, 69.9 million from China, and 60.7 million from the Philippines. Legal immigrants do not of course include the large numbers of undocumented immigrants who enter the country each year.

Immigrants and refugees seeking asylum can be found in nearly every state of the country, although different ethnicities seem to congregate in different regions. For example, 52.7 percent of Central American and 44.5 percent of Asian immigrants settled in the west. Immigrants from Cuba preferred Florida, whereas immigrants from other Caribbean countries such as Puerto Rico, Jamaica, the Dominican Republic, and Haiti settled in the mid-Atlantic states of New York, New Jersey, and Pennsylvania. The projections are that by the year 2020, the population of the United States will be more than 40 percent racial and ethnic minorities, and by 2050 what is now the majority will be the minority (U.S. Census Bureau, 2004).

It is important not to simplify the diversity of residents in this country by looking solely at the broad categories used in the census. Each of the groups identified by the census has tremendous heterogeneity. To say that 0.1 percent of the population is Native American ignores the fact that each of the more than 560 federally recognized tribal governments in the country has its own beliefs and values. There are 296 indigenous languages spoken in North America. Although most tribal groups are declining in number, there are twenty-three tribes with 10,000 or more members living throughout the United States. The largest tribal groups in the United States are the Cherokee and Navajo, followed by the Chippewa and Sioux. There are Native Americans in every state, either living on reservations or in urban and rural communities (U.S. Census Bureau, 2007).

To classify Asians as one group is also to ignore the diversity among those classified as Asian, which include persons from Afghanistan, Cambodia, China, Hong Kong, Japan, Laos, Philippines, Thailand, and Vietnam, to name a few. The same can be said for the various cultures included under the classification of Hispanic or Latino, which includes people from Mexico, Puerto Rico, Cuba, Jamaica, Haiti, Colombia, Venezuela, and the many other countries of Central and South America and the Caribbean. Each country has its own culture and its own language or dialect. Although most Hispanic or Latin countries speak Spanish as their primary language, the primary language of Brazil is Portuguese. Any understanding of cultural diversity in the United States must include the full scope of diversity, with the many cultures and languages beyond those classified by census data.

By welcoming immigrants and refugees from around the world, the nation has become culturally diverse. Currently, one in ten U.S. citizens was born outside the United States. These immigrants bring with them cultural values that are often different from the cultural foundation of the original European settlers who forged what came to be understood as American culture. This diversity of cultures, beliefs, and values shape the language and language development of young children. Patterns of development will be affected by cultural traditions and history and length of residence in the United States, as well as immigration patterns to communities in the United States. Other factors, such as socioeconomic status, amount and type of formal education, and degree of language proficiency in the home language as well as in English, add to the complexity of cultural influences in the United States (Langdon, 1996).

As could be expected, the cultural and linguistic diversity of children in the schools has increased dramatically. Many immigrant and refugee children in the public schools speak little or no English or use a language other than English at home. This presents a tremendous challenge for those charged with their education. Among the 262.5 million people surveyed over the age of 5 years, 47 million (18%) spoke a language other than English in the home (U.S. Census Bureau, 2000). There were also approximately 47 million children aged 5 to 17 who spoke a language other than English at home. In 2004, 8.1 percent of children aged 5 and over spoke English less than very well. Although Spanish, used by over 28 million children, continues to be the most commonly used language other than English, other languages are increasing. Chinese is the second most common language other than English spoken at home (2 million) followed by French (1.6 million) and German (1.4 million). Other languages used vary with the population; some school districts report as many as 100 different languages being used by children and their families at home.

Language Disorders and Diversity

The American Speech-Language-Hearing Association (ASHA, 2008) and the National Institution for Deafness and Other Communication Disorders (1991) estimate that between 10 and 15 percent of the U.S. population has a speech-language or hearing disorder. The prevalence of speech-language disorders among culturally and linguistically diverse populations is difficult to determine. Using current population figures and estimates of prevalence, it would be expected that 27 million persons in the country have a communication disorder. Based on this figure, 7.56 million persons from culturally and linguistically diverse groups have a disorder of speech, language, or hearing, including 6 million children under the age of 18 years. However, these estimates are probably low because there is believed to be a greater risk for disorders among persons from low-income families, and low-income families are disproportionately represented among immigrants and refugees in this country. According to the 2000 census, of the 28.4 million immigrants, 16.6 percent were living at or below the poverty level, compared to 11.5 percent of U.S.-born residents. More than 25 percent of immigrants were receiving public assistance (versus 16.7 percent of U.S.-born residents) and 33.4 percent were uninsured (versus 12.8 percent of U.S.-born residents). Many immigrants are underemployed according to their home country professional training. For example, a person trained as a dentist in the home country may not be able to obtain employment in this country because of licensing and language requirements. They may instead be employed at unskilled labor positions if they are employed at all. The socioeconomic status of the immigrants or refugees may be very different from the status they enjoyed in their home country (Portes & Rumbaut, 2001). Low-income groups, including recent immigrants and refugees, are more likely to have disorders related to trauma, poor prenatal care, poor health care, poor access to preventive care, high lead levels, drug and alcohol abuse, and a higher incidence of medical conditions associated with stroke, such as high blood pressure. The children may not have attended school at all or may be functioning below the age level expectations of American schools. Combinations of such factors may lead to depression and other mental health concerns that may hinder acculturation to the country.

To understand the factors associated with language and language disorders in culturally and linguistically diverse populations, it is necessary to understand (1) the relationship between culture and language, (2) the meaning of language dialects, (3) the nature of language development in monolingual and bilingual populations, (4) the issues related to the identification of language disorders, and (5) appropriate interventions to foster language development.

LANGUAGE AND CULTURE

The values, beliefs, attitudes, folkways, behavioral styles, and traditions of a people define culture. Culture encompasses a set of behaviors, institutions, and worldviews passed on and maintained by an identifiable group, linked to form an integrated whole that functions to identify a society. Language is the primary mode of communication used by members of a cultural group to express their fundamental thoughts, principles, and attitudes. It is developed within a cultural group and is defined by the rules governing language form, content, and use. It is the fabric that serves to both bind and unify members of a society and to separate the group from others. Language helps to shape a culture, and a culture is shaped by its language. Cultural values influencing speech-language behavior include ethnic origin, race, place of birth, immigration pattern, age, gender, socioeconomic status, educational level (particularly that of the mother), language or dialects spoken, religious beliefs, health care practices and beliefs, and family and community networks. For example, most of the early immigrants to this country were of European descent and came to this country seeking religious freedom within Christianity. There are now at least 36 Christian faiths practiced in this country. However, changes in immigration patterns has meant a significant increase in the non-Christian religions practiced in this country, as practiced by

Muslims, Buddhists, Hindus, Bahais, Sikhs, and Taoists, to name the most prominent ones. Persons practicing non-Christian religions in the United States more than doubled from 1990; in 2001, there were more than 1 million persons practicing Islam and Buddhism and nearly as many people practicing Hinduism in this country. The implications of the various religions are broad, influencing the way holidays are identified and celebrated, the foods people eat or do not eat, the clothes they wear, and the social practices within families and communities. They also impact family understanding of the cause of disability and roles in treatment.

CULTURE, FAMILY, AND LANGUAGE

Culture strongly influences family dynamics. Children acquire language in the context of the family. The language system used by the family is passed to the child. The structure of the family, the roles of individual members within the family, and the expectations of family members are important variables in the development of language. These variables differ across cultural groups (Lynch & Hanson, 2003, 2004). Each culture has its own communication rules and accepted ways of communicating within the group and with others who are not part of the group. Children learn the importance of language in their culture as a medium for interacting with others and for transmitting information to others. Cultural information is transmitted to the child through daily interaction with primary caretakers and significant others in a variety of situations. These daily interactions, including preferred language patterns and modes of interaction, influence the number and type of communication functions that the child will develop.

In some middle-class families, mothers or primary caretakers structure their children's language learning environment. The children are encouraged to engage in two-way conversations and exchanges with other individuals, especially the primary caretaker. The interchange begins in infancy during daily caretaking routines and continues throughout childhood. Caretakers see the teaching of language as one of their primary responsibilities. In some cultures and socioeconomic groups, however, children are often passive observers of the conversations of others. They are indirect participants in conversations and are encouraged to speak only when spoken to. Children learn through observation or gradual participation in adult tasks rather than involvement in child-centered activities (Harris, 1998; Heath, 1983b; Kayser, 1998; Owens, 2003).

It is difficult to make specific cross-cultural comparisons of the role of the family in language development because of the pattern of intercultural and interethnic marriage. There may be various cultural backgrounds within a single family. The 2000 U.S. census tallied more than 2.5 million interracial marriages (approximately 4.9% of all marriages) in the United States. Intergroup marriages in 1998 included white/African American (9 percent), white/Native American (12 percent), white/Asian (19 percent), and white/Hispanic (52 percent). The number of interethnic marriages is also increasing, such that nearly one in six Asian Americans is married to an Asian of a different ethnic background, such as Chinese/Japanese. Interethnic and interracial marriages are shaping the cultural values of families (U.S. Census Bureau, 2000). Intercultural and interethnic families make it challenging to determine the culture of the home. This underscores the need to view each family as an individual culture with its own beliefs, values, and thoughts about childrearing and development.

As stated by Schieffelin and Ochs (1986), "little is known about how caretakers and children speak and act toward one another and how that is linked to cultural patterns that extend and have consequences beyond specific interactions observed" (p. 116). According to more recent work by Hammer & Weiss (2000), African American mothers from low and middle socioeconomic groups believed that children learn to talk by experiencing (watching, listening, imitating, and participating in communicative interactions). The mothers varied, however, in the extent to which they expected their children to participate in the interactions to learn how to communicate. They also found that, in general, the views of the African American mothers did not differ from the views of western European middle-class mothers with respect to their role in their child's language development. They support the view of Crago (1992) that particular language socializing practices "are not the unique holding of any one culture" (p. 30). However, specific form and discourse patterns used by caretakers when interacting with young children is likely to have cultural differences. For example, Inuit parents are less likely to encourage their children to talk than western European parents (Crago, 1992). Japanese mothers are more likely to focus on affect than reference interacting with their infants. Chinese mothers differ from western European mothers in their beliefs about childrearing and verbal interactions with their preschool children. Although they may believe in the importance of nurturing their children, they are less likely to prompt their children for speech about personal narratives or talk about non-shared events of the day and are less likely to engage their children in frequent book reading (Johnston & Wong, 2002). Depending on the degree of acculturation into the mainstream of western European cultures, Mexican mothers may be more authoritarian and more likely to look to extrinsic causes for any impairment than western European mothers (Rodriquez & Olswang, 2003). West African families living in the United Kingdom believe that children need explicit instruction to learn to speak (Law, 2000). Although there are variations across cultures as to particular format, in most cultures children learn language according to the cultural rules governing interactions among family members, receiving verbal stimulation from the members of the family through storytelling, rhyming, poetry, and the encouragement of communication from early ages (Lynch & Hanson, 2003, 2004).

Another variable is family size. Many families are structured as nuclear families, usually defined as parents and their children. There are over 12 million children who live in one-parent homes (U.S. Census Bureau, 2000). This is an increase from 9 to 16 percent of all homes from 1990 to 2000, with more than 85 percent of them being with the mother. The increase in the number of single-parent homes and blended families, in which the child has both parents and stepparents, siblings and stepsiblings, has changed the perception of the nuclear family and the roles that individual family members play in language development. In traditional nuclear families, the parents are the primary caretakers participating in providing a language environment for the child. Other families are known as extended families, which include not only parents and children but other relatives or close friends living in the same household or very nearby and who play a role in the development and rearing of the child. In extended families, the persons responsible for language development may include grandparents, aunts, or older siblings.

In some western European families, but not all, families' cultural and linguistic behaviors are transmitted by the primary caretaker in two-way conversations in which the child is encouraged to be an active participant. The child is expected to engage in social communication, and the role of the caretaker is to encourage and facilitate that engagement. In some families, children learn language through the efforts of extended family caretakers and language is learned through nonverbal instructions rather than direct conversations (Kayser, 1998; Owens, 2003). Children are not expected to engage in social conversation with parents but rather are expected to observe or engage in conversation with age peers until they are competent to engage in interactions with adults. However, differences that may have been observed in the past seem to have been eradicated by increased contact between the cultural groups and exposure to effective childrearing practices through the media. In addition, previously perceived differences related to race may not be as strong as those related to socioeconomic status (Hammer & Weiss, 2000).

Hall, Nagy, and Linn (1984) audiotaped middle-class and working-class parents talking to their preschool children. The middle-class parents used nearly 30 percent more words while talking to their children than the working-class parents. The middle-class children used more words per hour in their conversations than did the working-class children. Hart and Risley (1995), who compared the language experiences of infants and toddlers in professional, working-class, and welfare families, obtained similar results. The children from working-class and professional homes had significantly more language experiences than the children from welfare families. In addition, the types of language and feedback to the children were different across the socioeconomic groups. When the socioeconomic factors are added to the variation in cultures within and between families, the exact role of language development in an individual family must be examined or considered on an individual basis.

Language Development, Dialects, and Language Disorders

DIALECTS AND LANGUAGES

The type of English spoken in the United States is commonly referred to as Mainstream American English (MAE). MAE is the variety of English most used in the conduct of commerce and is fostered in the schools as most acceptable. It can vary somewhat from one region of the country to another. There is an MAE spoken in Boston that sounds different from the MAE of Mississippi. Yet both are considered mainstream since they represent the "mainstream" of those respective communities (Seymour, Roeper, deVilliers, & deVilliers, 2003).

Languages are invariably manifested through their dialects. To speak a language is to speak some dialect of that language. A **dialect** is any variety of a language that is shared by a particular speech community for the purposes of interaction (Taylor, 1986; Wolfram, 1991). Dialects reflect variations in almost every aspect of language, including phonology, semantics, syntax, and pragmatics. Dialects reflect basic behavioral differences between groups within a society and are a cultural manifestation of the group. Dialects of the same language may differ in form, pronunciation, vocabulary, or grammar from each other; however, they are enough alike to be mutually understood by speakers of different dialects of the same language. Although each dialect of a language has distinguishing characteristics, all share a basic core of grammatical features that are common to all varieties of the language.

Dialects of a language vary by geography. Dialects of Mainstream American English include, but are not limited to, African American English (AAE), Appalachian English, Southern White English, and numerous other regional dialects. They are spoken by groups of people who came together by geography and social history and serve as primary identifiers of the particular group. When one dialect comes into contact with another, dialects may merge, one dialect may replace the other, or both dialects may coexist (Chen, 1999). It is important to understand that there is a considerable range of language diversity within each dialectal community; individual speakers vary their language use in accordance with sociolinguistic dynamics. For example, not all African Americans use African American English in the same way. Some do not use the dialect at all, while others use the dialect in individual ways (ASHA, 2003).

Because of the relationship between social history and the development of a dialect, certain dialects carry with them social stigma. African American dialects, for example, are often associated with persons of lower social class because of the history of slavery in this country. Spanish dialects are often associated with poverty and immigration because of the large number of undocumented immigrants from Central and South America. However, New England dialects, especially Boston dialects, are considered prestigious because of their association with European culture, literature, and education (Taylor, 1999).

Dialects of Spanish are spoken by persons with historical roots in as many as twenty different countries. The vocabulary and pronunciations of certain words may vary, but the underlying principles of the language allow the dialects to be understood by most speakers of Spanish. They are considered to be mutually intelligible. Mutual intelligibility resulting from contact of individuals using different dialects is eventuated when short-term accommodation of one dialect leads to a more long-term adjustment to that dialect (Penny, 2003). For example, although there may be vocabulary and pronunciation differences between the dialect of Spanish spoken in Cuba and the dialect spoken in Mexico, the people in these countries are able to communicate with each other and be understood while each uses his own dialect.

Some dialects of a language are not understood by speakers of the same language. They are considered mutually unintelligible. For example, there are 87 mutually unintelligible languages and dialects spoken in the 7,107 islands that make up the Philippines. Arabic, the sixth most common language spoken in the world and the primary language in eighteen countries of the Middle East, has many dialects that are so different as to preclude communication across dialectical boundaries unless Standard Arabic is used. The 500 Native American tribal entities in the United States speak as many as 200 distinct languages and dialects, some of which are mutually intelligible, but most of which are mutually unintelligible to other Native American speakers (Harris, 1998).

Most speakers of a dialect choose to speak the dialect to identify themselves as a member of a cultural group. Some users of a dialect use all of the usual dialect markers while others use relatively few. The number of dialect features used is known as *dialect density*. Speakers of a dialect vary their dialect density depending on the social or communicative context. They may switch from high dialect density to a low density or even to no features of the dialect. This is known as **code switching.** For example, speakers of African American English are able to switch to the use of Mainstream American English depending on the context, the message, or the communication partner. Children who use African American English have been shown to use fewer features of the dialect when talking to their teachers than when talking to their age peers. They have been shown to use fewer features of the dialect when retelling a story than when reporting an event (Wyatt, 1991). It is important to recognize the use of a dialect as a social, linguistic, and cultural bond between people and not to form a judgment of the value of the people or their ability to use language based on their use of a dialect. This is particularly important in making judgments about the language proficiency of children who use language dialects.

DIALECTS AND LANGUAGE DISORDERS

The American Speech-Language-Hearing Association (ASHA) defines a language disorder as "impaired comprehension and/or use of spoken, written, and/or other symbol systems. The disorder may involve (1) the form of language (phonology, morphology, or syntax), (2) the content of language (semantics), and/or (3) the function of language in communication (pragmatics in any combination)" (ASHA, 2008). Since language is embedded in culture, any definition of a language disorder must be defined by the parameters established by the community of which the child is a member. As culturally defined, a language disorder is impaired comprehension and/or use of a spoken, written, and/or other symbol system used by the child's indigenous culture and language group (Taylor, 1986).

According to the ASHA Position Paper on Social Dialects (ASHA, 1983), "No dialectal variety of English (or any other language) is a disorder or pathological form of speech or language. Each social dialect is adequate as a functional and effective variety of English. Each serves a communication function as well as a social solidarity function. It maintains the communication network and the social construct of the community of speakers who use it" (pp. 23–24).

The identification of language disorders among children who are in the process of developing language is difficult. Distinctions have to be made between what is expected of the child at a particular age. When considering a child from a culturally and linguistically different background, the task is even more challenging. Distinction must be made between what is expected of the child in his language or dialect, in his culture, and at his stage of language development. Much is known about the development of language by children developing Mainstream American English (Bloom & Lahey, 1978; Brown, 1973). Less is known about the development of language by children learning African American English, Spanish-influenced English, or English being developed by children who speak other languages.

LANGUAGE DEVELOPMENT, DIALECTS, AND DISORDERS IN SPEAKERS OF AAE

African American English (AAE) is the dialect of English spoken by many, but not all, persons in working-class African American families. It reflects the complex social history of persons of African heritage in the United States and patterns of migration from the rural South to the urban North (Dillard, 1972). Because of its historical roots, the use of African American English carries a negative social stigma to persons in economic power in the country. Many attempts have been made to eradicate or eliminate the use of the dialect by schoolchildren, spurred by the feeling that its use will delay the development of literacy in Mainstream American English. However, members of the African American community continue to use the dialect in certain social situations, particularly when they are among their social and cultural peers. Most are able to code switch to the use of Mainstream American English forms when educational, social, and economic mobility considerations require it (Rickford, 1999, 2000)

The major contrasts between Mainstream American English and African American English occur in phonology, morphology, syntax, and in the pragmatic and non-linguistic features of language. There are few assessment measures that are sensitive to the cultural and linguistic differences between the dialects of American English and disorders. The Diagnostic Evaluation of Language Variation (DELV) was recently developed by speech-language pathologists and linguists to distinguish disorders among ordinary dialectical differences by focusing on the features of syntax, semantics, and phonology that do not distinguish between the dialects (Seymour & Roeper et al., 2003).

Development of Phonology

All of the phonetic sounds of English are used by speakers of AAE. The early development of phonology and phonological patterns in infants and toddlers from homes where MAE and AAE is used is similar. At 36 months, the conversational speech of children exposed to African American English includes the same sounds and patterns as those used by speakers of Mainstream American English (e.g., /n/, /m/, /b/, /d/, /t/, /g/, /k/, /f/, /h/, and /w/) (Bland-Stewart, 2003; Caig, Thompson, Washington & Potter, 2003; Seymour & Ralabate, 1985; Seymour & Seymour, 1981; Steffersen, 1974; Stockman, 1998).

Some differences in the use of sounds occur among those sounds that develop after age 5 years. Differences occur in the use of /f/ for /θ/ in words such as *thumb* and the use of /b/ for /v/ in words such as *valentine*. Although there are other differences that become evident among later-developing phonological forms, the consonants that distinguish between AAE and MAE are not usually evident until after the age of 5 years. According to Bleile and Wallach (1992), the features that do not contrast between AAE and MAE are useful in distinguishing between AAE that is developing normally and that which may be delayed. These features include the following: the use of more than one or two stop errors (e.g., /p/, /t/, /k/, /g/); initial-word position errors; errors in /r/ or /l/ in children over the age of 4 years; more than a few cluster errors (e.g., /t/ for /st/); and fricative errors other than /θ/ (e.g., /f/) (Craig & Washington, 2002, 2004; Laing, 2003). The phonological patterns used most frequently by 3-year-old children in studies by Bland-Stewart (2003) were cluster reduction (77%), final consonant deletion (41%), stopping of affricates (25%), gliding of liquids (24%), and vowelization of /r/ (22%). The patterns were not unlike those of children of the same age who speak Mainstream American English.

Development of Semantics and Pragmatics

Infants and toddlers in homes where AAE is spoken develop communication intent and semantic meanings in the same manner as has been described for children in homes where MAE is spoken (Bridgeforth, 1984; Davis, Williams, & Vaughn-Cooke, 1992–1993; Stockman, 1998; Vaughn-Cooke & Wright-Harp, 1992). The number of language functions used increases with age through the preschool years. Young children from homes where AAE is spoken imitate, ask questions, express their needs both verbally and nonverbally, answer questions, and are interested in both telling and listening to stories in the same manner as children in other homes (Stockman, 1996).

The development of oral language skills and literacy are important in both African American and European American children (Craig & Washington, 2002). Differences in narrative production are a by-product of sociocultural differences, individual differences and preferences, and individual experiences (McGregor, 2000). Consequently, cultural expectations and patterns influence the manner in which narrative style and literacy are developed. The expectations for the involvement of the children may be different in different families, depending on the culture and the family members' understanding of their role in the development of language (Thompson, Craig, & Washington, 2004). For example, in some working-class homes, storybooks and other forms of children's literature are not prominent. Although stories are often told, comprehension is not negotiated through questions and expectation of feedback. In some families, the children may be expected to engage in conversations with peers and give recounts of the day. However, recall and discussion of past experiences may be rare among children in other families. For example, talking about events of the day begins early in Asian and European American families but is less likely to occur in Hispanic and African American families. The differences observed and frequently reported across cultural groups may be more related to social class and the education and expectations of family members than racial or ethnic identity.

There has been much discussion about the differences in narrative styles across cultural groups. For example, the narratives of some Japanese speakers are considered succinct and unelaborated. The narratives of children from Latin or Hispanic families do not appear to pay attention to sequencing of events. They are usually related to family and family events rather than out-of-context events. The narratives of working-class African American speakers are characterized by accounts that allow the speaker to share information with the listener. The children use more descriptions and have a complex organization and structure (Champion, Seymour, & Camarata, 1995). Speakers from European American families frequently use descriptions or explanation of events and past experiences (Heath, 1986). Selection of narrative style reflects cultural values as well as individual preferences, task demands, and linguistic experiences (Hester, 1996). It is important to distinguish between a narrative that reflects a speaker's cultural style and personal preferences and one that reflects disordered communication (McCabe, 1995).

Preferences for narrative style and for organization of discourse had been thought to be related to cultural and racial differences. There are generally two types of narrative styles: topic associative and topic centered. In *topic-associative style* the narrative moves from one topic to another linked by covert semantic or thematic associations related to the main topic. Frequent shifts in temporal, locative, and character references, as well as multiple experiences, are told in one story (Gee, 1989; Hyon & Sulzby, 1994). In *topic-centered narratives,* component events are linked in explicit chronological or sequential order, with consistent use of temporal, locational, and character references; beginnings and ends are clearly marked (Hyon & Sulzby, 1994). The narrative styles are evident in both oral language and in writing in school children.

Early research on the cultural differences in the use of narratives indicated that speakers of MAE were more likely to use topic-centered narratives and that speakers of AAE used the topic-associative style (Campbell, 1994; Gutierrez-Clellan & Quinn, 1993). More recent research has shown that children who use AAE use both topic-centered and topic-associative narrative styles, depending on the communicative context. Hester (1996) found that children switch narrative styles according to the discourse task, such as a conversation, story retelling, or fictional storytelling. The narratives produced by African American children from low-income families aged 6 to 10 years have a complex organization and structure (Champion et al., 1995). It is therefore necessary to distinguish between narratives that reflect a speaker's cultural style or preference in a given communication event from those that reflect disordered communication.

There are cross-linguistic/cross-cultural variations in narrative production. Narrative ability depends on the cultural background and experiences of speakers and listeners. Mexican American children are more likely to produce accounts of stories, retelling of family events, or descriptive information about family or personal relationships. They are less likely to use event casts than children from western European families. Bilingual children may produce different narratives in each of their languages (Fiestas & Peña, 2004; Rodriguez & Olswang, 2003).

Differences in cultural background may influence the interpretation of the narrative produced by the child. Differences in narrative style between the speaker and the listener may result in communication breakdown. When listening to a child who uses a topic-associative style, the listener may interrupt with questions and comments to seek clarification. The interruptions may result in a communication breakdown and frustrate the child's further attempts to communicate (Bliss, Covington, & McCabe, 1999).

Development of Morphology

The morphological development of children who speak AAE is similar to that of children who use MAE up to the age of 3 years (Blake, 1984; Stockman, 1986). By the age of 18 months, children in homes where AAE is used make one- and two-word utterances similar to those of children from homes where MAE is used (Blake, 1984; Steffersen, 1974; Stockman & Vaughn-Cooke, 1992). The morphological features of plural *-s,* possessive *'s,* past tense *-ed,* and third-person singular *-s* are acquired in the same pattern as in children using MAE. (See Chapter 1 for information on normal language development.) Similarly, the features marking tense, mood, aspect markers of the verb phrase, and negation develop in the later preschool years. At the age of 3 years, children from homes where AAE is used produce well-formed multiword constructions, simple declaratives, questions, and a few complex sentences. As the children develop through the preschool years, a variety of complex sentences including coordinated, subordinate, and relative clause sentences are used (Craig & Washington, 1994, 1995). Thus, in the preschool years, the morphological development of children in homes where AAE is used is similar to that of children in homes where MAE is used. Lack of the past tense marker (*-ed*), absence of possessive *'s*, and inflection of *be* are all common morphological features of AAE. Absence of plural *-s* marker (with nouns of measure such as numbers) has been noted as a salient feature in AAE as a means of reducing redundancy (Bland-Stewart, 2005).

The features that differ AAE from MAE involve the later-developing morphological forms. Forms used by speakers of AAE after the age of 5 years include the use of *at* in questions (e.g., "Where my shoes at?"); *go* as a copula (e.g., "There go my shoes"); deletion of *be* (e.g., "He working"). The use of other forms such as habitual *be* (e.g., "She be working"), and the use of *what* in embedded clauses (e.g., "He the one what ate it") also develop later in the preschool years.

Speakers who use African American English do not use all features of the dialect in all contexts. Some children use only a few features, whereas others use more. The patterns of variability for particular features have important implications for understanding the use of AAE. For example, a child may omit the copula in some contexts ("She a girl"), but use it in others ("Mary is a girl"). Wyatt (1995) reported that school-age children used more features of the dialect when talking to their age peers and when excited about the topic than when retelling a story or talking to their teacher. Failure to use the copula or any form when it is expected in both MAE and AAE may be an indicator of a communication disorder. It is important to consider the content and the context of the communication event to distinguish between morphology that is developing normally and that which may be disordered.

Language Disorders

The linguistic features of AAE can appear to be identical to symptoms that are found in children with language disorders. Utterances that feature noncontrastive elements of both MAE and AAE may be ambiguous and may draw concern over acceptability (Seymour, Roeper, deVilliers, & deVilliers, 2003). Differences in phonology and morphology as described above between AAE and MAE can be identified as a disorder in a child who does not use AAE. They can be identified as normal features of AAE when the child is actually exposed to AAE at home. For example, an 8-year-old child who uses /f/ for /θ/ may be thought to be using AAE when his home language is actually MAE. He might be considered to be developing normally, although he actually has a disorder (Seymour, Bland-Stewart, & Green, 1998). The same can be said for a child who appears to omit copula verb forms as used in AAE. Considering that AAE has some within-feature variability, a child who omits the copula verb forms may do so in one context and not another. Within-feature variability is governed by social and linguistic constraints that are intrinsic to AAE grammar (Seymour et al., 2003). The omission of the copula is frequently cited as a feature of AAE. However, research has shown that the omission of the copula by AAE speakers decreases between the ages of 5 and 7 years, and its use in younger children is dependent on the linguistic context (Wyatt, 1991). An older speaker of AAE who omits the copula may be considered to be developing normally when in actuality he may have a disorder. These differences can extend to pragmatics and semantic areas as well.

Differentiating between normal language development, the development of linguistic features of a dialect, and a language disorder requires considerable expertise. It may be more beneficial to focus on the features that are shared between MAE and AAE than to make distinctions between them in determining the presence of a disorder. Regardless of the use of a dialect, children with language disorders use fewer prepositions, articles, conjunctions, locatives *(here, there)*, complex sentences, and modals *(want, will, could, can)* than do children without disorders. However, there do not appear to be significant differences between MAE and AAE in the use of pronouns, present progressive verbs *(-ing)*, or demonstratives *(this, that, these, those)*. Determination of a language disorder in children who are thought to use AAE should focus on those forms that are shared between the two dialects, rather than on those that are different (ASHA, 2003; Seymour, Bland-Stewart, & Green, 1998). Contrastive analysis (Craig & Washington, 2000; McGregor, Williams, Hearst & Johnson, 1997; Seymour, Roeper, deVilliers & deVilliers, 2003) focuses on the nondialect features of languages to allow the distinction between dialect and disorders in speakers of African American English.

LANGUAGE DEVELOPMENT AND DISORDERS IN HISPANIC/LATINO CHILDREN

Development of Phonology

Spanish is the most common language other than English spoken in the United States. There are many dialects of Spanish spoken in the United States; however, the most common are southwestern (e.g., Mexican) and Caribbean (e.g., Puerto Rican and Cuban). Spanish phonology has 18 consonants, 4 semivowels, and 5 vowels, compared to 24 consonants, 3 semivowels, and 12 to 14 vowels in MAE. There are thus several English consonants that are not present in Spanish, including /v/, /w/, and /sh/. There are consonants in Spanish that are not present in English, such as the trilled /r/, the flap /rr/, and /ñ/. In addition, some Spanish consonants are not aspirated, giving the perception of a near-voiced sound for an unvoiced sound, such as *baber* for *paper* or *pad* for *pat*. Typically developing Spanish-speaking children use the dialect features of their community with mastery of the vowel system and most of the consonant system (Goldstein, 2001; Goldstein & Cintron, 2001). In spite of differences in the sounds of the language, the course of normal development of phonology in children learning Spanish parallels that of children learning English. Most researchers agree that by the age of 4 to 4.5 years children learning Spanish have mastered all consonant sounds except the liquids /j/, /l/, /ch/, /s/, /rr/, and sometimes /ñ/. By the age of 6 years, all of the later-developing sounds are learned (Acevedo, 1989; Eblen, 1982; Jimenez, 1987; Linares, 1982). According to Ambert (1986) and Kamhi, Hodson, Becker, Diamond, and Meza (1989), unintelligible 4-year-old children who use Spanish make the same types of errors in Spanish as unintelligible 4-year-old children using English, namely omitting, distorting, or reversing the order of sounds in words; shortening the length of words (i.e., *nana* for *banana*); and making sound errors primarily involving /s/, /r/, /l/, and /rr/. They also show reduction of consonant sequences (e.g., *epexo* for *espejo*), liquid deviation (e.g., *ádbol* for *árbol*), and stridency deletion (e.g., *lápi* for *lápiz*). These patterns are similar to those reported by Bleile and Wallach (1992), Stockman (1996), and Bland-Stewart (2003) for children learning AAE.

Morphological Development and Disorders

The development of Spanish morphology has been studied by several researchers (Echeverria, 1975; Gudemar, 1981; Keller, 1976; Merino, 1982, 1992; Paradis, 2005). Spanish is classified as a "pro-drop" language. This means that subjects do not need to be overtly marked if the referents are clear in context (Bedore & Leonard, 2001). Although they used different methods of investigation and different criteria for acceptance of the form being acquired, the age of acquisition of the various morphological forms differed by one or two years at the most. The studies indicated that children learning to use Spanish morphology acquire morphological forms at ages similar to those of children learning English. Similar to children learning English, children learning Spanish learn specific morphological forms in Spanish earlier than others. Present progressive verb form (-*ing*), plural (-*s*), and past tense verbs (-*ed*) are mastered before passives, subjunctives, and indirect objects. In addition, verbs must agree with their subject in person and number. Children learning Spanish learn plural forms and first- and second-person pronouns before the age of 2.5 years. Before the age of 3 years, they have learned present progressive, present indicative, simple preterit, present indicative, direct imperative, singular object nouns, third-person subject pronouns, and plural clitic pronouns. Before entry to school they have mastered complex forms involving tense and mood, similar to children learning English.

There are several differences between English and Spanish morphology. Because of these differences, it is challenging to make comparisons between all aspects of morphological development. The differences occur in noun and gender agreement and in linguistic complexity. The use of articles in Spanish is different from that in English. Spanish speakers must use the correct gender of the article for the noun that is to be expressed. For example, in English the article *the* is used to modify all nouns. In Spanish, the language learner must distinguish between masculine and feminine nouns so that the proper article can be used. For example, in the phrase "the red car" the child must learn that *car* is masculine and therefore takes a masculine article: "el carro rojo." If the noun is plural, the child must mark the plural on the article, the adjective, and the noun (e.g., "los carros rojos"). Children learning Spanish have difficulty with gender and number agreement as late as 6 years of age (Bedore & Leonard, 2001; Garcia, Maez, & Gonzalez, 1984). For example, gender of nouns and noun adjectives is marked in Spanish but not in English (e.g., "un niño cortés" versus "una niña cortĕsa"—a polite boy versus a polite girl). Children learning English do not have to learn the gender of nouns except when a pronoun is used (e.g., *she* is used for ships and *it* is used for other gender-neutral nouns). In Spanish, the adjective is placed after the noun, such as *The house big*. The adverb follows the verb, such as *He drives very fast his car*. Apostrophe *s* is not used to mark plural and possessives, such as *The boy ball is red* and *Juan car is fast*. Past tense is also not marked, such as *We walk yesterday*. Superiority is marked by using *más*, such as *the dog is more (más) big*.

Spanish-speaking children learning English have difficulties producing grammatical morphemes that mark tense, like the auxiliary verb and verb inflections with the exception of -*ing*. Omissions are generally made rather than substitutions. Because of

Table 12.3   **Morphological Contrasts between Mainstream American English (MAE) and Spanish-English**

	Spanish-English	MAE
Possession	"hat of my brother"	"my brother's hat"
Plural	"The boy are here."	"The boys are here."
Regular past	"I walk yesterday."	"I walked yesterday."
Third-person regular	"He run fast."	"He runs fast."
Negation	"He no eat."	"He does not eat."
Question inversion	"Carlos is coming?"	"Is Carlos coming?"

the morphological contrasts between Mainstream American English and Spanish, children learning English as a second language may be perceived as having a language disorder. Prior research indicates that Spanish-speaking children learning English as a second language are often mistaken as being language impaired (Paradis, 2005). It is also common for true disorders in Spanish to be taken as language differences rather than disorders. As seen in Table 12.3, differences in the order of morphological markers may be mistaken for language disorder. The differences involve, for example, the placement of noun modifiers, absence of plural noun markers, and placement of negation markers. These difficulties become even greater challenges when the child is learning English as a second language.

SECOND LANGUAGE ACQUISITION: BILINGUALISM OR MULTILINGUALISM

The terms *bilingual* or *multilingual* are defined by the level of competence a speaker has in two or more languages. A bilingual or multilingual speaker is one who has native or near-native language proficiency in two or more different languages. When a child is in an environment where two languages are used, the child is expected to develop two linguistic systems, with a gradual differentiation of the two occurring over time (Vihman, 1986). While the child is in the process of developing language, the two systems interact with each other and affect the acquisition of each language. The age of exposure to the languages affects the way the child will develop the languages.

Baetens Beardsmore (1986) identified two types of bilinguals: natural bilinguals and academic bilinguals. A *natural bilingual* is one who has learned the second language without any formal training. An *academic bilingual* is one who learns the second or third language through formal instruction, such as in an academic program. Natural bilinguals may be either simultaneous or successive second language learners. That is, the acquisition of two or more languages can occur either simultaneously or in succession.

Simultaneous bilingualism occurs when a child is exposed to two or more languages from the onset of the development of language, usually before the age of

3 years. Children learning two or more languages at the same time acquire both languages at the same rate, according to normal expectations (Patterson & Pearson, 2004). Although there may be some initial interference with syntactic organization, choice of lexical forms, or phonology, simultaneous bilingual learners are able to use both languages with equal proficiency with minimal interference between the languages. They are able to code switch (switch between the languages) depending on the language of their communication partner or the situation. Code switching may also occur when a concept is more accurately expressed in one language than the other (Brice & Rosa-Lugo, 2000). Code switching may come with a price, however. According to Price, Green, and von Studnitz (1999), the level of energy required to inhibit one language in order to excite another may result in processing delays.

Successive or sequential bilinguals are children who learn a single minority language from birth (L1) and begin to learn a second, majority language (L2) sometime during early childhood (Jia, Kohnert, Colladoo, & Aquino-Garcia, 2006; Kayser, 2002; Kohnert, 2002;). The forms learned in the second language are learned in an order similar to the forms learned in the first language. There is usually interference of the first language when the new language is being learned with variation in the rates and stages of language acquisition. Common influences include omission and overextension of morphological markers, double marking, and changes in the ordering of words or sentence components. In addition to the interference of one language with the other, the development and use of a second language may result in the loss of the first language or a slowing of development of the first language, particularly when the first language is not used at home. This may give the perception of language disorder or delay, since the child may not be using either language at the level expected. Clinicians may believe that the child has a disorder of delay because the first language is not well developed. It is thus very important to understand fully the history of the child with both languages in order to distinguish whether the difference from the expected level in either language is a result of the normal course of bilingual language development (Kohnert, 2002; Kohnert & Goldstein, 2005).

Internationally adopted children may be simultaneous bilinguals or sequential bilinguals or monolinguals, depending on the age of adoption, their prior experience with a language, and the use of the language in the adoption home (Glennen, 2002; Glennen & Masters, 2002). Bilingual children become proficient in the language that they use the most. Children may become more proficient in the second language as they progress through the school years. Studies involving lexical comprehension and production reveal that the second language emerges as the dominant language and outpaces the first language in skills by the teenage years (Kohnert & Bates, 2002). This shift in second language dominance occurs earlier for comprehension than for production, revealing that a clear notion of language dominance at critical stages of development cannot be ascertained. This gray area calls into question the practical implications of assessment materials used in both educational settings and clinical settings. Since most academic material and new concepts are presented in the second language the child may develop advanced proficiency in the second language while either not using the first language or using it only for social rather than academic purposes. Vocabulary, morphology, and syntax may become more advanced in the language used in the school than in the language used at home for social communication. This is particularly the case when the child decides not to use the home language at all in order to advance more rapidly in the language of the school. Any testing in the home language in these cases may not provide an accurate assessment of the child's true language ability.

Bilingualism and Language Disorders

When a child uses the school language as his primary language and development of proficiency in the first language, which may be the language of the home, slows or stops, the child may be misidentified as having a disorder in the first language. The child may be perceived as having a disorder in both the first and the second languages. The first language may not have developed beyond basic communication skills and may not be at the level expected for chronological age. The child may not have developed the language proficiency in the second language to be able to use the language for complex academic tasks. As children enter school and are expected to use language for literacy such as reading and writing, it is critical that they have a firm foundation in the ability to use complex language skills in a language. This is usually the language of the home.

Language proficiency for academic tasks must consider the cognitive level of the material being presented and the amount of contextual support available to the child to assist in understanding the material or activity (Cummins, 1984). Contextual support may be in the form of pictures and interactive, multimodal exposure to presentations to assist the child in putting the material into a frame of reference. A child learning a second language may require two to three years to achieve social proficiency in basic interpersonal communicative skills (BICS) in the second language. This includes learning vocabulary, morphology, syntax, and the pragmatic rules necessary to express ideas and thoughts and to understand the ideas and thoughts of others—to share information. It may take five to seven years to develop the language skills necessary for the cognitive tasks expected in the academic environment. Cognitive academic language proficiency (CALP) requires the child to use language to analyze, synthesize, and evaluate information in the academic curriculum in oral communication and in reading and writing. In the lower grades, textbooks and classroom activity provide support through extensive use of pictures and hands-on activities. As the child advances in the academic program, the amount of contextualized support is reduced. In upper grades the textbooks may not include pictures to support the text material. The material may refer to events in the past that are not subject to observation or hands-on activities. The child may be expected to generate the concept from verbally presented material in written format. Students may have the basic communication skills necessary for conversation or for understanding highly contextualized material, but they may not have the cognitive academic language skills to perform more complex abstract academic tasks expected in upper elementary and middle school grades. This may contribute to the very high failure rate of Hispanic youth in middle and secondary school (Langdon & Cheng, 1992).

The development of complex language skills in the first language is necessary while the child learns the basic forms in the second language. Failure to provide early academic instruction in reading and writing in the first language may result in language deficits throughout the academic program. Mercer (1987) and Damico, Oller, and Storey (1983) have suggested that certain indicators of learning disabilities may be characteristic of students in the process of learning a second language, including the following:

- a discrepancy between verbal and nonverbal performance measures on intelligence tests
- academic learning difficulty, particularly with the abstract concepts required in upper elementary and secondary grades
- inability to perceive and organize and remember information when such information is based on different experiences, different cultural values, or different linguistic backgrounds
- social and emotional difficulties related to difficulty in ability to communicate or to problems related to adjustment to a new culture and cultural expectations in a new academic environment
- the appearance of attention-deficit problems because of difficulty comprehending information presented
- delays in responding to questions, or silence or not responding, which may be the result of difficulty understanding the second language rather than a word-finding or expression problem

Nonlinguistic behaviors of second language learners or children from different cultures may also contribute to the identification of language disorders. Eye-contact behavior is culturally determined. Use of averted or indirect eye contact, while expected in some cultures, may give the appearance that the child is not paying attention in others. In some cultures it is considered disrespectful for a child or person in a subordinate position to establish or maintain eye contact with a superior or elder. In other cultures a more sustained direct eye contact may be perceived as defiance or disrespect. For example, looking a person in the eyes while talking or listening is considered to be very aggressive in Japan, where it is appropriate to look at a person's cheek, not at the eyes while in conversation. Second language/second culture children are sometimes perceived as being disorganized, lacking responsibility, arriving late or not using time wisely, or having difficulty changing activities. These behaviors can often be explained by cultural differences in the perception of time across cultures, difficulty adapting to a new culture, or failure to understand the directions, especially those given indirectly or using advanced syntactic structures.

A child learning a second language is often also learning a second culture. This is even more important if the child arrives in the new culture at an age when she is expected to enter the academic environment. Both the neighborhood culture and the school culture may be different from the environment of her first culture. In addition to learning the new language, the child must learn new rules for communicating, interacting, and learning in the new culture. The adjustment to the new culture may be further complicated by frequent trips back to the home country, when the child must shift again to the home culture and then shift back to the new culture, often in yet another new neighborhood and a new school. This may also lead to a perception of slower language development or a disorder. It thus becomes critical to obtain a full history of the child's opportunity to learn the new language before a diagnosis of language disorder can be made.

There are sociocultural factors that must be considered when determining that a second language learner has a language disorder or learning disability. Children in a new and different language environment frequently do not respond when spoken to or prefer to be alone. The child may be hesitant to speak with less than adequate language skills. When learning a second language and placed in a strange learning environment, the child may go through a silent period of three to six months during which he listens to the language and observes the behavior of others. This may be particularly true of children from cultures where they are encouraged to observe until they are competent to participate. Care must be taken to understand the social history, the cultural history, and the language history of the child, so that all factors affecting language development can be considered.

When the child is determined to have a language disorder, the clinical decisions for intervention are challenging. Most questions revolve around decisions about the appropriate language of instruction for a child whose primary language is not English. Should instruction be in the language of the home or in the language of the school? Current literature stresses the need to develop a firm language base in the child's first language before teaching a second language (Hamayan, 1992; Wong-Fillmore, 1991a, b). Teaching the language of the home allows the family to continue to be involved in the development of language. Once the language base is established in the first language, the child will more readily learn the second language. If the second language is begun before a firm base in language is established, the child may forever be delayed in the ability to develop the higher-level cognitive skills required for academic work and literacy.

Assessment of Language in Culturally and Linguistically Diverse Children

According to the Individuals with Disabilities Education Improvement Act (2004), all testing and evaluation procedures for the purpose of determining the presence of a disorder must be administered in a nondiscriminatory manner. To the extent possible, the testing and evaluation must be provided in the language or mode of communication with which the child is most proficient. The tests must accurately reflect the child's ability in the areas being tested rather than the child's impaired language or the child's proficiency with English. Finally, no single procedure may be used as the sole criterion for determining the presence of an impairment of the need for special education. The law does not require standardized measures, nor does it exclude subjective or qualitative measures. Speech-language pathologists are able to use a variety of assessment methods to determine the presence of a communication impairment and the need for special education.

It is essential that the assessment of language skills of culturally and linguistically diverse children distinguish between the opportunity to develop language, the use of language dialect, and a true disorder. To make this distinction, alternative assessment techniques must be used in addition to or in place of norm-referenced assessment techniques.

NORM-REFERENCED ASSESSMENT

Because language is a sociocultural phenomenon, the assessment of language abilities must occur in a sociocultural context. The language skills of children from culturally and linguistically diverse backgrounds are often assessed using tests and procedures that are not culturally relevant to their needs. There are few tests of language abilities that are not inherently biased against culturally and linguistically diverse backgrounds. Test taking itself is a cultural phenomenon and thus by its very nature is biased against children who do not have family backgrounds that frequently ask the child to perform or respond to an item out of context. For example, if a child does not have experience naming pictures in books, the child will not do well on a picture-naming task on a test. Likewise, if the child has little experience identifying pictures, telling stories, or describing pictures, the child will not do well on tests in those formats. These problems in assessment are in addition to the obvious ones of expecting the child to identify pictures, places, and events with which he has had limited experience.

Most formal standardized norm-referenced language tests are biased against children from culturally and linguistically diverse backgrounds because they are not included in the normative sample. Although some tests may indicate that the test was standardized on a representative sample of the population of the United States, there is no assurance that the child being tested is "representative" of children in the United States. The bias of vocabulary tests against children from culturally and linguistically diverse backgrounds has been well documented in the literature (see Scarborough, 2001, for a comprehensive review). Champion, Hyter, McCabe, and Bland-Stewart (2003) showed that even though the widely used Peabody Picture Vocabulary Test (Dunn & Dunn, 1997) included a representative sample of minority children in the standardization group, an item analysis showed that few items were missed by most of the 3- to 5-year-old African American children in their study group. Instead, their performance was reflective of socioeconomic and ethnic patterns of vocabulary usage and word knowledge based on their cultural experiences and language use in their communities as expressed by Stockman (2000).

Each child has unique cultural and language experiences different from any other child and cannot be assumed to be represented in the sample in sufficient manner for the data to serve as a comparative baseline of normal behavior for the child. Every formal standardized test score obtained on a child from a culturally and linguistically diverse background must be considered suspect. The question must be asked whether the child had the opportunity to develop the skills being tested, whether the child had experience with the format of the test or the items used in the assessment, and whether the child had opportunity to be exposed to the content of the test at the level of children in the standardization sample.

Vaughn-Cooke (1983) and Musselwhite (1983) present several questions that may be useful in evaluating whether norm-referenced assessment instruments are appropriate for children from culturally and linguistically diverse families.

1. Has the child had the opportunity to become familiar with the underlying assumptions in the format of the test?
2. Is the child represented in the normative sample in a meaningful way?

3. Has the child had experience with the content of the test at a level similar to children in the standardization sample?
4. Has the child had an opportunity to learn the content of the test similar to that of children in the standardization sample?
5. Does the test allow a reliable determination of whether the child is developing normally in the child's own linguistic and cultural community?
6. Can the test distinguish between normal development, dialectal differences, and disorders?
7. Does the test provide an opportunity for the child to express ideas without structural constraints on form?
8. Does the test allow the child to demonstrate understanding of an idea or concept in alternative ways with alternative linguistic formats?
9. Does the format of the test include an opportunity to obtain a sample of the child's spontaneous language?
10. Can the test provide an adequate description of the child's language ability as an integrated whole?

If the answer to any of these questions is "no," the test should not be used as a valid indicator of the child's ability to understand and use language. It should not be used to make educational judgments about the presence of a disorder or the need for special education or related services. If the test is used, the report of the results should carry a disclaimer about the interpretation of the validity of results.

There are several commercial norm-referenced tests that have been translated into Spanish. Caution must be taken when using these tests with children who speak Spanish. First, unless the test giver is fluent in the language of the test, the pronunciation of items in the test protocol may be incorrect. Translations do not usually take into account the opportunity of the child to be exposed to the cultural and linguistic items on the test in the same manner or at the same level as children in the English version of the test. They usually do not take into account regional differences in vocabulary or pronunciation of test items.

Two widely used English norm-referenced tests have been developed for use with children who speak Spanish. The *Clinical Evaluation of Language Function-4 Spanish* (CELF-4 SP) (Secord, Wiig, & Semel, 2006) and the *Preschool Language Scale-4 Spanish* (PLS-4SP) (Zimmerman, Steiner, & Pond, 2002) have been developed using the basic construct of the English versions; however, they are not translations. They have been developed based on the Spanish cultural experiences appropriate to the age of the child and include alternate vocabulary for regional differences. Because the tests have different components, test tasks, and scaling and research design, scores on the Spanish versions of these tests cannot be compared with the English versions. The Test of Phonological Awareness in Spanish (TAPAS) (Riccio, Imhoff, Hasbruck, & Davis 2004) was developed using a large sample of children who speak Spanish in several regions of the country.

The literature has suggestions for using standardized tests with culturally and linguistically diverse children (Roseberry-McKibbon, 2007, 2008; Wyatt, 2002). The suggestions usually include extending the time limits for the test and allowing the child more time to respond to items, rewording or providing additional explanations for instructions, providing additional practice items, allowing the child to explain incorrect answers, and continuing to test beyond the usual ceiling.

When altering the administration of a standardized test, several precautions must be taken. The primary consideration, before the test can be administered even with alterations, is the appropriateness of the test format, test content, and mode of responding of the test. If these factors are not considered, then no alteration in test administration can render the test valid. The normative scores cannot be used because the test was not administered in the standardized manner. When any alteration in the test format is used, the test scores cannot be used in interpretation or represented or interpreted as valid indicators of the child's language ability. There must be a record of the alterations that were made in the formal report.

Because of the limitations of verbal standardized tests, culturally and linguistically diverse children are often assessed using nonverbal assessments (Hamayan & Damico, 1991). Although nonverbal tests do not require verbal ability, there are cultural variables that may affect the child's performance on these tests as well. Nonverbal aspects of assessment including perception and use of time, display learning, competitiveness, and sociolinguistic dimensions such as cross-racial relationships between the child and the adult may also affect the child's ability to perform on nonverbal tests.

ALTERNATE ASSESSMENT TECHNIQUES

Because of the limitations of norm-referenced assessment procedures with culturally and linguistically diverse children, alternate assessment techniques offer an opportunity to obtain a clearer distinction between language development and language disorder.

Criterion-Referenced Assessment

Criterion-referenced assessment allows the "comparison of a child's performance on a specific skill, grammatical structure or linguistic concept to an independently predetermined criteria" (Laing & Kamhi, 2003, p. 46.) Criterion-referenced assessment is usually more appropriate than norm-referenced assessment for determining the presence of a language disorder in culturally and linguistically diverse children because it allows a description of the child's performance on specific, independently defined criteria rather than comparison against an artificially established and culturally irrelevant group. The assessment results are interpreted by comparison against predetermined criteria rather than against norm-based scores (Scriven, 1991). Criterion-referenced assessment has limitations in defining the specific criteria that should be used; however, it is far superior to norm-referenced testing because it allows for full consideration of the child's cultural and linguistic background.

There are few assessment instruments that have been developed to provide criterion-referenced assessment of language development with consideration of the linguistic and cultural variation in children. The *Developmental Evaluation of Language Variation* (DELV) (Seymour, Roeper, deVilliers, & deVilliers, 2001) was developed to distinguish variations due to normal developmental changes and to regional and cultural patterns of language difference from the markers of language disorder or delay. The assessment which is appropriate for children aged 4 to 9 years provides criteria in the areas of pragmatics, syntax, semantics, and phonology which are noncontrastive across language dialects and is thus appropriate for language assessment of all children.

Ethnographic Assessment

Ethnography is the qualitative study of culture often used in the study of language and communication in societies (Ochs & Schieffelin, 1995). Ethnographic assessment techniques are also very important in assessing children from culturally and linguistically diverse backgrounds (Westby, 1990). The ethnographic techniques consider the experiences of the child and family as members of their society as the focal point of the assessment rather than on individual performance within cultural and language contexts different from that of the child or family. It is very important to consider that the socioeconomic status of immigrant children may be very different from their former status both economically and socially in their home country. While they may have had opportunities to learn through language enrichment in their home country, they may not have had a similar opportunity in their new country. They may also have had just the reverse, depending on the situation. By using open-ended questions rather than dichotomous questions that require a certain response, an ethnographic approach allows the client and the family to describe their experiences, their daily activities, and the objects and people in their lives without the constraints placed on them by more formal norm-referenced or criterion-referenced techniques. Parents have been shown to be able to give valid reports of the vocabulary and syntax of their children in both English and Spanish (Thal, Jackson-Maldonado, & Acosta, 2000; Thal, O'Hanlon, Clemmons, & Fralin, 1999). Their understanding of their child's ability to communicate at home should be considered as an important and valid contribution to the assessment.

Criterion-referenced assessment should include a family-centered ethnographic interview and an analysis of the child's speech and communication skills in natural contexts. It involves the triangulation of cultural, linguistic, and experiential factors of communication. It considers the social context in which communication occurs and how language is used in a particular culture to share knowledge and establish order (Cheng, 1990; Crago & Cole, 1991). The family-centered ethnographic interview allows the evaluator to consider the environmental influences on the development of language in the home and the perception of the child's communication competence by the family (Westby, 1990). The family-centered interview allows investigation of the child's communication with age peers, siblings, and adult communication partners against the background of the familiar social context. Items addressed in a family-centered ethnographic interview include the following:

1. What language(s) do the parents use in speaking to the child?
2. What language(s) do the parents use in speaking to each other?
3. What language does the child use in speaking to age peers? Adults?
4. How does the child express needs to the primary caretakers at home?
5. Does the child initiate conversations at home? With whom?
6. How does the child interact with the caretakers? With age peers? With siblings?
7. What is the parent's perception of the child's language ability?
8. Do members of the family understand the child?

9. Do other children use language with the child in the same manner that they do with his age peers?
10. Does the child understand language and instructions at home as expected for her age?
11. Does the family communicate to the child with gestures or simplified speech as compared to the child's age peers?
12. Is the child interested in objects and toys at the level expected in his home and by his cultural age peers?

The following guidelines can be used to conduct a criterion-referenced ethnographic assessment.

- Interview members of the family to collect information on the child's language skills in the home environment and the family's perception of his or her overall development.
- Obtain information concerning the child's language history, including the opportunity to learn the language of the home and community and to participate in language-enrichment experiences.
- Observe and describe the child's use of language in conversation with familiar partners, with familiar objects, and in familiar situations.
- Observe the child over time in different contexts with different communication partners.
- Interact with the child, considering the child's frame of reference, life experiences, and familiarity with unfamiliar communication partners.
- Observe the child's attempts to communicate and to problem solve in familiar and unfamiliar situations.
- Collect narrative samples using books, pictures, toys, and objects that are familiar to the child and that have low cognitive demand.

Dynamic Assessment

Despite the use of criterion-referenced assessment and other "nonbiased assessments," many children from culturally and linguistically different backgrounds have not had an opportunity to learn the mode of assessment nor the content of the assessment materials. As a result they are often misdiagnosed as children with a disability. Dynamic assessment is an assessment approach that focuses on the ability of the child to learn rather than what the child has had an opportunity to learn. Dynamic assessment is most often a pretest–intervention–posttest format. The clinician actively intervenes during the course of the assessment with the goal of intentionally inducing changes in the child's performance in the area being assessed. During the dynamic assessment, the clinician provides a mediated learning experience (MLE) to facilitate the child's learning of the concept expected for the assessment. The clinician focuses on the child's processes of problem solving and attempts to communicate. The clinician gains information about the client's responsiveness to intervention attempts and information on what intervention strategies promoted a change in the speech-language behavior being assessed.

Dynamic assessment (DA) has been advocated as an alternative or supplemental approach to traditional standardized testing with children who are culturally and linguistically diverse (Guitérrez-Clellen & Peña, 2001; Peña, 2000; Peña, Iglesias & Lidz, 2001). Peña, Igleias, and Lidz (2001), in a study of word-learning ability by Latino and African American children in a bilingual Head Start program for preschool children found that the children with typical language development benefited the most from a short-term intervention within a dynamic assessment framework. The children made significant gains from pretest scores on assessment tests that required labeling. The intervention from the dynamic assessment showed that the children had normal capacity to learn language and were thus not identified as having a language disorder from low performances on tests requiring labeling, such as the Expressive One-Word Vocabulary Test (Gardner, 1990). Modifiability, or responsiveness to intervention during the assessment process, is especially important for children from diverse cultural and linguistic backgrounds. The clinician can make judgments about the child response to the intervention by observing the time, amount of input, and type of instructional strategies it took for the child to learn the intervention target. This information can be compared with that obtained from children of similar cultural and linguistic background and language history to determine the presence of an impairment.

The assessment of language in culturally and linguistically diverse children should be comprehensive and dynamic, including child-centered free play language sample analyses with included mean length of communication units (MLCU), frequencies of complex syntax, numbers of different words, measures of language comprehension, responses to requests for information in the form of *wh*-questions, and responses to probes of active and passive sentence constructions (Craig & Washington, 2000; Gilliam & Peña, 2004; Guitérrez-Clellen & Peña, 2001).

Language Sample

A language sample is an opportunity to observe the child's use of language in natural contexts without the constraints of either norm-referenced or criterion-referenced assessment techniques. A language sample should be collected through observation of the child in multiple contexts and with multiple communication partners in environments that are familiar to the child, with objects that are culturally relevant and familiar to the child. Cheng (1990) suggests collecting the language sample using several different tasks, including relating past events, describing objects, describing pictures, retelling culturally familiar stories, asking for assistance, or other tasks that are appropriate for the child's age and level of language development. The sample should be analyzed using criteria established for the phonology, syntax, morphology, and pragmatics of the child's language and dialect. Because language parameters differ in various languages, analysis should consider normal development in the child's language and dialect and the child's language history. A recently available reference, the *International Guide to Speech Acquisition* (McLeod, 2007), provides a summary of the major developmental factors in thirty-five languages other than English, an invaluable aid in understanding the language development of children from various linguistic backgrounds.

Determining the Existence of a Language Disorder versus Language Development

The following criteria can be used as a guide in determining the existence of a language disorder within the parameters established for the culture and linguistic environment of the child:

- rarely initiates verbal interactions or activities with peers or family members
- does not respond verbally when verbal interactions are initiated by peers or family members
- has difficulty using language at the level used by age peers of the same cultural and linguistic background
- has a smaller vocabulary than expected for age, regardless of the language used
- uses shorter, less complex sentences than would be expected by age
- has difficulty communicating verbally with parents or cultural and linguistic age peers
- relies heavily on gestures and nonverbal means to communicate
- requires frequent repetition and rephrasing of instructions by parents and language peers
- is inordinately slow in responding to questions or instructions
- has difficulty with the noncontrastive elements of language form
- rarely has opportunity for peer-initiated verbal exchanges or only with a notably lower level of verbal communication with the child than with age peers
- has difficulty being understandable to peers
- does not attempt to repair communication failures
- does not comment on the actions of others or express feelings verbally
- does not take turns or maintain conversations with peers
- does not ask for clarification or assistance verbally
- uses false starts, self-interruptions, or revisions
- makes frequent use of *it, thing, this,* or *that*
- does not learn new concepts or vocabulary or forgets material assumed to be learned (Kayser, 1990; Mattes & Omark, 1991)

Combining a comprehensive review of the child's language history and life experiences, observation of the child's use of language, an ethnographic interview with the family, and criterion-referenced and dynamic assessment, the speech-language pathologist can make a judgment about the presence or absence of a speech-language disorder. Information gathered in multiple ways in multiple contexts can provide a comprehensive picture of the child in order to better understand his or her language status. These procedures may also influence recommendations for management.

Using Interpreters in Assessment

When the clinical service provider does not have native or near-native proficiency in the language of the child or the family, it is difficult to make judgments about the language proficiency of the child. In these cases the service provider should seek the services of an interpreter to assist in assessment and possible intervention. According to ASHA (1985), the interpreter must be trained in speech-language development and must be trained to work with families and children. The interpreter should be familiar with the language, dialect, and culture of the child and family and should be able to assist the service provider in selecting the appropriate assessment techniques and materials considering the culture of the child and family. Besides being able to interpret the speech and language of the child and parents, the interpreter should also be a cultural informant able to provide guidance on other phenomena affecting the situation. Assessment should be performed to determine both the social and academic language abilities of the child. Social language proficiency may develop within the first three years, while academic language proficiency may take an additional five years (ASHA, 2000). The trained interpreter/ translator can also be used to report results of the assessment to the family.

The clinician should discuss with the interpreter the items and questions to be used in the assessment in advance of the session to determine their cultural appropriateness. The interpreter should be instructed in advance to provide a translation and an interpretation of the meanings and feelings expressed by the client. During the session the interpreter should also be able to alert the clinician to any verbal and nonverbal cues that may be misunderstood and thus affect the interaction. After the session, the interpreter and the service provider should debrief to determine whether there were any verbal or nonverbal issues that were particularly relevant to the session.

Language Intervention in Culturally and Linguistically Diverse Children

Appropriate language intervention is challenging for any clinician. Providing appropriate intervention for culturally and linguistically diverse children with language disorders is particularly challenging. Many clinicians use a normative or developmental approach to intervention. Because the developmental norms may not be appropriate for the culture and language of the child, it may be more appropriate to use a functional approach to intervention. Using the International Classification of Functioning (ICF) Model (WHO, 2001), intervention should help the child participate in the activities needed in the primary environment in which he or she will function. These include learning and applying knowledge for listening, reading, and thinking; communication in the environments important to daily functioning, such as home and school; and interpersonal interactions and relationships including both home and school. Emphasis should be placed on teaching function and the use of language and semantics before emphasis on form. Stress should be given to helping the child develop a means of communicating from the level where he is and building according to individual need.

There is considerable concern about the language of intervention with children who are monolingual in a language other than English or are English language learners (ELLs). The language of intervention is particularly challenging for monolingual clinicians, or for clinicians who do not speak the language of the child and family. It is critical for children learning a language to have a firm foundation of oral language before transitioning to print or written language. This is especially important for children learning English prior to entry to school. Intervention should be presented in the child's first language until a firm foundation in language is established. The child must develop basic interpersonal communication skills (BICS) in a first language before a second language is introduced. The child then can make advances toward cognitive academic language proficiency (CALP) to achieve academic success (Cummins, 1992, 2000). There may be as much as a two-year discrepancy between the child's interpersonal skills and the child's abilities to function academically. It is essential that the child have proficiency in the BICS of the first language prior to attempting to succeed in an academic environment using a language the child is learning.

Intervention must be at the level of the child's cognitive and linguistic level. The child must be able to function in a language environment with highly embedded concrete context and familiar environment and social constraints and progress in stages to where the context is progressively more abstract and cognitively more demanding. Intervention must begin at the child's level in the primary language and progress to the language expected for his age peers. The language intervention should be additive, or in addition to the primary language, rather than eliminating or reducing the primary language.

In creating a culturally appropriate intervention process, the clinician should establish a collaborative relationship with the family within their cultural boundaries. There are cultural differences in the families' perception of the extent of their role in intervention. Some families expect the clinician to be the teacher while they just observe. Others welcome the opportunity to be fully involved in the intervention program. In developing an intervention plan, it is critical to incorporate practices that are culturally comfortable for the family. Intervention goals, objectives, and anticipated outcomes should be consistent with the concerns, priorities, and expectations of the family. Intervention materials should be based on experiences and situations that are familiar to the child and family and that will be functional in the child's life. Familiar concepts of family, housing, foods, art, music, dress, religious experiences, and cultural holidays and celebrations should be appropriate to the child and family. When the familiar base is established and coded in the language of the child, new experiences can be added to enrich the language used.

Roseberry-McKibbon (2007) provides the following useful guidelines for matching intervention to second-language acquisition and intervention:

- Focus on comprehension of basic routines, especially for school-aged children.
- Focus on yes-no responses and progress to one- or two-word responses in routines.
- Focus on vocabulary and on labeling items that are functional in the environment.
- Use visualization, copying, and drawing.
- Engage the child in basic literacy skills appropriate to their academic level.

The following suggestions are useful in guiding clinical intervention for children with communication disorders from culturally and linguistically diverse populations.

1. View each clinical interaction as a socially situated communicative event that is influenced by the rules of culture and language of both the clinician and the client.
2. Present clear explanations of objectives, goals, and expected outcomes using language, concepts, and cultural values that are appropriate and understood by the family.
3. Adapt materials and experiences to the client's individual needs and the life experiences of the child.
4. Preview materials and strategies to be used to determine whether they are culturally relevant and appropriate.
5. Review the lessons to determine whether the child's inability to acquire the concepts could be explained by cultural or linguistic factors.
6. Incorporate content from the child's culture while helping the child learn new concepts; review and expand familiar structures and concepts with new experiences.

7. Present materials and information using timing, pacing, and manner of communication appropriate for the culture. Expect responses according to those expected in the child's culture and language.
8. Use speech and language appropriate for the child's level of comprehension. Repeat and rephrase instructions to increase the likelihood that the instruction or concept is understood.
9. Use multiple modes to support the language being developed.
10. Use small-group sessions of age peers to encourage supportive, cooperative interactions along with individual sessions to teach particular skills and functions.

Summary

More than three decades of research on the acquisition of language and language disorders in culturally and linguistically diverse children has resulted in increased understanding of the complexity of the issue. The more we come to understand about the great diversity among and between children and groups of people, the more we see what we do not know. While we have learned much about the language development of children from European American middle-class homes, we have yet to understand all we need to know about differential diagnoses of children from other cultures, other socioeconomic groups, those who speak another language or dialect, and those who live in different cultures. As we learn, diversity in the United States continues to increase at remarkable rates, such that soon there will be no minority or majority culture. The clinical skills necessary to provide appropriate clinical service and education to children with disorders and to assist them in the development of language will provide challenges and opportunities for new discoveries for years to come.

The International Classification of Functioning, Disability, and Health (ICF) (WHO, 2001) identifies several important components to understanding disability—body function, body structures, ability to participate in activities, environmental, and personal factors. All of the components are related to language development and disorders in children of different cultural and linguistic backgrounds. Consideration of the family understanding of impairment, consideration of the family's social and educational context, and the language history of the child and family are necessary considerations in determining the limitations and expectations of all children, especially those from culturally and linguistically different backgrounds.

Study Questions

1. What is the responsibility of the monolingual English-speaking speech-language pathologist in providing clinical service to a monolingual Spanish-speaking child and family? How can the speech-language pathologist work with other members of the educational team to assist the child in learning language?

2. What resources can the speech-language pathologist use to assist with providing culturally and linguistically relevant clinical services to a culturally and linguistically different child with a speech-language disorder?

3. What resources are available in your area to help you understand the culture and language of the children and families likely to require clinical services?

4. What opportunities are there for continuing education to prepare speech-language pathologists for serving culturally and linguistically diverse children and families?

5. What is the ethical responsibility of the speech-language pathologist in providing clinical services for a culturally and linguistically diverse child and family with a language disorder?

References

Acevedo, M. (1989, November). Typical speech misarticulations of Mexican-American preschoolers. Paper presented at the annual meeting of the American-Speech-Language-Hearing Association, St. Louis, MO.

Ambert, A. (1986). Identifying language disorders in Spanish speakers. In A. C. Willig & H. F. Baetens-Beardsmore (Eds.), *Bilingualism: Basic principles* (2nd ed.). San Diego, CA: College Hill.

American Speech-Language-Hearing Association. (1983). Position paper on social dialects. *ASHA, 25*(9), 23–24.

American Speech-Language-Hearing Association. (1985). Clinical management of communicatively handicapped minority language populations. *ASHA, 27*(6), 29–32.

American Speech-Language-Hearing Association. (2000). *Guidelines for the roles and responsibilities of school-based speech-language pathologist.* Rockville, MD: Author.

American Speech-Language Hearing Association. (2003). American English Dialects. [Technical Report], *ASHA Supplement 23*, pp. 45–46.

American Speech-Language-Hearing Association. (2008). Incidence and prevalence of communication disorders and hearing loss in children. Retrieved April 2, 2008, from www.asha.org/members/research/reports/children.htm.

Baetens Beardsmore, H. (1986). *Bilingualism: Basic principles* (2nd ed.). Clevedon, UK: Tieto.

Bedore, L., & Leonard, L. (2001). Grammatical morphology deficits in Spanish speaking children with SLI. *Journal of Speech Language Hearing Research 44*(4), 905–924.

Blake, I. (1984). Language development in working class black children: An examination of form, content and use. Doctoral dissertation, Columbia University, New York.

Bland-Stewart, L. (2003). Phonetic inventories and phonological patterns of African American two-year-olds: A preliminary investigation. *Communications Disorders Quarterly, 24*(3), 109–120.

Bland-Stewart, L. M. (2005, May 3). Difference or deficit in speakers of African American English: What every clinician should know . . . and do. *The ASHA Leader,* 6–7, 30–31.

Bleile, K., & Wallach, H. (1992). A sociolinguistic investigation of the speech of African American preschoolers. *American Journal of Speech Language Pathology 1*(2), 54–62.

Bliss, L. S., Covington, Z., & McCabe, A. (1999). Assessing the narratives of African American children. *Contemporary Issues in Communication Sciences and Disorders, 26,* 160–167.

Bloom, M., & Lahey, M. (1978). *Language development and disorders.* New York: Wiley.

Brice, A., & Rosa-Lugo, L. T. (2000). Code switching: A bridge or barrier between two languages? *Multiple Voices for Ethnically Diverse Exceptional Learners, 4*(1), 1–12.

Bridgeforth, C. (1984). The development of language functions among black children from working class families. Paper presented at the presession of the 35th Annual Georgetown University Round Table on Language and Linguistics, Washington, DC.

Brown, R. (1973). *A first language, the early stages.* Cambridge, MA: Harvard University Press.

Campbell, L. (1994). Discourse diversity and Black English vernacular. In D. Ripich & N. Creaghead (Eds.), *School discourse problems* (pp. 93–131). San Diego, CA: Singular.

Champion, T., Hyter, Y., McCabe, A., & Bland-Stewart, L. (2003). "A Matter of Vocabulary": Performances of low-income African American Headstart children on the Peabody Picture Vocabulary Test-III. *Communication Disorders Quarterly, 24*(3), 121–127.

Champion, T., Seymour, H., & Camarata, S. (1995). Narrative discourse in African American children. *Journal of Narrative and Life History, 5,* 333–352.

Chen, P. (1999). *Modern Chinese: History and Sociolinguistics* (pp. 50–53). New York: Cambridge University Press.

Cheng, L. L. (1990). Identification of communicative disorders in Asian-Pacific students. *Journal of Childhood Communication Disorders, 13*(1), 113–119.

Cole, L. (1980). A development analysis of social dialect features in the spontaneous language of preschool black children. Doctoral dissertation, Northwestern University, Evanston, IL.

Crago, M. B. (1992). Ethnography and language socialization: A cross-cultural perspective. *Topics in Language Disorders, 12*(3), 28–39.

Crago, M. B., & Cole, E. (1991). Using ethnography to bring children's communicative and cultural words into focus. In T. M. Gallagher (Ed.), *Pragmatics of language: Clinical practice issues* (pp. 99–132). San Diego, CA: Singular.

Craig, H., & Washington, J. A. (1994). The complex syntax skills of poor, urban, African-American preschoolers at school entry. *Language, Speech, and Hearing Services in Schools, 25*(2), 181–190.

Craig, H., & Washington, J. A. (1995). African-American English and linguistic complexity in preschool discourse: A second look. *Language, Speech, and Hearing Services in Schools, 26*(1), 87–93.

Craig, H. K., Thompson, C. A., Washington, J. A., & Potter, S. L. (2003). Phonological features of child African American English. *Journal of Speech, Language, and Hearing Research, 46*(3), 623–635.

Craig, H. K., & Washington, J. A. (2000). An assessment battery for identifying language impairments in African American children. *Journal of Speech, Language, and Hearing Research, 43*(2) 366–379.

Craig, H. K., & Washington, J. A. (2002). Oral language expectations for African American preschoolers and kindergartens. *American Journal of Speech-Language Pathology, 11*(1), 59–70.

Craig, H. K., & Washington, J. A. (2004). Grade related changes in the production of African American English. *Journal of Speech, Language, and Hearing Research, 47,* 450–43.

Cummins, J. (1984). *Bilingualism and special education.* San Diego, CA: College-Hill.

Cummins, J. (1992). The role of primary language development in promoting educational success or language minority students. In C. Leyba (Ed.), *Schooling and language minority children: A theoretical framework* (pp. 3–50). Los Angeles, CA: California State University, Los Angeles.

Cummins, J. (2000). *Language, power and pedagogy: Bilingual children in the crossfire.* Clevedon, England: Multicultural Matters.

Damico, J. S., Oller, J. W., & Storey, M. E. (1983). The diagnosis of language disorders in bilingual children: Surface-oriented and pragmatic criteria. *Journal of Speech and Hearing Disorders, 46,* 385–394.

Davis, P., Williams, J., & Vaughn-Cooke, F. (1992–1993). A comparison of lexical development in a child with normal language development and in a child with language delay. *National Student Speech-Language-Hearing Association Journal, 20,* 63–77.

Department of Homeland Security, Office of Immigration Statistics. (2005). *Yearbook of immigration statistics: 2005.* Washington, DC: Author.

Dillard, J. (1972). *Black English: Its history and usage.* New York: Random House.

Dunn, L. M., & Dunn, L. M. (1997). Peabody Picture Vocabulary Test III. Circle Pines, MN: American Guidance Service.

Eblen, R. E. (1982). A study of the acquisition of fricatives by 3 year old children learning Mexican Spanish. *Language and Speech, 25,* 201–220.

Echeverria, M. (1975). Late stages in the acquisition of Spanish syntax. Doctoral dissertation, University of Washington, Seattle.

Fiestas, C. E., & Peña, E. D. (2004). Narrative discourse in bilingual children: Language and task effects. *Language, Speech, and Hearing Services in Schools, 35*(3), 155–168.

Garcia, E. E., Maez, L. F., & Gonzalez, G. (1984). *A national study of Spanish/English bilingualism in young Hispanic children of the United States.* Los Angeles: California State University, National Dissemination and Assessment Center.

Gardner, M. F. (1990). *Expressive One-Word Picture Vocabulary Test.* Novato, CA: Academic Therapy Publications.

Gee, J. P. (1989). Two styles of narrative construction and their linguistic and educational implications. *Discourse Processes, 12,* 287–307.

Gillam, R. B. & Peña, E. D. (2004). Dynamic assessment of children from culturally diverse backgrounds. *Newsletter of the ASHA Special Interest Division 1: Perspectives on Language, Learning and Education, 11*(2), 2–5.

Glennen, S. (2002). Language development and delay in internationally adopted infants and toddlers: A review. *American Journal of Speech Language Pathology, 11,* 333–339.

Glennen, S., & Masters, G. (2002). Typical and atypical language development in infants and toddlers adopted from East-Europe. *America Journal of Speech-Language Pathology, 11,* 417–433.

Goldstein, B. (2001). Assessing phonological skills in Hispanic/Latino children. *Seminars in Speech and Language, 22,* 39–49.

Goldstein, B., & Cintron, P. (2001). An investigation of phonlogical skills in Puerto Rican Spanish-speaking 2-year-olds. *Clinical Linguistic and Phonetics, 15,* 343–361.

Gudeman, R. H. (1981). Learning Spanish: A cross-sectional study of imitation, comprehension and production of Spanish grammatical forms by rural Panamanians. Doctoral dissertation, University of Minnesota, Minneapolis.

Gutiérrez-Clellen, V., & Quinn, R. (1993). Assessing narratives of children from diverse cultural/linguistic groups. *Language, Speech, and Hearing Services in Schools, 24*(1), 2–9.

Gutiérrez-Clellen, V. F., & Peña, E. (2001). Dynamic assessment of diverse children: A tutorial. *Language, Speech, and Hearing Services in Schools, 32*(4), 212–224.

Hall, W., Nagy, W., & Linn, R. (1984). *Spoken words: Effects of stimulation and social group on oral word usage and frequency.* Hillsdale, NJ: Erlbaum.

Hamayan, E. (1992, September). Meeting the challenge of cultural and linguistic diversity in the schools: Best practices in language intervention. Paper presented at the Broward County Exceptional Student Education In-Service, Ft. Lauderdale, FL.

Hamayan, E. V., & Damico, J. S. (1991). *Limiting bias in the assessment of bilingual students.* Austin, TX: Pro-Ed.

Hammer, C. S., & Weiss, A. L. (2000). African American mothers' views of their infants' language development and language-learning environment. *American Journal of Speech-Language Pathology, 9,* 126–140.

Harris, G. (1998). American Indian culture: A lesson in diversity. In D. Battle (Ed.), *Communication disorders in multicultural populations* (pp. 78–113). Newton, MA: Butterworth-Heinemann.

Hart, B., & Risley, T. (1995). *Meaningful differences in the everyday experiences of young American children.* Baltimore: Paul H. Brookes.

Heath, S. B. (1983). Sociocultural contexts of language development. In *Beyond Language.* Los Angeles: Evaluation, Dissemination and Assessment Center.

Heath, S. B. (1986). Taking a cross cultural look at narratives. *Topics in Language Disorders, 7*(1), 84–89.

Hester, E., & Westby, C. (1996). Using oral narratives to assess communicative competence. In A. G. Kamhi, *Communication disorders in African American children: Research, assessment and intervention* (pp. 227–245). Baltimore: Paul H. Brookes.

Hyon, S., & Sulzby, L. (1994). Black kindergarteners' spoken narratives: Style, structure and task. *Linguistics and Education, 6*(2), 121–152.

Individuals with Disabilities Education Improvement Act of 2004 (IDEA 2004). Public Law 108-446, Stat. 2647 (December 3, 2004).

Jia, G., Kohnert, K., Collado, J., & Aquino-Garcia (2006). *Journal of Speech, Language, and Hearing Research, 49*(3), 588–602.

Jimenez, B. C. (1987). Acquisition of Spanish consonants in children aged 3–5 years. *Language, Speech, and Hearing Services in Schools, 18*(4), 357–363.

Johnson, J. R., & Wong, M.-Y. A. (2002). Cultural differences in beliefs and practices concerning talk to children. *Journal of Speech, Language, and Hearing Research, 45*(5), 916–926.

Kamhi, A. G., Hodson, B., Becker, M., Diamond, F., & Meza, P. (1989). Phonological analysis of unintelligible children's utterances: English and Spanish. In *Occasional papers on linguistics: The uses of phonology.* Carbondale: Southern Illinois University Press.

Kayser, H. (1990). Social communicative behaviors of language-disordered Mexican-American students. *Child Language Teaching Therapy, 6*(3), 255–269.

Kayser, H. (1998). Hispanic cultures and language. In D. E. Battle (Ed.), *Communication disorders in multicultural populations* (2nd ed., pp. 157–196). Boston: Butterworth-Heinemann.

Kayser, H. (2002). Bilingual language development and disorders. In D. E. Battle (Ed.), *Communication disorders in multicultural populations* (3rd ed., pp. 205–232) Woburn, MA: Butterworth-Heinemann.

Keller, G. (1976). Acquisition of the English and Spanish passive voices among bilingual children. In G. D. Keller, R. V. Teschner, & S. Viera (Eds.), *Bilingualism in the bicentennial and beyond* (pp. 161–168). New York: Bilingual Press.

Kohnert, K. (2002). Picture naming in early sequential bilinguals: A 1-year follow-up. *Journal of Speech, Language and Hearing Research, 45,* 759–771.

Kohnert, K., & Bates, E. (2002). Balancing bilinguals II: Lexical comprehension and cognitive processing in children learning Spanish and English. *Journal of Speech, Language and Hearing Research, 45*(2), 347–359.

Kohnert, K., & Goldstein, B. (2005). Speech, language, and hearing in developing bilingual children: From practice to research. *Language, Speech, and Hearing Services in Schools, 36*(3), 169–171.

Laing, S. P. (2003). Assessment of phonology in preschool African American Vernacular English speakers using an alternate response mode. *American Journal of Speech-Language Pathology, 12*(3), 273–281.

Laing, S. P., & Kamhi, A. (2003) Alternate assessment of language and literacy in culturally and linguistically diverse populations. *Language, Speech and Hearing Services in Schools, 34*(1), 44–55.

Langdon, H. W. (1996). English language learning by immigrant Spanish speakers: A United States perspective. *Topics in Language Disorders, 16,* 38–53.

Langdon, H. W. (2002). Language interpreters and translators: Bridging communication with clients and families. *The ASHA Leader, 7*(6), 14–15.

Langdon, H. W., & Cheng, L. (Eds.). (1992). *Hispanic children and adults with communication disorders: Assessments and intervention.* Gaithersburg, MD: Aspen.

Law, J. (2000). Factors affecting language development in West African Children: A pilot study using qualitative methodology. *Child Care, Health & Development, 26*(4), 289–308.

Linares, T. A. (1982). Articulation skills of Spanish-speaking children. *Ethnoperspectives in bilingual education, series vol III: Bilingual education technology* (pp. 363–387). Ypsilanti, MI: Eastern Michigan University.

Lynch, E. W., & Hanson, M. J. (2003). *Understanding families: Approaches to diversity, disability, and risk.* Baltimore: Paul H. Brookes.

Lynch, E. W., & Hanson, M. J. (2004). *Developing cross-cultural competence: A guide for working with young children and their families* (4th ed.). Baltimore: Paul H. Brookes.

Mattes, L. J., & Omark, D. R. (1991). *Speech and language assessment for the bilingual handicapped* (2nd ed.). San Diego, CA: College Hill.

McCabe, A. (1995). Evaluation of narrative discourse skills. In K. N. Cole, P. S. Dale, & D. J. Thal (Eds.), *Assessment of communication and language* (pp. 121–142). Baltimore: Paul H. Brookes.

McGregor, K. K. (2000). The development and enhancement of narrative skills in a preschool children: Towards a solution to clinical-client mismatch. *American Journal of Speech-Language Pathology, 9*(1), 55–71.

McGregor, K. K., Williams, D., Hearst, S., & Johnson, A. C. (1997). The use of contrastive analysis in distinguishing difference from disorder: A tutorial. *American Journal of Speech Language Pathology, 6,* 45–56.

McLeod, S. (2007). *The international guide to speech acquisition.* Clifton Park, NY: Delmar.

Mercer, C. D. (1987). *Students with learning disabilities* (3rd ed.). New York: Merrill.

Merino, B. J. (1982, October–November). Language development in Spanish as a first language: Implications of assessment. Paper presented at the National Conference on the Exceptional Bilingual Child, Phoenix, AZ.

Merino, B. J. (1992). Acquisition of syntactic and phonological features in Spanish. In H. W. Langdon & L. L. Cheng (Eds.), *Hispanic children and adults with communication disorders* (pp. 57–98). Gaithersburg, MD: Aspen.

Musselwhite, C. (1983). Pluralistic assessment in speech-language pathology: Use of dual norms in the placement process. *Language, Speech and Hearing Services in Schools, 14,* 29–37.

National Deafness and Other Communication Disorders Advisory Board. (1991). *Research in human communication,* Annual report (NIH Publication No. 92-3317). Bethesda, MD: National Institutes of Health.

Ochs, E., & Schieffelin, B. (1995). The impact of language socialization on grammatical development. In P. Fletcher & B. MacWhinney (Eds.), *The handbook of child language* (pp. 73–94). Oxford: Blackwell.

Owens, R. (2003). *Language disorders: A functional approach to assessment and intervention.* New York: Allyn & Bacon.

Paradis, J. (2005). Grammatical morphology in children learning English as a second language: Implications of similarities with specific language impairment. *Language, Speech, and Hearing Services in Schools, 36,* 172–187.

Patterson, J., & Pearson, B. (2004). Bilingual lexical development: Influences, contexts, and processes. In B. A. Goldstein (Ed.), *Bilingual language development and disorders in Spanish-English speakers* (pp. 77–104). Baltimore: Paul H. Brookes.

Peña, E. D. (2000). Measurement of modifiability in children from culturally and linguistically diverse backgrounds. *Communication Disorders Quarterly, 21*(2), 87–97.

Peña, E., Iglasias, A., & Lidz, C. (2001). Reducing test bias through dynamic assessment of children word learning ability. *American Journal of Speech Language Pathology, 10*(3), 138–154.

Penny, R (2003). *History of the Spanish language* (2nd ed.). New York: Cambridge University Press.

Portes, A., & Rumbaut, R. (2001). *Legacies: The story of the immigrant second generation.* Berkeley, CA: University of California Press.

Price, C. J., Green, D. W., & von Studnitz, R. (1999). A functional imaging study of translation and language switching. *Brain, 122,* 2221–2235.

Roseberry-McKibbon, C. (2007). *Language disorders in children: A multicultural and case perspective.* Boston: Pearson Education.

Roseberry-McKibbon, C. (2008). *Multicultural students with special needs: Practical strategies for assessment and intervention* (3rd ed.). Oceanside, CA: Academic Communication Associates.

Rickford, J. R. (1999). *African American vernacular English.* Malden, MA: Blackwell.

Rickford, J. R. (2000). *Spoken soul: The story of Black English.* New York: John Wiley.

Rodriguez, B. L., & Olswang, L. B. (2003). Mexican-American and Anglo-American mothers' beliefs and values about child rearing, education, and language impairment. *American Journal of Speech-Language Pathology, 12*(4), 452–462.

Scarborough, H. (2001). Connecting early language and literacy to later reading (dis)abilities: Evidence, theory, and practice. In S. B. Neuman & D. K. Dickon (Eds.), *Handbook of early literacy research* (pp. 97–110). New York: Guilford Press.

Schieffelin, B., & Ochs, E. (1986). Language socialization. *Annual Review of Anthropology, 15,* 163–191.

Scriven, M. (1991). *Evaluation thesaurus* (4th ed.). New York: Sage.

Secord, W., Wiig, E., & Semel, E. (2006) *Clinical Evaluation of Language Function Spanish.* San Antonio: Harcourt Assessment, Inc.

Seymour, H., Bland-Stewart, L., & Green, L. J. (1998). Difference versus deficit in child African American English. *Language, Speech, and Hearing Services in Schools, 29,* 96–108.

Seymour, H., & Ralabate, P. (1985). The acquisition of a phonological feature of Black English. *Journal of Communication Disorders, 18,* 139–148.

Seymour H., Roeper, T. W., deVilliers, J., & deVilliers, P. (2003). *Diagnostic Evaluation of Language Variation (DELV).* San Antonio: Harcourt Assessments, Inc.

Seymour, H., & Seymour, C. (1981). Black English and Standard English contrasts in consonantal development of four- and five-year old children. *Journal of Speech and Hearing Disorders, 46,* 274–280.

Steffersen, M. (1974). The acquisition of Black English. Doctoral dissertation, University of Illinois, Evanston.

Stockman, I. (1986). Language acquisition in culturally diverse populations: The black child as a case study. In O. Taylor (Ed.), *Nature of communication disorders in culturally and linguistically diverse populations* (pp. 117–155). San Diego, CA: College Hill.

Stockman, I. (1996). Phonological development and disorders in African American children. In A. Kamhi, K. Pollock, & J. Harris, *Communication development and disorders in African American children: Research, assessment, and intervention* (pp. 117–154). Baltimore: Paul H. Brookes.

Stockman, I. (1998). The promises and pitfalls of language sample analysis as an assessment tool for linguistic minority children. *Language Speech and Hearing Services in Schools, 27*(4), 355–365.

Stockman, I. (2000). The new Peabody Picture Vocabulary Test III: An illusion of unbiased assessment? *Language, Speech and Hearing Services in Schools, 31,* 340–353.

Stockman, I., & Vaughn-Cooke, F. (1992). Lexical elaboration in children's locative action expressions. *Child Development, 63,* 1104–1125.

Taylor, O. (1986). *Nature of communication disorders in culturally and linguistically diverse populations.* San Diego, CA: College Hill.

Taylor, O. T. (1999). Cultural issues and language acquisition. In O. T. Taylor & L. B. Leonard (Eds.), *Language acquisition across North America: Cross-cultural and cross linguistic perspectives.* San Diego, CA: Singular.

Thal, D., Jackson-Maldonado, D., & Acosta, D. (2000). Validity of a parent report measure of vocabulary and grammar for Spanish-speaking toddlers. *Journal of Speech, Language, and Hearing Research, 43,* 1087–1100.

Thal, D., O'Hanlon, L., Clemmons, M., & Fralin, L. (1999). Validity of parent report measure of vocabulary and syntax for preschool children with language impairment. *Journal of Speech, Language Hearing Research, 42,* 482–496.

Thompson, C. A., Craig, H. K., & Washington, J. A. (2004). Variable production of African American English across oracy and literacy contexts. *Language, Speech, and Hearing Services in Schools, 35*(3), 269–282.

U.S. Census Bureau. (2000). *American Indian and Alaskan Native tribes in the United States* (revised June 30, 2004). Washington, DC: U.S. Department of Commerce.

U.S. Census Bureau. (2003). *Census 2000 brief language use and English speaking ability.* Washington, DC: Department of Commerce.

U.S. Census Bureau. (2004). *U.S. Interim projections by age, sex, race, and Hispanic origin.* Washington, DC: U.S. Department of Commerce.

U.S. Census Bureau. (2007). *Statistical abstract of the United States* (126th ed.) Washington, DC: U.S. Department of Commerce.

U.S. Census Bureau. (2008). SC-EST2006-6RACE: Annual state population estimates with sex, 6 race groups (5 race alone groups and one group with two or more race groups) and Hispanic origin: April 1, 2000 to July 1, 2006. In U.S. Census Bureau, *Statistical Abstract of the United States* (p. 23). Washington, DC: Author.

Vaughn-Cooke, F. (1983). Improving language assessment in minority children. *ASHA, 9,* 29–34.

Vaughn-Cooke, F., & Wright-Harp, W. (1992). *Lexical development in working-class Black children.* National Institutes of Health Grant #RR08005-23.

Vihman, M. M. (1986). More on language differentiation. *Journal of Child Language, 13,* 595–607.

Westby, C. (1990). Ethnographic interviewing. *Journal of Childhood Communication Disorders, 13*(1), 110–118.

World Health Organization (2001). *International classification of functioning, disability and health.* Geneva: Author.

Wolfram, W. (1991). *Dialects and American English.* Englewood Cliffs, NJ: Prentice Hall.

Wong-Fillmore, L. (1991a). Second language learning in children: A model of language learning in social context. In E. Bialystok (Ed.), *Language processing in bilingual children* (pp. 49–69). Cambridge, UK: Cambridge University Press.

Wong-Fillmore, L., (1991b). When learning a second language means losing the first. *Early Childhood Research Quarterly, 6,* 323–346.

Wyatt, T. (1991). Linguistic constraints on copula production in Black English child speech. *Dissertation Abstracts International, 523*(2), 781B (University Microfilms No. DA9120958).

Wyatt, T. (1995). Language development in African American child speech. *Linguistics and Education, 7,* 7–22.

Wyatt, T. (2002). Assessing the communicative abilities of clients from diverse cultural and language backgrounds. In D. E. Battle (Ed.), *Communication disorders in multicultural populations* (3rd ed., pp. 415–459). Boston: Butterworth-Heinemann.

Zimmerman, I. A., Steiner, V. G., & Pond, R. E. (2002). *Preschool Language Scale-4 Spanish.* San Antonio, TX: Harcourt Assessments, Inc.

About the Contributors

Susan Antonellis is the clinical supervisor of audiology at the St. John's University Speech and Hearing Center in Queens, New York. She has practiced in the field of audiology for the past 24 years and has supervised hundreds of students who are pursuing a career in audiology. Dr. Antonellis has worked at St. John's University for the past 17 years. Dr. antonellis recently received her doctoral degree in audiology (AuD) from the Arizona School of Health Sciences–A.T. Still University of Health Sciences. She serves on several committees, including The Long Island Hearing Screening Program Board and the Executive Board of the Long Island Speech-Language Hearing Association as audiology councilor. She also served on the regional planning committee to help develop early intervention services for young children.

Dolores E. Battle is a professor of speech-language pathology at Buffalo State College, Buffalo, New York. She is also senior advisor to the president for Equity and Campus Diversity. Dr. Battle is president of the International Association of Logopedics and Phoniatrics and former president of the American Speech-Language-Hearing Association. Dr. Battle received her PhD in communication sciences and disorders from the State University of New York at Buffalo. She has published widely in communication disorders in multicultural populations and college students with disabilities and has made over 100 presentations to national and international professional organizations.

Sylvia Diehl is a professor at the University of South Florida, where she teaches courses in autism, augmentative and alternative communication, research, developmental disabilities, and language disorders. She has served as a consultant in the area of autism spectrum disorders for the National Education Association and the American Speech-Language-Hearing Association (ASHA) along with numerous school districts. Dr. Diehl has created online coursework for ASHA and the Florida Department of Education as well as a master clinician series for ASHA. She has published numerous articles in peer-reviewed journals related to communication disorders in children with developmental disabilities. Her research and publication interests focus on consistent frameworks to support children with developmental disabilities in classroom settings.

Sandra Levey is an associate professor in the department of speech-language-hearing sciences at Lehman College of the City University of New York, with degrees in linguistics and speech-language pathology. She is a member of the Lehman College chapter of the Scientific Research Society and a board recognized specialist in child language. Dr. Levey has received grants for research in Nigeria and the Slovak Republic, where she delivered lectures and worked with linguists from Bratislava and the Ukraine. She was the conferences coordinator of the seventeenth annual Stanford Child Language Research Forum at Stanford University and an editorial consultant for the *Journal of Speech-Language-Hearing Sciences* and the *Texas Journal of Audiology and Speech Pathology*. Dr. Levey's research interests and publications address phonetics, phonology, and perception. Her publications and presentations at international conferences focus on the perception and reading skills of bilingual Spanish/English and English children and adults.

Robert E. Owens, Jr. ("Dr. Bob") is Distinguished Teaching Professor of Speech-Language Pathology at the State University of New York at Geneseo. He has authored two texts, *Language Development, An Introduction*, and *Language Disorders, A Functional Approach*; created the Program for Acquisition of Language with the Severely Impaired (PALS); co-authored *Introduction to Communication Disorders, A Life Span Perspective*; and authored *Help Your Baby Talk*, a guide for parents, and *Queer Kids*, about the trials and triumphs of gay youth. He has also written several book chapters and articles, presented approximately 150 professional papers and workshops in both the United States and abroad, and authored two novels, which will no doubt win the Nobel Prize posthumously. He teaches language development and disorders courses. His clients are primarily preschoolers, as are some of his closest friends. And he's a grandpa.

Christine Radziewicz is the director of the School for Language and Communication Development, a special education school for children age 2 through 21 in New York. She has been working in the areas of deaf education and speech language pathology for more than 30 years. Dr. Radziewicz received her doctoral degree in speech language pathology from Adelphi University. Dr. Radziewicz has instituted the inclusion program at SLCD, which integrates children with language disorders with typical peers. In addition, she has served as a consultant to several public school districts providing in-service training to their speech teachers and assessing students. Today her clinical/educational interests focus on enhancing educational environments to better support academic learning for children in educational settings and working directly with children in her private practice. Dr. Radziewicz has been a contributing author in several books and has coauthored *Collaborative Decision Making: The Pathway to Inclusion* (1998) and *Language Disorders in Children: Real Families, Real Issues, and Real Interventions* (2007) with her friend and colleague, Dr. Ellenmorris Tiegerman-Farber.

Nancy B. Robinson holds a faculty appointment at San Francisco State University in the communicative disorders program, where she is currently the program coordinator. She teaches in the areas of augmentative and alternative communication (AAC), early intervention, and language disorders in children. She completed her doctoral studies at the University of Washington in Seattle in 1987. For many years, Dr. Robinson assisted in the development of the Center on Disability Studies at the University of Hawaii and personnel development in American Samoa, the Federated States of Micronesia, and the Republic of Palau. Her areas of research include family support in multicultural contexts, collaboration and interdisciplinary team development, early intervention, and AAC. She continues to teach and consult at the University of Hawaii and most recently at the University of Canterbury in New Zealand.

Liat Seiger-Gardner is an assistant professor in the department of speech-language-hearing sciences at Lehman College, the City University of New York and a faculty member in the PhD program of speech and hearing sciences at the Graduate Center of the City University of New York. Dr. Seiger-Gardner is an ASHA certified and a New York state licensed speech-language pathologist. She received her PhD from the Graduate Center, CUNY. Her area of specialty is child language development and disorder. Her current research focuses on lexical access and word-finding difficulties in children with SLI.

Cheryl Smith Gabig is an assistant professor in the department of speech-language-hearing sciences at Lehman College/CUNY. Dr. Smith Gabig received her PhD in speech pathology from the University of Connecticut. She has many years of university teaching experience as well as over 25 years of clinical experience in both educational and hospital settings serving school-age and adolescents with language based learning disabilities. Her research interests include diagnosis and classification of language disorders in children with an emphasis on clinical profiles, particularly in the area of memory, language, and reading.

Amy L. Weiss is a professor in the department of communicative disorders at the University of Rhode Island. An ASHA fellow, Dr. Weiss is the current coordinator of ASHA's Special Interest Division 1: Language Learning and Education. Dr. Weiss teaches courses in language disorders in infants and toddlers, preschoolers, and school-age children. She also teaches a course in fluency disorders and multicultural issues in language assessment and intervention. A frequent presenter at local, national, and international conferences, she is also secretary of the International Fluency Association.

Index